D0478605

Coronary Artery Disease
Essentials of Prevention and Rehabilitation Programs

Peter H. Brubaker, PhD
Wake Forest University
Winston-Salem, North Carolina

Leonard A. Kaminsky, PhD
Mitchell H. Whaley, PhD
Ball State University
Muncie, Indiana

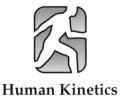

Human Kinetics

Library of Congress Cataloging-in-Publication Data

Brubaker, Peter H., 1961-
     Coronary artery disease : essentials of prevention and rehabilitation / Peter H. Brubaker,
Leonard A. Kaminsky, Mitchell H. Whaley.
          p. ; cm.
     Includes bibliographical references and index.
     ISBN 0-7360-2795-5
     1. Coronary heart disease--Prevention. 2. Coronary heart disease--Treatment. I.
Kaminsky, Leonard A. 1955- II. Whaley, Mitchell H., 1955- III. Title.
     [DNLM: 1. Coronary Disease--prevention & control. 2. Coronary
Disease--rehabilitation. WG 300 B886c 2002]
     RC685.C6 .B77 2002
     616.1'23--dc21

                                                                  2001039466

ISBN-10: 0-7360-2795-5
ISBN-13: 978-0-7360-2795-3

Acquisitions Editor: Loarn D. Robertson, PhD; **Developmental Editor:** Myles Schrag; **Assistant Editors:** Jennifer L. Davis, Amanda S. Ewing, J. Gordon Wilson; **Copyeditor:** Joyce Sexton; **Proofreader:** Pamela Johnson; **Indexer:** Craig Brown; **Permission Manager:** Dalene Reeder; **Graphic Designer:** Stuart Cartwright; **Graphic Artist:** Dawn Sills; **Photo Manager:** Leslie A. Woodrum; **Cover Designer:** Jack W. Davis; **Art Managers:** Carl D. Johnson, Craig Newsom; **Medical Illustrator:** Jason M. McAlexander, MFA/Interactive Composition Corporation; **Printer:** Sheridan Books

Printed in the United States of America   10   9   8   7   6   5   4   3   2

Human Kinetics
Web site: www.humankinetics.com

United States: Human Kinetics
P.O. Box 5076
Champaign, IL 61825-5076
800-747-4457
e-mail: humank@hkusa.com

Canada: Human Kinetics
475 Devonshire Road Unit 100
Windsor, ON N8Y 2L5
800-465-7301 (in Canada only)
e-mail: orders@hkcanada.com

Europe: Human Kinetics
107 Bradford Road
Stanningley
Leeds LS28 6AT, United Kingdom
+44 (0) 113 255 5665
e-mail: hk@hkeurope.com

Australia: Human Kinetics
57A Price Avenue
Lower Mitcham, South Australia 5062
08 8372 0999
e-mail: info@hkaustralia.com

New Zealand: Human Kinetics
Division of Sports Distributors NZ Ltd.
P.O. Box 300 226 Albany
North Shore City
Auckland
0064 9 448 1207
e-mail: info@humankinetics.co.nz

To Lisa, Ryan, Ashley, and Colin: For countless sacrifices,
boundless love, and unwavering support. You keep
me balanced and make my life complete!
P.H.B.

To Jesus Christ, my Lord and Savior who has so bountifully filled
my life with blessings. To my wife Mary and my daughters Lauren
and Bonnie. Your love makes my life complete. To my parents for all the love
and sacrifices you made for me and all the lessons you so ably taught me.
L.A.K.

To my daughters, Liz and Rachael. You continually validate
my belief in what's good about this world. Thank you
for your love and support throughout this project.
M.H.W.

CONTENTS

                 Artery Disease**

                 Detection and Prevention of CAD in Youth   84
                 Risk Factor Management for Adults   85
                 Risk Factor Reduction and Regression of CAD   97
                 Surgical and Interventional Procedures for CAD   100
                 Summary   107
                 Case Studies   107
                 Glossary   108
                 References   109

**Part II   Practical Applications to Coronary Artery   111
              Disease Prevention and Rehabilitation**

        Chapter 5   Electrocardiography   111

                 Electrocardiogram Fundamentals   112
                 Systematic Approach to Interpretation   122
                 Abnormal Cardiac Rhythms   127
                 Chamber Enlargement   141
                 Myocardial Ischemia, Injury, and Infarction   142
                 Summary   147
                 Case Studies   151
                 Glossary   159
                 References   159
                 Suggested Readings   159

        **Chapter 6   Physical Fitness Assessment   161
                         and Interpretation**

                 What is Physical Fitness?   162
                 Basic Body Composition Measurement   162
                 Advanced Body Composition Measurement   165
                 *Muscular Strength and Endurance   168
                   and Flexibility Measurement*
                 Cardiorespiratory Fitness   171
                 Summary   186
                 Case Studies   187
                 Glossary   198
                 References   198

        **Chapter 7   Exercise Prescription in Coronary Artery   201
                         Disease Prevention and Rehabilitation
                         Programs**

                 *Principles of Exercise Prescription—   202
                   Primary Prevention*
                 *Principles of Exercise Prescription—   224
                   Secondary Prevention*

PREFACE

The last quarter of the 20th century produced tremendous advances in the prevention and treatment of coronary artery disease (CAD) that have resulted in a decline in the prevalence of CAD and an improved survival rate from coronary events. However, CAD remains the leading cause of death in the United States and will continue to impose a tremendous financial burden on our health care system long into the 21st century. Lifestyle modification in the prevention and rehabilitation of CAD has only recently been widely embraced and promoted as conventional medical treatment of this disease. The first formal programs to promote lifestyle modification were initiated approximately 30 years ago at a few U.S. universities, including our institutions, Wake Forest University and Ball State University.

While these programs were traditionally called "adult fitness" or "prevention" programs when they focused on apparently healthy individuals and/or those with risk factors for cardiovascular disease, and were called "cardiac rehabilitation" when their interventions were for individuals with known cardiovascular disease, their objectives were in fact very similar. In practice, the type of intervention provided to an individual who participated in an "adult fitness/prevention" program to reduce risk factors would not be any different from the intervention provided to a post-myocardial infarction patient with elevated risk factors participating in a cardiac rehabilitation program. In either setting, management of the individual's risk factors is first attempted with lifestyle modifications including regular exercise, proper nutrition, weight and stress management, and smoking cessation. If individuals do not achieve goals through lifestyle modification, then medications are prescribed. Although these lifestyle modification programs have traditionally been dichotomized into prevention versus rehabilitation programs based purely on the presence or absence of overt CAD manifestations (myocardial infarction, angina, revascularization), a more contemporary perspective considers the risk of CAD to be on a continuum, ranging from low risk (in persons who are younger with few risk factors), to moderate risk (in persons who are older or who have multiple risk factors), to subclinical atherosclerosis (small lesions in the coronary arteries that are not easily detectable), to atherosclerotic manifestations and overt CAD (angina, myocardial infarction, need for revascularization). Furthermore, as technological advances lead to earlier detection and recognition of subclinical CAD, the line between those with and those without CAD becomes less clear. Consequently, it seems appropriate to view programs as lying on a continuum from prevention (for those without overt CAD) to rehabilitation (for those with clinical manifestations of CAD), recognizing the potential for many to fall in between. While there are some important differences between prevention and rehabilitation programs, in reality there are more similarities. Thus throughout the book we present primary and secondary prevention programs as one entity. When unique features do exist between these programs, we clearly point out these features in the text.

Guidelines have been developed by the American College of Sports Medicine (*Guidelines for Exercise Testing and Prescription*) and the American Association of Cardiovascular and Pulmonary Rehabilitation (*Guidelines for Cardiac Rehabilitation and Secondary Prevention Programs*) to enhance and standardize the "practice" of CAD prevention and rehabilitation. These books were written for professionals and were not designed as texts for students. In our opinion, there is no single comprehensive resource devoted to providing the foundational information required for the student preparing to enter the CAD prevention and rehabilitation field. Rather than duplicating the content of these essential resources for the student, our goal throughout this book is to describe when and how to apply these guidelines in the practice of CAD prevention and rehabilitation and why we should practice that way. Although not required for successful use of this book, we highly recommend these two guideline texts as companion resources for this book. This book is primarily designed for the upper-level undergraduate or entry-level graduate student in an exercise science curriculum, yet individuals crossing over from other allied health professions (i.e., nurses, physical therapists, medical students, and residents) to CAD prevention and rehabilitation programs will also find this book very useful in building a solid educational foundation. Regardless of the reader's prior education or career background, this textbook provides a clear and concise resource on the essential issues in CAD prevention and rehabilitation.

The practice of clinical exercise physiology is rapidly expanding as the medical community and consumers appreciate the value of exercise and physical activity in the management of many chronic diseases. Other chronic diseases and conditions for which exercise or physical activity has been shown to be efficacious include chronic pulmonary disease, certain metabolic and hematologic disorders, and many neuromuscular and musculoskeletal disorders. Rather than attempting to cover the *breadth* of knowledge required for the contemporary clinical exercise physiologist, our objective with this book is to present the appropriate *depth* of knowledge needed by the individual training for a career in a CAD prevention or rehabilitation setting. We do, however, recognize that CAD is not always an isolated disease process and that it can be accompanied by other, sometimes more limiting, medical conditions (commonly called comorbidities). To this end, we have dedicated an entire chapter of this book (chapter 9) to address the "complex" CAD patient, in whom the impact of common comorbidities (chronic obstructive pulmonary disease, diabetes, congestive heart failure, hypertension, obesity, and peripheral arterial disease) must be considered. Additionally, a section of chapter 11 describes specific credentials offered by professional organizations that, in addition to college degrees, are generally recommended or required for employment in preventive and rehabilitative exercise programs.

The authors of this text all have extensive experience in teaching this material to undergraduate and graduate students and allied health professionals, as well as in administering CAD prevention and rehabilitation programs. As mentioned earlier, our universities have long been widely recognized for offering high-quality undergraduate and graduate education programs as well as successful Adult Fitness and cardiac rehabilitation programs. We have had the good fortune to follow in the footsteps of several of the pioneers and leaders in our field, including Leroy "Bud" Getchell, PhD; Paul M. Ribisl, PhD; and Henry S. Miller, Jr., MD. Moreover, all the authors are certified by the American College of Sports

Medicine as Preventive/Rehabilitative Program Directors$_{SM}$ and have been involved in writing various guidelines and manuals for that organization. Our combined educational and professional experience allows us to understand the needs of the student preparing for a career in CAD prevention and rehabilitation in the 21st century.

To help meet these needs in the book, we use numerous tables, figures, and photographs to emphasize important points and apply concepts. We also frequently present clinical experiences and research findings from studies conducted at our institutions. Furthermore, we present three extensive case studies (a low-risk primary prevention participant, a high-risk primary prevention participant, and a secondary prevention/cardiac rehabilitation participant) to help readers learn the material presented in the text. The three cases were selected to demonstrate how the information presented in this text can be applied at different stages of the CAD disease continuum. Thus, we have elected to introduce the case studies in the first chapter and build on each case with information presented in subsequent chapters.

We have arranged the text in an order that we have found to be appropriate for an undergraduate or graduate course in CAD prevention/rehabilitation. However, each chapter can stand alone and thus be used in other related courses. The text is divided into three parts: Introduction to Coronary Artery Disease Prevention and Rehabilitation, Practical Applications to Coronary Artery Disease Prevention and Rehabilitation, and Organization and Administration of Coronary Artery Disease Prevention and Rehabilitation Programs. These three parts are further divided into 11 chapters that cover a variety of topics relevant to primary and secondary CAD prevention. To assist with learning, each chapter begins with a list of behavioral objectives and an introduction to guide the reader. Each chapter ends with a summary, a glossary of key terms, and references. Where appropriate, case studies are included to help readers integrate the information. We believe this textbook is unique because it is comprehensive yet foundational, and therefore appealing to individuals preparing for or crossing over to a career in CAD prevention and rehabilitation. Moreover, our textbook presents the contemporary view that CAD prevention and rehabilitation programs are not dichotomous, but instead represent similar lifestyle interventions that are offered at different stages of the disease continuum.

ACKNOWLEDGMENTS

First, I want to acknowledge my parents for raising me in a loving and supportive environment. Thank you for providing me with a solid foundation and a value system that continues to serve me well. I am grateful that you instilled me in the desire to be the best that I can regardless of what I chose to do. Also, thanks to the Bross family for their endless support and generosity. Secondly, I am extremely fortunate to work at Wake Forest University where I have the support of numerous administrators, faculty, and staff. Because of you, I have the best job in the world and the opportunity to write this book! Finally, I would also like to acknowledge numerous mentors and colleagues, undergraduate and graduate students, as well as the cardiac rehabilitation program participants, all of whom have taught me so much. Through you I have learned what, how, and why to teach the information contained in this book.

P.H.B.

I want to express my appreciation to my co-authors Mitch Whaley and Pete Brubaker. You are both great professors and great men. I am fortunate to count both of you as friends. I also want to thank all of my colleagues and the staff of the American College of Sports Medicine for providing such a solid professional family to grow up in. Additionally, I want to thank my mentor Ronald G. Knowlton. I consider it an honor to have had the opportunity to study with you. Finally, I want to express my gratitude to all of the graduate and undergraduate students and the patients and participants who I have been blessed to work with.

L.A.K.

I want to express a deep appreciation to several of my professional mentors. First, thanks to Dr. Michael Bobo, Professor at Texas Tech University, who saw something in me and encouraged me to think about graduate school in exercise science. Short of his influence, I would probably have been a very successful high school football coach right now. I also want to thank Dr. Leroy "Bud" Getchell, who introduced me to the fields of adult fitness and cardiac rehabilitation and provided me the opportunity to study in his program at Ball State. Finally, I would like to thank Dr. Thomas Woodall, professor at Eastern Illinois University, who took a chance on a young, green exercise physiologist and allowed me to learn on the job, providing me significant guidance and friendship along the way. These men were major influences in my professional and personal life, and I owe them a debt of gratitude that I will never be able to repay. Much of their influence has found its way into the pages of this text. Thanks, Gentlemen!

M.H.W.

PART I

Introduction to Coronary Artery Disease Prevention and Rehabilitation

CHAPTER 1

Coronary Artery Disease: The Role of Prevention and Rehabilitation Programs

BEHAVIORAL OBJECTIVES

- To be able to describe the prevalence of coronary artery disease in the U.S. population and identify risk factors for the development of coronary artery disease
- To be able to describe the role that physical activity or cardiorespiratory fitness plays in the primary and secondary prevention of coronary artery disease
- To be able to identify and use current coronary artery disease risk prediction models for both primary and secondary prevention

Recent data from the American Heart Association (AHA) suggest that the number of deaths from cardiovascular diseases (CVDs) has declined approximately 20% in the U.S. population in recent years (between 1988 and 1998) (1). While this appears to be good news in the fight against CVD, the AHA also estimates that 60 million Americans currently have some form of coronary artery disease (CAD). In addition, CVDs remain the leading cause of death in adult Americans (figure 1.1)—accounting for approximately 41% of all U.S. deaths in 1998—and, according to recent estimates, cost our society close to $300 billion annually (figure 1.2). Within the broad spectrum of

CVDs, mortality from CAD ranks number one for both adult men and women (figures 1.1 and 1.3). However, CAD mortality is not the only concern, as this disease is also the leading cause of permanent disability in the U.S. labor force.

An accumulation of data from epidemiological studies has led to the identification of various risk factors associated with development of CAD. Along with the more generally accepted CAD risk factors of cigarette smoking, hypertension, and hyperlipidemia, both physical inactivity and obesity have recently been recognized as major heart disease risk factors (2, 3). In addition, researchers in the field of CAD prevention

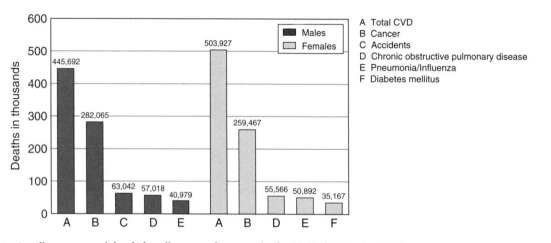

Figure 1.1   Leading causes of death for all men and women in the United States in 1998.
Note: There is no C listing for females because accidents were not among the top five causes of death for women; there is no F listing for men because DM was not among the top five for men.
Reproduced with permission, *2001 Heart and Stroke Facts, AHA* ©2000, Copyright American Heart Association.

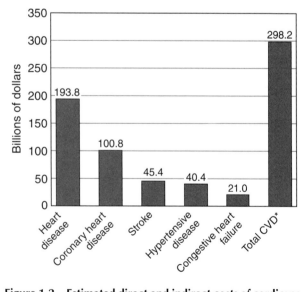

Figure 1.2   Estimated direct and indirect costs of cardiovascular diseases and stroke in the United States in 1998.
Reproduced with permission, *2001 Heart and Stroke Facts, AHA* ©2000, Copyright American Heart Association.

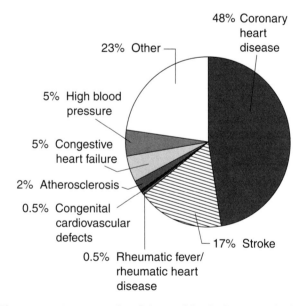

Figure 1.3   Percentage breakdown of deaths from CVD in the United States in 1998.
Reproduced with permission, *2001 Heart and Stroke Facts, AHA* ©2000, Copyright American Heart Association.

continue to identify new potential physiological markers of heart disease risk. This chapter presents an overview of CAD **epidemiology,** identifies traditional and emerging risk factors for the disease, and discusses the scientific evidence that links inactivity or low fitness to risk for CAD. In addition, the chapter discusses professional organizations that have guided the evolution of exercise-based primary and secondary prevention programs.

PREVALENCE OF CORONARY ARTERY DISEASE

Coronary artery disease has reached nearly epidemic proportions in our society and is the cause of more deaths, disability, and economic loss than any other group of diseases. A look at recent CAD statistics from the AHA reveals a mixed message. On the one hand, death rates from CAD appear to be declining in the United States (figure 1.4); but in contrast, both diagnostic and revascularization pro-

cedures for heart diseases are on the rise (figure 1.5). Therefore, we seem to be making progress in one area (decreased CAD mortality), but one could argue that the actual burden of the disease within our society remains quite high. The combined figures show a plateau in CAD mortality (figure 1.4) but an increase in CAD **morbidity** (figure 1.5), which reflects the high burden of the disease.

Consider these staggering statistics from the AHA (1):

- Coronary artery disease caused 459,841 deaths in the United States in 1998—1 of every 5 deaths.

- About every 29 seconds an American will experience a coronary event, and about every minute someone will die from a coronary event.

- This year an estimated 1,100,000 Americans will have a new or recurrent coronary attack (defined as myocardial infarction or fatal CAD). About 650,000 of these will be first attacks, with the remainder representing recurrent attacks. Over 40% of the people experiencing these attacks will die of them.

- Among people alive today, 12.4 million have a history of heart attack, angina pectoris (chest pain), or both. This breaks down to approximately 6,000,000 males and 6,300,000 females.

- In 1998, there were approximately 553,000 coronary artery bypass graft surgeries and 539,000 angioplasty procedures performed on Americans. From 1979 to 1998, the number of cardiovascular operations and procedures increased by 384%.

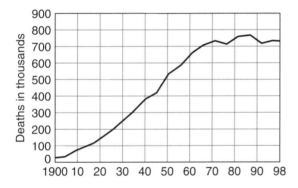

Figure 1.4   Deaths from heart diseases in the United States between 1900 and 1998.

Reproduced with permission, *2001 Heart and Stroke Facts, AHA* ©2000, Copyright American Heart Association.

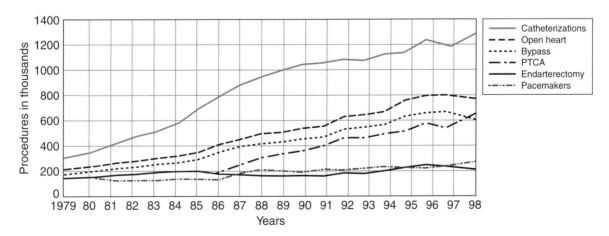

Figure 1.5   Trends in cardiovascular operations and procedures in the United States between 1979 and 1998.

Reproduced with permission, *2001 Heart and Stroke Facts, AHA* ©2000, Copyright American Heart Association.

- Coronary artery disease is the leading cause of premature, permanent disability in the U.S. labor force, accounting for 19% of disability allowances by the Social Security Administration.

What can we conclude from these statistics? They show that despite an increased public awareness of various genetic and lifestyle risk factors for CAD, as well as significant advances in medical therapies aimed at reducing CAD risk, the burden of the disease remains extremely high within our society. Therefore, national and local campaigns aimed at educating the general public about both established and emerging risk factors and their modification must continue in an effort to significantly reduce the burden of CAD on our population. Furthermore, as the number of individuals within our society who have experienced a myocardial infarction (MI) and/or undergone coronary revascularization procedures continues to grow (see figure 1.5), efforts within the medical community directed toward secondary prevention programs are more important than ever.

CORONARY ARTERY DISEASE RISK TERMINOLOGY

Before considering CAD risk factors, we need to define several terms used in describing an individual's chronic disease risk. The terms *absolute* and *relative* risk are often used for this purpose. An individual's absolute risk (AR) is the probability of developing CAD in a certain period of time (e.g., 5 or 10 years). Absolute risk is typically presented as a percentage such as 3% to 4% over the next 10 years. For example, an individual with several CAD risk factors (e.g., elevated cholesterol, elevated systolic blood pressure, and cigarette smoking) might have an AR for developing disease of 8% during the next 10 years. This would mean that 8 of 100 individuals with that particular set of risk factors would likely develop CAD by the end of the 10th year. Now, at issue is how to interpret this statistic. Should 8 out of 100 chances for developing disease be viewed as high risk, low risk, or somewhere in between? That would likely depend on one's frame of reference and the ultimate consequences of incurring the event (i.e., having a heart attack). Some might argue that an event that occurs only 8 times out of 100 is a rare event with a low probability of occurrence. However, if the event (i.e., CAD) could be fatal, then an 8% risk for the event

might be considered unacceptably high within our society. So health care professionals debate when and how to interpret absolute disease risk estimates. Consequently many health care professionals advocate the use of another statistic called the relative risk (RR) to provide insight into an individual's risk for developing a chronic disease. In a general sense, an individual's RR for a disease compares the person's AR to the AR for the disease within some type of reference group. The most commonly used reference group is a gender- and age-matched population. In this context the individual's risk is compared to the *average* risk for persons of the same age and gender. This RR can be calculated by dividing the individual's absolute risk (%) by the *average absolute* risk (%) within the population. Let's return to our hypothetical individual who has an AR of 8% for developing CAD within the next 10 years. Let's assume that the individual is a 35-year-old male. National CAD statistics suggest that the average AR of developing CAD during a 10-year period for 35- to 39-year-old U.S. males is approximately 5%. Using the two AR scores—the individual's and the average—we can estimate the individual's RR for CAD. Within this context, we calculate the RR by dividing the individual's risk by the reference or average risk as follows:

RR for CAD in 10 years = 8%/5% = 1.6

An RR of >1.0 means that the individual's risk is greater than the reference or average risk, whereas an RR of <1.0 would mean that the individual's risk is lower than the average risk within the population. Obviously, when we're referring to risk of CAD, it would be better to have an RR of <1.0—in other words, to have a lower-than-average risk. How do we interpret the 1.6 RR for our hypothetical male? This number indicates that the individual is 1.6 times more likely to develop the disease within a 10-year period than age-matched men within the population. Now, let's pause to reflect for a moment. Our hypothetical male had an 8% AR and a 1.6 RR for developing CAD. Is the RR statistic superior to the AR statistic as a means of quantifying this person's risk for developing CAD? That's a matter of opinion and beyond the scope of this brief discussion of risk estimates. Needless to say, there is considerable debate among health care professionals regarding which statistic better reflects an individual's risk. Fortunately, you don't have to pick one or the other method at this point. We simply define these terms within the context of estimating risk of CAD, and use the hypothetical example to set the stage for our discussions of CAD risk factors and the application of CAD risk prediction models presented in the rest of the chapter.

And finally, a different form of RR is often used to conceptualize the risk associated with a specific risk factor. In this context, RR is defined as the ratio of the likelihood of developing the disease (i.e., CAD) in persons with and without the risk factor (e.g., hypertensive vs. normotensive) or at a given amount of the risk factor (e.g., 120 vs. 140 mmHg systolic blood pressure). The major CAD risk factors have estimates of RR associated with them (e.g., RR of cigarette smokers 2-3 times that of nonsmokers), and these RR can serve as a crude way to compare the relative potency of each of the risk factors.

CORONARY ARTERY DISEASE RISK FACTORS

Researchers of the famous Framingham Heart Study (4) coined the term **risk factor** years ago as they identified characteristics that appeared to be associated with the development of heart disease in residents of Framingham, Massachusetts. Both observational (5-7) and interventional (8-10) studies have confirmed the notion that selected lifestyle and genetic factors predispose an individual to premature CAD. The AHA currently lists nine major CAD risk factors, divided into two categories—modifiable and non-modifiable (table 1.1).

The concept of risk factor identification and modification is based on the premise that exposure to certain host (e.g., hypercholesterolemia, hypertension) and environmental factors (e.g., physical inactivity) increases the statistical risk for developing the disease, and that alteration of these conditions decreases the risk (11). However, a given factor may not stand in a cause-and-effect relationship to the disease but simply be a nonspecific marker of the disease process. Most risk factors are not evaluated using randomized clinical trials.[1] Although this approach would clearly identify cause-and-effect relationships, it is generally not feasible (cost, time), nor would it be ethical. Rather, risk factors are usually initially identified from observational studies [2] in which the likelihood of causation is implied on the basis of the strength of the association, the exposure preceding disease onset, dose dependency, consistency of the relationship under diverse circumstances, specificity of the association, and the biological plausibility (12). The identification of risk factors provides a means for formulating treatment decisions through more accurate determination of overall risk status, as well as for decreasing CAD risk through the reduction of modifiable risk factors.

Risk factors for CAD are typically classified based on their positive or negative association with the presence of the disease and based on whether they are modifiable or non-modifiable (table 1.1). Furthermore, the defining criteria for certain risk factors vary depending on whether the context is primary or secondary prevention of CAD. The purpose of the following section is to identify the known risk factors for CAD, briefly describe their biological mechanisms, and identify their defining criteria. Appropriate treatment strategies for modifiable risk factors are outlined in detail in chapter 4.

Non-Modifiable Coronary Artery Disease Risk Factors

Several risk factors have been shown to be associated with an increased risk for CAD but cannot be modified through lifestyle changes or pharmacotherapy. Although non-modifiable, age, gender, and family history of early disease can help define the CAD risk profile of individuals and alter their treatment course.

Table 1.1
Major CAD Risk Factors

Non-modifiable	Modifiable
Increasing age	Cigarette or tobacco smoking
Male sex	High blood cholesterol
Heredity	High blood pressure
	Physical inactivity
	Obesity and overweight
	Diabetes

From American Heart Association (1).

---

1 Randomized clinical trials are considered the most rigorous type of experimental design available to assess a cause-and-effect relationship. Within this type of study, subjects are randomly assigned to either receive or not receive a proposed therapeutic intervention, and then both groups are followed for a period of time to assess the effectiveness of the procedure in lowering the incidence of disease.

2 Observational studies are those in which one or more variables (i.e., risk factors) are measured within a sample of individuals and then the entire group is followed to assess the association between the risk factors and incidence of disease.

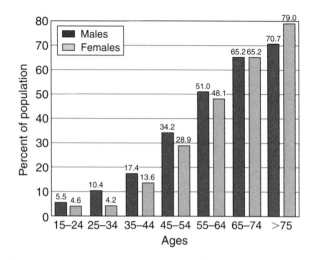

Figure 1.6   Estimated prevalence of cardiovascular diseases by age and sex within the United States between 1988 and 1994. Reproduced with permission, *2001 Heart and Stroke Facts, AHA* ©2000, Copyright American Heart Association.

Age

It is well known that advancing age is associated with an increased risk for CVD (figure 1.6). However, age is not associated with a specific mechanism for increasing CAD in the way that cigarette smoking or elevated low-density lipoprotein cholesterol (LDL-C) is; rather the contribution of age as a risk factor relates to the issue of exposure. The older an individual is, the longer his arteries have been exposed to development of CAD lesions, so there is a clear association between advancing age and increased risk. In fact, about four of every five CAD deaths occur in patients 65 and older (1). Despite these statistics, elderly patients can still benefit from reduction of modifiable risk factors. In fact, because of the short-term risk for CAD events in patients who are middle-aged and elderly, reduction of modifiable risk factors in this population is more likely to decrease CAD events in a shorter period of time than in younger patients with otherwise similar risk factors. The decision to aggressively treat risk factors in patients who are elderly should not be made on the basis of age alone, but rather on the basis of the overall health status and the potential benefit of the intervention.

Gender

While CAD continues to be the leading cause of death in both men and women, there is clearly a gender difference in the incidence of CAD. Between the ages of 45 and 49, the incidence of CAD in men is 4 times that of women. By ages 65 to 69, the incidence ratio declines to about 2. By the age of 85, the incidence ratio is about 1 (i.e., CAD is equal in men and women) (13).

The onset of symptomatic CAD is typically about 10 years earlier in men, but CAD incidence in women increases rapidly after menopause. Differences in CAD rates observed between men and women at younger ages may be due, at least in part, to the protective effect of estrogen (14). The earlier onset of CAD in males has led to a widespread misconception that the disease is less prevalent in women. However, according to data from the American Heart Association (1) (see figure 1.1), the number of deaths attributed to cardiovascular disease in the United States in 1998 was higher for women than it was for men (503,927 vs. 445,692) when considering all age groups collectively. Therefore, the burden of cardiovascular diseases within the female population of the United States is clearly a significant one that needs to be addressed in both primary and secondary prevention settings. Surprising to most is the sobering fact that 1 in 25 women will die from breast cancer, whereas 1 of 3 women will die from heart disease (1). Despite these grim statistics, a recent Gallup poll showed that 46% of women perceived breast cancer to be their major health risk, while only 4% believed this to be the case for heart disease (13).

Family History

It is said that the best way to avoid CAD is to choose one's parents wisely! It is widely recognized that CAD tends to aggregate in families. In studies controlling for other risk factors, a family history of CAD has been shown to be a strong independent risk factor for CAD. The association between CAD and a positive family history may be mediated by genetic effects on other risk factors such as obesity, hypertension, dyslipidemia, and diabetes (15).

However, there is recognized potential for other "family" factors—such as the home environment, adverse behaviors, and as yet to be described genetic syndromes—that may influence the development of CAD as decisively as currently known single-gene mutations (16).

Modifiable Coronary Artery Disease Risk Factors

The majority of the risk factors associated with CAD can be modified through lifestyle changes or pharmacotherapy. These risk factors, some of which are behaviors (e.g., use of tobacco products, sedentary lifestyle) while others are considered diseases (e.g., hypercholesterolemia, hypertension, obesity, diabetes mellitus, and so on), should be targets for aggressive intervention when identified.

Tobacco

The use of tobacco products, including smoking cigars or cigarettes and using smokeless tobacco, continues to be a major public health hazard in the United States and many other countries. Recent figures set the cost of medical care for smoking-related illnesses for Americans at approximately $50 billion annually. Although smoking is declining in the United States, more than 46 million adults, or 25% of the population 18 years and older, currently smoke; and some 4 million adolescents ages 12 to 17 years are smokers. Between 1990 and 1994, as estimated by the Centers for Disease Control (CDC), an average of 430,700 Americans died annually of smoking-related causes, with the majority of these deaths from cardiovascular causes (1). Smoking appears to multiply the effect of other CAD risk factors and is estimated to be the cause of approximately 20% of all cardiovascular deaths in the United States. Despite the high incidence of heart disease in smokers, one study showed that only 29% of current smokers thought their risk of an MI was higher than that of nonsmokers the same age (17). This points to the need for continual efforts to educate the general public on the harmful effects of smoking. The Framingham study revealed that for each 10 cigarettes smoked per day, cardiovascular mortality increased by 18% in men and 31% in women (18). In addition, the risk of vascular disease is magnified in women using oral contraceptives who also smoke cigarettes (19). It appears that mortality is increased regardless of how many cigarettes are smoked and regardless of whether smokeless tobacco products are used. A 12-year observational study of 135,000 men (20) demonstrated that the age-adjusted RR (nonsmokers' RR = 1.0) for death due to CVD was 1.4 in users of smokeless tobacco, 1.8 in those who smoked less than 15 cigarettes per day, and 1.9 in those who smoked more than 15 cigarettes per day.

What about the risk of cigarette smoking for those who've already had a coronary event or a revascularization procedure? Patients who continue to smoke after an MI have a 22% greater subsequent risk of death and a 47% greater risk of reinfarction compared to patients who have not smoked following their MI. Furthermore, continued cigarette smoking after coronary artery bypass graft surgery appears to double a patient's risk of death (21).

Cigarette smoking has both acute and chronic effects on the cardiovascular system. Acutely, cigarette smoking accentuates risk for cardiac

events (e.g., MI and cardiac arrest) by elevating heart rate and blood pressure, thereby increasing myocardial demand, reducing the oxygen-carrying capacity of the blood, lowering the threshold for cardiac arrhythmias, causing coronary artery vasospasm, and increasing platelet aggregation. The chronic effects of cigarette smoking include decreases in high-density lipoprotein levels, oxidation of LDL-C, increases of blood fibrinogen levels (increased potential for blood clotting), damage to the vascular endothelium, and increases in blood viscosity through polycythemia (increased red blood cell production) (12). Although an MI has been the traditional marker of CAD in most observational studies assessing the association between smoking and CAD, the effects of cigarette smoking on the progression of CAD lesions is also important. The Atherosclerosis Risk in Communities Study (22) used the change in the size of the intimal-medial thickness of the carotid artery to measure the progression of **atherosclerosis** among 10,914 participants during a three-year period. This study revealed that current smokers (n = 2956) had a 50% increase in the rate of progression of atherosclerosis compared to individuals who had never smoked. Former smokers (n = 1849) still had a 25% greater rate of progression than those who had never smoked. Thus, even though an individual with CAD quits smoking, the apparent residual risk for disease progression indicates the importance of aggressive intervention on the other modifiable risk factors.

What about the CAD risk associated with passive or "secondhand" smoke exposure? According to the AHA (1), 48% of nonsmoking, working adults age 17 and older reported some exposure to environmental tobacco smoke in the home or workplace. Furthermore, according to results of a recent survey analyzed by the CDC, 43% of American children under age 11 are exposed to environmental tobacco smoke in the home. In an analysis of nine epidemiologic studies, the RR for death due to heart disease among individuals who had never smoked was as much as 3.0 in subjects who lived with current or former smokers compared with those who lived with nonsmokers (23). In the Atherosclerosis Risk in Communities Study already described, the rate of progression of atherosclerosis in the 2449 individuals who had never smoked but who had been exposed to secondhand smoke was 20% higher than for those who had never smoked and never been exposed to smoke (22). Passive or secondhand smoke exposure increases the risk of CAD in individuals who have never smoked by as much as 30% and is estimated to cause 53,000 heart disease deaths per year in the United States (24).

Dyslipidemia

Lipids are fats transported in the blood plasma in structures called lipoproteins. Lipoproteins are complex water-soluble molecules that consist of a core of cholesterol ester and triglyceride covered by a monolayer surface of phospholipids, free cholesterol, and apolipoproteins. The major plasma lipoproteins—chylomicrons, very low density lipoprotein (VLDL), intermediate-density lipoprotein (IDL), low-density lipoprotein (LDL), and high-density lipoprotein (HDL)—are distinguished by density, mobility, lipid content, and surface proteins (25). The lipoproteins vary in their contribution to atherosclerotic risk. Figure 1.7 presents an overview of the current understanding of the metabolic pathway for lipids important in the atherosclerotic process. The triglyceride-rich chylomicrons and VLDL are not thought to be **atherogenic** (i.e., to lead to progression of CAD), but the remnants of their lipolysis or breakdown (e.g., chylomicron remnants and IDL) are believed to be atherogenic.

The metabolic end point of VLDL is LDL, which, along with lipoprotein(a), is thought to be highly atherogenic. In contrast, HDL is known to have a cardioprotective effect. The dyslipidemia most clearly associated with increased risk for CAD is hypercholesterolemia, particularly elevated plasma levels of cholesterol carried in LDL. Low-density lipoprotein contains approximately

70% of the cholesterol in the blood and is the primary target of intervention in the guidelines of the third Adult Treatment Panel of the National Cholesterol Education Program (NCEP) (26).

Total cholesterol

According to a recent estimate from the CDC (National Health and Nutrition Examination Survey, NHANES III) , approximately 52% of American adults have total cholesterol levels of >200 mg/dl, and 20% have levels of ≥240 mg/dl. These total cholesterol levels represent the NCEP borderline-high and high-risk categories, respectively (table 1.2). These data suggest that elevated total cholesterol is a very prevalent risk factor within the U.S. population.

The association between elevated blood cholesterol and CAD, established in observational and interventional epidemiologic studies, clearly supports the hypothesis that an increase in serum cholesterol results in an increased risk of CAD. A continuous and graded positive relationship was demonstrated between total cholesterol level and CAD mortality in the more than 350,000 men screened for the Multiple Risk Factor Intervention Trial (MRFIT) (11) (figure 1.8). Furthermore, the Seven Countries Study (27) demonstrated that in areas of the world where the intake of satu-

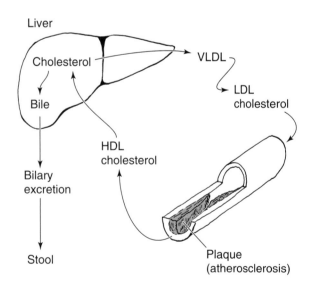

Figure 1.7 Overview of lipoproteins and lipoprotein pathways.
Reprinted, by permission, from D.C. Nieman, 1998, *Exercise testing and prescription: A health related approach*, 4th ed. (Mountain View: Mayfield Publishing Company), 373.

Table 1.2
Classification of Total Serum Cholesterol and Serum Low- (LDL) and High-Density Lipoprotein (HDL) Cholesterol Concentrations

Total cholesterol	Classification
< 200 mg/dl	Desirable
200-239 mg/dl	Borderline high
≥ 240 mg/dl	High
LDL cholesterol	**Classification**
< 100 mg/dl	Optimal
100-129 mg/dl	Near optimal/above optimal
130-159 mg/dl	Borderline high
160-189 mg/dl	High
≥190 mg/dl	Very high
HDL cholesterol	**Classification**
< 40 mg/dl	Low
> 60 mg/dl	High

From the National Cholesterol Education Program (26).

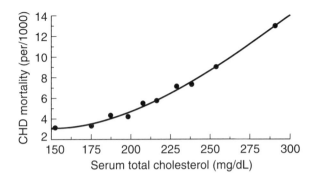

Figure 1.8 Relationship between serum total cholesterol and CAD mortality in the Multiple Risk Factor Intervention Trial.
Data from J. Stamler, et al., 1986.

rated fat was low and the average plasma cholesterol levels were relatively low, such as Japan and countries around the Mediterranean Sea, the **mortality rate** for CAD was also low. In contrast, in countries where the average serum cholesterol was higher, such as the United States and Finland, the mortality from CAD was also higher. Similarly, the Ni-Hon-San study (28) showed that men of Japanese descent living in the United States consumed a diet higher in fat and cholesterol than Japanese men living in Japan. The men living in the United States had higher total cholesterol levels and higher age-adjusted increase in MI and CAD death. The NCEP recommends that adults maintain a total serum cholesterol of less than 200 mg/dl across the life span (table 1.2).

Low-density lipoproteins
Recent data from the CDC (NHANES III) suggest that the prevalence of borderline-high (130-159 mg/dl) and high LDL-C (>160 mg/dl) within the U.S. adult population is only slightly less than the percentages for total cholesterol already described. Published treatment guidelines strongly recommend the evaluation of LDL in both primary and secondary CAD prevention settings because of strong evidence from epidemiologic, genetic, animal, and clinical investigations indicating a causal link between elevated LDL and CAD risk (12). Low-density lipoprotein is the major carrier of cholesterol to the periphery, and it supplies cholesterol essential for the integrity of nerve tissue and cell membranes, as well as for steroid synthesis. However, LDL promotes atherogenesis by affecting the influx of lipids into the vessel wall through the injured or dysfunctional endothelium. Low-density lipoprotein becomes more atherogenic as it becomes oxidized from exposure to endothelial cells, smooth muscle cells, or macrophages (foam cells). The oxidized LDL then attracts circulating monocytes, causing

them to adhere to the arterial wall and precipitating their activation as macrophages. Macrophages liberate a large number of products, including cholesterol, that can further damage the endothelium and contribute to the lesion formation (16). In addition to the LDL level, LDL composition appears to influence CAD risk. Smaller, denser LDL particles (known as LDL subclass pattern B) have been shown to be associated with a threefold-increased risk for MI (29). Small dense LDL frequently occurs in conjunction with an elevated triglyceride level, low HDL cholesterol level, obesity, and hypertension. The mechanism by which small dense LDL confers increased risk of CAD has not been clearly defined.

High-density lipoproteins
Numerous epidemiologic studies have shown a strong inverse relationship between HDL and CAD. The Framingham Heart Study and other large studies have shown that for every 1 mg/dl increase in HDL, there is a 2% to 3% decrease in CAD risk (30). This effect is seen even after adjusting for other risk factors and in both men and women. According to recent data from the CDC (NHANES III), the prevalence of low high-density lipoprotein cholesterol (HDL-C) less than 35 mg/dl among adult American males is 18%, 15%, and 9% in non-Hispanic whites, Mexican Americans, and non-Hispanic blacks, respectively. The prevalence of HDL-C less than 35 mg/dl in the respective female groups is 6%, 6%, and 3%.

High-density lipoproteins are secreted by the liver and intestines as precursor particles composed of phospholipids, cholesterol, and apolipoproteins. The activity of lecithin:cholesterol acetyltransferase helps create HDL_3 from the precursor particles. The HDL_3 acquires additional phospholipid and cholesterol and is eventually converted to HDL_2. The HDL_2, larger and more cholesterol rich than HDL_3, is thought to be the more cardioprotective of the two. Women have significantly higher levels of the larger, less dense HDL_2, which may be partially responsible for the reduced CAD risk in premenopausal women (25). It appears that HDL_2 prevents entry of cholesterol into the atherosclerotic process and that it may even remove cholesterol from established atherosclerotic lesions (so-called reverse cholesterol transport). Other potential mechanisms by which HDL may confer cardioprotection include enhancement of endothelial function, rapid clearance of triglyceride-rich particles, and protection against the oxidative effects of LDL (25). In addition to targeting LDL, NCEP has recommended the addition of HDL to initial cholesterol testing. This organization has designated a high HDL (>60 mg/dl) as a negative risk factor and a low HDL (<40 mg/dl) as a positive risk factor for CAD (table 1.2).

Triglycerides

Observational studies have consistently shown a strong association between increased triglyceride levels and CAD. However, when these studies are subjected to multivariate analyses, controlling for LDL-C or total cholesterol and other risk factors such as blood pressure, physical activity, and obesity, the role of triglycerides is diminished. The addition of indicators of abnormal glucose metabolism (i.e., elevated blood glucose) or low HDL eliminates or significantly reduces the role of triglycerides as an independent predictor of CAD risk (29). A combination of high triglycerides and low HDL does appear, however, to be a highly atherogenic pattern and is often seen in patients with CAD who have otherwise normal lipid profiles (i.e., normal total cholesterol and LDL) (91). Table 1.3 presents the NCEP classifications for serum triglyceride levels.

Within the context of **hyperlipidemia** and CAD risk, blood lipids have been measured with the subject in the fasted state (i.e., 8-12 h following the last meal). Thus, the majority of the scientific evidence linking abnormal lipids to CAD has been based on this type of measurement. However, because of our typical eating patterns, we spend a majority of each day in the nonfasted state, and scientists have often debated whether or not fasting blood lipids truly represent the arterial milieu that we ought to be studying. More recently, researchers have begun to assess the association between elevated triglycerides following a meal, referred to as postprandial lipemia, and atherogenesis. Data suggest that those with elevated triglyceride concentrations in the postmeal state may possess a metabolic disorder that is likely atherogenic.

Hypertension

The **prevalence** of **hypertension** in the United States and other Western countries continues to be high, and increases with age. The most recent National Health and Nutrition Examination Survey (NHANES III) (31), conducted between 1988 and 1991, documented an overall prevalence of hypertension in Americans of 24% (or 43 million people). The prevalence of hypertension was only 4% in ages 18 to 29, but it rose progressively with each age group and reached a peak of 65% in Americans over the age of 80. According to the Sixth Report of the Joint National Committee on Prevention, Detection, Evaluation, and Treatment of High Blood Pressure (JNC VI) (32), about one-third of persons with hypertension are unaware that they have it, and only about half of those who are taking medications to control their blood pressure have their pressure under control.

Blood pressure levels are classified by the JNC VI (32) and are outlined in table 1.4. Hypertension is believed to increase the risk for CAD both through direct injury to the vascular endothelium and through adverse effects on the heart. The increased blood pressure represents an increase in afterload, which in turn causes an increase in myocardial wall stress and ultimately an increased myocardial oxygen demand (16).

Physical Inactivity

Regular physical activity has been shown to reduce the risk for CAD events in numerous observational epidemiologic studies, although the pre-

Table 1.3
Classification of Fasting Serum Triglyceride Concentrations

Serum triglycerides	Classification
<150 mg/dl	Normal
150-199 mg/dl	Borderline high
200-499 mg/dl	High
≥500 mg/dl	Very high

From The National Cholesterol Education Program (26).

Table 1.4
Classification of Blood Pressure for Adults Aged 18 Years and Older

Systolic (mmHg)	Diastolic (mmHg)	Category
<130	<85	Normal
130-139	85-89	High normal
140-159	90-99	Mild (Stage 1)
160-179	100-109	Moderate (Stage 2)
180-209	110-119	Severe (Stage 3)
≥210	≥120	Very severe (Stage 4)

These data represent the classification of blood pressure for adults aged 18 years and older when they are not taking antihypertensive medication and are not acutely ill. When SBP and DBP fall into different categories, the higher of the two categories should be selected.
From The Joint National Committee on Detection, Evaluation, and Treatment of High Blood Pressure (32).

cise amount of activity for optimal protection remains unclear (33). Unfortunately, nearly 25% of adult Americans reported no leisure-time physical activity (LTPA), and approximately 60% of adults do not accrue even the minimal recommended amount of activity (34). Because physical inactivity is considerably more prevalent in our society than are the more traditional risk factors of smoking, dyslipidemia, and hypertension, some have postulated that increasing activity levels within our society could have a larger overall impact on reducing CAD than interventions aimed at the other risk factors we have discussed (12, 35).

Research study designs

Before we review the results from recent prospective epidemiological studies on physical activity/fitness and CAD, a brief primer on basic design features of these studies will be helpful. Figure 1.9 illustrates a generic design for epidemiological studies of LTPA and/or cardiorespiratory fitness (CRF). The overall importance of a particular study depends on how the researchers designed the study, and one should evaluate the features illustrated in figure 1.9 before placing any importance on the study conclusions. Obviously, well-designed studies provide the best information regarding the association between physical activity or CRF and CAD. A basic requirement for this type of study is a rather large sample (often referred to as a cohort) of men and/or women who can be followed for a period of years (i.e., 5 to 20 years) for the incidence of CAD. The sample needs to be sufficiently large to allow for enough disease end points to occur (typically >1000 subjects). In addition, characteristics such as the age and general health status of the sample at the beginning of the study should be evaluated. As CAD is a chronic disease that

often takes years to develop, studies are generally conducted on samples of middle- or older-age adults (≥35 years of age). The sample is then followed for an appropriate amount of time to allow for the disease to develop. In addition, within the context of primary prevention, it is important for the researchers to document that the sample was healthy (i.e., free of CAD) at the beginning of the study.

Perhaps the most important design feature in epidemiological studies of LTPA/CRF is the measurement of the exposure to the risk factor for the disease in question (i.e., CAD). The measure of LTPA and/or CRF defines each individual's exposure to this risk factor during the study. The majority of studies to date used a single self-reported measure of activity or fitness at baseline as the exposure variable, although a few of the more recent studies included measures of LTPA or CRF at both baseline and some point during the follow-up period. We will look more closely at this design feature later in this section. The measurement of LTPA has varied among the studies from as little as a single multiple-choice question describing current physical activity habits to more extensive individual interviews designed to quantify physical activity habits throughout the previous year. The measurement of CRF is usually derived from the results of an exercise test. The stronger studies used a maximal exercise test to quantify fitness. Information on physical activity habits is usually converted for analysis either to an estimate of total energy expenditure (e.g., kilocalories per day or week) or to a physical activity index with individuals assigned to LTPA categories based on a combination of type, amount, and intensity of self-reported physical activity. Within the better epidemiological studies, CRF is usually quantified as either a measured or a predicted $\dot{V}O_2$max or some sort of physical work capacity. When one is evaluating studies that quantified risk exposure using a measure of CRF, it's important to remember the genetic component associated with $\dot{V}O_2$max. In a review of this topic, Bouchard et al. (36) concluded that the genetic component probably lies between 10% and 50%. Therefore, it is appropriate to view measures of fitness within these studies as a consequence of both hereditary factors and habitual physical activity.

Needless to say, the variability in LTPA or CRF assessment within the studies makes it difficult to compare results among them in any more than a qualitative way. For a more detailed discussion of the design features and results of recent LTPA/

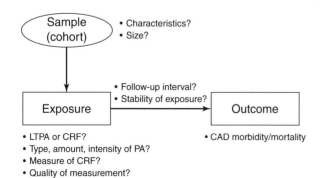

Figure 1.9　Basic research design used in epidemiological studies of physical activity/fitness and coronary artery disease risk.

CRF studies, readers may refer to more extensive reviews on the topic (33, 37, 38). Now, with a basic understanding of design features within epidemiologic studies, we can proceed to a discussion of the evidence linking sedentary lifestyle and low physical fitness with increased risk for CAD.

Studies of male cohorts

A summary of the results from several recent epidemiological studies (39-43) of LTPA or CRF and CAD/CVD is presented in figure 1.10. Although the studies shown in the figure are only a few of those available, they are all well designed, and they represent a variety of LTPA survey instruments and fitness measures. The message that the figure depicts is that as one moves from the lower to the higher end of the physical activity or fitness continuum, the risk for CAD decreases.

But let's take a closer look at each of these frequently cited studies. Leon et al. assessed LTPA and both fatal and nonfatal CAD in 12,132 high-risk men from the MRFIT (41). During a seven-year follow-up period there was an approximate 65% reduction in CAD mortality for those men expending ≥1500 kcal per week in mostly light-to moderate-intensity LTPA. While this is clearly good news, remember that the end point in the analysis was a fatal MI. As discussed earlier in the chapter, individuals survive close to two-thirds of the 650,000 new MIs each year. So, what do the results of the MRFIT suggest about protection from a nonfatal MI? These data from the MRFIT are shown in figure 1.10. When the broader end point for CAD of combined fatal and nonfatal MI was used in the analysis, only the most active men—those expending >4400 kcal per week in LTPA—received protection, and the amount of protection was modest compared to that shown in other studies (17% reduction). Therefore, the results of the MRFIT suggest that if one of the goals of participation in a physical

activity program is preventing the first heart attack (whether fatal or nonfatal), a higher volume of exercise may be necessary.

In a study from the British Civil Service cohort, Morris et al. (42) reported that men who participated in regular vigorous aerobic exercise (>7.5 kcal · min^{-1} or >65% of maximal oxygen uptake) had 63% and 75% lower CAD morbidity and mortality, respectively, when compared to men who reported no vigorous aerobic exercise. This finding was stronger for the younger men (45-54 years) compared to the older men (55-64 years), suggesting that the absolute energy expenditure threshold (>7.5 kcal · min^{-1}) used by Morris et al. might not be as important in older men as the relative intensity of the activity (>65% of maximal oxygen uptake). Why would this be the case? The answer relates to the general notion that $\dot{V}O_2$max declines across the life span. In theory, a given absolute exercise intensity (e.g., 8 METs or 7.5 kcal · min^{-1}) would represent a higher percentage of an older person's $\dot{V}O_2$max compared to a younger person's, because the older person has a lower $\dot{V}O_2$max to begin with. Therefore, if we are attempting to translate the results from the study by Morris et al. into exercise recommendations for older individuals, expressing exercise intensity in relative terms (percentage of $\dot{V}O_2$max) would be most important. Morris et al. also reported that after excluding vigorous aerobic exercise, they observed no relation between the total quantity of less intense physical activity and CAD. Similarly, Lakka et al. (40) reported that Finnish men who engaged in greater than 2.2 h per week of "conditioning" activities (e.g., mostly aerobic activities with intensities ≥6 METs) had a 66% lower rate of combined fatal and nonfatal CAD compared to those with lesser amounts; but "nonconditioning" activities were not associated with protection regardless of the amount.

Do the results from Lakka et al. (40) and Morris et al. (42) conflict with those of Leon et al. (41)? In fact, these studies may not be all that different. Leon et al. found that less than 5% of the MRFIT men reported 1 h or more of "vigorous" exercise per week, and concluded that their study lacked the statistical power to test whether more vigorous exercise would have further lowered the risk of CVD mortality. So the larger reductions in CAD risk reported in the British and Finnish studies in relation to more vigorous activity may simply reflect the concept of dose response within the context of the intensity of LTPA. The other two studies shown in figure 1.10 used a measure of CRF as the exposure variable. Blair et al. (39) used a maximal treadmill test to quantify CRF within the 10,224 men of the Aerobics Center Longitudi-

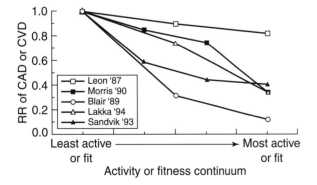

Figure 1.10 Relative risk of CVD morbidity/mortality across the physical activity or fitness continuum from recent epidemiological studies of men.

Adapted from R. R. Pate, et al., 1995.

nal Study. The men were divided into fitness quintiles based on their maximal treadmill time during the test. There was a sevenfold-greater risk for CVD mortality during eight years of follow-up for the men within the cohort whose fitness was low compared to the men whose fitness level was highest. Sandvik et al. (43) used a maximal leg cycling test to quantify CRF in 1960 Norwegian men who were followed for 16 years. The men with the highest fitness level had a significant reduction in risk of CAD mortality (RR of 0.41) compared to the men whose fitness was lowest.

In summary, when viewed collectively, the studies in figure 1.10 show an inverse dose-response relationship between the amount of physical activity or fitness and CAD/CVD. In other words, the more you do, up to a point, the lower your risk for disease.

Studies of female cohorts

Although the link between CAD and inactivity or low fitness is firmly established for men, the scientific evidence for this relationship in women has been lacking until recently. Early prospective studies on women were not clearly supportive of a protective effect for a more active lifestyle (44-47). Despite this lack of evidence, public health messages strongly encouraged women to be more physically active primarily on the strength of the evidence for a protective effect seen in studies of men. However, results from more recent physical activity and fitness studies on women bring this issue into clearer focus (39, 48-50). Results from these studies are illustrated in figure 1.11. In the report from the Aerobics Center Longitudinal Study, Blair et al. (39) assessed CVD risk in 3120 women using maximal treadmill test time as a marker of CRF.

The women were followed for mortality for an average of eight years after the exercise test. As the figure shows, increasing fitness level was associated with a significant reduction in CVD mortality within this cohort. Lissner et al. (49) studied the effects of leisure-time activity in a group of 1267 Swedish women followed for 20 years for all-cause mortality. The investigators reported that the most active women had less than half the risk of death during the follow-up period compared to the least-active women. Kushi et al. (48) reported similar results from the Iowa Women's Health Study. This study included over 32,000 women followed for CVD for seven years. Once again, the most active group had about half the risk for CVD compared to the least-active women. And finally, in one of the largest epidemiological studies on women to date (72,000 women within the Nurses' Health Study), Manson et al. (50) reported a significant reduction in both fatal and nonfatal CAD risk for several measures of physical activity.

In this study, Manson et al. (50) first assessed the relationship between LTPA and CAD across quintiles of MET-hours per week. This measure captures both the quantity (i.e., amount) and quality (i.e., intensity) of physical activity during leisure time. Those women in the most active quintile had a 34% reduction in CAD risk during the follow-up period compared to the least-active groups. As illustrated in figure 1.11, women in the middle quintiles also experienced a reduction in risk compared to the least-active women. The authors also assessed the protective effect of increasing amounts of walking within women who reported no vigorous activity. In other words, what's the protective effect for *moderate*-intensity activity? The results were quite similar to those shown in figure 1.11. The women who walked the most each week had the lowest risk of CAD. And further, the authors also observed a gradient across walking pace, with the faster walkers having lower risk than the slower walkers. All the studies included in figure 1.11 showed an inverse dose-response relationship between physical activity or CRF and either CAD or all-cause mortality. Therefore, current public health recommendations encouraging women to be more active are clearly supported by recent epidemiological studies.

Important interpretative issues

Several aspects of the physical activity/fitness studies presented here warrant further explanation. First, it might seem logical to try to compare the degree of protection afforded men or women among the studies (e.g., Leon et al. [41] vs. Blair

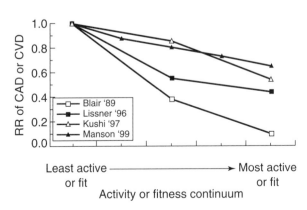

Figure 1.11 Relative risk of CVD morbidity/mortality across the physical activity or fitness continuum from recent epidemiological studies of women.

et al. [39]). In this regard, the data in figures 1.10 and 1.11 would appear to suggest that the protective effect for a given quantity (amount of activity or fitness) or quality (intensity) of activity varied considerably across the studies. However, because of significant differences among the studies in measures of physical activity or fitness and the specific disease end points assessed, the observed variability in the protective effect of activity/fitness across the studies would be expected, and the figure should not be interpreted to mean that the data are unclear. The important message within the figure is that each study shows a decline in disease incidence across activity or fitness categories, which strongly supports the notion that sedentary habits or a low CRF serves to increase one's CAD risk. Second, each study in figures 1.10 and 1.11 was based on a single measure of physical activity or fitness taken at the beginning of the research. This type of epidemiological research design assumes a stable pattern of activity throughout the study period (see figure 1.9). The problem with this type of epidemiological research design is that if the subjects altered their activity habits during the follow-up period, the initial measure of activity or fitness might not reflect their true risk exposure during the study. This concern—referred to by epidemiologists as misclassification bias—could influence one's confidence in the ability of these studies to truly define the relationship between the risk factor under investigation (i.e., physical activity/fitness) and the disease end point (i.e., CAD). The next section describes several more recent studies that attempted to lessen the impact of this sort of bias by including information about an individual's change (or lack thereof) in physical activity or CRF within the analysis.

Studies incorporating changes in physical activity or fitness

Several recent studies of men (51-55) and women (49, 50) included research designs that, to a degree, lessen the impact of potential misclassification bias by incorporating multiple measures of physical activity or fitness during the course of the follow-up period. This type of research design differs from the one presented in figure 1.9, in which only a baseline exposure measure of activity or fitness is used to assess CAD risk. When two or more assessments of LTPA or CRF are incorporated into the follow-up period, studies can better assess the impact of changes in physical activity habits (increases or decreases) on the risk of CAD. For example, let's say that a 45-year-old man who's been sedentary for years takes our advice about increasing his activity level

and starts a regular exercise program. Can he expect to benefit from a reduction in CAD risk as much as his neighbor who has maintained an active lifestyle throughout his adult life? Needless to say, it's a very important question within the context of lifestyle modification recommendations. In other words, can we get up off the couch after 20 years of sedentary living and reduce our risk by becoming more active? Recent studies using multiple activity or fitness assessments across time suggest that the answer is yes.

Results from the Harvard Alumni Study are presented in figure 1.12. Paffenbarger et al. (54) followed 14,786 men from the early 1960s through to 1988. They assessed physical activity levels at the beginning of the study (baseline) just as those studies summarized in figure 1.10 did. However, what makes this study and others like it unique is that the investigators reassessed activity levels again in 1977 (reassessment) and then followed the men for another nine years to determine the effect of change in activity (i.e., becoming more or less active) on CAD risk. The bars in figure 1.12 represent the RR of CAD for each of the four study groups. Those who reported less than 1500 kcal per week of leisure-time activity at both assessments—labeled Stable Sedentary in the figure—represent the least-active group of men in the study and were assigned an RR of 1.0. The three other groups were compared to this most sedentary group. The two middle bars represent men who reported a significant change in LTPA by the time of the reassessment. The men who became less active (labeled Decreased) during the follow-up period actually experienced an increase in CAD risk when compared to those who were considered the most sedentary. However, either the adoption (Increased) or maintenance (Stable Active) of a more active lifestyle significantly lowered CAD risk.

Other recent investigations have supported the results from the Harvard Alumni Study

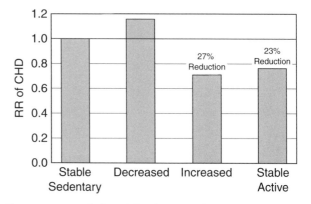

Figure 1.12 Relative risk of CAD related to changes in physical activity habits within the Harvard Alumni.
Data from R.S. Paffenbarger, et al., 1994.

shown in figure 1.12. Wannamethee, Shaper, and Walker (55), following 4311 British men from the British Regional Heart Study for three years after a second assessment of LTPA, reported that the most active men at each of the two assessments were at 60% lower risk for CVD mortality compared to the least-active men. However, those who increased their activity during the follow-up period (i.e., got up off the couch!) were at 50% lower risk for CVD compared to the least active men within the study. Two other studies that assessed changes in CRF during follow-up periods also support the notion that getting up off the couch in midlife pays off. Results from the Aerobic Center Longitudinal Study by Blair et al. (51) showed that men who were considered aerobically fit at both assessments were at 78% lower risk of CVD mortality compared to those men who were the least fit at both exams. In addition, CVD mortality risk for those who changed their level of fitness between the clinic exams (an increase or decrease) was approximately 50% less than for those who were unfit at both exams. Similar results were observed within subgroups of healthy and unhealthy men and across all the age categories studied. One might wonder why the group that experienced a decline in fitness (as defined within the study) had a mortality risk during the follow-up period similar to that for the people who improved their CRF. The answer may be that men who experienced a change in their fitness level (again, either an increase or decrease) spent part of the follow-up period more physically fit than those men who were not considered fit at either examination. Thus, by virtue of being more fit for part of the study period, the men who experienced a change in fitness level during the follow-up period had a lower CVD risk than the men who were chronically less fit. And finally, in a recent study with Norwegian men, Erikssen et al. (52) reported an approximate 50% reduction in risk of CVD mortality for men who increased their fitness level the most when compared to men who had a decline in fitness during seven years of follow-up.

Once again, it appears that most of the evidence showing a benefit for increasing activity or fitness comes from studies on men. Does this benefit apply to women as well? Two recent reports have assessed the effect of changes in activity on CAD risk in women (49, 50). In the study on Swedish women reviewed earlier, Lissner et al. (49) also reassessed physical activity habits during the follow-up period and found that women who decreased their physical activity levels (i.e., became less active after the initial assessment) had a modest increase in mortality compared to women who maintained higher levels or increased their activity. In addition, data by Manson et al. (50) from the Nurses' Health Study also support the notion that initially sedentary women who increase their activity levels can reduce their risk of CAD. Figure 1.13 illustrates this reduction in risk across quintiles of increased activity for the nurses who were mostly sedentary at the beginning of the study. Those who increased their activity the most (i.e., quintiles 4 and 5) had about a 30% reduction in risk compared to the nurses who remained more sedentary throughout the study period.

In summary, results from studies on men and women that included assessment of a change in LTPA or CRF strengthen findings from earlier reports based solely on baseline measures of activity or fitness (figures 1.10 and 1.11). The findings provide needed encouragement to adults who've been sedentary for years and who perhaps perceive midlife efforts at lifestyle modification as a waste of time. These studies contain a message for the general public—it's never too late to adopt a more active lifestyle! This is precisely the message contained within recent public health communications (34, 37) and national exercise guidelines (56, 57).

The plausible mechanisms by which aerobic exercise and increased fitness may decrease risk for CAD events include improvements in risk factors such as HDL, insulin resistance, body weight and fat, and blood pressure (3). Furthermore, exercise may favorably affect known triggers for cardiac events such as platelet aggregation, prevent clot formation (fibrinolysis), improve endothelial function, and decrease the threshold for malignant arrhythmias (12).

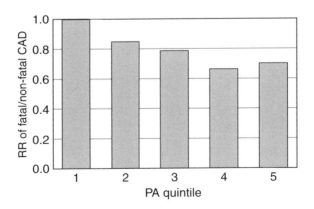

Figure 1.13 Relative risk of CAD related to increases in physical activity for initially sedentary women within the Nurses' Health Study. Quintile 1 are those who increased their activity the least and quintile 5 are those who increased the most.

Data from J.E. Manson, et al., 1999.

Obesity

According to NHANES III, approximately 58 million U.S. adults, or one-third of Americans over the age of 20, are estimated to be overweight (defined by a body mass index [weight in kilograms/height in meters squared] greater than 27.8 in men and 27.3 in women). For years, health care professionals viewed obesity as a risk factor that exerted its influence through other traditional risk factors such as hypertension and hyperlipidemia. However, the AHA adopted obesity as a major risk factor for heart disease in 1998 (2), and defined overweight as body mass index (BMI) >25 but <30 and obesity as BMI >30. Obesity-related conditions are estimated to contribute to 300,000 deaths annually in the United States (58). The health risks of obesity not only increase with its severity but also appear to be affected by the distribution of body fat. Abdominal adiposity, characterized by excessive fat in the abdomen (apple shape), appears to impart greater risk of CAD than increased adiposity around the hips (pear shape). Consequently, the waist:hip ratio has been used to define risk of CAD, but precise thresholds are elusive (56). However, the Expert Panel on obesity and health risk recommends use of the waist circumference alone (the numerator in the waist:hip ratio) as the most convenient and accurate measure of abdominal adiposity (59).

Gender-specific values greater than 40 in. (102 cm; men) and 35 in. (88 cm; women) were cited by the panel as associated with increased health risk (table 1.5). We should note, though, that other waist circumference risk thresholds have been advocated (60, 61). Chapter 6 discusses in more detail issues concerning which measure of fatness/obesity to use for risk assessment.

The metabolic linkage of visceral obesity, high triglyceride levels, low HDL levels, insulin resistance (with subsequent **hyperinsulinemia**), and hypertension has been termed the metabolic *syndrome X* and is associated with a dramatically increased risk for CAD. This clustering of CAD risk factors has also been associated with low CRF (62)—an additional risk factor for CAD. The mechanism by which obesity increases the risk for CAD is not well understood, but it relates at least in part to the association between obesity and other CAD risk factors (physical inactivity, hypertension, hyperlipidemia, and diabetes). However, in the Framingham study, obesity was found to be an "independent" risk factor for CAD in both men and women (63).

Diabetes Mellitus

According to the American Diabetes Association (64), nearly 14 million individuals in the United States are estimated to have diabetes mellitus (the term roughly translates to "sweet urine"), but surprisingly, more than half of these individuals have not been diagnosed. Among persons with diabetes, only 5% to 10% have insulin-dependent diabetes mellitus (IDDM), which is often referred to as type I diabetes since it usually occurs before the

Table 1.5

Classification of Disease Risk Based on BMI and Waist Circumference*

	BMI (kg/m²)	Disease risk[†] relative to normal weight and waist circumference[‡]	
		Men (≤102 cm) Women (≤88 cm)	Men (>102 cm) Women (>88 cm)
Underweight	<18.5	. . .	. . .
Normal[§]	18.5–24.9	. . .	. . .
Overweight	25.0–29.9	Increased	High
Obesity, class			
I	30.0–34.9	High	Very high
II	35.0–39.9	Very high	Very high
III	≥40	Extremely high	Extremely high

*Modified from Expert Panel. Executive summary of the clinical guidelines on the identification, evaluation, and treatment of overweight and obesity in adults. Arch Intern Med 1998; 158:1855-1867.

[†]Disease risk for type II diabetes, hypertension, and cardiovascualar disease. Ellipses indicate that no additional risk at these levels of BMI was assigned.

[‡]A gender neutral value for waist circumference (>100 cm) has also been suggested as an index of obesity.

[§]Increased waist circumference can also be a marker for increased risk even in persons of normal weight.

Reprinted, by permission, from Expert Panel, 1998, "Executive summary of the clinical guidelines on the identification, evaluation, and treatment of overweight and obesity in adults," *Archives of Internal Medicine* 158:1855-1867.

age of 30. In this condition, the pancreas produces inadequate amounts of insulin, thus necessitating exogenous administration of insulin. The form of diabetes that affects the other 90% to 95% of individuals with diabetes is non-insulin-dependent diabetes mellitus (NIDDM), called type II diabetes. This condition usually occurs after the age of 40 and often goes unrecognized for many years. The prevalence of diabetes increases with age and is higher in blacks and Hispanics than in whites (64). Coronary artery disease is a major complication of both IDDM and NIDDM. The Rancho Bernardo Study (65) followed 334 men and women with NIDDM, as well as 2137 men and women without diabetes, for 14 years. The RR for CAD death was 1.9 in diabetic men and 3.3 in diabetic women compared with nondiabetic men and women (whose RR = 1.0) after other CAD risk factors were adjusted for. More sobering is the finding that CAD, cerebrovascular disease, or peripheral vascular disease is the cause of death in 75% to 80% of adults with diabetes. Diabetes frequently exists in the presence of other, often modifiable, CAD risk factors. Hypertension and obesity, as well as the atherogenic combination of high triglycerides and low HDL levels, are commonly seen in patients with diabetes. In addition to these risk factors, chronic **hyperglycemia** results in a number of complex vascular alterations that increase the risk for atherosclerosis and thrombosis (blood clotting) (16).

Psychosocial Factors

The role of personality type and emotional stress in the risk stratification for CAD has been debated for many years, but recent prospective studies have shown that "type A" personality, hostility, depression, and stress caused by "high demand-low control" situations increase the risk for CAD (12). The mechanisms by which personality types may predispose to increased risk are not known but may include increased sympathetic nervous system activity, which increases heart rate and blood pressure, and increased cardiovascular reactivity, which may lead to endothelial injury and platelet aggregation (66).

It is estimated that depression affects more than 17 million Americans. Unfortunately, nearly two-thirds of those who experience depression don't receive proper treatment because of misdiagnosis, a misunderstanding of the condition, or the patient's inability to seek help. Therefore, depression represents a risk factor that is likely underappreciated within the general population. Is there solid evidence that clinical depression is associated with increased risk of CAD? Two recent prospective studies have assessed the relationship between depression and CAD (67, 68). The Johns Hopkins Precursor Study followed 1190 male medical students for depression and incidence of MI. The cumulative incidence of clinical depression during 40 years of follow-up was 12% in these men. There were no differences in blood pressure, serum cholesterol levels, smoking status, physical activity, obesity, or family history of CAD between depressed and nondepressed men. Men with a history of clinical depression had a doubling of risk (RR = 2.1) for subsequent coronary heart disease, defined as MI, angina, or coronary revascularization (surgery or angioplasty) (68). Depression was also associated with greater risk of total and CVD mortality (i.e., death) within the study. Another prospective study, involving 5007 women and 2886 men enrolled in the first National Health and Nutrition Examination Survey (NHANES I), assessed depression using the Center for Epidemiologic Studies Depression Scale (67). After adjusting for poverty rates, race, hypertension, BMI, and smoking, the investigators found a 1.7 RR of incident CAD for depressed men and women compared to their nondepressed counterparts. These and other studies confirm an association between depression and CAD. The investigations suggest that clinical depression is an independent risk factor for incident CAD and that perhaps we should place more emphasis on screening and treatment for this disorder as a means to lower CAD risk.

Emerging and Controversial Risk Factors for Coronary Artery Disease

As with any chronic disease on which there is an evolving body of science, research into the pathophysiological mechanisms underlying the development of CAD is constantly being updated with new studies that identify various new or emerging risk factors for the disease, or perhaps modify understanding of the role that existing risk factors play in the disease process. This section provides information about several emerging risk factors for CAD.

Lipoprotein(a)

Lipoprotein(a) or Lp(a), pronounced "L P little a," is an LDL-like lipoprotein that has been identified as a genetic risk factor for CAD. Elevated Lp(a) is present in 10% to 15% of the white population and appears to exert its pathologic effect at levels above 20 mg/dl. Modified Lp(a) can be taken up by macrophages, much like LDL, leading to foam cell formation, which contributes to the atherosclerotic process. Furthermore, Lp(a) may also prevent clots from dissolving (69). Although lowering Lp(a) is theoretically appealing, the clinical impact has not been determined (25).

Because Lp(a) measurement is not a widely available laboratory procedure and the clinical significance of altering Lp(a) is not known, NCEP does not recommend the routine measurement of this lipoprotein at this time.

Hemostatic Factors

Several hemostatic determinants, particularly fibrinogen, have been associated with an increased risk of CVD. Although elevated plasma fibrinogen occurs in conjunction with other CAD risk factors such as age, cigarette smoking, hypertension, and obesity, fibrinogen has been demonstrated to be an independent CAD risk factor (70). In a six-year follow-up study, mean plasma fibrinogen level was significantly higher in men who had coronary events (2.88 gm/L) than in men who did not have events (2.63 gm/L) (71).

Left Ventricular Hypertrophy

Chapter 5 presents a detailed discussion of left ventricular hypertrophy (LVH) and related electrocardiographic changes. In brief, LVH is a concentric thickening of the left ventricular chamber that occurs in response to chronic pressure and/or volume overloading. One prospective study has demonstrated a reduced risk with the reversal of electrocardiographic evidence of LVH (72). Appropriate treatment for LVH centers primarily on effective blood pressure control, which can be accomplished by lifestyle changes, pharmacotherapy, or both (see discussion of antihypertensive drugs in chapter 4).

Homocysteine

Homocysteine is an amino acid found in the body as the result of the breakdown of methionine, which is an amino acid derived from foods including dairy products. Normally, homocysteine is converted into nondamaging amino acids by folacin (often called folate or folic acid) and vitamins B_6 and B_{12}. However, in some individuals, these processes are impaired, and homocysteine accumulates in greater quantity than it would normally. Elevated levels of homocysteine appear to increase the risk for vascular disease through endothelial damage and alterations in blood coagulation (73). On the basis of this link, homocysteine is now being recognized as an independent risk factor for CAD and cerebrovascular and peripheral vascular disease (73). A European study of 1500 men indicated that those ranked in the top 20% for homocysteine levels had double the risk of heart disease—a risk similar to that from cigarette smoking or hypercholesterolemia (25). Unfortunately, the blood assay for homocysteine is expensive and not widely available. Moreover,

specific criterion levels of homocysteine have not been clearly defined, although most studies have used an "at-risk" value of approximately 14 nmol/ml. Patients with known CAD are encouraged to reduce homocysteine levels to <10 nmol/ml.

C-Reactive Protein

C-reactive protein, a marker of systemic inflammation, was recently evaluated as a potential risk factor for CAD in both the Physician's Health Study (74) and the Nurses' Health Study (75). Increased blood levels of C-reactive protein were associated with increased risks of subsequent MI and stroke for both men and women. In addition, within the Physician's Health Study, the use of aspirin was associated with a significant reduction (50%) in the risk of MI among men with high levels of C-reactive protein. These findings raise the possibility that anti-inflammatory agents such as aspirin may have a clinical benefit in preventing CVD. Low doses of aspirin (e.g., a "baby" aspirin or 75 mg per day) are recommended for patients with known CAD who are not taking other anticoagulants and do not have other contraindications to aspirin. Furthermore, it appears that middle-aged individuals with moderate to low risk for CAD may also benefit from low-dose aspirin therapy. One study showed that aspirin combined with warfarin (a potent prescription anticoagulant) was more effective than either agent alone at decreasing cardiovascular events (i.e., death, MI, stroke) in men at high risk for CAD (92).

Oxidative Stress

Blood concentration of antioxidants may affect the susceptibility of LDL and Lp(a) to oxidation, making these compounds less atherogenic. Consequently, decreased levels of substances that protect against oxidation may increase the risk of atherosclerosis (25). Observational epidemiologic studies have demonstrated an inverse relationship between vitamin E intake and risk for CAD. In the very large Health Professionals Follow-up study (76), 39,910 American male health professionals, aged 40 to 75 years, were followed for four years. Risk for CAD events (death, MI, heart surgery) in the subjects with the highest vitamin E intake (median of 419 IU per day) was 41% lower than in the subjects with the lowest vitamin E consumption (6.4 IU per day). A similar reduction in CAD events for females with vitamin E use was observed in the Nurses' Health Study (77). Although these observational studies are promising and suggest that the use of antioxidants (specifically vitamin E) may reduce the risk of CAD, until more conclusive data are available, NCEP does not support the use of antioxidants to reduce the risk for CAD. Furthermore, antioxidants do not appear to be beneficial in the secondary prevention of CAD. A Finnish study failed to detect any benefit of vitamin E or beta-carotene in limiting progression to severe symptomatic angina or MI among men with established CAD. The low dose of vitamin E (50 mg per day) may have contributed to the negative findings of this study (78).

Alcohol Consumption

The role of alcohol in CAD risk is complicated by difficulties in obtaining accurate data on individual alcohol consumption. Several studies have shown that moderate alcohol intake (1.3 drinks per day) is associated with a 50% reduction in CAD risk (12). Alcohol consumption at mealtime appears to provide more protection than other patterns of consumption. The protective effect of alcohol consumption may be mediated by an increase in the HDL cholesterol, changes in blood coagulation, or both (25). In France, CAD incidence is relatively low despite mean plasma HDL cholesterol levels similar to those in other countries and fairly high intakes of saturated fat. Suggested explanations for this so-called French paradox include alcohol-induced inhibition of platelet aggregation and antioxidant effect of red wine (79). In contrast, excessive alcohol consumption (more than three drinks per day) is associated with an increased risk for CAD mortality, secondary to arrhythmias, hypertension, and/or alcoholic cardiomyopathy (weak heart muscle) (12). Thus, the potential benefits of moderate alcohol consumption may have to be weighed against the risks of excessive alcohol intake. Recent evidence indicates that similar benefits can be obtained from grape juice or red wine, suggesting that the benefit may come from substances (phenols) in the grape skin, not the alcohol.

Viral and Bacterial Infections

Recently, attention has been directed to the potential for either viral or bacterial infections to play a role in the development of CAD. Although the two most highly suspected viruses (cytomegalovirus and herpes) have been found to be present in atherosclerotic lesions, it is not known whether they are culprits or mere bystanders. Some have postulated that the virus itself, or the body's immune response to the virus, might injure the vascular endothelium and initiate the atherosclerotic process. Cardiac transplant patients who take large doses of immune-suppression drugs not only are frequently infected by the cytomegalovirus but also have a very high incidence of rapid atherosclerosis. Likewise, it has been hypothesized that bacterial infections can cause inflammatory reactions in coronary arteries, possibly initiating or contributing to the atherosclerotic process (80). British researchers reviewed the records of 3315 patients who had experienced an MI but had no known risk factors for heart disease. Compared to the more than 13,000 who had never had an MI, the patients who had had an MI were 70% as likely to have used a tetracycline antibiotic and 45% as likely to have used a quinolone antibiotic (Cipro) in the previous three years. No effect was seen for other types of antibiotics such as penicillin, erythromycin, or sulfonamides. These findings seemed to support the proposed hypothesis, since the germ suspected of causing artery inflammation, *Chlamydia pneumonie*, is effectively treated with tetracycline and quinolones. The strong positive relation between poor dental hygiene and increased incidence of CAD is often used to support the bacterial hypothesis. Although it has always been assumed that aspirin reduces the risk of MI by suppressing platelet aggregation, now it is postulated that aspirin may also reduce the inflammatory action of the bacterial infection.

Predicting Coronary Artery Disease Risk for Primary Prevention

As presented in the previous section, a variety of risk factors can lead to the development of CAD. In the context of primary prevention, health care professionals often attempt to quantify an individual's excess risk [3] for CAD based on available data for selected CAD risk factors. The most commonly used method for estimating CAD risk is the Framingham risk score (FRS), which is based on data and outcomes from the well-known Framingham Heart Study. Risk prediction equations are available for both primary (81, 82) and secondary (83) prevention applications. These individual risk estimates can be used for educating patients, guiding decisions regarding treatment options, and quantifying the potential for CAD risk reduction based on risk factor modification. A recent version of the Framingham CAD risk factor prediction chart, designed for use in the primary prevention setting, is presented in figure 1.14, *a* and *b* (82). As you can see from reviewing the chart, the process involves collecting data on selected risk factors, assigning a point value to each risk factor,

---

3 Excess risk for CAD is the amount of risk above that which an individual with favorable levels of all the major CAD risk factors would have.

Step 1

Age		
Years	LDL pts	Chol pts
30-34	−1	[−1]
35-39	0	[0]
40-44	1	[1]
45-49	2	[2]
50-54	3	[3]
55-59	4	[4]
60-64	5	[5]
65-69	6	[6]
70-74	7	[7]

Step 2

LDL-C		
(mg/dL)	(mmol/L)	LDL pts
<100	<2.59	−3
100-129	2.60-3.36	0
130-159	3.37-4.14	0
160-190	4.15-4.92	1
≥190	≥4.92	2

Cholesterol		
(mg/dL)	(mmol/L)	Chol pts
<160	<4.14	[−3]
160-199	4.15-5.17	[0]
200-239	5.18-6.21	[1]
240-279	6.22-7.24	[2]
≥280	≥7.25	[3]

Step 3

HDL-C			
(mg/dL)	(mmol/L)	LDL pts	Chol pts
<35	<0.90	2	[2]
35-44	0.91-1.16	1	[1]
45-49	1.17-1.29	0	[0]
50-59	1.30-1.55	0	[0]
≥60	≥1.56	−1	[−2]

Step 4

Blood pressure					
Systolic	Diastolic (mm Hg)				
(mm Hg)	<80	80-84	85-89	90-99	≥100
<120	0 [0] pts				
120-129		0 [0] pts			
130-139			1 [1] pts		
140-159				2 [2] pts	
≥160					3 [3] pts

Note: When systolic and diastolic pressures provide different estimates for point scores, use the higher number

Step 5

Diabetes		
	LDL pts	Chol pts
No	0	[0]
Yes	2	[2]

Step 6

Smoker		
	LDL pts	Chol pts
No	0	[0]
Yes	2	[2]

Step 7 (sum from steps 1-6)

Adding up the points	
Age	_____
LDL-C or chol	_____
HDL-C	_____
Blood pressure	_____
Diabetes	_____
Smoker	_____
Point total	_____

Step 8 (determine CHD risk from point total)

CHD risk			
LDL pts total	10 yr CHD risk	Chol pts total	10 yr CHD risk
<−3	1%		
−2	2%		
−1	2%	[<−1]	[2%]
0	3%	[0]	[3%]
1	4%	[1]	[3%]
2	4%	[2]	[4%]
3	6%	[3]	[5%]
4	7%	[4]	[7%]
5	9%	[5]	[8%]
6	11%	[6]	[10%]
7	14%	[7]	[13%]
8	18%	[8]	[16%]
9	22%	[9]	[20%]
10	27%	[10]	[25%]
11	33%	[11]	[31%]
12	40%	[12]	[37%]
13	47%	[13]	[45%]
≥14	≥56%	[≥14]	[≥53%]

Step 9 (compare to average person your age)

Comparative risk			
Age (years)	Average 10 yr CHD risk	Average 10 yr hard* CHD risk	Low** 10 yr CHD risk
30-34	3%	1%	2%
35-39	5%	4%	3%
40-44	7%	4%	4%
45-49	11%	8%	4%
50-54	14%	10%	6%
55-59	16%	13%	7%
60-64	21%	20%	9%
65-69	25%	22%	11%
70-74	30%	25%	14%

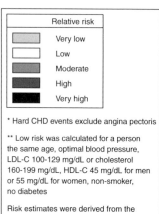

Relative risk	
	Very low
	Low
	Moderate
	High
	Very high

* Hard CHD events exclude angina pectoris

** Low risk was calculated for a person the same age, optimal blood pressure, LDL-C 100-129 mg/dL or cholesterol 160-199 mg/dL, HDL-C 45 mg/dL for men or 55 mg/dL for women, non-smoker, no diabetes

Risk estimates were derived from the experience of the Framingham Heart Study, a predominantly Caucasian population in Massachusetts, USA

Figure 1.14a   Framingham Risk Score worksheet for men. When LDL-C data are available, assess points in the chart based on LDL-C; when not available, use the column labeled "chol points" to determine the points associated with each risk factor.

Reprinted, by permission, from Wilson et al., 1998, "Prediction of coronary heart disease," *Circulation* 97:1837-1847.

Step 1

Age		
Years	LDL pts	Chol pts
30-34	−9	[−9]
35-39	−4	[−4]
40-44	0	[0]
45-49	3	[3]
50-54	6	[6]
55-59	7	[7]
60-64	8	[8]
65-69	8	[8]
70-74	8	[8]

Step 2

LDL-C		
(mg/dL)	(mmol/L)	LDL pts
<100	<2.59	−2
100-129	2.60-3.36	0
130-159	3.37-4.14	0
160-190	4.15-4.92	2
≥190	≥4.92	2

Cholesterol		
(mg/dL)	(mmol/L)	Chol pts
<160	<4.14	[−2]
160-199	4.15-5.17	[0]
200-239	5.18-6.21	[1]
240-279	6.22-7.24	[1]
≥280	≥7.25	[3]

Step 3

HDL-C			
(mg/dL)	(mmol/L)	LDL pts	Chol pts
<35	<0.90	5	[5]
35-44	0.91-1.16	2	[2]
45-49	1.17-1.29	1	[1]
50-59	1.30-1.55	0	[0]
≥60	≥1.56	−2	[−3]

Step 4

Blood pressure					
Systolic	Diastolic (mm Hg)				
(mm Hg)	<80	80-84	85-89	90-99	≥100
<120	−3 [−3] pts				
120-129	0 [0] pts				
130-139		0 [0] pts			
140-159				2 [2] pts	
≥160					3 [3] pts

Note: When systolic and diastolic pressures provide different estimates for point scores, use the higher number

Step 5

Diabetes		
	LDL pts	Chol pts
No	0	[0]
Yes	4	[4]

Step 6

Smoker		
	LDL pts	Chol pts
No	0	[0]
Yes	2	[2]

Step 7 (sum from steps 1-6)

Adding up the points	
Age	_____
LDL-C or chol	_____
HDL-C	_____
Blood pressure	_____
Diabetes	_____
Smoker	_____
Point total	_____

Step 8 (determine CHD risk from point total)

CHD risk			
LDL pts total	10 yr CHD risk	Chol pts total	10 yr CHD risk
≤−2	1%	[≤−2]	[1%]
−1	2%	[−1]	[2%]
0	2%	[0]	[2%]
1	2%	[1]	[2%]
2	3%	[2]	[3%]
3	3%	[3]	[3%]
4	4%	[4]	[4%]
5	5%	[5]	[4%]
6	6%	[6]	[5%]
7	7%	[7]	[6%]
8	8%	[8]	[7%]
9	9%	[9]	[8%]
10	11%	[10]	[10%]
11	13%	[11]	[11%]
12	15%	[12]	[13%]
13	17%	[13]	[15%]
14	20%	[14]	[18%]
15	24%	[15]	[20%]
16	27%	[16]	[24%]
≥17	≥32%	[≥17]	[≥27%]

Step 9 (compare to average person your age)

Comparative risk			
Age (years)	Average 10 yr CHD risk	Average 10 yr hard* CHD risk	Low** 10 yr CHD risk
30-34	<1%	<1%	<1%
35-39	<1%	<1%	1%
40-44	2%	1%	2%
45-49	5%	2%	3%
50-54	8%	3%	5%
55-59	12%	7%	7%
60-64	12%	8%	8%
65-69	13%	8%	8%
70-74	14%	11%	8%

Relative risk	
	Very low
	Low
	Moderate
	High
	Very high

* Hard CHD events exclude angina pectoris

** Low risk was calculated for a person the same age, optimal blood pressure, LDL-C 100-129 mg/dL or cholesterol 160-199 mg/dL, HDL-C 45 mg/dL for men or 55 mg/dL for women, non-smoker, no diabetes

Risk estimates were derived from the experience of the Framingham Heart Study, a predominantly Caucasian population in Massachusetts, USA

Figure 1.14b   Framingham Risk Score worksheet for women. When LDL-C data are available, assess points in the chart based on LDL-C; when not available, use the column labeled "chol points" to determine the points associated with each risk factor.
Reprinted, by permission, from Wilson et al., 1998, "Prediction of coronary heart disease," *Circulation* 97:1837-1847.

and then summing the points associated with each risk factor to predict the individual's absolute risk of CAD. The concept of AR was defined earlier in this chapter.

The past two decades have seen several iterations of the prediction equations upon which the risk score is based, each using updated risk factors and CAD outcomes from the Framingham Heart Study. It should be mentioned at this point that not all the CAD risk factors presented earlier are part of the Framingham risk prediction model. Notably, physical inactivity and obesity are not used to predict CAD risk within the models shown in figure 1.14, *a* or *b*. This would seem contradictory to the message presented earlier. If obesity and sedentary lifestyle have significant adverse associations with CAD, why aren't they included in the Framingham risk charts for predicting heart disease? In an endorsement of the Framingham risk charts, the AHA's Task Force on Risk Reduction (84) made the following statement:

> *Certainly it is possible that some of the increased risk imparted by obesity and physical inactivity results from mechanisms unrelated to the major risk factors. However, these mechanisms are not well understood, and it is difficult to define the risk imparted by these two factors independent of their influence on the major risk factors. [p. 1877]*

Therefore, while obesity and physical inactivity are clearly positive risk factors, the Framingham researchers did not feel that their inclusion in the risk charts would improve the prediction accuracy over the traditional risk factors of age, lipids, hypertension, smoking, and diabetes. In summary, then, a number of risk factors considered earlier in this chapter are not incorporated into the Framingham risk charts. Readers should not interpret their omission from the risk charts to mean they are not risk factors. Furthermore, obesity and physical inactivity are clear targets for intervention in both the primary and secondary prevention settings.

The following section presents several case study examples showing how to calculate the Framingham risk score and how it is used in both the primary and secondary prevention settings. The cases included in this book were selected in an attempt to span the continuum from low to high risk for CAD. As mentioned in the preface, these cases serve throughout the course of the book to illustrate and amplify concepts discussed in each chapter. We begin here by presenting each case to illustrate the use of the Framingham risk scores (82, 83) for estimating CAD risk in both the primary and secondary prevention settings. Modified versions of the Framingham risk scores are available online through the National Heart, Lung, and Blood Institute's Web site at **www.nhlbi.nih.gov/**. The online version uses total cholesterol rather than LDL-C and does not use diabetes as a risk factor in the 10-year CAD risk estimate. Therefore, the FRS version from Wilson et al. (82) is used with the case studies in chapter 1.

SUMMARY

In this chapter we've presented recent data from the AHA showing that although mortality from CAD appears to be declining, the disease remains the leading cause of death in adult Americans, and the burden of the disease remains a significant public health problem. We've reviewed known and emerging risk factors for coronary disease and summarized the scientific data supporting habitual physical activity's role in reducing CAD risk in both the primary and secondary prevention settings. There is no doubt that as we proceed into the 21st century, our knowledge of risk factors and ways to most effectively modify such risk factors will become more focused. However, it is very unlikely that advanced knowledge of risk factors and newer treatments emerging in the future will lessen the important role of habitual physical activity in the primary and secondary prevention of CAD. Therefore, professionals trained in clinical aspects of exercise science will continue to be an important entity in the battle against CAD. The remainder of this text provides state of the art information to help students who are interested in physical fitness and cardiac rehabilitation gain the knowledge and skills necessary to enter the field.

Case Study 1
Primary Prevention: Low Risk

The original use of the Framingham risk score was to estimate an individual's risk of developing CAD in the primary prevention setting. Table 1.6 contains CAD factor data on a middle-aged, asymptomatic male who joined the Ball State University Adult Physical Fitness Program. In addition to the risk factors listed in table 1.6, this 38-year-old man reported no regular physical activity on his health history questionnaire and had a body composition assessment that revealed a BMI of 28.0 (i.e., overweight), a percent body fat of 24.0, and a waist girth of 37.7 in. (95.8 cm). Chapter 6 has more on the fitness assessment for this case.

As shown in table 1.6, the first step is to assign each of the risk factors in the Framingham risk score a point value. This man accumulated points for high LDL-C [4] (1 point) and elevated blood pressure (3 points, based on diastolic ≥100 mmHg). Our case did not accumulate points for age, HDL-C, diabetes, or smoking. The point total of 4 for this man equates with an AR for CAD of 7%. This means that 7 out of 100 men with this combination of risk factors would be predicted to have diagnosed CAD within 10 years. However, as discussed earlier in the chapter, some professionals find the AR lacking in interpretive value and suggest using the

---

4 When LDL-C data are available, assess the points in the chart based on LDL-C. When LDL-C data are not available, use the column labeled "chol pts" to determine the points associated with each risk factor.

Table 1.6
Framingham CAD Risk Score—Case Study 1

Steps 1–7 on Framingham Score Sheet: Determine point values for risk factors.

Risk factor	Raw data	Framingham points
Age (years)	38	0
LDL-cholesterol (mg/dl)*	169	1
Total cholesterol (mg/dl)	238	-
HDL cholesterol (mg/dl)	45	0
Blood pressure (mmHg)	144/100	3
Diabetes (yes/no)	No	0
Smoking (yes/no)	No	0
Total points		**4**

Step 8 on Framingham Score Sheet: Determine individual's *absolute* risk for CAD over 10 years.

- Absolute risk of CAD within 10 years for individual with 4 points = 7% (see figure 1.14a)

Step 9 on Framingham Score Sheet: Determine average and low *absolute* 10 year CAD risks for males age 35–39 years.

- Average 10 yr risk of CAD = 5%
- Average 10 yr risk for hard CAD endpoints[1] = 4%
- Low[2] 10 yr risk for CAD = 3%

(continued)

Table 1.6 *(cont.)*
Framingham CAD Risk Score—Case Study 1

Calculate individual's relative risk for CAD over 10 years.

- Individual's relative risk compared to average age-/gender-matched persons

- 7%/5% = 1.4x average risk

- Individual's relative risk compared to low risk age-/gender-matched persons

- 7%/3% = 2.3x low risk

---

*The LDL-C value was used in the prediction model, thus eliminating points for total cholesterol.
[1]Hard CAD endpoints exclude angina pectoris.
[2]Low risk was calculated for a person the same age, optimal blood pressure, LDL-C 100-129 mg/dl or total cholesterol 160-199 mg/dl, HDL-C 45 mg/dl for men or 55 for women, non-smoker, no diabetes.

RR statistic. As table 1.6 illustrates, compared to the average risk for men his age within the Framingham cohort, our subject has an RR of 1.4. This indicates that due to his collection of risk factors, our subject has a 40% greater risk for CAD compared to the average man his age in the Framingham Heart Study cohort. And to take it one step further, he has 2.3 times the risk of CAD when compared to men his age with optimal risk factors (using an AR of 3% for those in the low-risk category). Clearly, our subject has an excess risk for CAD based on his Framingham risk score and would appear likely to benefit from a risk factor modification regimen targeting his abnormal lipids, moderately elevated blood pressure, obesity, and sedentary lifestyle.

An additional use of the Framingham risk score within the context of primary prevention is to estimate the projected reduction in CAD risk based on risk factor modification (84). Let's take a look at how this would theoretically apply within the context of the case study presented in table 1.6. Through lifestyle measures (i.e., adoption of a more physically active lifestyle and modification of nutritional habits), our case study subject could begin to normalize his lipid profile and blood pressure. His physician might also choose to start him on a lipid-lowering medical regimen. More likely, though, the combination of the various lifestyle

modifications could result in lower systolic and diastolic blood pressure and a normalization of the LDL-C. Hypothetically, this would eliminate, or at least reduce, the number of points in table 1.6 for elevated blood pressure and perhaps eliminate the point for elevated LDL-C. Would these changes in blood pressure and lipids be possible with aggressive risk factor modification? The answer is a definite yes! Chronic exercise training and body fat reduction could effect a reduction in resting blood pressure of 10 mmHg (85). This would lower our case's resting blood pressure to close to the normal range. In addition, a review of our case's LDL-C data indicates that he would need a 17% reduction in LDL-C to reach an initial goal of <160 mg/dl or a 24% reduction to reach the more optimal level of <130 mg/dl. He could achieve the changes through the combination of progressively increased physical activity and reductions in dietary fat and total calories. The results of this man's participation in the structured exercise program at Ball State are discussed in chapter 8. We encourage you to stay tuned for the rest of the story! However, remember that the process of predicting risk is not an exact science and therefore the actual reduction in risk achieved by this man via modification of his risk factors may be more or less than our hypothetical example indicates.

Case Study 2
Primary Prevention: High Risk

Our second case study is a middle-aged, asymptomatic man who joined the exercise program at Wake Forest University. Coronary artery disease risk factor data for this individual are presented in table 1.7. This man joined the program at Wake Forest to get help modifying his lifestyle and improving his overall physical fitness level. His medical evaluation and clinical assessment are described in more detail in the case study sections of chapters 3 and 4. Here, we will describe his risk for developing CAD using the Framingham risk score concept presented in figure 1.14a.

We start by assigning a point value to each of the risk factors used in the prediction scheme. Our man is 50 years of age, which equates with 3 points. His blood lipid concentrations—before initiation of antihyperlipidemic medications—resulted in 2 more points (1 point each for LDL-C and HDL-C). His blood pressure—again, before initiation of antihypertensive medication—was significantly elevated, and he was assigned 3 points for hypertension (based on the systolic blood pressure of 170 in figure 1.14a). And finally, he was assigned 2 points for being diagnosed with diabetes at the time of the assessment. Thus, his risk factor profile was worth 10 points from the Framingham risk score chart in figure 1.14a. This gentleman received points for each risk factor in the Framingham risk score except cigarette smoking. Contrast this with our first case, who received points for only one of the lipids (LDL-C) and blood pressure. It would appear that our second case study has a higher risk for developing CAD than Case 1.

Following the rest of the steps in table 1.7, you'll note that our second case's AR for developing CAD within 10 years is 27%. When translating his CAD risk into relative terms, we have to use the average AR for men his age (i.e., 50 years)

within the Framingham Heart Study. The average AR for 50- to 54-year old men is estimated to be 14%. Therefore, our second case's *relative* risk is almost double that of the average man his age (27/14 = 1.9). And furthermore, when we compare this man's risk to the lowest possible risk for men his age (again by hypothetically normalizing all his modifiable risk factors), he has a 4.5 times greater risk of developing CAD during the next 10 years.

This man is clearly a candidate for risk factor modification. His physician would likely consider treating his elevated lipids and would definitely consider treating his hypertension and diabetes. As previously mentioned, neither physical activity nor body composition status is used in estimating CAD risk within the Framingham risk score concept. This second case study was both sedentary and obese (BMI at 43.9) at the time he joined the program. So, in addition to treatment strategies for his hyperlipidemia, hypertension, and diabetes, his sedentary lifestyle and obesity would be targets for intervention. And it stands to reason that a regular exercise program and body fat reduction would contribute in an important way to the treatment of his other modifiable risk factors. The hypothetical analysis presented at the end of the first case—recalculating the AR based on normalization of that person's risk factors—would apply with this case as well; our second case could clearly lower his CAD risk with aggressive management of his risk factors. More details on this man's complete medical evaluation, treatment options, and physical fitness assessment are provided in subsequent chapters. In addition, the results of his participation in the structured exercise program at Wake Forest are reviewed in chapter 8. Again, keep reading to find out how successful this man was at modifying his risk factors!

Table 1.7
Framingham CAD Risk Score—Case Study 2

Steps 1–7 on Framingham Score Sheet: Determine point values for risk factors.

Risk factor	Raw data	Framingham points
Age (years)	50	3
LDL-cholesterol (mg/dl)*	178	1
Total cholesterol (mg/dl)	243	-
HDL cholesterol (mg/dl)	35	1
Blood pressure (mmHg)	170/90	3
Diabetes (yes/no)	Yes	2
Smoking (yes/no)	No	0
Total points		**10**

Step 8 on Framingham Score Sheet: Determine individual's *absolute* risk for CAD over 10 years.

- Absolute risk of CAD within 10 years for individual with 10 points = 27%

Step 9 on Framingham Score Sheet: Determine average and low *absolute* 10 year CAD risks for males age 50–54 years.

- Average 10 yr risk of CAD = 14%

- Average 10 yr risk for hard CAD endpoints[1] = 10%

- Low[2] 10 yr risk for CAD = 6%

Calculate individual's relative risk for CAD over 10 years.

- Individual's relative risk compared to average age-/gender-matched persons

- 27%/14% = 1.9x average risk

- Individual's relative risk compared to low risk age-/gender-matched persons

- 27%/6% = 4.5x low risk

---

*The LDL-C value was used in the prediction model, thus eliminating points for total cholesterol.
[1]Hard CAD endpoints exclude angina pectoris.
[2]Low risk was calculated for a person the same age, optimal blood pressure, LDL-C 100-129 mg/dl or total cholesterol 160-199 mg/dl, HDL-C 45 mg/dl for men or 55 for women, non-smoker, no diabetes.

Summary

In summary, we've reviewed documented and emerging risk factors for CAD and provided a context that allows the use of risk factors collectively to estimate an individual's risk for developing CAD in the primary prevention setting. The Framingham risk charts are not the only CAD prediction models available. However, because they are the most widely recognized and because they are endorsed by the AHA (84), we felt it appropriate to use them in our discussions here. And finally, even though the Framingham risk predic-tions are reasonably accurate, they are not perfect; professionals using the charts should bear in mind that the scores derived from the charts are only estimates based on a predominantly Caucasian American sample of adults.

Secondary Prevention

Rehabilitation regimens for patients with documented CAD have evolved extensively during the past few decades, and current guidelines stress the importance of an aggressive approach to risk factor reduction for cardiac patients (86, 87).

Within the context of secondary prevention, two major goals of cardiac rehabilitation programs are (1) to reduce the morbidity/mortality associated with recurrent MI and (2) to slow or reverse the progression of CAD lesions in patients. Therefore, one obvious question becomes, "Does participation in a cardiac rehabilitation program decrease CAD morbidity/mortality?" Oldridge et al. (88) combined the results of 10 randomized clinical trials of cardiac rehabilitation that included exercise training and multiple risk factor interventions to assess the efficacy of such programs for reducing CAD morbidity/mortality. Collectively, the studies included 4347 CAD patients—mostly male—who were randomly assigned to either an exercise-based cardiac rehabilitation program or to usual care (i.e., less focused medical care). Analyses from the pooled studies revealed a 25% reduction in risk of cardiovascular death in the patients who participated in the rehabilitation programs compared to those who didn't. However, the results did not reveal such a protective effect for recurrent nonfatal MI. One should note that most of these studies were conducted in the 1970s, and therefore it might be reasonable to assume that today's more aggressive approach to the management of post-MI patients (i.e., increased use of coronary revascularization, increased use of hyperlipidemia medications, etc.) would result in lower CAD morbidity in future studies. Needless to say, this is a very active area of clinical research as we embark on the 21st century.

Another important goal within the context of secondary prevention of CAD is to slow the *progression* of CAD lesions. Obviously, all cardiac patients would benefit from this. Better still would be a reversal of the disease process (i.e., shrinking of the lesion), often referred to as *regression*. Evaluating the potential for disease regression requires clinical trials that employ multiple cardiac catheterizations (e.g., before, during, and after the intervention program) to assess changes in CAD lesions over several years. Within such studies, an increase in a lesion's size across time would document progression of CAD, whereas a decrease in a lesion's size would demonstrate regression of disease. A number of well-designed clinical trials have addressed this topic in recent years, and there is evidence that aggressive risk factor intervention, especially from studies in which elevated LDL-C is lowered with medications, can slow disease progression and in some instances produce a regression of the plaque within the artery. Results from several of these

studies are reviewed in detail in chapter 4. The following section serves as an introduction to the concept of *risk reduction* in the secondary prevention setting. More detailed discussions of risk reduction strategies appear in the later chapters of the book.

Secondary Coronary Artery Disease Risk Reduction

The global risk estimates derived from the Framingham risk score pertain to the prevention of CAD in the primary setting—in those individuals who are free of CAD at the time risk factors are assessed. Once an individual has been diagnosed with CAD, her risk for future MI is greatly increased, and efforts to lower this risk are very important. Data from the Framingham Heart Study show that the risk of reinfarction is definitely associated with elevations of many of the same risk factors that contributed to the initial infarction (89). Wong et al. (89) followed 459 MI survivors from the Framingham cohort for an average of 9.7 years after their initial cardiac event. The risk of subsequent MI or CAD death was associated with elevations in systolic blood pressure, total cholesterol, blood sugar, relative body weight, and the presence of diabetes. On the basis of this and other studies, the AHA and American College of Cardiology have published guidelines (87) for preventing MI in individuals who already have CAD; these guidelines promote assessment and modification of many of the risk factors discussed in this chapter. The recommendations from this report are presented in chapter 4, where risk factor modification concepts are presented and discussed. Professionals working in the secondary prevention setting (i.e., cardiac rehabilitation programs) should be familiar with these risk reduction guidelines and stay abreast of newer guidelines as they are published.

There are several methods for estimating risk of subsequent CAD events in persons with established coronary disease (83, 86). Most of these models provide qualitative distinctions such as low- versus high-risk status as it relates to early mortality following the cardiac event or procedure, or to complications that could occur during participation in an exercise program. This type of information would certainly be useful for the clinician in evaluating treatment options after the event. The American Association of Cardiovascular and Pulmonary Rehabilitation (AACVPR) has published just such risk stratification guidelines based on clinical data such as symptoms, left ventricular function indexes, and exercise test responses. These guidelines for risk stratification are reviewed in detail in chapter 7 (table 7.11) in relation to a patient's entry into a cardiac rehabilitation exercise program. The AACVPR has also provided risk stratification guidelines aimed at classifying cardiac patients for risk of progression of disease based on their respective risk factor levels (i.e., lipids, blood pressure, smoking status, etc.), with the purpose of establishing treatment goals within each risk factor. These guidelines are also presented and discussed in chapter 7 (table 7.12). Once again, this information would be useful in guiding the treatment of abnormal risk factors in cardiac patients.

But what about the concept of predicting the risk of a subsequent cardiac event for those with documented CAD? Researchers from the Framingham Heart Study have recently published a means of estimating AR for subsequent events (CAD or stroke) in persons with documented CAD. The Framingham models for estimating future risk for cardiac patients are illustrated in figure 1.15a (men) and 1.15b (women). There are several differences between the mod-

els for primary prevention that we have discussed and those used for secondary prevention. First, once an individual has been diagnosed with coronary disease, he has a greater likelihood for a subsequent event compared to the general population. Therefore, the follow-up interval used to estimate subsequent events is typically much shorter (e.g., 1-4 years as opposed to 5-10 years for primary prevention models). The Framingham risk estimates shown in figure 1.15, a and b, are based on a two-year time frame—in other words, they indicate the risk that the individual will have another cardiac event within the next two years. That's considerably different from estimating one's risk over the next 10 years. Second, you will notice that the list of risk factors used in the prediction models is much narrower. For example, in figure 1.15a, age, lipids, and diabetes are the only risk factors used to estimate CAD risk. What happened to cigarette smoking, hypertension, and sedentary lifestyle? The fact that they don't appear in the prediction model as variables should not be interpreted to mean that they are not important risk factors in the secondary

Age			HDL-C									Diabetes
35-39	0	Total-C	25	30	35	40	45	50	60	70	80	No = 0
40-44	1	160	10	9	7	6	5	4	3	1	0	Yes = 4
45-49	3	170	11	9	8	7	6	5	3	2	1	
50-54	4	180	11	10	8	7	6	5	4	2	1	
55-59	6	190	12	10	9	8	7	6	4	3	2	
60-64	7	200	12	11	9	8	7	6	5	3	2	
65-69	9	210	13	11	10	9	7	7	5	4	2	
70-74	10	220	13	11	10	9	8	7	5	4	3	
		230	13	12	10	9	8	7	6	4	3	
		240	14	12	11	10	9	8	6	5	4	
		250	14	13	11	10	9	8	6	5	4	
		260	15	13	12	10	9	8	7	5	4	
		270	15	13	12	11	10	9	7	6	5	
		280	15	14	12	11	10	9	7	6	5	
		290	16	14	13	11	10	9	8	6	5	
		300	16	14	13	12	11	10	8	7	6	

Pts	2-yr Probabilities	Pts	2-yr Probabilities	Pts	2-yr Probabilities
0	3%	14	9%	28	25%
2	4%	16	11%	30	29%
4	4%	18	13%		
6	5%	20	14%		
8	6%	22	17%		
10	7%	24	19%		
12	8%	26	22%		

Figure 1.15a Probability of subsequent coronary heart disease within 2 years for men aged 35 to 74 with prior history of CHD or stroke.

Reprinted, by permission, from R.B. D'Agostino et al., 2000, "Primary and subsequent coronary risk appraisal: new results from the Framingham Study," *American Heart Journal* 139:272.

Age	
35-39	0
40-44	1
45-49	2
50-54	3
55-59	4
60-64	5
65-69	6
70-74	7

Total-C	HDL-C 25	30	35	40	45	50	60	70	80
160	10	9	7	6	5	4	3	1	0
170	11	9	8	7	6	5	3	2	1
180	11	10	8	7	6	5	4	2	1
190	12	10	9	8	7	6	4	3	2
200	12	11	9	8	7	6	5	3	2
210	13	11	10	9	7	7	5	4	2
220	13	11	10	9	8	7	5	4	3
230	14	12	11	9	8	7	6	4	3
240	14	12	11	10	9	8	6	5	4
250	14	13	11	10	9	8	7	5	4
260	15	13	12	10	9	9	7	6	4
270	15	13	12	11	10	9	7	6	5
280	15	14	12	11	10	9	8	6	5
290	16	14	13	12	10	10	8	7	5
300	16	14	13	12	11	10	8	7	6

Diabetes	Cigs
No = 0	No = 0
Yes = 8	Yes = 4

SBP	
<110	0
110-114	1
115-124	3
125-134	4
135-144	5
145-154	6
155-164	7
165-184	8
185-194	9
195-214	10
215-224	11
225-244	12
245+	13

Pts	2-yr Probabilities	Pts	2-yr Probabilities	Pts	2-yr Probabilities
0	1%	14	3%	28	9%
2	1%	16	3%	30	11%
4	1%	18	4%	32	13%
6	1%	20	5%	34	16%
8	2%	22	5%	36	19%
10	2%	24	7%	38	22%
12	2%	26	8%		

Figure 1.15b Probability of subsequent coronary heart disease within 2 years for women aged 35 to 74 with prior history of CHD or stroke.

Reprinted, by permission, from R.B. D'Agostino et al., 2000, "Primary and subsequent coronary risk appraisal: new results from the Framingham Study," *American Heart Journal* 139:272.

prevention setting. They clearly are important targets for intervention when present. However, in the statistical world, when one is developing a mathematical equation that predicts an outcome (i.e., CAD), variables (i.e., risk factors) that do not contribute in an independent way are often eliminated from the mathematical equation in an attempt to simplify the equation. So, in short, the fact that a risk factor is not used to predict the event doesn't mean it's not related to the event in a causal way, only that it's expendable in a mathematical sense.

From statistical theory, let's move on to the important practical message within this discussion: how to use the Framingham risk model to predict CAD events for those with documented disease.

Case Study 3
Secondary Prevention

Our third case study is a patient in the Cardiac Rehabilitation Program at Wake Forest University. At the time he presented for entry into the program he was 61 years of age and had a recent history of MI. Detailed discussion of his medical history, assessment, diagnostic procedures, exercise prescription, and training outcomes appears in subsequent chapters. Here we focus on use of the Framingham prediction model to estimate his risk for a future event, using the risk factor data at the time he entered the program. At this point it is important to understand that most cardiac patients are started on several cardiovascular medications prior to hospital discharge. In fact, our case was taking aspirin, Lipitor, atenolol, vitamin E, nitroglycerin, and Plavix at the time he presented to the Wake Forest program. Although more detailed discussion of the indications for these medications is provided in chapter 4, it is relevant here that our case's lipid profile and blood pressure are being treated by his physician. So the risk factor data we present for this case study had already been favorably altered by the time the man enrolled in the program.

Our case's risk factor data, along with the point equivalents for the various risk factors, are presented in table 1.8. As shown, our cardiac patient receives 7 points for being 61 years of age and 8 points for having the total cholesterol and HDL-C combination of 186 and 36 mg/dl, respectively. Thus, our case has a total of 15 points from the risk factor analysis. The next step is to determine the risk associated with 15 risk factor points in figure 1.15a. As you can see from the chart, 15 points equates with a two-year AR for CAD of 10%. Now remember, this is an *absolute* risk estimate, meaning that 1 in 10 men this man's age, with his risk factor profile, would likely have another cardiac event within the next two years.

You'll note that we don't discuss an estimate of this man's RR compared to that of other cardiac patients his age. The observational nature of the Framingham Heart Study implies that research-ers must wait until enough cardiac patients have subsequent events before these events can be predicted with reasonable accuracy. The study cohort has not evolved to the point at which this type of information is readily available. As more follow-up data within the Framingham cohort become available, it may be possible to make better, more reliable risk estimates. However, another way to evaluate our case study's RR for another event would be to assess, albeit in a qualitative way, his CAD risk following some intervention. Remember, he's already being treated for hyperlipidemia, and you'll note that his LDL-C is currently at 131 mg/dl (LDL treatment goal as discussed in later chapters of this text is <100 for cardiac patients). While a further reduction in LDL-C would be prudent, clinical trials show that he's reduced his risk by lowering his LDL-C (87, 90). In addition, he is being treated for hypertension, and his blood pressure is currently within the optimal range according to the AACVPR (86). So within the context of our case's risk factor profile, he's lowered his risk of a subsequent event with appropriate risk factor interventions. We will be providing considerably more detail on the concept of risk factor modification in later chapters of the text. Stay tuned!

Table 1.8
Framingham CAD Risk Score—Case Study 3

Step 1: Determine point values for risk factors.*

Risk factor	Raw data	Framingham points
Age (years)*	61	7
LDL-cholesterol (mg/dl)	131	-
Total cholesterol (mg/dl)*	186	Points for lipids combined reported with HDL-C
HDL cholesterol (mg/dl)*	36	8
Blood pressure (mmHg)	118/62	-
Diabetes (yes/no)	No	0
Smoking (yes/no)	No	-
Total points		**15**

Step 2: Determine individual's *absolute* risk for recurrent CAD over two years using the chart in figure 1.15a.

• Absolute risk of CAD within 2 years for individual with 15 points = 10%

*Only variables used in prediction model for recurrent events.

GLOSSARY

Arteriosclerosis: a chronic disease characterized by abnormal thickening and hardening of the arterial walls

Atherogenic: a process relating or contributing to degenerative changes in arterial walls leading to atherosclerosis

Atherosclerosis: an arteriosclerosis characterized by atheromatous deposits in and fibrosis of the inner layer of the arteries

Epidemiology: a branch of medical science that deals with the incidence, distribution, and control of disease in a population

Hyperglycemia: abnormally high blood glucose concentration, usually defined in either the fasting state or after a standardized glucose feeding

Hyperinsulinemia: abnormally high insulin concentration within the blood, usually defined in either the fasting or postabsorptive state

Hyperlipidemia: excess fat or lipids in the blood; usually defined by measures of cholesterol or triglycerides

Hypertension: abnormally high blood pressure

Morbidity rate: the number of occurrences of a disease within a population over a specified period of time (e.g., per year)

Mortality rate: the number of deaths within a population over a specified period of time (e.g., per year), usually expressed for a given disease (e.g., cardiovascular disease)

Prevalence: the percentage of a population that is affected by a particular disease or risk factor for a disease at a given time

Risk factor: a characteristic (i.e., smoking or elevated cholesterol) that is associated with the development of a health problem (i.e., cardiovascular disease)

REFERENCES

1. American Heart Association. 2001. *Heart and stroke statistical update.* Dallas: American Heart Association.
2. Eckel, R.H., and R.M. Krauss. 1998. American Heart Association call to action: Obesity as a major risk factor for coronary heart disease. *Circulation* 97:2099–2100.
3. Fletcher, G.F., S.N. Blair, J. Blumenthal, C. Casperson, B. Chaitman, S. Epstein, et al. 1992. Statement on exercise: Benefits and recommendations for physical activity programs for all Americans. *Circulation* 86:340–344.
4. Dawber, T.R. 1980. *The Framingham Study: The Epidemiology Of Atherosclerotic Disease.* Cambridge: Harvard University Press.
5. Kannel, W.B., D. McGee, and T. Gordon. 1976. A general cardiovascular risk profile: The Framingham Study. *Am. J. Cardiol.* 38:46–52.
6. Pooling Project Research Group. 1978. Relationship of blood pressure, serum cholesterol, smoking habit, relative weight and ECG abnormalities to incidence of major coronary events: Final report of the Pooling Project. *J. Chron. Dis.* 31:202–306.
7. Ragland, S.W., and R.J. Brand. 1988. Coronary heart disease mortality in the Western Collaborative Group Study: Follow-up experience of 22 years. *Am. J. Epidemiol.* 127:462–475.
8. Hjermann, I., I. Holme, B.K. Velve, and P. Leren. 1981. Effect of diet and smoking intervention on the incidence of coronary heart disease. *Lancet*:1303–1310.
9. Lipid Research Clinics Program. 1984. The Lipid Research Clinics Coronary Primary Prevention Trial results. I. Reduction in incidence of coronary heart disease. *J.A.M.A.* 251:351–364.
10. Multiple Risk Factor Intervention Research Group. 1982. Multiple Risk Factor Intervention Trial: Risk factor changes and mortality results. *J.A.M.A.* 248:1465–1477.
11. Stamler, J., D. Wentworth, J.D. Nelson, et al. 1986. Is the relationship between serum cholesterol and risk of premature death from coronary heart disease continuous and graded? Findings in 356,222 primary screenees of the Multiple Risk Factor Intervention Trial (MRFIT). *J.A.M.A.* 256:2823–2828.
12. Gordon, N.F. 1998. Conceptual basis for coronary artery disease risk factor assessment in *ACSM's Resource Manual For Guidelines For Exercise Testing And Prescription.* 3rd ed., ed. J.L. Roitman, 3–12. Baltimore: Williams & Wilkins.
13. Eaker, E.D., J.H. Chesebro, F.M. Sacks, et al. Special Report: Cardiovascular disease in women. *Circulation.* 1993; 88:1999-2009.
14. Goldstein, F., and M. Stampler. 1995. The epidemiology of coronary heart disease and estrogen replacement in postmenopausal women. *Progressive Cardiovasc. Dis.* 38:199–210.
15. Slyper, A., and G. Schectman. 1994. Coronary artery disease risk factors from a genetic and developmental perspective. *Arch. Intern. Med.* 154:633–638.
16. Fuster, V., A.M. Gotto, P. Libby, J. Loscalzo, and H.C. McGill. 1996. 27th Bethesda Conference: Matching the intensity of risk factor management with the hazard for coronary disease events. Task Force 1. Pathogenesis of coronary disease: The biologic role of risk factors. *J. Am. Coll. Cardiol.* 27:964–976.

17. Ayanian, J.Z., and P.D. Cleary. 1999. Perceived risks of heart disease and cancer among cigarette smokers. *J.A.M.A.* 281:1019–1021.

18. Kannel, W.B., and M. Higgins. 1990. Smoking and hypertension as predictors of cardiovascular risk in population studies. *J. Hypertension* 8:S3–8.

19. Slone, D., S. Shapiro, L. Rosenberg, D.W. Kaufman, S.C. Hartz, A.C. Rossi, et al. 1978. Relation of cigarette smoking to myocardial infarction in young women. *N. Engl. J. Med.* 298:1273–1276.

20. Bolinder, G., L. Alfredsson, A. Englund, and U. deFaire. 1994. Smokeless tobacco use and increased cardiovascular mortality among Swedish construction workers. *Am. J. Public Health* 84:399–404.

21. Pasternak, R.C., S.M. Grundy, D. Levy, and P.D. Thompson. 1996. 27th Bethesda Conference: Matching the intensity of risk factor management with the hazard for coronary disease events. Task Force 3: Spectrum in risk factors for coronary artery disease. *J. Am. Coll. Cardiol.* 27:978–990.

22. Howard, G., L.E. Wagenknecht, G.L. Burke, A. Diez-Roux, G.W. Evans, P. McGovern, et al. 1998. Cigarette smoking and progression of atherosclerosis: The Atherosclerosis Risk in Communities (ARIC) Study. *J.A.M.A.* 279:119–124.

23. Steenland, K. 1992. Passive smoking and the risk of heart disease. *J.A.M.A.* 267:94–99.

24. Glantz, S.A., and W.W. Parmley. 1996. Passive and active smoking: A problem for adults. *Circulation* 94:596–598.

25. Braunwald, E., ed. 1997. *Heart Disease: A Textbook Of Cardiovascular Medicine.* 5th ed. Philadelphia: Saunders.

26. National Cholesterol Education Program. 2001. Summary of the Third report of the National Cholesterol Education Program (NCEP) Expert Panel on Detection, Evaluation, and Treatment of High Blood Cholesterol in Adults (Adult Treatment Panel III). *J.A.M.A.* 285:2486–2497.

27. Keys, A. Coronary heart disease in seven countries. 1970. *Circulation* 41 (suppl. 1):1.

28. Robertson, T.L., H. Kato, T. Gordon, A. Kagan, G.G. Rhoads, C.E. Land, et al. 1977. Epidemiologic studies of coronary heart disease and stroke in Japanese men living in Japan, Hawaii, and California. *Am. J. Cardiol.* 39:244–249.

29. Austin, M.A., J.L. Breslow, C.H. Henneken, J.E. Buring, W.C. Willett, and R.M. Krauss. 1988. Low density lipoprotein subclass patterns and risk of myocardial infarction. *J.A.M.A.* 260:1917–1921.

30. Gordon, T., W.P. Castelli, M.C. Hjortland, W.B. Kannel, and T.R. Dawber. 1977. High-density lipoprotein as a protective factor against coronary artery disease. *Am. J. Med.* 62:707–714.

31. Burt, V.L., P. Whelton, E.J. Roccella, C. Brown, J.A. Cutler, M. Higgins, et al. 1995. Prevalence of hypertension in the US adult population: Results from the Third National Health and Nutrition Examination Survey, 1988-1991. *Hypertension* 25:305–313.

32. Joint National Committee. 1997. Joint National Committee on Detection, Evaluation and Treatment of High Blood Pressure. The sixth report (JNC). *Arch. Intern. Med.* 157:2413–2446.

33. Whaley, M.H., and S.N. Blair. 1995. Physical activity, physical fitness and coronary heart disease. *J. Cardiovasc. Risk* 2:289–295.

34. Pate, R.R., M. Pratt, S.N. Blair, W.L. Haskell, C.A. Macera, C. Bouchard, et al. 1995. Physical activity and public health: A recommendation from the Centers for Disease Control and Prevention and the American College of Sports Medicine. *J.A.M.A.* 273:402–407.

35. Paffenbarger, R.S., R.T. Hyde, A.L. Wing, and C.C. Hsieh. 1986. Physical activity, all-cause mortality, and longevity of college alumni. *N. Engl. J. Med.* 314:605–613.

36. Bouchard, C., F.T. Dionne, J. Simoneau, and M.R. Boulay. 1992. Genetics of aerobic and anaerobic performances. In *Exercise and Sports Science Reviews,* ed. J.O. Holloszy. 20:27–58. Baltimore: Williams & Wilkins.

37. U.S. Department of Health and Human Services. 1996. *Physical activity and health: A report of the Surgeon General.* Atlanta: U.S. Department of Health and Human Services, Centers for Disease Control and Prevention, National Center for Chronic Disease Prevention and Health Promotion.

38. Whaley, M.H., and L.A. Kaminsky. 2001. Epidemiology of physical activity, physical fitness and selected chronic diseases. pp. 17-33. In *ACSM's Resource Manual For Guidelines For Exercise Testing And Prescription.* 4th ed., ed. J. Roitman. Baltimore: Williams & Wilkins.

39. Blair, S.N., H.W. Kohl, R.S. Paffenbarger, D.G. Clark, K.H. Cooper, and L.W. Gibbons. 1989. Physical fitness and all-cause mortality: A prospective study of healthy men and women. *J.A.M.A.* 262:2395–2401.

40. Lakka, T.A., J.M. Venalainen, R. Rauramaa, R. Salonen, J. Tuomilehto, and J.T. Salonen. 1994. Relation of leisure-time physical activity and cardiorespiratory fitness to the risk of acute myocardial infarction. *N. Engl. J. Med.* 330:1549–1554.

41. Leon, A.S., J. Connett, D.R. Jacobs, and R. Rauramaa. 1987. Leisure-time physical activity levels and risk of coronary heart disease and death. The Multiple Risk Factor Intervention Trial. *J.A.M.A.* 258:2388–2395.

42. Morris, J.N., D.G. Clayton, M.G. Everitt, A.M. Semmence, and E.H. Burgess. 1990. Exercise in leisure time: Coronary attack and death rates. *Br. Heart J.* 63:325–334.

43. Sandvik, L., J. Erikssen, E. Thaulow, G. Erikssen, R. Mundal, and K. Rodahl. 1993. Physical fitness as a predictor of mortality among healthy, middle-aged Norwegian men. *N. Engl. J. Med.* 328:533–537.

44. Arraiz, G.A., D.T. Wigle, and Y. Mao. 1992. Risk assessment of physical activity and physical fitness in the Canadian Health Survey Mortality Follow-up Study. *J. Clin. Epidemiol.* 45:419–428.

45. Blair, S.N., H.W. Kohl, and C.E. Barlow. 1993. Physical activity, physical fitness, and mortality in women: Do women need to be active? *J. Am. Coll. Nut.* 12:368–371.

46. Powell, K.E., P.D. Thompson, C.J. Caspersen, and J.S. Kendrick. 1987. Physical activity and the incidence of coronary heart disease. *Annu. Rev. Public Health* 8:253–287.

47. Sherman, S.E., R.B. D'Agostino, J.L. Cobb, and W.B. Kannel. 1994. Physical activity and mortality in women in the Framingham Heart Study. *Am. Heart J.* 128:879–884.

48. Kushi, L.H., R.M. Fee, A.R. Folsom, P.J. Mink, K.E. Anderson, and T.A. Sellers. 1997. Physical activity and mortality in postmenopausal women. *J.A.M.A.* 277:1287–1292.

49. Lissner, L., C. Bengtsson, C. Bjorkelund, and H. Wedel. 1996. Physical activity levels and changes in relation to longevity. A prospective study of Swedish women. *Am. J. Epidemiol.* 143:54–62.

50. Manson, J.E., F.B. Hu, J.W. Rich-Edwards, G.A. Colditz, M.J. Stampher, W.C. Willett, et al. 1999. A prospective study of walking as compared with vigorous exercise in the prevention of coronary heart disease in women. *N. Engl. J. Med.* 341:650–658.

51. Blair, S.N., H.W. Kohl, C.E. Barlow, R.S. Paffenbarger, L.W. Gibbons, and C.A. Macera. 1995. Changes in physical fitness and all-cause mortality: A prospective study of healthy and unhealthy men. *J.A.M.A.* 273:1093–1098.

52. Eriksssen, G., K. Liestol, J. Bjornholt, E. Thaulow, L. Sandvik, and J. Erikssen. 1998. Changes in physical fitness and changes in mortality. *Lancet* 352:759–762.

53. Paffenbarger, R.S., R.T. Hyde, A.L. Wing, I.M. Lee, D.L. Jung, and J.B. Kampert. 1993. The association of changes in physical-activity level and other lifestyle characteristics with mortality among men. *N. Engl. J. Med.* 328:538–545.

54. Paffenbarger, R.S., J.B. Kampert, I.M. Lee, R.T. Hyde, R.W. Leung, and A.L. Wing. 1994. Changes in physical activity and other lifeway patterns influencing longevity. *Med. Sci. Sports Exerc.* 26:857–865.

55. Wannamethee, S.G., A.G. Shaper, and M. Walker. 1998. Changes in physical activity, mortality, and incidence of coronary heart disease in older men. *Lancet* 351:1603–1608.

56. American College of Sports Medicine. 2000. *ACSM's Guidelines For Exercise Testing And Prescription.* 6th ed., ed. B.F. Franklin, M.H. Whaley, and E.T. Howley. Baltimore: Lippincott, Williams & Wilkins.

57. American Heart Association. 1992. Statement on exercise. Benefits and recommendations for physical activity programs for all Americans. *Circulation* 86:340–344.

58. Pi-Sunyer, F.X. 1993. Medical hazards of obesity. *Ann. Intern. Med.* 100:655–660.

59. Expert Panel. 1998. Executive summary of the clinical guidelines on the identification, evaluation, and treatment of overweight and obesity in adults. *Arch. Intern. Med.* 158:1855–1867.

60. Despres, J.P., and A. Marette. 1994. Relation of components of insulin resistance syndrome to coronary disease risk. *Curr. Opin. in Lipidol.* 4:274–289.

61. Pouliot, M.C., J.P. Despres, S. Lemieux, S. Moorjani, C. Bouchard, A. Tremblay, et al. 1994. Waist circumference and abdominal sagittal diameter: Best simple anthropometric indexes of abdominal visceral adipose tissue accumulation and related cardiovascular risk in men and women. *Am. J. Cardiol.* 73:460–468.

62. Whaley, M.H., J.B. Kampert, H.W. Kohl, and S.N. Blair. 1999. Physical fitness and clustering of risk factors associated with the metabolic syndrome. *Med. Sci. Sports Exerc.* 31:287–293.

63. Hubert, H.B., M. Feinlieb, P.M. McNamara, and W.P. Castelli. 1983. Obesity as an independent risk factor for cardiovascular disease: A 26-year follow-up of participants in the Framingham Heart Study. *Circulation* 67:968.

64. American Diabetes Association. 1998. Report of the Expert Committee on the Diagnosis and Classification of Diabetes Mellitus. *Diabetes Care* 21 (suppl. 1):S5–S19.

65. Barrett-Conner, E.L., B.A. Cohn, D.L. Wingard, and S.L. Edelstein. 1991. Why is diabetes mellitus a strange risk factor for fatal ischemic heart disease in women more than in men? Rancho Bernardo Study. *J.A.M.A.* 265:627–631.

66. Matthews, K.A., and S.G. Haynes. 1986. Type A behavior pattern and coronary disease risk: Update and critical evaluations. *Am. J. Epidemiol.* 123:923–960.

67. Ferketich, A.K., J.A. Schwartzbaum, D.J. Frid, and M.L. Moeschberger. 2000. Depression as an antecedent to heart disease among women and men in the NHANES I study. National Health and Nutrition Examination Survey. *Arch. Intern. Med.* 160:1261–1268.

68. Ford, D.E., L.A. Mead, P.P. Chang, L. Cooper-Patrick, N.Y. Wang, and M.J. Klag. 1998. Depression is a risk factor for coronary artery disease in men. The Precursors Study. *Arch. Intern. Med.* 158:1422–1426.

69. Loscalzo, J. 1990. Lipoprotein (a): A unique risk factor for atherothrombotic disease. *Atherosclerosis* 10:672–679.

70. Ernst, E. 1990. Plasma fibrinogen: An independent cardiovascular risk factor. *J. Internal Med.* 227:365–372.

71. Heinrich, J., L. Balleisen, H. Schultz, G. Assmann, and J. van de Loo. 1994. Fibrinogen and factors VII in the prediction of coronary risk. Results from the PROCAM study in healthy men. *Arterioscler. Thromb.* 14:54–59.

72. Kannel, W.B., T. Gordon, W.P. Castelli, and J.R. Margolis. 1970. Electrocardiographic left ventricular hypertrophy and risk factors for coronary heart disease. The Framingham Study. *Ann. Intern. Med.* 72:813–822.

73. Clarke, R., L. Daly, K. Robinson, E. Naughten, S. Cahalane, B. Fowler, and I. Graham. 1991. Hyperhomocysteinemia: An independent risk factor for vascular disease. *N. Engl. J. Med.* 324:1149–1155.

74. Ridker, P.M., M. Cushman, M.J. Stampfer, R.P. Tracy, and C.H. Hennekens. 1997. Inflammation, aspirin, and the risk of cardiovascular disease in apparently healthy men. *N. Engl. J. Med.* 336:973–979.

75. Ridker, P.M., C.H. Hennekens, J.E. Buring, and N. Rifai. 2000. C-reactive protein and other markers of inflammation in the prediction of cardiovascular disease in women. *Circulation* 342:836–843.

76. Rimm, E.B., M.J. Stampfer, A. Ascherio, E. Giovannucci, G.A. Colditz, and W.C. Willett. 1993. Vitamin E consumption and the risk for coronary heart disease in men. *N. Engl. J. Med.* 328:1450–1456.

77. Stampfer, M.J., C.H. Hennekens, J.E. Manson, G.A. Colditz, B. Rosner, and W.C. Willett. 1993. Vitamin E consumption and the risk of coronary disease in women. *N. Engl. J. Med.* 328:1440–1449.

78. Virtamo, J., J.M. Rapola, S. Ripatti, O.P. Heinonen, P.R. Taylor, D. Albanes, and J.K. Huttunen. 1998. Effect of vitamin E and beta carotene on the incidence of primary nonfatal myocardial infarction and fatal coronary heart disease. *Arch. Intern. Med.* 158:668–675.

79. Renaud, S., and M. de Lorgeril. 1992. Wine, alcohol, platelets, and the French paradox for coronary heart disease. *Lancet* 339:1523–1526.

80. Meier, C.R., L.E. Derby, S.S. Jick, C. Vasilakis, and H. Jick. 1999. Antibiotics and risk of subsequent first time acute myocardial infarction. *J.A.M.A.* 281:427–431.

81. Anderson, K.M., P.W.F. Wilson, P.M. Odell, and W.B. Kannel. 1991. An updated coronary risk profile: A statement for health professionals. *Circulation* 83:356–362.

82. Wilson, P.W.F., R.B. D'Agostino, D. Levy, A.M. Belanger, H. Silbershatz, and W.B. Kannel. 1998. Prediction of coronary heart disease using risk factor categories. *Circulation* 97:1837–1847.

83. D'Agostino, R.B., M.W. Russell, D.M. Huse, R.C. Ellison, H. Silbershatz, P.W. Wilson, and S.C. Hartz. 2000. Primary and subsequent coronary risk appraisal: New results from the Framingham study. *Am Heart J.* 139:272–281.

84. American Heart Association. 1998. Primary prevention of coronary heart disease: Guidance from Framingham: A statement for healthcare professionals from the AHA Task Force on Risk Reduction. *Circulation* 97:1876–1887.

85. Gordon, N.F. 1997. Hypertension. In *ACSM's Exercise Management For Persons With Chronic Diseases,* ed. J.L. Durstine, 269. Champaign, IL: Human Kinetics.

86. American Association of Cardiovascular and Pulmonary Rehabilitation. 1999. *Guidelines For Cardiac Rehabilitation And Secondary Prevention Programs.* 3rd ed. Champaign, IL: Human Kinetics.

87. Smith, S.C., S.N. Blair, M.H. Criqui, G.F. Fletcher, V. Fuster, B.J. Gersh, et al. 1995. American Heart Association consensus statement: Prevention of heart attack and death in patients with coronary artery disease. *Circulation* 92:2–4.

88. Oldridge, N.B., G.H. Guyatt, M.E. Fischer, and A.A. Rimm. 1988. Cardiac rehabilitation after myocardial infarction: Combined experience of randomized clinical trials. *J.A.M.A.* 260:945–950.

89. Wong, N.D., L.A. Cupples, A.M. Ostfeld, D. Levy, and W.B. Kannel. 1989. Risk factors for long-term coronary prognosis after initial myocardial infarction: The Framingham Study. *Am. J. Epidemiol.* 130:469–480.

90. Smith, S.C. 1996. Risk reduction therapy: The challenge to change. *Circulation* 93:2205–2211.

91. NIH Concensus Development Panel on Triglyceride, High-Density Lipoprotein, and Coronary Heart Disease. 1993. Triglyceride, high-density lipoprotein, and coronary heart disease. *J.A.M.A.* 269:505–510.

92. The Medical Research Council's General Practice Research Framework. 1998. Thrombosis prevention trial: randomised trial of low-intensity oral anticoagulation with warfarin and low-dose aspirin in the primary prevention of ischaemic heart disease in men at increased risk. *Lancet 351*:233–241.

SUGGESTED READINGS

American Association of Cardiovascular and Pulmonary Rehabilitation. 1999. *Guidelines For Cardiac Rehabilitation And Secondary Prevention Programs.* 3rd ed. Champaign, IL: Human Kinetics.

Gordon, N.F. 1998. Conceptual basis for coronary artery disease risk factor assessment in *ACSM's Resource Manual For Guidelines For Exercise Testing And Prescription*. 3rd ed., ed. J.L. Roitman, 3-12. Baltimore: Williams & Wilkins.

Report of the United States Surgeon General. Physical Activity and Public Health, 1996.

Whaley, M.H., and L.A. Kaminsky. 2001. Epidemiology of physical activity, physical fitness and selected chronic diseases. In *ACSM's Resource Manual For Guidelines For Exercise Testing And Prescription*. 4th ed., ed. J. L. Roitman, 17-33. Baltimore: Williams & Wilkins.

Whaley, M.H., and S.N. Blair. 1995. Physical activity, physical fitness and coronary heart disease. *J. Cardiovasc. Risk* 2:289–295.

CHAPTER 2
Cardiovascular Physiology and Pathophysiology

BEHAVIORAL OBJECTIVES

- To be able to describe the basic anatomy of the heart and the vascular system

- To be able to describe how cardiac output is regulated at rest and during exercise

- To be able to describe how blood pressure is regulated at rest and during exercise

- To be able to describe the basic aspects of the development of coronary atherosclerosis and the pathophysiology of myocardial ischemia and infarction

Physiology is the study of how a living organism functions. In this chapter we focus specifically on the function of the major aspects of the human cardiovascular system that form a basis for many of the topics presented in subsequent chapters. We emphasize key mechanisms associated with the normal control of the cardiovascular system. The student will apply this information throughout the text in discussions evaluating both normal and abnormal physiological responses observed in prevention and rehabilitation programs. In addition, the chapter provides a brief overview of the pathophysiology of cardiovascular disease.

Students can certainly benefit from reviewing the appropriate sections in their anatomy and physiology textbooks for more detailed information on this topic. We begin here with an overview of the basic anatomy of the cardiovascular system and then discuss how the heart and blood vessels function to supply blood to all tissues in the body. We review the response of the cardiovascular system to the stress of exercise and the ways in which this may differ in an individual with coronary artery disease. The chapter concludes with a brief overview of the pathophysiology of coronary artery disease.

BASIC ANATOMY OF THE CARDIOVASCULAR SYSTEM

In this section a brief overview of the anatomy of the heart and circulatory system is provided. Specific anatomical features key to understanding cardiovascular physiology will be reviewed.

Heart

The heart is composed of a specialized type of muscle called **myocardium** that is housed within a protective structure called the **pericardium** (figure 2.1). The pericardium has a fibrous outer layer, which functions primarily to prevent overdistension of the myocardium. The thin inner layer of the pericardium, the epicardium, attaches to the myocardium, forming the outer wall of the heart. The space between these two pericardial layers contains a small amount of fluid, pericardial fluid, which allows the myocardium to move smoothly when contracting within the pericardium. The myocardium is the thick (middle) layer of the heart, which provides the contractile function. The inner wall of the heart, the **endocardium,** is composed of both a layer of endothelium and a layer of connective tissue.

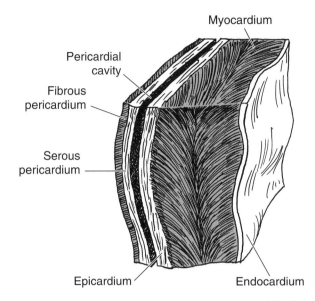

Figure 2.1 The structure of the pericardium and the heart wall.

The myocardium is structured to create two sides of the heart, a right and a left, with both sides having two interior chambers, an atrium and a ventricle, which hold the blood that the heart circulates to the body (figure 2.2). The atria and ventricles are connected by two valves, the tricuspid valve on the right side and the mitral valve on the left side, which allow blood to flow only in the direction from atrium to ventricle. Similarly, during ventricular relaxation, one-way valves prevent blood flow from the pulmonary artery (pulmonic valve) and aorta (aortic valve) to the right and left ventricles, respectively.

Myocardium has characteristics similar to those of skeletal muscle in that it contains actin and myosin myofilaments that attach via crossbridges and function to create tension while shortening the myofibril. In comparison to skeletal muscle, though, myocardium has a higher density of mitochondria (>33% of cell volume) and a higher myofiber-to-capillary ratio (1.0). The most distinct difference in myocardium is the presence of intercalated discs, which are specialized portions of the cell membranes that connect individual cardiac muscle cells. The intercalated discs allow an action potential to pass from one cell to the next-adjoining cell to allow the myocardium to contract as a functional unit, or actually two functional units—the atria and the ventricles.

The stimulus for myocardial contraction comes from a specialized structure called the sinoatrial (SA) node, commonly referred to as

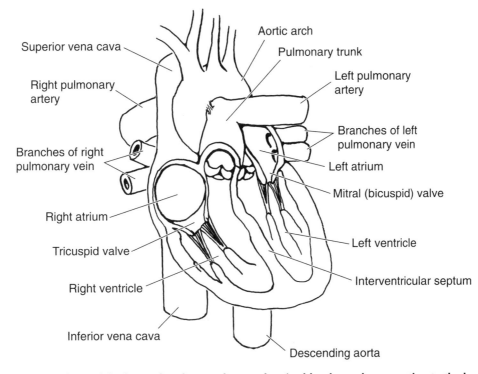

Figure 2.2   The four chambers of the heart, four heart valves, and major blood vessels connecting to the heart.

the pacemaker of the heart. From the SA node the stimulatory impulse spreads through the heart via its electrical conduction system, which includes the atrioventricular (AV) node, the bundle of His, right and left bundle branches, and finally the diffuse terminal structures known as the Purkinje fibers (figure 2.3). The primary feature of the heart's conduction system is its intrinsic ability to generate a stimulatory impulse. Although the impulse is usually generated from the SA node, which typically has a rate of discharge of approximately 75 times per minute, other myocardial tissues also have the capability of self-excitability. A thorough discussion of these topics appears later in this chapter and in chapter 5.

Circulatory System

The heart functions as a pump to deliver blood to the various organs and tissues in the body and then to return blood to the heart via a continuous network of blood vessels called the circulatory system. These blood vessels can be divided into three basic types: arteries, which carry blood to the tissues under high pressure; capillaries, which allow diffusion of gases and other substances through their thin walls; and veins, which return

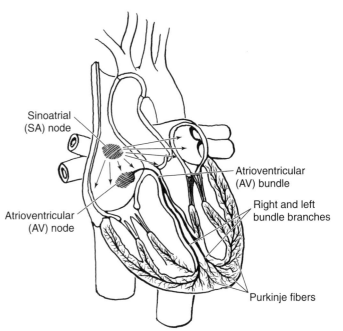

Figure 2.3   The electrical conduction system of the heart.

blood to the heart under low pressure. Both the arterial and venous parts of the circulation have smaller branches that deliver blood to (the arterioles) and collect blood from (the venules) the capillaries. The circulatory system functions primarily as a transportation network, carrying desired substances (e.g., oxygen, glucose, hormones) to the tissues throughout the body and concurrently allowing tissues to dispose of unwanted substances (e.g., carbon dioxide, lactic acid).

The circulatory system actually consists of two separate circulatory routes: the systemic circulation and the pulmonic circulation (figure 2.4). The pulmonic circulation carries blood from the right ventricle to the lungs via the pulmonary artery and then returns blood to the left atrium via the pulmonary vein. The pulmonic circulation serves the important functions of (a) removing carbon dioxide from the blood and (b) reoxygenating the blood via diffusion between the gases in the blood in the pulmonary capillaries and the gases in the alveoli. It is also important to recognize that in comparison to the systemic circulation, the pulmonic circulation requires less pressure to maintain blood flow due to the lower resistance in this branch of the circulation.

The systemic circulation carries blood from the left ventricle to the rest of the body via the aorta and then returns blood to the right atrium via the superior and inferior venae cavae. The aorta branches off numerous times to supply blood to all the regions of the body (with the exception of the lungs, which are supplied by the pulmonic circulation). The systemic circulation provides oxygenated blood and nutrients to the brain and to tissues throughout the body, and collects carbon dioxide and other waste products from these same areas.

The heart, like all other organs, has its blood supply delivered via two branches of the aorta (figure 2.5). The right coronary artery (RCA), which lies in the coronary sulcus, branches off to supply the right atrium and the right ventricle. Additionally, the right coronary artery supplies blood to the anterior portion of the SA node (in 50-60% of the population), the AV node (in 90% of the population), the ventricular septum, and the posterior wall of the left ventricle (in 70% of

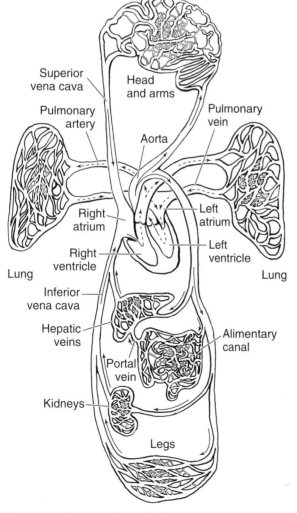

Figure 2.4   The systemic and pulmonic circulatory systems.

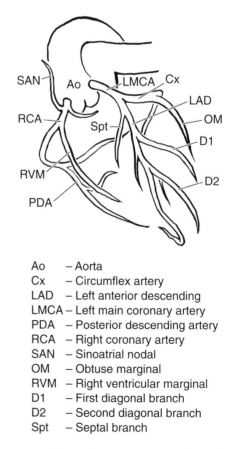

Ao	– Aorta
Cx	– Circumflex artery
LAD	– Left anterior descending
LMCA	– Left main coronary artery
PDA	– Posterior descending artery
RCA	– Right coronary artery
SAN	– Sinoatrial nodal
OM	– Obtuse marginal
RVM	– Right ventricular marginal
D1	– First diagonal branch
D2	– Second diagonal branch
Spt	– Septal branch

Figure 2.5   The main coronary arteries and significant branches.

the population). The left coronary artery (LCA) immediately branches into two main divisions—the left circumflex artery (Cx) and the left anterior descending artery. The Cx, which lies in the anterior interventricular sulcus, provides the blood supply for the SA node (40-50% of the population), the left atrium, and the lateral wall of the left ventricle; and it contributes to the supply of the posterior wall of the left ventricle. In approximately 10% of the population, the Cx is the dominant supplier of blood to the posterior wall of the left ventricle, and in approximately 20% of hearts, it shares equally in the supply of blood to this region. The left anterior descending artery principally supplies blood to the wall of the left ventricle and the ventricular septum, with an additional role in providing some of the supply to the anterior wall of the right ventricle. After being distributed via an extensive capillary bed, blood drains from the thebesian veins (which then primarily empty into the right and left atria) and the anterior cardiac veins and coronary sinus (which both empty into the right atrium).

One other important anatomical feature of the circulatory system is the layer of **endothelium** that lines the blood vessels. It is important to note that endothelium also lines the endocardium and the coronary blood vessels. Until recently, the function of endothelium was not well understood. However, current research is revealing a number of important physiological roles of endothelium. Some of these functions, which are related to coronary disease and or an exercise response, are discussed later in the book.

CARDIOVASCULAR PHYSIOLOGY

The heart will beat approximately 3 to 4 billion times during the average human's life span. With each beat of the heart, blood is ejected both to the lungs (pulmonic circulation) and to the rest of the body (systemic circulation) and serves as the medium to transport substances throughout the body. It is essential that students interested in the primary and secondary prevention of heart disease have a complete understanding of the physiological events that occur with each cycle of the heart. The first comprehensive diagram of the events of the cardiac cycle was developed in 1915, and figure 2.6 presents a modification of that diagram. This figure describes the changes in pressure (aortic, ventricular, and atrial), left ventricular volume, and the electrocardiogram over the time period of one complete cardiac cycle (note that although this figure presents events oc-

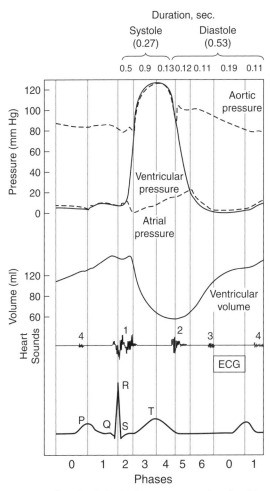

Figure 2.6 **The physiological events associated with one cardiac cycle.**

curring in the left side of the heart, corresponding events are happening on the right side).

For the purpose of describing these events, we will begin with the period toward the end of ventricular diastole that is labeled phase 0. During this period, blood continues to flow into the left ventricle as noted by the increase in ventricular volume as the mitral valve is open (atrial pressure > ventricular pressure) and the aortic valve is closed (aortic pressure > ventricular pressure). It is vital to remember that in order for the myocardium to contract it must first be stimulated. The stimulation of each beat of the heart usually originates from the SA node; and as the impulse spreads across the atria, we can observe a P wave on the electrocardiogram. Note the short time delay from the onset of the P wave to the beginning of the atrial contraction, which is labeled phase 1. This phase, often described as the atrial kick, functions to increase the flow of blood into the left ventricle prior to its contraction. The AV node, which functions to delay the stimulatory impulse, provides adequate time for this to take place as noted by the PR interval on the electrocardiogram. Phase 1 ends with the stimulation of the ventricles (QRS complex on the electrocardiogram), which precedes the beginning of the ventricular contraction. Phase 2 is termed isovolumic contraction—no change in ventricular volume is occurring, since both the mitral and aortic valves are closed. However, the contraction of the ventricles creates a large and rapid increase in ventricular pressure. When ventricular pressure exceeds aortic pressure, the aortic valve opens and phase 3 begins; this is termed the rapid ejection phase. Note that during this phase, the stimulation of the ventricles is completed and the repolarization period (T wave) begins. As the ventricles begin to relax, phase 4 begins (reduced ejection). This phase continues until the left ventricular pressure drops below that of the aortic pressure, which results in closure of the aortic valve. Notice the large decrease in ventricular volume (i.e., the stroke volume) that occurs during phases 3 and 4. Phase 5, isovolumic relaxation, is associated with the time period when ventricular pressure remains higher than atrial pressure, resulting in a static left ventricular volume. As the relaxation period continues, left ventricular pressure eventually drops below that of atrial pressure, the mitral valve opens (phase 6), and the rapid filling of the left ventricle begins again.

Cardiac Output

Since the tissues depend on the heart to provide a continuous flow of fresh blood via the systemic circulation, it is important to understand the factors that allow this to happen and the ways these factors change in response to different demands of the tissues, such as those that occur during exercise. Cardiac output is defined as the total amount of blood that is ejected from the ventricle (usually measured from the left ventricle) into the circulation in 1 min. Although this review concentrates on cardiac output, it is important to remember that in order to maintain blood flow, an equal volume of blood must be returned (i.e., the venous return) to the heart each minute. The two primary determinants of cardiac output are heart rate and stroke volume.

$$\text{cardiac output (CO)} = \text{heart rate (HR)} \times \text{stroke volume (SV)}$$

Thus, the heart can meet increased demands for blood flow from the tissues by increasing heart rate, stroke volume, or both. At rest, cardiac output averages about 5 L·min^{-1} for an adult. Two primary

characteristics that affect cardiac output are body size and age. Generally, cardiac output is directly related to body size (e.g., CO increases as body size increases), which accounts for most of the difference between the genders. Also, after maturity, cardiac output is inversely related to age (e.g., as age increases, CO decreases). Thus, the expected cardiac output for any given person should be adjusted based on that individual's characteristics.

Measurement of Cardiac Output

The classic method for determining cardiac output is based on the Fick equation:

$$\text{cardiac output (CO)} = \frac{\text{oxygen uptake } (\dot{V}O_2)}{\text{arteriovenous oxygen difference (a-}\bar{v}O_2 \text{ diff)}}$$

This method requires invasive measures of arterial and mixed venous blood samples, with subsequent measurement of the O_2 content using a blood gas analyzer. $\dot{V}O_2$ is measured via open-circuit spirometry. Because of the risks associated with the invasive measurements this technique employs, its use is typically limited to clinical research settings. Other similarly invasive techniques include the dye-dilution and thermal dilution methods.

In the clinical setting, reasonable estimates of cardiac output are made during echocardiographic exams. Cardiac output can also be determined noninvasively through use of a modification of the Fick equation with measures of carbon dioxide instead of oxygen.

$$\text{cardiac output (CO)} = \frac{\text{carbon dioxide production } (\dot{V}CO_2)}{\text{venoarterial carbon dioxide difference (}\bar{v}\text{-a } CO_2 \text{ diff)}}$$

$\dot{V}CO_2$ is measured via open-circuit spirometry. Estimates of mixed venous and arterial CO_2 contents are estimated from gas-exchange measurements during rebreathing from a container that has either a high or a low CO_2 concentration.

Control of Heart Rate

As mentioned earlier, the stimulation of the heart is intrinsically generated by the SA node. However, the rate of this stimulation can be affected by both neural and hormonal factors. The SA node is innervated by both the parasympathetic (cholinergic) and sympathetic (adrenergic) divisions of the autonomic nervous system. At rest, the heart rate is controlled by the relative dominance of the parasympathetic vagus nerve activity. The vagus nerve releases acetylcholine, which binds to the muscarinic receptors of the SA node membrane, which in turn causes the membrane to become hyperpolarized. In the membrane's hyperpolarized state, more time is needed for the membrane potential to reach the threshold required for an action potential, thus resulting in a slowed rate of firing. Chapter 5 provides an in-depth review of cardiac electrophysiology.

One of the primary mechanisms to obtain an increase in heart rate is to reduce or remove the activity of the vagus nerve (i.e., parasympathetic withdrawal). Without the influence of acetylcholine, the intrinsic rate of firing of the SA node can increase by up to 50%. Further increases in heart rate result from the adrenergic release of norepinephrine, which binds to the beta 1 (β_1) receptors on the SA node and causes reduced membrane potential. This allows for an earlier depolarization of the SA node and also a more rapid repolarization. There can also be an indirect influence of adrenergic stimulation on heart rate. This response, which occurs during exercise, results from the release of the hormone epinephrine into the blood from the adrenal medulla, which is located on the kidney. The adrenal medulla is stimulated by the sympathetic nervous system as part of the body's reaction to stressful situations. The β_1 receptors on the SA node can also bind with epinephrine from the circulation; this leads to further stimulation and a more rapid rate of firing. Any factor that influences the heart rate is sometimes referred to as a **chronotropic** factor. These factors are described as having a positive or a negative effect, depending whether they increase or decrease heart rate, respectively.

Control of Stroke Volume

The other means the heart has to increase its output is by increasing the volume of blood ejected with each contraction (i.e., the stroke volume). Similar to control of heart rate, changes in stroke volume result both from intrinsic mechanisms and from neural and hormonal stimulation. At this point it would be helpful to introduce some commonly used terminology related to stroke volume. **Preload** is the load on the heart, measured as the pressure in the left ventricle immediately prior to ventricular contraction. The corresponding volume in the left ventricle at this time is termed the end-diastolic volume. **Afterload** is the force against which the left ventricle is working during contraction, measured as the pressure in the aorta at the end of diastole. Recall that in order for the aortic valve to open, pressure in the left ventricle must exceed that in the aorta. Another common term that readers need to understand is end-systolic

volume, which is defined as the volume of blood remaining in the left ventricle immediately following ventricular contraction. Stroke volume (SV) represents the difference between end-diastolic volume and end-systolic volume. Finally, **ejection fraction** refers to the amount of blood ejected from the left ventricle as a percentage of the total volume in the left ventricle prior to contraction (i.e., the end-diastolic volume).

$$\text{ejection fraction} = \frac{\begin{array}{c}\text{end-diastolic volume} -\\ \text{end-systolic volume}\\ \text{(or SV)}\end{array}}{\text{end-diastolic volume}} \times 100$$

The intrinsic mechanism for increasing stroke volume is understood on the basis of observations made by two physiologists approximately one century ago and thus is named the Frank-Starling law. The underlying physiological mechanism that explains this response is the known effect of sarcomere length on the ability of both skeletal and cardiac muscle to develop tension. You will recall from your physiology class that as sarcomeres are lengthened (up to an optimal distance), more actin binding sites become available to the myosin cross-bridges to allow greater tension development. Thus, as ventricular volume is increased (principally via increased venous return, but also due to atrial contraction), the wall of the ventricles becomes stretched, and this lengthens the sarcomeres (figure 2.7). Essentially, the heart responds to an increase in ventricular volume by increasing its force of contraction, thereby generating a greater stroke volume.

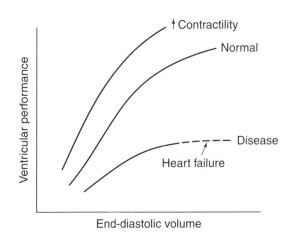

Figure 2.7 Left ventricular performance (stroke volume) as a function of end-diastolic volume. Stroke volume can also change positively because of increased contractility or negatively because of disease.

Increasing the contractility of the ventricles via adrenergic stimulation brings about additional increases in stroke volume. This response, also known as a positive **inotropic** effect, results from a cascade of events in the myocardium that ultimately leads to an increase in the contractile force of the myocardium. Thus, at any given ventricular volume, increased contractility via adrenergic stimulation results in a decreased end-systolic volume. The same indirect effect of adrenergic stimulation (i.e., release of epinephrine into the circulation by the adrenal medulla) mentioned earlier, in relation to control of heart rate, will also enhance contractility.

The density of adrenergic (β_1) receptors within the ventricles is second in the entire heart only to that in the SA node. Thus, adrenergic stimulation provides both positive chronotropic and inotropic effects.

Myocardial Oxygen Uptake

One of the most common measures made by exercise physiologists is that of oxygen uptake ($\dot{V}O_2$), which is used to describe the energy expended by the body in meeting the demands to perform work. Similarly, the demands placed on the heart to perform its work can be quantified by the measure of myocardial oxygen uptake ($m\dot{V}O_2$).

Skeletal muscle can increase its uptake of oxygen both by increasing its extraction of oxygen from the blood and by obtaining a greater blood flow. Myocardium, on the other hand, extracts almost all of the oxygen from the blood when functioning at its basal level (i.e., resting cardiac output). Thus, when cardiac output increases, and thus the work of the heart, all of the additional oxygen must come from increasing the rate of blood flow via the coronary arteries.

Unlike the measurement of whole-body $\dot{V}O_2$, which can be obtained via the noninvasive method of open-circuit spirometry, determination of $m\dot{V}O_2$ would require invasive procedures to measure coronary blood flow and the difference between the amount of oxygen in the coronary arteries and the coronary veins (i.e., the ateriovenous oxygen difference [a-$\bar{v}$ O_2 diff]). Since these invasive procedures are not practical, other indicators of myocardial work demands become important. Essentially, the two components of cardiac output (heart rate and stroke volume) determine the $m\dot{V}O_2$. Obviously, heart rate is easy to measure and quantify; however, stroke volume—or more precisely the factors that determine stroke volume—is more difficult to ascertain. Remember that preload, afterload, and contractility influence stroke volume. Opie (1)

explains how these factors contribute to the wall stress or tension of the myocardium via the following relationship:

$$\text{wall stress} = \frac{\text{pressure} \times \text{radius}}{2 \times \text{wall thickness}}$$

where pressure = end-diastolic pressure, radius = radius of the left ventricular chamber, and wall thickness = thickness of the left ventricular wall. Wall thickness changes only as a result of chronic adaptations over time; thus, on an acute basis it is not a contributing factor to demand of the heart. Pressure and radius, on the other hand, both respond to stimulation to increase the stroke volume or to maintain the stroke volume against a greater afterload. Increases in either or both of these result in greater wall stress and therefore a higher $m\dot{V}O_2$. Various disease processes (e.g., hypertension) or pathological conditions (e.g., congestive heart failure) can result in changes in pressure, radius, and/or wall thickness and thus cause changes in $m\dot{V}O_2$ (see table 2.1).

Measurements obtained by a variety of clinical tests (see chapter 3) can help define the components of $m\dot{V}O_2$. However, a simple indicator of myocardial oxygen demand is the rate-pressure product (also called the **double product)**, which is derived from the product of heart rate and systolic blood pressure. In patients with angina, in which myocardial demand exceeds myocardial blood supply, the rate-pressure product is commonly used for clinical correlation.

Hemodynamics

Although it is the heart that is responsible for pumping the blood, it is the circulatory system that actually delivers the blood to the various tissues throughout the body. From a "central" perspective, blood flow to the body is dictated by the cardiac output, whereas blood flow to the individual tissues in the periphery is determined by the blood pressure (or actually the change in pressure along a segment of the blood vessels) and the resis-

Table 2.1

Factors That Influence Myocardial Oxygen Uptake

Heart rate	Preload
Stroke volume	Afterload

tance within the blood vessels. An understanding of the following relationship is important:

$$\text{flow (Q)} = \frac{\Delta \text{ pressure}}{\text{resistance}}$$

We can easily understand some of the key features related to circulation of blood by applying this relationship. One important feature is the difference in pressures throughout the systemic circulation. In order for flow to take place, blood moves according to pressure gradients (i.e., from higher pressure to lower pressure) (figure 2.8). Since the systemic circulation is a complete circuit, we can see that the pressure at the origin of the circuit (i.e., the aorta) is the highest, averaging ≈100 mmHg in the basal state, and that the pressure at the end of the circuit (i.e., the right atrium) is the lowest, where it falls to ≈0 mmHg. To allow perfusion to all parts of the body, mean pressure is maintained at relatively high values (>95 mmHg) throughout all of the arteries. This is partially attributable to the elastin component of the arterial vessel walls. The greatest drop in pressure within the systemic circulation occurs in the smaller arterioles, allowing these vessels to have the greatest impact on blood flow to the tissues they supply.

The second important feature of the circulation to understand is the dramatic effect that changing the size of the vessel has on the flow of blood to a tissue. A component of the vascular wall of all blood vessels, with the exception of capillaries, is smooth muscle. Contraction of this smooth muscle reduces the size of the blood vessel, an effect called **vasoconstriction.** Relaxation of this smooth muscle allows the vessel to enlarge, an effect called **vasodilation**. Changes in the size of the blood vessel, measured as the radius of the opening, have a fourfold effect on the resistance to blood flow. This effect, which is known as Poiseuille's law, is the major determinant of blood flow to individual tissues and organs in the body.

Control of Blood Pressure

When one is discussing factors that influence blood pressure, it is important to understand the different ways this variable can be measured. Systolic blood pressure is the resulting pressure in the arteries during the contractile phase of the heart. Diastolic blood pressure is the pressure that remains in the arteries during the period of relaxation between ventricular contractions. The mathematical difference between systolic and diastolic pressure is called the pulse pressure. Finally, the average pressure in the arteries is called the mean arterial pressure. Since time spent for systole is less than time spent in diastole, the mean arterial pressure is a weighted average, generally estimated by the following formula:

$$\text{mean arterial pressure} = \frac{\text{pulse pressure}}{3} + \text{diastolic pressure}$$

The mean arterial pressure is the primary measure used in determining regulation of blood pressure.

Rearranging the relationship just described demonstrates the two factors that determine arterial blood pressure.

$$\text{blood pressure} = \text{cardiac output} \times \text{peripheral vascular resistance}$$

Thus, anything that affects cardiac output or peripheral vascular resistance (PVR) will also affect blood pressure. Certainly students should be aware that all the factors discussed so far in relation to control of heart rate and stroke volume are important for their potential effects on blood pressure. This section also reviews other mechanisms that create a change in cardiac output and consequently affect blood pressure. In addition, we review mechanisms that create a change in PVR. In essence, all these latter mechanisms result primarily in neural stimulation of the vascular smooth muscle to induce either vasoconstriction or vasodilation. In a process similar to stimulation of the myocardium, the vascular smooth muscle is excited to contract by the release of norepinephrine from sympathetic nerve endings, with vasoconstriction being the end result. However, it is important to realize that the vascular smooth muscle has different receptors that bind with the norepinephrine known as alpha (α) receptors. Another important concept to understand is that vasodilation effects are created mainly by inhibition of the sympathetic stimulation rather than via direct neural stimulation. Although there are some parasympathetic nerves that stimulate vasodilation, they do not play a significant role in the regulation of blood pressure.

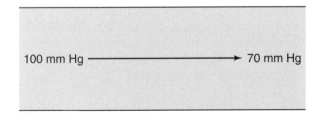

100 mm Hg ⟶ 70 mm Hg

Figure 2.8 Blood flow always moves in the direction from higher to lower pressure throughout the circulatory system.

Unlike some variables of the body that are tightly regulated within a small range of values (e.g., body temperature or blood pH), blood pressure can be quite variable throughout a day in response to numerous stimuli. This does not mean that blood pressure is poorly regulated. Indeed, the control of blood pressure is quite complex, with some mechanisms that respond quite rapidly when the body senses an increase or decrease in blood pressure and other mechanisms that attempt to provide longer-term regulation of blood pressure within a desirable range.

Control of blood pressure by the vasomotor center

Most of the rapid control of blood pressure is regulated through the vasomotor center located in the reticular formation of the brain. A primary function of the vasomotor center is to provide a continual stimulation of the smooth muscle cells lining the arterioles to produce a basal level of vasomotor tone. Another important function of the vasomotor center is to translate afferent impulses received from higher centers in the brain, as well as from various sensory receptors throughout the body.

Signals from the higher centers in the brain can result in either increases or decreases in blood pressure. For example, when the cerebral cortex is aroused, in association with some emotions like anger, it can stimulate the vasomotor center to send more excitatory impulses, resulting in an increased blood pressure. On the other hand, some extreme emotions may cause the vasomotor center to send inhibitory impulses, which would immediately lower blood pressure and in some cases result in fainting. Chemoreceptors, along with their primary function of providing the respiratory center of the brain with regulatory information, also provide impulses to the vasomotor center. These receptors, which are located in both the aorta and the carotid arteries, respond to increases in carbon dioxide, decreases in pH, and decreases in oxygen in the arterial blood. The response of the vasomotor center to afferent signals from the chemoreceptors is to send excitatory impulses, resulting in an increased blood pressure. Other factors that also lead to increases in blood pressure include the Bainbridge reflex (which responds to stretch of mechanoreceptors in the atria) and the central nervous system ischemic response (which responds principally to accumulation of carbon dioxide and possibly lactic acid). It is important to be aware of the influence of these factors on blood pressure; however, one should view them as secondary responses and not truly fac-

tors that regulate blood pressure. The primary control mechanisms were to enhance circulation (regulate flow) of blood to a region of the body.

Two other receptor mechanisms operate to truly regulate blood pressure: the baroreceptors (baro means "pressure"), sometimes referred to as high-pressure receptors, and the low-pressure receptors in the pulmonary arteries and the atria. The designation of high vs. low pressure with these receptors signifies their location in either the systemic (high-pressure) or pulmonic (low-pressure) circulations. Both these receptors respond to stretch and thus are really mechanoreceptors. The baroreceptors are located in both the aorta and the carotid arteries, as are the chemoreceptors, and can rapidly respond to either increases or decreases in arterial blood pressure. The response of the baroreceptors to an increase in blood pressure is to immediately send inhibitory signals to the vasomotor center to cause vasodilation (i.e., decrease PVR) and to excite the vagus nerve, which results in a decrease in heart rate (i.e., decreased CO). The result of this baroreceptor response is an immediate reduction in blood pressure. There are obviously some situations in which the body requires a higher blood pressure to allow greater blood flow to tissues (e.g., any stressful situation, including exercise). In these situations the baroreceptors serve to buffer the increase in blood pressure—in other words they prevent exaggerated responses. Interestingly, the rate of impulse firing of the baroreceptors is much higher in response to an acutely changing arterial pressure than it is to a slower increase or static elevation of arterial pressure. The baroreceptors also respond to a reduced stretch or lowered arterial blood pressure. The most common example of this occurs when a person changes from a sitting or supine posture to an upright position, causing an immediate lowering of arterial blood pressure due to gravitational effects. In this situation, the baroreceptors immediately send excitatory signals to the vasomotor center to cause vasoconstriction (i.e., increase PVR) and to inhibit the vagus nerve, resulting in an increased heart rate (i.e., increased CO). The low-pressure receptors primarily respond to increases in blood volume in the pulmonic circulation, which could result from a blood transfusion or via increased venous return. The response to the afferent impulses sent by these receptors is inhibitory signals to the arteriole smooth muscle, resulting in vasodilation (i.e., decreased PVR).

Influence of hormones on blood pressure control

The regulation of blood pressure within reasonable physiological limits is essentially the function of the vasomotor center. Many functions of the body require changes in blood flow, and these are often mediated by changes in PVR and hence blood pressure. As discussed earlier, some of these functions create a change in blood pressure via neural pathways. However, many hormones also influence blood pressure.

One hormonal response—the release of epinephrine and norepinephrine from the adrenal medulla—was touched upon in the section on control of cardiac output. Circulating epinephrine, which binds with the α receptors on the vascular smooth muscle, has the same vasoconstrictive effect that neural stimulation does. However, circulating norepinephrine is not thought to play a major role, as its concentrations are usually quite low and neural stimulation is already occurring when this hormone is released into the bloodstream. Epinephrine, on the other hand, functions through vascular α and β receptors. The fact that α receptor stimulation requires higher concentrations of epinephrine probably serves only to magnify the already present vasoconstrictive neural effect. Circulating epinephrine stimulation of the β receptors occurs at lower concentrations and results in vasodilation to specific organs—for example, skeletal muscle during exercise.

Angiotensin II is another hormone that affects blood pressure through a variety of actions, both direct and indirect. The process of angiotensin II formation and its multitude of actions are a prime example of the tremendous complexity of the organization and function of the human body. The process of producing angiotensin II begins with the release of the enzyme renin from the kidneys. The kidneys are stimulated to release renin as a response to direct adrenergic stimulation, a reduction in renal arterial pressure, or a decrease in the renal tubular sodium reabsorption. Once present in the circulation, renin catalyzes a reaction that results in the formation of angiotensin I. Then, angiotensin I quickly undergoes an additional reaction to form angiotensin II. This latter reaction is catalyzed by an enzyme called angiotensin-converting enzyme that is found in the vascular epithelium, particularly of the lungs. Angiotensin II is a powerful vasoconstrictor; however, it has a very short existence (usually only 1-2 min) in the circulation. Angiotensin II exerts its direct effect to increase blood pressure by stimulation of smooth muscle contraction via a specific vascular angiotensin II receptor. Angiotensin II also exerts a number of indirect effects to increase blood pressure, including stimulating the release of aldosterone (an adrenal cortical hormone that

promotes sodium reabsorption), promoting decreased elimination of sodium and water in the renal tubules, increasing sympathetic nervous system activation, promoting the release of endothelin, and preventing the baroreceptor-mediated lowering of heart rate. It is important to recall that blood volume and blood pressure are directly related; that is, as blood volume increases, so does blood pressure (and vice versa). Thus we should view any mechanism of the body that influences blood volume as a factor that will affect blood pressure.

Another hormone that produces effects similar to those of angiotensin II is vasopressin (or antidiuretic hormone). Vasopressin is secreted by the posterior pituitary gland when its osmoreceptors sense a decrease in blood volume or blood pressure. Vasopressin is a powerful vasoconstrictor as it can stimulate smooth muscle contraction via a specific vascular (V_1) receptor. This hormone can also promote blood pressure increases via increasing blood volume, as its more descriptive name, antidiuretic hormone, would suggest. This effect of vasopressin is exerted at the kidneys, where it increases the reabsorption of water in the renal tubules.

Atrial natriuretic factor is a peptide hormone released by the atria when they are stretched due to increased volumes. Atrial natriuretic factor can act as a compensatory mechanism to reduce blood volume via its influence in inhibiting renin release by the kidneys and vasopressin release by the posterior pituitary gland, which results in increased sodium and water excretion, respectively. Another role of atrial natriuretic factor is to produce vasodilation via a direct effect on the vascular smooth muscle. Thus, atrial natriuretic factor can play an important role in regulation by decreasing blood pressure.

Local control

Tissues have an intrinsic mechanism that allows them to increase blood flow under certain conditions. The increased blood flow is brought about by vasodilation of the arterioles supplying this tissue. During situations resulting in an imbalance between demand of the tissues and the supply of blood, the concentration of substances in the interstitial space between the tissue and the capillaries changes. For example, when the metabolism of a tissue increases, the immediate result is an increased use of oxygen and increased production of carbon dioxide. Thus, the concentrations of oxygen and carbon dioxide in the interstitial space will change. The arterioles will directly react by vasodilating to increase blood flow, thereby supplying more oxygen and carrying away the excess carbon dioxide. Other substances released by the tissues that can increase blood flow are hydrogen ions, potassium ions, and adenosine. Substances that cause this direct effect on the arterioles are generically referred to as vasodilating factors.

Vascular endothelium is also known to release some factors that can control blood flow to a tissue. The two best-understood factors are nitric oxide and endothelin. Nitric oxide produces vasodilation, whereas endothelin release results in vasoconstriction of the arterioles. As research on the role and function of endothelium continues to expand, so does our understanding of its important physiological roles. Presently it is known that acetylcholine, bradykinin, histamine, serotonin, and vasopressin can all stimulate endothelium to release nitric oxide, whereas hypoxia, thrombin, and free radicals all result in endothelin release (1). It is also known that damaged endothelium releases endothelin, which can be of consequence to a number of pathological conditions.

Factors involved in local control of blood flow are not stimulated for the purpose of regulating blood pressure. However, since they involve vasodilation of the arterioles, which in turn can have a dramatic effect on blood pressure, it is important to understand their function. These factors do play an important role in blood pressure control in situations such as exercise that involves large-muscle groups and in certain disease states.

RELATED EXERCISE PHYSIOLOGY

During physical activity, skeletal muscles have an increased requirement for oxygen, as well as other nutrients, and an increased need to eliminate by-products of metabolism such as carbon dioxide and lactic acid. It is well known that the amount of oxygen taken up by the body ($\dot{V}O_2$) is highly correlated with the amount of heat energy dissipated. Thus, since measuring $\dot{V}O_2$ is much easier than determining heat energy given off by the body, it is the principal measure used to quantify energy expenditure. Since the body requires energy for all work, measurement of both maximal and submaximal $\dot{V}O_2$ has many applications.

One of the principal outcome measures from exercise testing is that of maximal oxygen uptake ($\dot{V}O_2$max, sometimes referred to as $\dot{V}O_2$peak). Bruce (2) used the term functional capacity to describe the importance of $\dot{V}O_2$max, since this measure defines the capabilities of the body to produce energy for work (i.e., function) over the long term. Additionally, $\dot{V}O_2$max is considered a

whole-body measure, as it reflects the function of many organs and systems in the body (e.g., cardiac, vascular, pulmonary, skeletal, muscular).

The importance of the cardiovascular system in determining $\dot{V}O_2$max can be observed from the Fick equation. The ability of the body to use oxygen is determined by both central factors (cardiac output) and peripheral factors (arteriovenous oxygen difference [a-$\bar{v}$ O_2 diff]). The Fick equation shown in figure 2.9 clearly demonstrates the vital role the cardiovascular system has in determining $\dot{V}O_2$, in relation to both central and peripheral factors. The contribution of the cardiovascular system to the peripheral side of the equation is sometimes not appreciated by those who think of this factor only in relation to the skeletal muscle (i.e., the ability of the muscle to take up and utilize oxygen). As we will see, the vascular system plays an essential role in supporting the skeletal muscle's use of oxygen.

Cardiac Output During Exercise

Earlier in the chapter we considered factors that control heart rate and stroke volume. These factors obviously are responsible for the large increase in cardiac output that occurs during aerobic exercise. Most of the discussion that follows relates to aerobic or dynamic exercise versus isometric or static exercise. There are only minor changes in cardiac output during static exercise. Typically, aerobic exercise can increase cardiac output between three and six times above the resting level of $\approx$5 L·min^{-1} in healthy adults. This is brought about by increases in both heart rate and stroke volume. To understand the magnitude of these increases, it is helpful to have average resting values as a reference point. Thus, for the purpose of this discussion, average resting heart rate

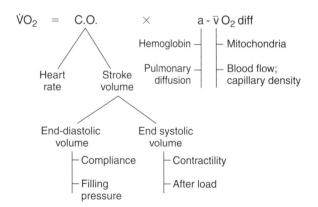

Figure 2.9 The Fick equation describes the determinants of oxygen uptake.

and stroke volume are 70 bpm and 70 ml·beat⁻¹, respectively.

When exercise begins, the initial increase in cardiac output is brought about principally by an increase in heart rate as a result of release from parasympathetic vagal dominance. This mechanism alone can cause an increase in heart rate of approximately 50% of the resting value. Often a pre-exercise, anticipatory rise in heart rate is also stimulated by the cerebral cortex. Stroke volume also begins to increase as exercise commences. The increase in stroke volume is created via the pumping action of the muscles on the veins to induce a greater venous return, thus activating the Frank-Starling mechanism. This effect takes place when muscles are repeatedly stimulated to alternately contract and relax as occurs during dynamic types of activity. As muscles contract, they squeeze the veins that pass through the muscles, forcing blood to move forward in the circulatory system toward the heart and thereby give the heart a boost in filling volume that occurs naturally with exercise. As exercise continues, further increases in cardiac output result from additional elevations of both heart rate and stroke volume. These result primarily from the activation of the sympathetic nervous system during exercise, which directly stimulates the SA node to increase its rate of discharge as well as increase the contractility of the heart.

The contributions of both heart rate and stroke volume to increasing cardiac output continue until the individual reaches ≈50% to 60% of her $\dot{V}O_2$max. At this point the individual's stroke volume is at its maximal level, and further increases in cardiac output are obtained solely from increasing heart rate (figure 2.10). When one considers the effectiveness of further increases in cardiac output, the peaking of stroke volume at a relatively

low percentage of the individual's maximal capacity makes more sense. To generate a greater stroke volume would require either a greater filling or a more complete emptying of the left ventricle. Either of these conditions would require more time and would have other potentially unfavorable consequences, which would adversely influence the ability to increase heart rate. Thus, the intended gains in cardiac output by further increases in stroke volume would be compromised by the necessity to reduce the heart rate. This does not suggest that the contractile work of the heart peaks at 50% to 60% of maximal capacity. Indeed, when one considers that stroke volume remains stable as the heart rate continues to increase past 50% to 60% of capacity, it is clear that the heart must be working harder to continue to maintain peak levels of stroke volume.

Maximal stroke volume values vary considerably between individuals. A major factor in determining maximal stroke volume is the size of the heart—large hearts are capable of holding a larger volume and thus of generating a greater stroke volume. It is this factor that accounts for most of the gender difference in stroke volume (i.e., since, in general, men are larger than women, they have larger hearts and thus greater stroke volumes at both resting and maximal levels). Age also influences maximal stroke volume: values are lower by approximately 20% in elderly compared to younger individuals. This reduction in stroke volume with age is associated with a number of physiological age-related changes including increased myocardial stiffness (e.g., decreased end-diastolic volume), an increased afterload due to vascular stiffness, and fewer myocardial adrenergic receptors. These differences in stroke volume due to heart size/gender and age can be viewed as fixed differences—that is, they are not modifiable. Exercise training, on the other hand, is a factor that is modifiable and that can affect stroke volume. Among the training-induced adaptations that contribute to augmenting stroke volume are increased blood volume, increased heart chamber size, and increased contractility. Although training responsiveness varies between individuals, one would generally expect to observe increases in maximal stroke volume in the magnitude of 15% to 20%. Thus, keeping in mind the various factors that can influence maximal stroke volume, we can use reference values of 90 and 110 ml for sedentary 45-year-old women and men, respectively.

As exercise intensity increases above moderate levels, defined as >60% of $\dot{V}O_2$max, heart rate increases continue to produce higher cardiac outputs until maximal heart rate is reached. These

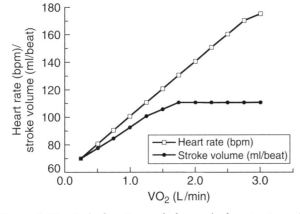

Figure 2.10 Typical pattern of change in heart rate and stroke volume from rest to maximal exercise. Note that the heart rate responds linearly throughout the entire range but that stroke volume plateaus at approximately 60% of $\dot{V}O_2$max.

increases in heart rate are brought about primarily by increased adrenergic stimulation of the SA node, with some additional support from circulating catecholamines. Although maximal heart rate is quite variable between individuals, in general it has a strong inverse relationship with age. This is discussed in more detail in chapter 6; here it is important to understand that age plays a major role in setting the limits on cardiac output, primarily through its influence on maximal heart rate. Many regression equations have been developed to describe the inverse relationship between age and maximal heart rate. The regression coefficient associated with age in most of these equations ranges between 0.7 and 1, suggesting that on average, maximal heart rate declines ≈7 to 10 beats per decade. The most commonly used estimation suggests the following:

maximal heart rate (bpm) =
220 – age (years) ± 10-15 bpm

The most notable feature of this and other regression equations to predict maximal heart rate is the large standard of error of the estimate, which points to the wide degree of variation in maximal heart rate between individuals. Indeed, a study completed with the Ball State University Adult Physical Fitness Program cohort indicated that the maximal heart rate of approximately one in four individuals varies by at least 15 bpm from the age-predicted value (3) (figure 2.11, a and b). Irrespective of the inaccuracy of predictions of maximal heart rate from age, the general characteristic of a decline in maximal heart rate with age applies to all. The only other factor that may influence maximal heart rate is exercise training status. Some studies have indicated that maximal heart rate may actually decline slightly (≈5-10 bpm) as an adaptation to an aerobic exercise training program, but other studies have shown no significant change. The explanation for the decline in maximal heart rate following an exercise-training program relates to the minimal time needed to fill and then empty the left ventricle at maximal exercise. In order to maintain the training-augmented maximal stroke volume, the heart rate is limited slightly. To increase heart rate further would result in a reduction in stroke volume and thus a reduction in cardiac output.

Blood Pressure and Distribution During Exercise

From the preceding discussion one would expect that since cardiac output increases significantly during dynamic exercise, blood pressure would

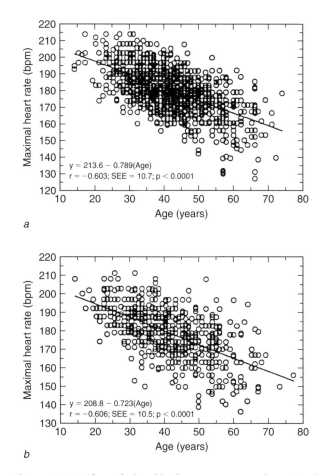

Figure 2.11 The relationship between age and maximal heart rate for *(a)* men and *(b)* women. Note that although maximal heart rate generally declines with increasing age, wide variability exists at any age.

Reprinted, by permission, from M.H. Whaley et al., 1992, "Predictors of over-and underachievement of age-predicted maximal heart rate," *Medicine and Science in Sport and Exercise* 24(10):1176.

also increase. While it is true that systolic blood pressure increases in a linear fashion with increases in exercise intensity, diastolic blood pressure does not increase and may actually decrease during exercise. Thus, mean arterial pressure increases only slightly during exercise, suggesting that PVR must decrease during exercise.

The change in blood pressure during aerobic exercise essentially reflects the complementary actions of increasing cardiac output and the vascular actions to provide more blood to the active muscles. As shown in figure 2.12a, in the resting state, blood flow is distributed generously to many different tissues and organs in the body. Approximately 70% of the total resting blood flow is divided relatively equally among the kidneys, liver, and skeletal muscles; and the myocardium receives approximately 4% of the cardiac output. As discussed earlier, during exercise (figure 2.12b) the cardiac output increases to meet the heightened demand of skeletal muscles for oxygen. This re-

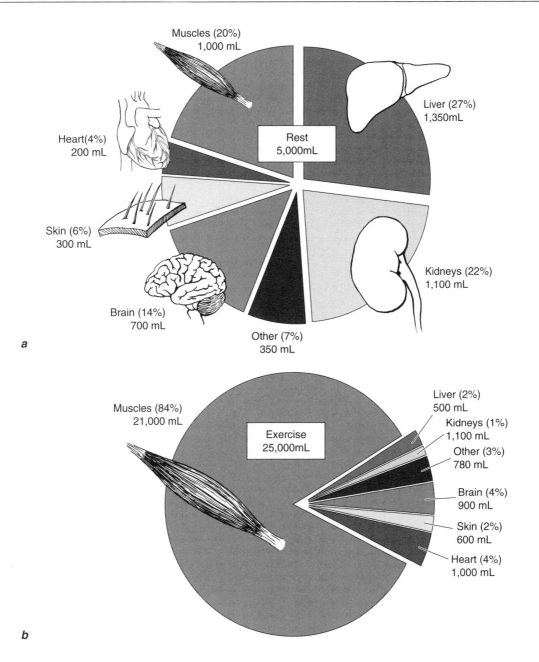

Figure 2.12 Although some of the increased blood flow to muscles during exercise is due to elevated cardiac output, much of the increase is due to a redistribution of the blood. Note that the proportion of flow to the muscle is increased approximately fourfold from the (a) resting state to (b) maximal exercise.

sponse results in an increased systolic blood pressure. The relative distribution of blood flow to the various tissues also changes during exercise. Part of this redistribution is mediated by neural stimulation of the vascular smooth muscle, which results in vasoconstriction of the arterioles supplying the gastrointestinal tract, kidneys, liver, and skin. Simultaneously, vasodilation of the arterioles supplying the skeletal muscles is occurring as a result of the potent effect of the many different vasodilator substances released by the muscles. These dual vascular effects obviously have opposite influences on PVR; however, because of the proportionally larger surface area of the skeletal muscles, the vasodilatory effect dominates and total PVR declines. The magnitude of this response can be observed by the dramatic increase in percentage of blood flow to the skeletal muscles and the reductions to the liver and kidneys.

Although the increased cardiac output plays a significant role in providing more blood to the skeletal muscles, oxygen delivery would be quite limited without the concurrent vascular changes. One way to observe this is to note the absolute volume of blood delivered to the skeletal muscles at rest and during maximal exercise. Since the skeletal muscles receive approximately 20% of the total cardiac output (1 L) at rest, a fourfold increase in cardiac output would result in a total blood flow of 4 L at maximal exercise. However, the actual blood supply is approximately 17 L—demonstrating the tremendous importance of the vascular system. To understand how this dramatic change in blood distribution can occur, the student should remember Poiseuille's law, which states that for every unit of change in the size of a blood vessel, there is a fourfold change in the resistance to flow through that vessel.

Blood pressure (systolic, diastolic, and mean) is substantially elevated during static exercise, such as straining to hold a heavy object in place. The magnitude of the elevation is directly related to the proportion of muscle mass that is actively contracting. The increase is almost entirely due to elevated PVR created by external compression of the blood vessels by the contracting skeletal muscles. Certainly, heightened stimulation of the sympathetic nervous system also contributes to this response. The resulting increased afterload creates increased myocardial wall stress and $m\dot{V}O_2$.

PATHOPHYSIOLOGY

As discussed in chapter 1, cardiovascular diseases are the leading cause of death in the United States. Although the disease processes are quite complex and our understanding of the pathophysiology is still developing, an introduction to this topic is important for people planning on working with patients who have these diseases.

Atherosclerosis is the pathological process whereby lesions or plaques form in the coronary arteries, creating a narrowed lumen and thus impaired ability for blood flow. Although the process also commonly takes place in the aorta, carotid, and femoral arteries, this review focuses on coronary atherosclerosis. The most commonly accepted theory on how atherogenesis takes place is the response-to-injury hypothesis. Students are referred to the comprehensive review paper written by Ross in 1993 (4) for a detailed explanation of this theory. The atherogenic process begins when damage to the coronary artery endothelium occurs. Many different factors have been associated with endothelial injury (table 2.2). The student should note that many of the major risk factors for coronary artery disease can directly promote endothelial damage. Once damage has occurred, circulating platelets adhere to this portion of the endothelium and are thereby stimulated to release a number of "growth factors" that trigger smooth muscle cell proliferation, monocyte binding, and low-density lipoprotein recep-

Table 2.2
Factors Associated With Endothelial Dysfunction and/or Injury

Low-density lipoprotein-cholesterol (LDL-C)
Hypertension
Cigarette smoking
Hyperinsulinemia
Homocysteine
Infections

tor activation. Monocytes are now able to infiltrate the damaged endothelium, where they become activated macrophages that accumulate cholesterol from low-density lipoprotein molecules. As the macrophages accumulate cholesterol, they are transformed into foam cells that are capable of holding large amounts of lipid. The smooth muscle cells also are stimulated to release additional growth factors that lead to further infiltration of cell materials including fibrous connective tissue. This entire process is summarized in figure 2.13. The end result is a plaque containing a variety of materials, characterized by an outer fibromuscular layer surrounding a cholesterol core. Initially, plaques can develop without affecting lumen size; but if the plaques continue to expand, they eventually result in narrowing of the coronary artery lumen (figure 2.14).

Plaque development can begin early in life, and atherosclerosis is generally thought to be a progressive disease. Lifestyle activity and dietary habits play an important role in determining the rate of atherogenesis. Plaques can remain stable for periods of time, or they may grow slowly, or they may grow quite rapidly. Once formed, plaques are more susceptible to damage than other areas within the vessel. Rupture of the plaque is known to be precipitated by hemodynamic shear forces, as well as by vasoconstriction and possibly by some circulating substances. A thrombus is formed at the site of the rupture; the thrombus may be incorporated into the plaque and/or may form a mural thrombus that partially protrudes into the lumen of the vessel.

These latter type (mural) may continue to stimulate thrombus development that can rapidly progress to completely occlude the artery (figure 2.15). In fact, plaque rupturing causes most myocardial infarctions. The size of the plaque does not seem to be linearly related to likelihood for rupture. We now know that plaques that take up 40% to 50% of the lumen are more likely to rupture than larger plaques (5) and that they quickly become totally occluded by a thrombus.

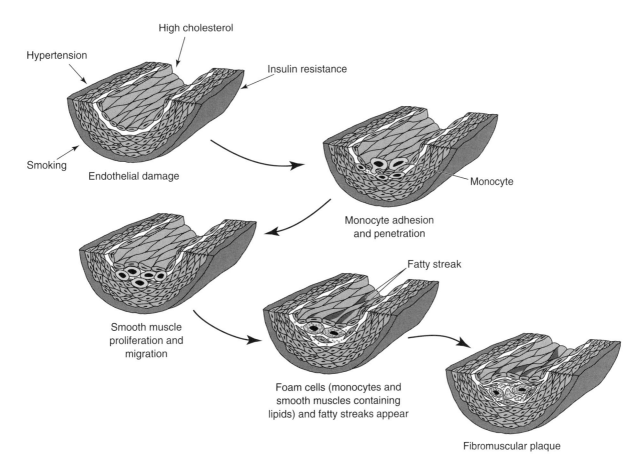

Figure 2.13 The sequence of events in the atherosclerotic process begins with an endothelial injury.

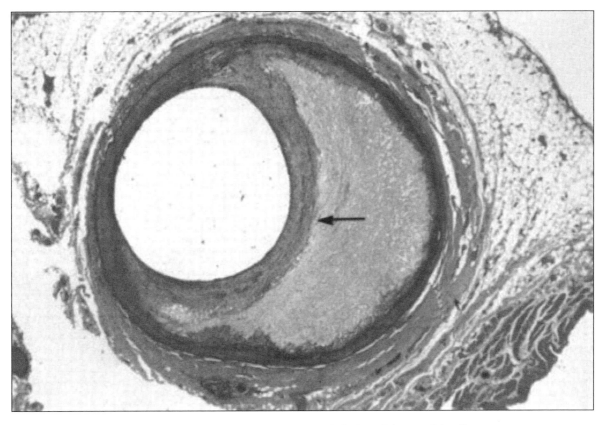

Figure 2.14 A cross section of a diseased coronary artery (eccentric lesion of the arterial wall).

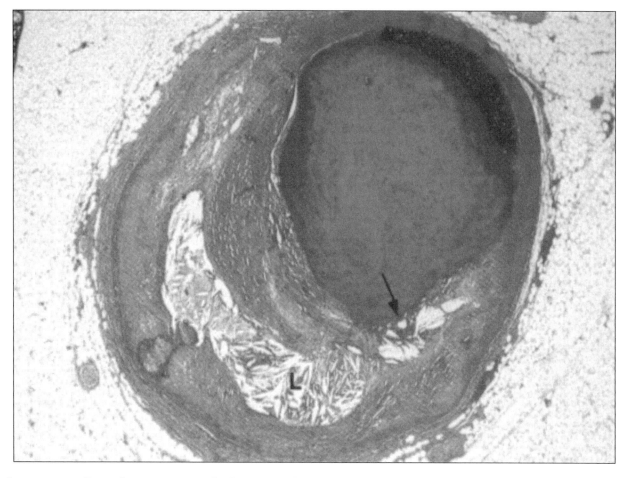

Figure 2.15   A diseased coronary artery that became totally occluded by a thrombus.

When a coronary artery becomes occluded to the point where oxygen supply cannot meet oxygen demand due to a blood flow limitation, the myocardium being supplied by this vessel is compromised. This condition is called myocardial **ischemia.** If blood flow is not quickly restored (within ≈60 min), irreversible damage will occur. When ischemia occurs, the myocardium must shift from its preferred aerobic energy production pathway to the anaerobic pathway and the resultant development of acidosis. The contractile ability of the myocardium becomes impaired, and systolic function deteriorates. This condition is rcognizable both by signs such as an abnormal electrocardiogram and by symptoms such as angina. Typically, ischemia does not occur until a coronary artery develops an obstruction of at least 50% of the luminal diameter, which is equivalent to a 75% reduction in cross-sectional area. Although ischemia is commonly associated with atherosclerotic plaques that have significantly narrowed a coronary artery, it can also occur in vessels with little to no atherosclerosis. This happens when the smooth muscles surrounding a portion of a coronary artery are stimulated to con-

tract intensely, resulting in a vasospasm. Although the exact mechanisms that precipitate a coronary vasospasm for any given individual are not known, endothelial dysfunction and greater sensitivity to both neural and hormonal vasoconstrictive substances are believed to be factors.

Generally, ischemia is first recognized by the affected person during some stressful situation (e.g., exercise, arousal, or anger). That is, at rest the blood supply can meet the myocardial demands; but as the myocardial work increases to meet the demands of the stress, the reduced coronary artery lumen size keeps sufficient blood from reaching the myocardium. Unfortunately, some people do not develop angina during ischemia and thus lack a major warning signal that they have a serious condition. This condition, which can only be detected by an exercise test or other diagnostic procedure, is termed **silent ischemia.** If the ischemia occurs acutely during resting, or occurs during activity and is not relieved with rest, it is possible that a thrombus has formed that has completely or almost completely occluded the coronary artery. Immediate emergency care is required in this situation to provide the patient with a thrombolytic agent (e.g., tissue plasminogen activator). The sooner this therapy begins, the more likely it is to eliminate or minimize the damage to the myocardium. Chapters 3 and 4 provide a more thorough explanation of the diagnosis and treatment of ischemic events.

When ischemia goes untreated for more than approximately 60 min, necrosis of myocardial cells begins; this is termed a myocardial infarction. The exact time frame for initiation of myocardial cell death depends on the severity of the ischemia (i.e., whether it is precipitated by an incomplete or a complete occlusion of a coronary artery) and the extent of collateral coronary arteries supplying the affected area. Typically, the infarction starts in the endocardium, as coronary blood supply to this area is most remote. If the portion of the myocardium that is ischemic is large enough and is left untreated, the infarction can spread through the entire wall of the heart (i.e., from endocardium to epicardium) and becomes what is termed a transmural myocardial infarction.

The irreversible nature of a myocardial infarction is characterized by the rupture of the myocardial sarcolemma. This damage can be observed diagnostically both from blood tests (chapter 3) and on the electrocardiogram (chapter 5).

SUMMARY

The anatomy and physiology of the cardiovascular system are wonderfully complex. Understanding the material presented in this chapter will help the student appreciate the reasons for the importance of various procedures used to evaluate and treat patients with coronary artery disease. Although we have attempted to review the fundamental principles of cardiovascular physiology, the student should realize that this chapter provides only a thumbnail sketch of this topic. Indeed, entire textbooks are devoted to cardiovascular physiology and even to subtopics like cardiac endothelium. Thus, students should do some of the reference reading to develop a more comprehensive knowledge of this topic as they become more involved in working with patients who are at risk for or who have coronary artery disease.

Case Study 1
Primary Prevention: Low Risk

We learned in chapter 1 that this 38-year-old man had elevated resting blood pressure. The obvious question for the clinician is why the resting blood pressure is elevated. This is where knowledge of normal physiology is important to help understand the potential causes of the elevated resting blood pressure. Recall that blood pressure is a function of cardiac output times peripheral vascular resistance. Start to think about all of the different control mechanisms that your body has to regulate blood pressure. What could be going wrong in this case? Now you are thinking like a clinician! Read on in the subsequent chapters to learn how this man's elevated blood pressure was diagnosed and treated.

Case Study 2
Primary Prevention: High Risk

As introduced in chapter 1, this 50-year-old man had hypertension (resting blood pressure of 170/90 mmHg). Let's consider a few of the physiological consequences of this elevated pressure. Comparing his elevated blood pressure to normal blood pressure (i.e., 120/80 mmHg) we can see a number of consequences. The increased blood pressure results in an increased afterload (diastolic pressure of 90 mmHg versus 80 mmHg) that could have a consequence of decreasing both stroke volume and cardiac output. Fortunately, the body's homeostatic control mechanisms operate to maintain cardiac output. However, to maintain cardiac output the heart must do more work. Applying the increased blood pressure values to the equations for wall stress and rate pressure product will demonstrate this. Although the homeostatic mechanisms maintain cardiac output, the long-term effects of increased demand on the heart (from uncontrolled resting blood pressure) can be deleterious. Read on in chapter 3 to see what happens to our 50-year-old man.

Case Study 3
Secondary Prevention

In chapter 1 we learned that this 61-year-old man had a myocardial infarction. We will see in chapter 3 the extent of his atherosclerosis. Note that he had two of the factors associated with endothelial injury (hypertension and hyperlipidemia). See figure 2.13 to review the process of how his atherosclerosis developed and figure 2.14 for an indication of how his distal circumflex coronary artery looked as this disease developed. Unfortunately in his case, the disease process was severe enough to cause necrosis of some of his myocardial cells. Read on in chapters 3 and 4 to learn how his disease was diagnosed and treated.

GLOSSARY

Afterload: the pressure in the pulmonary artery or aorta; pressure in the ventricles must become higher than the arterial pressure in order for blood to be ejected from the heart

Chronotropic: of or having to do with the rate of the heart's contractions (i.e., heart rate)

Double product: mathematical expression of the product of heart rate times systolic blood pressure; often used as an indicator of myocardial oxygen consumption

Ejection fraction: the amount of blood ejected from the ventricle expressed as a percentage relative to the amount of blood in the ventricle immediately prior to ejection (i.e., [end-diastolic volume – end-systolic volume]/end-diastolic volume)

Endocardium: the innermost layer of the heart wall, made up of a layer of endothelium

Endothelium: a specialized group of cells that serves a variety of purposes related to control of blood flow to tissues and protection of blood vessels

Inotropic: of or having to do with the forcefulness of the heart's contractions

Ischemia: a condition that results when blood supply to a tissue (e.g., myocardium) does not meet the demand of that tissue

Myocardium: cardiac muscle, the contracting tissue of the heart

Pericardium: the membranous structure that surrounds the heart

Preload: the pressure developed in the ventricle immediately prior to contraction (determined by the end-diastolic volume)

Silent ischemia: ischemia without a concurrent symptom (e.g., angina)

Vasoconstriction: process that results in a decrease of the lumen size of a blood vessel

Vasodilation: process that results in an increase of the lumen size of a blood vessel

REFERENCES

1. Opie, L.H. 1998. *The heart: Physiology from cell to circulation.* 3rd ed. Philadelphia: Lippincott-Raven, 637.

2. Bruce, R.A., F. Hosmer, and F. Kusumi. 1973. Maximal oxygen uptake and nomographic assessment of functional aerobic impairment in cardiovascular disease. *Am. Heart J.* 85:546–562.

3. Whaley, M.H., L.A. Kaminsky, G.B. Dwyer, L.H. Getchell, and J.A. Norton. 1992. Predictors of over and under achievement of age-predicted maximal heart rate in adult men and women. *Med. Sci. Sports Exerc.* 24:1173–1179.

4. Ross, R. 1993. The pathogenesis of atherosclerosis: A perspective for the 1990s. *Nature* 362: 801–809.

5. Little, W.C., M. Constantinesu, R.J. Applegate, M.A. Kutcher, M.T. Burrows, F.R. Kahl, and W.P. Santamore. 1988. Can coronary angiography predict the site of a subsequent myocardial infarction in patients with mild-to-moderate coronary disease? *Circulation* 78:1157–1166.

CHAPTER 3
Assessment and Diagnosis of Coronary Artery Disease

BEHAVIORAL OBJECTIVES

- To be able to identify physical findings suggestive of coronary artery disease
- To be able to describe laboratory procedures commonly used in the assessment of coronary artery disease
- To be able to identify the various noninvasive and invasive procedures used for diagnosing coronary disease and how they are used in clinical practice
- To be able to describe the indications, limitations, and cost effectiveness of specific cardiac diagnostic procedures

As outlined in chapter 1, CAD has reached nearly epidemic proportions in our society and is the cause of more deaths, disability, and economic loss than any other group of diseases (1). There has also been a widespread misconception that CAD is a male disease—a misconception that arises principally from an earlier disease onset in men. However, both in terms of absolute numbers and on a percentage basis, cardiovascular disease accounts for more deaths in women than in men when all ages are considered (2).

Clearly, more public education concerning the "pandemic" of cardiovascular disease is needed. However, the purpose of this chapter is to describe the methods and procedures used to diagnose the presence (or absence) of CAD.

MEDICAL HISTORY AND PHYSICAL EXAMINATION

Health care providers in the current era of medicine are often tempted to want to use the newest "high-tech" procedures to diagnose the presence of CAD. These procedures not only are costly but also can present substantial risk and discomfort to the patient. Often it is possible to diagnose CAD through a complete review of the patient's remote and recent medical history and a comprehensive physical examination. How and when this information is obtained may differ depending on how and when the individual enters the health care system (i.e., primary prevention vs. secondary prevention setting).

The medical history is typically obtained by a nurse, physician's assistant, physician, or in some settings, an exercise physiologist. It is essential that individuals performing this assessment have a basic understanding of why this information is gathered and how it will impact decisions regarding further diagnostic procedures or treatments. This information will be particularly valuable for identifying potential contraindications to exercise testing or training (refer to chapters 6 and 7). Although a detailed review on taking a medical history is beyond the scope of this text, several points are especially important to individuals working in a CAD prevention or rehabilitation setting. As table 3.1 shows, the key components of the medical history include diagnosing previous medical conditions including cardiac procedures; findings from a physical examination (discussed in more detail in the next section); presence of symptoms, particularly those related to the heart (e.g., discomfort, irregular heartbeat); recent illness or hospitalization; orthopedic problems; medication use

and drug allergies; other habits (caffeine, alcohol, tobacco, recreational drug use); exercise and physical activity habits; work history and requirements; and family history of disease. Careful history-taking may reveal important clues about the presence of CAD, which may be valuable for making decisions about further evaluation or treatment.

In most settings, the physical examination is performed by a licensed health care provider such as a physician, physician's assistant, or nurse practitioner. Again, the details of conducting a physical examination lie beyond the scope of this book; however, it is essential that individuals working in the preventive and rehabilitative ex-

Table 3.1
Key Components of the Medical History

Medical diagnosis
Cardiovascular diseases and conditions
Coronary artery disease (myocardial infarction, revascularization procedures, angina)
Valvular heart disease
Congenital heart defects
Arrhythmia and conduction defects
Left ventricular dysfunction (systolic or diastolic heart failure)
Peripheral and cerebral vascular disease
Non-cardiovascular diseases and conditions
Musculoskeletal/orthopedic problems
Gastrointestinal disorders
Pulmonary disease
Metabolic and hematologic disorders
Renal or hepatic disease
Cancer
Pregnancy
Physical exam and laboratory findings
Height, weight, body mass index, waist circumference
Blood pressure and pulse rate
Heart sounds (S1–S4)
Peripheral pulses (presence of bruits)
Peripheral or central edema
Pulmonary findings, i.e., breath sounds and pulmonary function studies
Chest X ray

Physical exam and laboratory findings
Electrocardiogram
Blood and urine glucose
Blood lipids and lipoproteins
History of symptoms
Chest pain/discomfort
Dyspnea
Palpitations
Dizziness, lightheadedness, or fainting (syncope)
Transient loss of vision or speech
Numbness and weakness
Fatigue
Medication, drug, and supplement use
Cardiovascular and non-cardiovascular medications
Illicit drugs
Vitamins, herbs
Other
Family history of cardiovascular, metabolic, and pulmonary diseases
Lifestyle habits
Dietary habits
Exercise and physical activity patterns
Vocational requirements
Use of tobacco products
Stress and other psychosocial disorders

ercise setting understand the role of the physical examination in evaluating the presence of CAD. Table 3.2 describes the basic components of a physical examination. The following sections address several key points related to the physical examination.

Angina Pectoris

From the perspective of diagnosing the presence of CAD, one of the most important goals of the medical history and physical examination is to identify potential signs and symptoms of myocardial ischemia. Inadequate perfusion of blood to the endocardial, myocardial, or epicardial layers of the heart results in myocardial ischemia and often leads to the symptom of angina pectoris (*angere* means "to choke"; *pectoris* refers to the chest). Angina pectoris, commonly called angina,

is a discomfort in the chest or adjacent areas that is often provoked by physical or emotional stress. While some patients will use very specific adjectives such as "crushing," "squeezing," or "burning" to describe their symptoms, others may convey only a vague feeling of pressure or numbness. Moreover, other patients, particularly those who are elderly, may experience an "anginal equivalent" (i.e., non-anginal symptom of myocardial ischemia), which can be **dyspnea** (shortness of breath), fatigue, or light-headedness. The site of the discomfort or sensation of typical angina is generally in the chest but can also be in the back, arms, and jaw (figure 3.1). Characteristics that are not suggestive of angina are fleeting, momentary chest pains (i.e., stabbing or sticking pain) or pain that is relieved by deep breaths, position or postural changes (i.e., sitting up vs. lying down), food, or drink. Pain that is localized to a small, specific area of the chest or that is associated with or reproduced by pressure on the chest is unlikely to represent angina pectoris. The typical episode of angina begins gradually and reaches its maximal intensity over a period of minutes before dissipating, and can be relieved with a reduction in effort, rest, or nitroglycerin use (see table 3.3 for a listing of anti-anginal medications).

It is important to distinguish between stable and **unstable angina.** The latter refers to a syndrome that is transient and reversible and intermediate in severity between chronic stable angina and myocardial infarction (MI), in which actual tissue damage occurs. The main feature and most common manifestation of unstable angina is dis-

Table 3.2
Basic Components of the Physical Examination

Body weight and anthropometric measurements (girths, body fat distribution)
Blood pressure (including postural changes)
Heart rate and rhythm
Auscultation of heart and lungs (heart and breath sounds)
Palpation of peripheral pulses (including carotid, abdominal, and femoral arteries)
Examination and palpation of abdomen (tenderness, masses)
Orthopedic evaluation (neck, back, limbs)
Neurologic assessment (reflexes, cognition)
Inspection for edema (heart failure), skin ulcers (diabetics), xanthomas (lipid pockets in skin and tendons due to hypercholesterolemia)

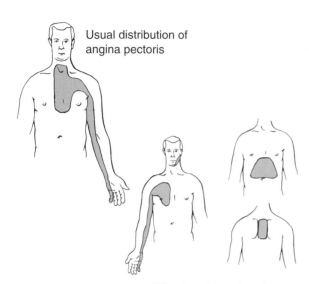

Usual distribution of angina pectoris

Other locations of angina

Figure 3.1   Patterns of angina pectoris. The usual distribution of angina pectoris is referral of pain or discomfort to all or part of sternal region, left side of chest, neck, and down left arm. Other sites sometimes involved are right arm, jaw, epigastrium, and back.

comfort or pain at rest, but angina that has had a recent onset or has a changing pattern should also be considered unstable.

Some patients may have angina at the onset of exertion and then experience relief of their symptoms as they continue to exercise. This phenomenon, typically referred to as "warm-up" or "walk-through" angina, is thought to be due to an exercise-mediated vasodilation that improves coronary blood supply and/or reduces afterload (i.e., reduced myocardial demand) through a reduction in peripheral vascular resistance (3).

Many individuals experience chest or abdominal discomfort after a large meal, especially during physical exertion after the meal. Often the cause is a gastrointestinal disorder such as esophageal reflux or hiatal hernia. However, recent studies have shown that **postprandial angina** (i.e., after a meal) can be a sign of significant multivessel CAD. Thus, postprandial angina should not be discounted and must be recognized as a potential sign of myocardial ischemia (3). Likewise, chest discomfort brought on by emotional stress or exposure to cold conditions can be an indicator of myocardial ischemia. Emotional stress can provoke myocardial ischemia by increasing myocardial demand as well as decreasing blood supply through coronary artery vasoconstriction. The latter is likely to occur especially in patients with established CAD in which endothelial dysfunction is present. In contrast to the "normal" coronary artery segment that dilates in

response to elevations of stress hormones, the diseased artery is more likely to constrict under these conditions, causing myocardial ischemia and associated symptoms. Patients with significant CAD often experience angina in cold, windy conditions, particularly during physical activity under these conditions. These conditions appear to cause coronary artery and/or peripheral artery vasoconstriction, which decrease myocardial blood supply and increase myocardial demand by increasing afterload, respectively (3).

A common cause of chest pain, particularly in women, is a condition that has been termed cardiac syndrome X. Chapter 1 describes a different syndrome X that is associated with metabolic disorders and represents increased risk for CAD. The term cardiac syndrome X has been used to characterize the 20% to 30% of patients who have classic symptoms of angina pectoris but are found to be free of "significant" CAD during diagnostic studies such as a cardiac catheterization (4). It is believed that the angina-like symptoms are caused by microvascular coronary disease (i.e., blockage in small vessels that cannot be visualized with cardiac catheterization), inadequate coronary artery **vasodilatory reserve** (i.e., inability to dilate and increase **myocardial perfusion** in the face of increased myocardial demand), or both. Patients with cardiac syndrome X are generally not good candidates for myocardial revascularization (i.e., coronary artery bypass graft surgery or catheter-based interventions), but do often benefit and get relief of their symptoms from anti-anginal medications (see table 3.3).

It is also important to note that a significant number of patients will have myocardial ischemia or infarction, or both, without ever experiencing an anginal symptom. This condition is referred to as silent ischemia or infarction. Population studies have indicated that 20% to 60% of patients who showed electrocardiographic evidence of a previous MI never experienced an anginal symptom (5). Patients with silent myocardial ischemia are of particular concern in the exercise setting, since they do not have an intrinsic mechanism to monitor myocardial ischemia (i.e., no symptoms) and thus may exercise at levels that provoke the condition.

Myocardial ischemia is not always the cause of chest pain or angina-like symptoms. The differential diagnosis of chest pain is a significant issue in medical management, since failing to recognize myocardial ischemia or infarction could lead to disastrous consequences (e.g., death and disability). In contrast, hospitalizing all patients with chest pain can be very costly, not to mention

Table 3.3
Common Anti-Anginal Agents by Class

Generic name	Brand name	Mechanism and benefit
Beta adrenergic antagonists (beta blockers)		
Atenolol	Tenormin	Competitively binds with
Bisoprolol	Zebeta	beta 1 receptors on
Esmolol	Brevibloc	myocardium and prevents
Metoprolol	Lopressor, Toprol	action of catecholamines,
Nadolol	Corgard	which results in decreased
Pindolol	Visken	heart rate and contractility and
Propranolol	Inderal	lowers myocardial
Sotolol	Betapace	oxygen demand and angina.
Timolol	Blocadren	
Calcium channel antagonists (calcium blockers)		
Amlopidine	Norvasc	Inhibits the entry of calcium
Diltazem	Cardizem, Dilacor	into vascular smooth muscle
Felodipine	Plendil	cells. Results in peripheral
Isradipine	DynaCirc	vascular dilation and
Nicardipine	Cardene	afterload reduction,
Nifedipine	Adalat, Procardia	which decreases myocardial
Verapamil	Calan, Isoptin	demand and angina.
Nitrates and nitroglycerine		
Short acting		Relaxes vascular smooth
Nitroglycerine (sublingual)	Nitrostat	muscle, which dilates arteries
Nitroglycerine (translingual)	Nitrolingual	and veins. The reduction
Nitroglycerine (transmucosal)	Nitrogard	in afterload and preload
Amyl Nitrate	Amyl Nitrate	results in lower myocardial
		demand. Unclear if able
Long acting		to dilate coronary arteries
Isosorbide mononitrate	Ismo, Imdur	and improve myocardial
Isosorbide dinitrate	Isordil, Sorbitrate	blood supply, particularly
Nitroglycerin (Transdermal)	Nitro-Dur, Transderm-Nitro	in atherosclerotic arteries.

inconvenient to patients. Many medical centers have created specific chest-pain centers to better diagnose and triage patients presenting with this often confusing symptomatology. Common noncardiac causes of angina-like symptoms include esophageal disorders (reflux, spasm), biliary or cystic duct obstructions, costosternal syndromes, degenerative changes of the cervical or thoracic vertebrae leading to impingement of nerves or blood vessels, and anxiety disorders (5). A careful history, physical exam, and risk factor assessment can often distinguish these noncardiac conditions from conditions caused by myocardial ischemia.

Cardiac Auscultation

Another important component of the physical exam is cardiac auscultation, which involves listening, by stethoscope, to the sounds made during the various phases of the cardiac cycle. Heart sounds are relatively brief, discrete auditory vibrations of varying intensity (loudness), frequency (pitch), and quality (timbre). The first heart sound identifies the onset of ventricular systole (i.e., contraction), and the second identifies the onset of diastole (i.e., relaxation). These two auscultatory events establish a framework within which other heart sounds and murmurs can be placed. The basic heart sounds are the first, second, third, and fourth. While the first and second normally occur, the third and fourth sounds do not occur in normal, healthy adults. Most other heart sounds, with few exceptions, are abnormal. The following discussion of heart sounds is limited to information that would be valuable to those working in preventive and rehabilitative exercise settings; Braunwald presents a more detailed description of heart sounds (5).

The relationship of the heart sounds to mechanical events during the cardiac cycle can be visualized from figure 2.6 in the previous chapter. In summary, the first heart sound (S_1) is initiated at the onset of ventricular systole and is related to the closure of the two atrioventricular valves, the mitral and tricuspid. Closure of these two valves results in oscillation of blood in the ventricular chambers and vibrations of the chamber walls. The vibrations are due in part to the abrupt rise of ventricular pressure with acceleration of blood back toward the atria, but are primarily caused by sudden tension and recoil of the valve leaflets. Although the mitral and tricuspid valves generally close at the same time, often there is a slight separation of the two events, resulting in a normal "splitting" of the S_1.

The second heart sound (S_2) occurs with closure of the two semilunar valves, aortic and pulmonic, and like the first heart sound, has two components. The sounds are the result of the valves' leaflets slamming shut; this initiates oscillations of the blood and tension on the nearby vessel walls. In the normal healthy adult, the aortic valve sound is louder than the pulmonic valve sound, resulting in a normal "splitting" of the second heart sound. Pathologic conditions that bring about a more rapid closure of the semilunar valves, such as increases in pulmonary artery or aortic pressure (i.e., pulmonary or systemic hypertension), increase the intensity of the second heart sound.

The third heart sound (S_3), while not commonly heard in healthy adults, is sometimes heard in children with thin chest walls or in patients with left ventricular dysfunction. The S_3 consists of low-intensity and low-frequency vibrations that occur early in diastole; these are believed to be caused by abrupt cessation of ventricular distension and deceleration of blood entering the ventricles. A third heart sound often occurs in a weakened, enlarged heart (referred to as a dilated cardiomyopathy), where the end-diastolic volume is very high and the ventricular walls are stretched to the point at which distensibility abruptly decreases. Presence of a third heart sound in a patient with heart disease portends a negative prognosis and reduced survival rate.

The fourth heart sound (S_4), also called the atrial sound, is occasionally heard in normal, healthy individuals but is usually present when there is an augmented atrial contraction. This occurs in situations in which an increased atrial contraction (often called atrial "kick") is needed to more adequately fill the left ventricle. Thus, the fourth heart sound is common with coronary disease, particularly with myocardial ischemia or infarction, when an increased atrial contribution is needed to assist with filling the stiffened ventricle. Moreover, patients with a condition known as diastolic dysfunction, in which the left ventricle does not relax appropriately and is resistant to filling, may demonstrate a fourth heart sound.

A variety of abnormal heart sounds and murmurs can occur during various phases of the cardiac cycle and are detectable by auscultation. Further description and discussion of these are beyond the scope of this text, and generally knowledge of these sounds is not essential for the CAD prevention or rehabilitation professional.

Evaluation of Peripheral Pulses

Evaluating the peripheral pulses is yet another valuable component of the physical examination and can indicate the presence of atherosclerotic disease in noncoronary vessels. However, it is now recognized that vascular disease rarely occurs in an isolated artery (e.g., just a coronary artery); rather, it usually appears in multiple arterial systems (coronary, cerebral, iliac, and femoral arteries) simultaneously. Thus, the presence of obstructive disease in peripheral arteries is highly suggestive of the presence of obstructive CAD. Examination of the arterial pulse is critically important in the diagnosis of obstructive arterial disease. Systematic bilateral palpation (i.e., feeling with fingers) of the common carotid, brachial, radial, femoral, popliteal, dorsal pedis, and posterior tibial arteries, as well as palpation of the abdominal aorta, should be conducted by a trained clinician (typically a physician or physician's assistant) on any patient suspected of having CAD. Absent or weak peripheral pulses usually signify obstruction in that artery. Furthermore, when a peripheral artery is partially obstructed, blood flow though the artery becomes nonlaminar, creating turbulence and a soft rumbling or blowing sound known as a **bruit**. One can detect bruits by placing a stethoscope over specific segments of the peripheral arteries and listening for these abnormal sounds. When the lumen of the artery is reduced by approximately 50%, a soft bruit can be auscultated. As the obstruction become more severe, the bruit becomes high-pitched, louder, and longer. Bruits in the carotid arteries suggest the presence of cerebrovascular disease and an increased risk for a transient ischemic attack, a cerebrovascular accident, or both. Transient ischemic attacks and cerebrovascular accidents involving the brain are analogous to ischemia and infarction to the heart, respectively. Whereas the transient ischemic attack passes and does not result in a permanent cerebral impairment, the cerebrovascular accident, commonly called a stroke, can cause permanent damage to specific areas of the brain. Much like what occurs with MI, the amount and location of the necrotic (dead) tissue generally dictate the prognosis and the extent of residual loss of bodily functions. Other important signs and symptoms of cerebrovascular disease include headaches, blurred vision or loss of vision, paralysis of one side of the face or one arm or leg, loss of motor skills, and/or an inability to speak or express thoughts (6).

Palpation of leg pulses during the physical exam can indicate the presence of peripheral vascular disease. Diminished or absent pulse waves in the femoral, popliteal, dorsal pedis, and posterior tibial arteries generally indicate obstruction in that particular artery. Blood pressure assessment in the lower limb can also be helpful in determining the presence of peripheral vascular disease. Changes to the pulse waves, as well as pressure changes at these locations in the lower limb, may become more obvious if the patient performs physical exertion. Patients with peripheral vascular disease are likely to describe discomfort (burning and/or cramping) in the lower extremity, particularly during exertion, that is known as **intermittent claudication** (from the Latin word *claudicare,* meaning "to limp").

LABORATORY TESTS

Depending on the outcome of the medical history and physical examination, a series of laboratory tests may be indicated. Laboratory tests commonly used to assess the individual with suspected CAD include a chest X ray, 12-lead electrocardiogram, and blood tests. The chest X ray is used to identify the presence of cardiomegaly (enlarged heart) and to obtain evidence of pulmonary edema, both associated with left ventricular dysfunction that can occur with an MI.

Although chapter 5 explains the 12-lead electrocardiogram (ECG) in greater detail, here we'll note several points relevant to the detection of CAD. The resting ECG can be used to identify a number of cardiac abnormalities—for example, to diagnose an acute MI and identify potentially lethal cardiac arrhythmias. Specifically, when an individual presents to the hospital or physician's office with signs and symptoms suggestive of CAD, the ECG is routinely used to help rule in or rule out an MI. Damage to the myocardial tissue often leads to profound changes on the ECG. Sur-

prisingly, though, approximately 50% of patients presenting with acute MI do not exhibit characteristic ECG changes with their myocardial injury (7). Often, patients having an MI experience ventricular arrhythmias, heart blocks, conduction defects, and/or bradyarrhythmias that the ECG can detect; all of these are described in chapter 5.

In light of the limited diagnostic value of patient symptoms and ECG changes, the measurement of blood serum "cardiac" enzymes becomes highly important in a patient suspected of having an MI. These markers are used to determine whether there has been actual heart muscle necrosis (i.e., cell death) versus transient, **reversible myocardial ischemia,** or whether the symptoms have another noncardiac cause. Persistent inadequate blood flow to the myocardial tissue results in a disruption of the cardiac cell membrane, allowing for a leaking of the cell constituents, including enzymes, into the extracellular fluid and eventually into the venous blood. Four main enzymes have been commonly used to identify actual myocardial damage (i.e., rule in for MI): aspartate transaminase, lactic dehydrogenase, and creatine kinase (CK) and the creatine kinase-MB (CK-MB) isoenzyme (5). However, elevations of aspartate transaminase, lactic dehydrogenase, and overall CK are not limited to cardiac injury, often occurring as a consequence of necrosis or trauma to liver, kidneys, brain, or skeletal muscle tissue. Consequently, to improve the sensitivity of these markers, particularly CK, it is necessary to access the CK-MB isoenzyme. Although three isoenzymes of CK have been identified (MM, BB, and MB), CK-MB is the most reflective of damage to cardiac muscle tissue; CK-MM and CK-BB are found mostly in the skeletal muscle and brain/kidney, respectively. When the CK-MB increases to more than 5% of the total CK, the diagnosis of MI can be made (5). Clinicians do not rely on measurements of CK or CK-MB at a single point in time, but instead evaluate the temporal rise and fall of serially obtained values. The time courses of the three common serum "cardiac" enzymes (lactic dehydrogenase, total CK, CK-MB), as well as two newer markers (myoglobin and troponin I), are shown in figure 3.2.

Although most hospitals obtain CK and CK-MB measurements when evaluating patients with suspected acute MI, this practice may change in the near future as assays for more rapidly released markers (such as myoglobin) and more cardiac-specific markers (such as troponin T and troponin I) become available clinically (5). Myoglobin is a protein that is released into circulation from injured myocardial cells and that can be observed

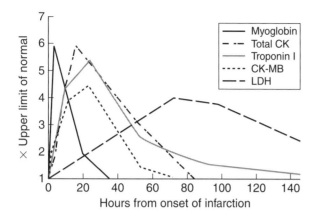

Figure 3.2   Time course of blood serum markers of acute myocardial infarction is shown. The figure summarizes the relative timing, rate of rise, peak values, and duration of elevation above the upper limits of normal for traditional markers: lactic dehydrogenase (LDH), total creatine kinase (CK), creatine kinase MB fraction (CK-MB), and newer markers—myoglobin and troponin I.

within a few hours after the onset of an acute infarction. Peak levels of serum myoglobin are reached significantly earlier (1-4 h) than peak values of CK. However, the clinical value of serial determination of myoglobin is limited by the brief duration of its elevation (<24 h) and by the lack of specificity (resulting from the fact that myoglobin is a constituent of skeletal muscle). Because of its lack of cardiac specificity, isolated elevation of myoglobin should not be relied upon to make the diagnosis of acute MI; a more cardiac-specific marker such as CK-MB, or the cardiac troponins, should also be used. Troponin T and troponin I are both part of the troponin complex that regulates the calcium-mediated contractile process of striated cardiac and skeletal muscle tissue (5). Recently, quantitative assays for cardiac-specific troponin T and troponin I have been developed and approved as diagnostic criteria for acute MI. Advantages of these new markers include, besides greater cardiac specificity, a shortened time to diagnosis. The development of improved markers of acute MI has important implications in terms of cost containment, allowing for shorter hospital stays for patients ruling out for an MI, as well as more rapid and focused treatment for those ruling in for an acute MI (5). Surprisingly, among patients admitted to the hospital with a chest pain syndrome, fewer than 20% are subsequently diagnosed with an MI (8). Thus, in the majority of these patients, clinicians must use serum marker measurements at periodic intervals (i.e., every 4-8 h) to either establish or exclude the

diagnosis of acute MI. Furthermore, the relative rise in these markers may also be used to quantify the size of the infarction (9).

Another recent approach to ruling in or ruling out an MI in patients who present to an emergency room with chest pain is the graded exercise test. This test, using 12-lead electrocardiography (discussed later in this chapter and in chapter 5), has been employed for more than 30 years to diagnose the presence of CAD in nonemergent conditions. However, use of the exercise test in the emergency department has recently been shown to be a safe and cost-effective method of assisting with the management of chest pain syndromes. Critical pathways have been developed that involve emergency department observation and exercise testing for the management of patients with chest pain who are at low risk for heart disease. Application of this pathway, with exercise testing as the first decision step, saves substantial money, since it has been associated with 17% fewer hospital admissions and 11% fewer hospital days (10).

DIAGNOSTIC PROCEDURES FOR CORONARY ARTERY DISEASE

All the information obtained from the patient's medical history, the physical examination, the laboratory tests, and the calculated risk for cardiac events (i.e., Framingham score; see chapter 1) is considered in determining the need for specific diagnostic procedures. The number and variety of cardiovascular diagnostic procedures available to the clinician have increased exponentially over the last quarter-century. The judicious and appropriate use of these tests in evaluating patients for CAD requires a balance of clinical judgment along with a clear understanding of the indications and limitations of each procedure. In the current era of medical practice, one must also consider the cost of the procedure. To assist with this often difficult decision-making process, the American College of Cardiology and the American Heart Association have developed practice guidelines that describe a range of generally acceptable approaches for the diagnosis, management, or prevention of cardiovascular disease (11). Typically the process of diagnosing the presence of CAD begins with the least costly and least invasive procedures. Abnormal or inconclusive findings of a particular procedure generally lead the clinician to the next level of testing. While each level of diagnostic testing potentially increases the diagnostic accuracy, it also increases the expense.

Also, as the testing becomes more invasive, the risk of complications increases. The following is a list of tests routinely used to diagnose the presence of CAD; subsequent sections will discuss each procedure in detail.

- Methods of stress testing
    - Exercise
    - Pharmacologic
- Noninvasive imaging approaches
    - Electrocardiography (ECG)
    - Echocardiography
    - Nuclear imaging (thallium-201 and technetium-99m)
    - Positron emission tomography (PET)
    - Electronic beam computed tomography (EBCT)
    - Magnetic resonance imaging (MRI)
- Invasive diagnostic methods
    - Coronary angiography
    - Left ventriculography
    - Intracoronary ultrasound
    - Hemodynamics (pressure and oxygen saturation)

It is essential that individuals working in CAD prevention and rehabilitation settings have a basic understanding of (1) the rationale for selecting a specific procedure, (2) the information generated by each procedure, and (3) the limitations and risks of each procedure. Often preventive and rehabilitative professionals are asked to describe a procedure or to explain the results of a test to patients in their program.

Selection of an Appropriate Diagnostic Procedure

Any test used to screen for CAD must be evaluated for its sensitivity and specificity. Sensitivity refers to the percentage of tests that correctly iden-

tify the presence of CAD, whereas specificity refers to the percentage of tests that correctly identify individuals without CAD. Sensitivity and specificity are inversely related. Furthermore, they vary with the population being tested, the definition of the disease, and the criteria used to determine an abnormal test. For example, if the population being tested is at risk for severe forms of CAD (e.g., three-vessel or left main coronary disease) or has known disease, the test will have a higher sensitivity. Likewise, the specificity will be highest in low-risk populations, such as a group of young, healthy subjects. We can more accurately determine the diagnostic value of a particular test by looking at its predictive value. The positive predictive value is the percentage of persons with known CAD who have an abnormal test result. The negative predictive value is the percentage of persons who do not have CAD and have a normal test result. Calculation of the predictive accuracy is based on the incidence of "true" and "false" test results and can be summarized as follows:

- In a true-positive test, the patient has CAD and the test is abnormal.
- In a true-negative test, the patient does not have CAD and the test is normal.
- In a **false-positive** test, the patient does not have CAD, but the test is abnormal.
- In a **false-negative** test, the patient has CAD, but the test is normal.

Table 3.4 presents the calculations used to determine sensitivity, specificity, and predictive values.

The information most important to the clinician attempting to diagnose CAD is the "probability" of the patient's having or not having CAD. Such probability is not only dependent on the outcome of the test (e.g., normal or abnormal) but is also dependent on the individual's pretest likelihood of having CAD (12). Bayes theorem indicates that the probability of a patient having the disease (in this case CAD) after a test is performed will be the product of the disease probability

Table 3.4
Terms Used to Describe the Diagnostic Value of a Test

Sensitivity	Specificity	Positive predictive value	Negative predictive value
True positives × 100 / True positives + false negatives	True negatives × 100 / True negatives + false positives	True positives × 100 / True positives + false positives	True negatives × 100 / True negatives + false negatives

before the test and the probability that the test provided a true result. Figure 3.3 shows how Bayes theorem can be used to calculate the probability for CAD. The pretest likelihood of having CAD can be estimated from table 3.5 and is determined by age, sex, and symptoms. By knowing the pretest likelihood of CAD, the clinician can determine whether the outcome (normal or abnormal) of the test, in this case an exercise ECG, will alter the posttest likelihood of the individual's having CAD. It should be apparent from figure 3.3 that the outcome of the exercise ECG (normal or abnormal) does very little to change the posttest likelihood of having CAD in the patient with either a very low or a very high pretest likelihood of CAD. In other words, you don't gain a great deal of information by performing the exercise ECG for diagnostic purposes in these very low or very high risk patients. However, for the individual with a moderate pretest likelihood of having CAD (e.g., a 55-year-old male with atypical chest pain who has a pretest probability of 58.9%), the exercise ECG would be very helpful in determining his posttest likelihood of CAD, depending on whether the outcome of the test was normal (posttest likelihood drops to 30%) or abnormal (posttest likelihood increases to 90%). Use of Bayes theorem, then, allows clinicians to effectively manage their patients by analyzing the diagnostic value of specific procedures. We used the exercise ECG test as an example, but any of the diagnostic procedures discussed in this chapter can be evaluated in this way.

Methods of Stress Testing

The detection of myocardial ischemia is one of the most important and fundamental goals of stress testing. To accomplish this goal, a test must

be capable of first inducing ischemia and then detecting some aspect of the ischemic event. Ischemia is generally induced through either exercise or pharmacologic means. The hallmark of myocardial ischemia is an imbalance between myocardial oxygen supply and demand. As described in chapter 2, CAD leads to epicardial coronary artery narrowing, which can limit coronary flow (i.e., decrease supply). While an obstructive lesion in a coronary artery may not be a problem at rest when the demand for oxygen is low, any increase in metabolic activity of the myocardial tissue (increased heart rate and/or blood pressure) will increase the myocardial demand. When the demand for oxygen exceeds the supply to the tissue, ischemia ensues. The temporally related sequence of events leading from myocardial oxygen supply-demand mismatch to the clinical marker of angina has been described as the ischemic cascade. This cascade of ischemic events progresses from subtle cellular changes (i.e., metabolic abnormalities in tissue) to mechanical changes in ventricular function, including diastolic and systolic dysfunction (inappropriate relaxation and diminished contractile response, respectively), to alterations in electrical conduction through the cardiac tissue (i.e., ECG changes), and ultimately to overt symptoms (i.e., angina) (13). Several diagnostic techniques are available, each one focusing on a different event in the ischemic cascade. The following sections describe tests commonly employed to detect these ischemic events.

Exercise Stress Testing

Exercise stress tests are among the most widely used tests in cardiology and when performed appropriately can yield valuable diagnostic, prognostic, functional, and therapeutic information at a relatively low cost and with minimal risk to the

Table 3.5
Estimate of Pretest Likelihood of Coronary Artery Disease

Age	Asymptomatic		Nonanginal chest pain		Atypical angina		Typical angina	
	Men	Women	Men	Women	Men	Women	Men	Women
35	1.9	0.3	5.2	0.8	21.8	4.2	69.7	25.8
45	5.5	1.0	14.1	2.8	46.1	13.3	87.3	55.2
55	9.7	3.2	21.5	8.4	58.9	32.4	92.0	79.4
65	12.3	7.5	28.1	18.6	67.1	54.4	94.3	90.6

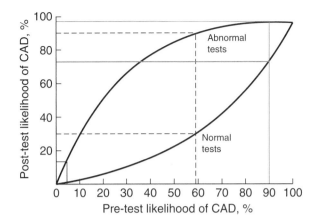

Figure 3.3 Use of Bayes theorem to calculate probability of CAD. Dotted line shows the impact of a 59% (from table 3.5—55-year-old man with atypical angina) pretest likelihood of CAD on posttest likelihood of having CAD. If the ECG is negative (i.e., no ST-segment changes), the posttest likelihood decreases to 30%. If the ECG is positive (i.e., ST segment changes during exercise), then the posttest likelihood increases to 90%. Thus, in the case of this 55-year-old male, the outcome of the stress test (positive vs. negative) has a significant impact on medical management. A low posttest likelihood of CAD would not warrant invasive assessment, whereas a high posttest likelihood would warrant further assessment and intervention (i.e., cardiac catheterization).

subject (11). Here we'll focus exclusively on the diagnostic and prognostic value of the exercise test, leaving the discussion of other important applications of exercise testing (particularly exercise prescription and functional assessment) for chapter 6. Similarly, chapter 5 discusses the specific electrocardiographic patterns associated with myocardial ischemia.

As outlined in chapter 2, unlike other tissue in the body, the myocardial tissue is at near-maximal oxygen extraction at rest. Thus, the only way to increase myocardial oxygen supply is by increasing blood flow through the coronary arteries. The exercise test provokes myocardial ischemia in a patient with coronary artery lesion because coronary blood flow is unable to meet the increasing demand for blood by the myocardial tissue. In the past, the degree of artery **stenosis** thought to significantly limit coronary artery blood flow—and ultimately result in myocardial ischemia during exertion—was approximately 60% to 70%. However, recent studies have shown that ischemia can occur with less severe coronary lesions and, conversely, that lesions greater than 60% may not cause ischemia (14). Despite a significant coronary lesion and reduced coronary blood flow, the

metabolic needs of the myocardial tissue may be met through an adaptive process called **collateralization.** Figure 3.4 shows that coronary collaterals are small dormant vascular channels that connect the coronary arteries. It appears that the difference in pressure between the obstructed and nonobstructed vessel is the stimulus to open these protective conduits and subsequently provide adequate blood flow to the myocardial tissue in question (5).

An often underutilized application of the exercise test is to stratify patients on the basis of their prognosis (i.e., risk for cardiac events such as death and MI). One of the strongest and most consistent prognostic markers identified from the exercise test is the maximal exercise capacity. Although several exercise parameters can be used as markers of exercise capacity, including maximal exercise duration and workload, directly measuring and/or estimating maximal oxygen consumption (often expressed as METs) appears to be the most prognostic (11). One study determined that patients with a <5-MET exercise capacity had an increased mortality and would clearly benefit from coronary artery bypass graft (CABG) surgery (15). Conversely, patients with a >10-MET capacity had equal survival rates with either conservative medical therapy (i.e., cardiac medications) or CABG surgery. Another study demonstrated that an incremental increase of just one MET unit was associated with a 20% and 25% reduction in all-cause mortality and cardiac events for men and women, respectively (16). A second group of prognostic exercise testing markers relates to exercise-induced ischemia. These markers include ST-segment elevation or depression, and exercise-induced angina.

Several recent studies have developed "prognostic scores" based on multiple exercise variables. Figure 3.5 shows the Duke nomogram to predict average annual mortality and five-year survival for patients with known or suspected disease (17). Prognosis based on the Duke model is determined by functional capacity (METs) and the presence of myocardial ischemia. Another group of investigators developed a prognostic score on patients from a Veterans Administration Hospital (18). This score includes two variables in common with the Duke model (METs and ST changes) and two other variables: drop in exercise systolic blood pressure below resting value, and a history of congestive heart failure (CHF) or use of digitalis (a drug to treat heart failure). The score is calculated in the following way:

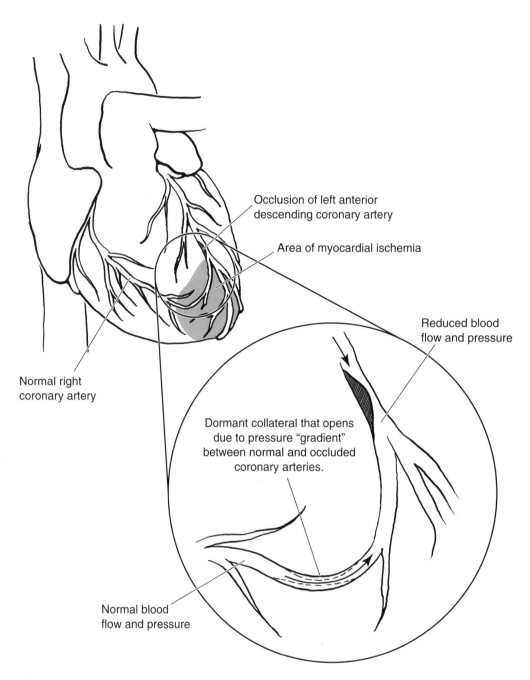

Figure 3.4   Collateral vessel formation secondary to myocardial ischemia.

$5 \times$ (CHF/Dig [yes = 1; no = 2]) +
exercise-induced ST depression in mm +
change in systolic blood pressure [0 = >40 mmHg,
1 = 31-40 mmHg, 2 = 21-30 mmHg,
4 = 0-11 mmHg, and
5 = a reduction below standing pre-exercise levels])

With use of this score, 77% of the Veterans Administration Hospital population were at low risk (<2% average annual mortality); 18% were moderate risk (average annual mortality = 7%); and 6% were at high risk (average annual mortality =

15%). Quantifying prognoses with these approaches allows the clinician to objectively determine which patients would benefit from interventional procedures, such as CABG surgery or others.

While it is widely accepted that exercise provides the "best" stress to provoke myocardial ischemia, it has been estimated that a significant number (21%) of patients are physically unable to perform an exercise test and that another 20% fail to achieve adequate levels of exertion (i.e., submaximal or nondiagnostic lev-

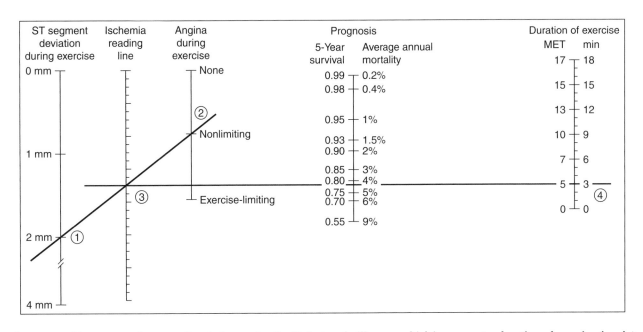

Figure 3.5 Nomogram of prognostic relations using the Duke treadmill score, which incorporates duration of exercise (in min) – (5 × maximal ST-segment deviation during or after exercise) (in mm) – (4 × treadmill angina index). Treadmill angina index is 0 for no angina, 1 for nonlimiting angina, and 2 for exercise limiting angina. The nomogram can be used to assess the prognosis of ambulatory outpatients referred for exercise testing. In this example, the obseved amount of exercise-induced ST-segment deviation (minus resting changes) is marked on the line for ST-segment deviation during exercise (1). The degree of angina during exercise is plotted (2), and the points are connected. The point of intersect on the ischemia reading line is noted (3). The number of METs (or min of exercise if the Bruce protocol is used) is marked on the exercise duration line (4). The marks on the ischemia reading line and duration of exercise line are connected, and the intersect on the prognosis line determines 5-year survival rate and average annual mortality for patients with these selected specific variables. In this example the 5-year prognosis is estimated at 78% in this patient with exercise-induced 2-mm ST-depression, nonlimiting exercise angina, and peak exercise workload of 5 METs.

els). Individuals in these two categories often have orthopedic, neurologic, pulmonary, or peripheral vascular disease or lack adequate motivation. Furthermore, a fairly large number of patients (24%) will have an exercise ECG that is classified as "uninterpretable" for myocardial ischemia. Consequently, some believe that exercise testing as a means of provoking and identifying myocardial ischemia may be appropriate for only 35% of patients commonly referred for diagnostic testing (19). Thus it is necessary to employ other approaches to stressing the heart for many patients referred for diagnostic testing for CAD.

Pharmacologic Stress Tests

Pharmacologic stress tests (commonly called non-exercise stress tests) have proven to be a reasonable alternative to elicit myocardial ischemia in those who cannot exercise adequately. Myocardial ischemia during a pharmacologic stress test is provoked through one of two mechanisms: coronary artery vasodilation or increased myocardial oxygen demand. Coronary artery vasodilation is accomplished by the intravenous administration of dipyridamole or adenosine. Both these agents work by relaxing coronary artery smooth muscle, which results in a decrease in coronary vascular resistance and increase in coronary blood flow (19). Coronary blood flow is compared in normal artery segments and those supplied by an occluded coronary artery. However, coronary arteries with a significant lesion, as an adaptive response to ischemia, have dilated to their maximal diameter. Consequently, infusion of dipyridamole or adenosine causes dilation only in the nondiseased artery, not in the diseased artery. This results in a physiologic phenomenon known as "coronary steal syndrome," in which blood flow through the normal segment is increased at the expense of the diseased vessel, where blood flow is actually diminished. Ischemia occurs as a result of a decreased perfusion to the myocardium served by the diseased artery. Use of these agents is generally well tolerated, although there may be occasional side effects including hypotension, light-headedness, headache, nausea, chest pain, and myocardial conduction problems (19).

Dobutamine and arbutamine are the two pharmacologic agents most commonly used to stress the heart by increasing the myocardial oxygen demand. These agents exert their influence by stimulating cardiac beta receptors that increase the rate and force of myocardial contraction. In the presence of a fixed coronary lesion, the myocardial blood supply cannot adequately meet the increased myocardial demand imposed by these agents, so myocardial ischemia results. Although dobutamine or arbutamine infusion is generally well tolerated, side effects include arrhythmia, chest pain, nausea, tremors, shortness of breath, headache, hypertension, or hypotension (19).

The involvement of different pathways to the development of myocardial ischemia with these pharmacologic stressors has led to their combined use. Furthermore, the addition of atropine (a vagolytic drug that increases heart rate) to either dipyridamole/adenosine or dobutamine/ arbutamine infusion has been shown to increase the heart rate as well as the sensitivity of the test. Also, the combination of dipyridamole and either isotonic (i.e., cycle ergometry) or isometric (i.e., hand-gripping) exercise has been used effectively (19). Pharmacologic stress testing through either mechanism (vasodilation or increased myocardial demand) is generally used in combination with a diagnostic technique other than electrocardiography. The mechanism of action of the vasodilators favors their use in combination with myocardial perfusion studies (to be discussed later). In contrast, the increase of myocardial oxygen requirements in response to dobutamine or arbutamine favors their use with echocardiography (also discussed later).

Noninvasive Techniques to Identify Myocardial Ischemia

As listed earlier, a number of techniques are now available to detect the presence of myocardial ischemia induced by either an exercise or a pharmacologic stress. This section provides a basic overview of these techniques, as well as their limitations.

Electrocardiography

The exercise test with recording of the ECG is often the first test used to diagnose the presence of CAD, primarily because of its relative safety and low cost. Conventional exercise testing uses exercise-induced ST-segment changes on the ECG to identify myocardial ischemia (described in more detail in chapter 5). However, as explained earlier, such electrical conduction changes tend to occur late in the ischemic cascade and consequently limit the diagnostic power of the exercise ECG. In a meta-analysis of 147 studies involving over 24,000 patients, the mean sensitivity and mean specificity of ST-segment changes for identifying angiographically defined CAD were 68% and 77%, respectively (20). The sensitivity of the exercise ECG does appear to increase with the number of diseased coronary arteries. In other words, the exercise ECG has only a 40% sensitivity for single-vessel CAD whereas its sensitivity improves to nearly 90% when three-vessel CAD is present. Furthermore, use of other clinical variables obtained during the exercise test, including blood pressure response and symptoms, improves the sensitivity of this diagnostic approach. Although the sensitivity of exercise ECG is considerably lower than that of other diagnostic procedures to be discussed (such as stress echocardiography and nuclear studies), the specificity of the technique is actually fairly good and is similar to that of the other procedures. We can improve the sensitivity of the exercise ECG by decreasing the number of false-negative tests and can improve the specificity by decreasing the false-positive tests. Factors known to lower the sensitivity and specificity of the exercise ECG are listed in table 3.6. Generally, the ECG is not used (for diagnostic purposes) in combination with a pharmacologic stress test because of the low sensitivity for detecting myocardial ischemia (19).

Echocardiography

The term echocardiography refers to a group of tests that utilize ultrasound to examine the heart and record information in the form of echoes, that is, reflected sonic waves. Ultrasonic waves are generated from a source (called the transducer) and applied to the chest wall of a subject (called transthoracic echocardiography or TTE) or from a tubular device placed in the esophagus (called transesophageal echocardiography or TEE). Since sound follows the principles of reflection or refraction, reflected waves return to the source (transducer), where they are processed to create an image. The standard echocardiographic examination encompasses M-mode, two-dimensional (2-D), conventional, and color-flow Doppler imaging. Additional applications include contrast echocardiography and stress (exercise or pharmacologic) echocardiography. The M-mode recording is sometimes called a one-dimensional or "ice-pick" view of the heart. This technique is very

Table 3.6
Factors That Lower the Sensitivity and Specificity of the Electrocardiogram During Exercise Testing

Factors that lower sensitivity (i.e., potential causes of false-negative tests)
Failure to reach ischemic threshold due to the following:
Reduced functional capacity or physical limitations (orthopedic)
Inadequate effort or motivation
Medications that decrease myocardial demand and/or increase myocardial blood supply (beta blockers, calcium blockers, nitroglycerine)
Inadequate monitoring of ECG changes such as the following:
Poor quality of recordings (artifact)
Inadequate number of ECG leads
Observer error
Failure to utilize "other" non-ECG signs and symptoms of ischemia, including:
Symptoms (e.g., angina)
Arrhythmia
Hypotensive blood pressure response
Single vessel CAD and/or collateral vessel compensation
Increased criteria for "significant" ST segment changes (e.g., 2 mv vs. 1 mv)
Factors that lower specificity (i.e., potential causes of false-positive tests)
Electrocardiographic abnormalities at rest or during exercise including:
Upsloping (vs. horizontal or downsloping) ST segments
Left bundle block and other conduction defects (such as Wolff-Parkinson-White)
Left ventricular hypertrophy
Digitalis and other medication "effect" on ST segments
Conditions of increased myocardial demand (with normal coronary supply):
Hypertension
Non-ischemic cardiomyopathy
Coronary artery vasospasm
Female gender
Mitral valve prolapse
Hypokalemia and anemia
Technical or observer error

good for determining chamber dimensions, wall thickness, and valve movement. The principle of 2-D echocardiography, depicted in figure 3.6a and b, can be used to obtain multiple two-dimensional images of the heart. Whereas M-mode and 2-D echocardiography essentially create ultrasonic images of the heart, Doppler echocardiography utilizes ultrasound to record blood flow within the cardiovascular system. Color Doppler can be used to identify the directional movement of blood within the 2-D or M-mode recording. Blood flowing through the heart away from the transducer will have a particular color (usually blue), whereas blood moving toward the transducer will be a different color (usually red). Turbulent blood flow within the heart appears as a mix or mosaic of colors. Color Doppler is very helpful in identifying valvular abnormalities including stenosis and

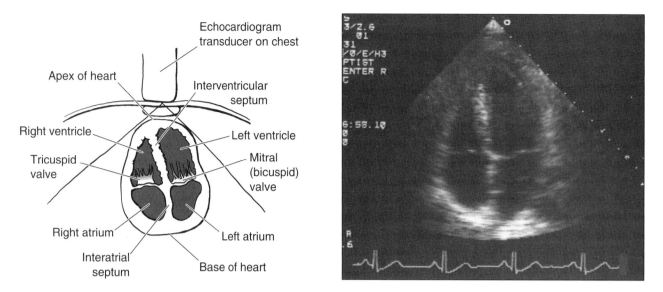

Figure 3.6 *(a)* Drawing of Apical four-chamber echocardiogram. *(b)* Actual echocardiogram was obtained on healthy young male; no abnormalities are present.

regurgitation. Ultrasound is also an extremely sensitive detector of intravascular bubbles. Thus, the injection of certain liquids (agitated saline solution is commonly used) into the blood introduces many microbubbles that travel to the heart and appear as a cloud on the echocardiogram. These so-called contrast echocardiograms can be very helpful for identifying cardiac shunts (blood moving inappropriately from chamber to chamber) and improving definition of chamber dimensions. Currently there are proposals for a variety of approaches to recording echocardiograms that are oriented in a three-dimensional space, and these approaches will likely move into clinical practice in the near future (5).

Stress-induced (exercise or pharmacologic) myocardial ischemia results in decreased regional wall motion and wall thickening. As discussed in relation to the ischemic cascade, these mechanical abnormalities of the left ventricle have been shown to appear before electrocardiographic changes or angina symptoms occur. Consequently, the sensitivity for detecting coronary lesions of greater than 50% stenosis is significantly higher with stress echocardiography than with exercise electrocardiography (average of 86% vs. 66%, respectively). However, the average specificity of exercise echocardiograpy, 81%, is only slightly higher than the average exercise ECG specificity of 77%. With exercise stress echocardiography, images are obtained before and immediately after (i.e., within 1-2 min) the completion of a standard exercise test. Commonly the user obtains and evaluates a quad-screen display of apical four-chamber (similar to the image in figure 3.6) and two-chamber views of left ven-

tricular systolic function at rest and during exercise. Obtaining this valuable information adds very little time and effort to a standard exercise ECG test. When electrocardiography is used with pharmacologic stress agents (generally dobutamine/arbutamine are preferred over the vasodilators), the echocardiographic images are obtained before and during the drug infusion.

Nuclear Imaging

The acquisition and display of a nuclear image of the heart result from the detection of radiation emitted from the patient following administration of a radionuclide (also called radioisotope). A radionuclide is an atom that disintegrates over time through emission of electromagnetic radiation. In radionuclide cardiac imaging, either the radionuclides are extracted by the myocardial tissue or they remain in the blood pool and enter the heart's chambers. Several components—including photomultiplier tubes, a collimator, and a scintillation camera that is interfaced with a computer—are needed to acquire the gamma rays emitted from the radionuclide and produce an image. Over the past several years, single-photon emission computed tomography (SPECT) has become the preferred imaging technique. With SPECT, a series of planar images are obtained over a 180° arc around the patient's thorax to form several images (short axis, horizontal and vertical long axis) (figure 3.7). The three major applications of nuclear imaging in the diagnosis of CAD are myocardial perfusion imaging, assessment of cardiac performance (i.e., left ventricular function), and positron emission tomography (PET). Myocardial perfusion imaging requires an intravenous injection of a radionuclide that is extracted only by normal cardiac cells. Cardiac cells that are ischemic will not take up the radionuclide. The images of the heart, obtained as described earlier, will appear bright (will light up) in areas that extract the radionuclide, but will not light up in areas where myocardial cells are ischemic (figure 3.7). Exercise-induced myocardial ischemia, until recently, has been most commonly visualized with a radionuclide called thallium-201. Newer compounds labeled with technetium-99m (currently technetium-99m sestamibi is most often used) have shown better characteristics for imaging myocardial perfusion abnormalities. Because of these compounds' differing properties, including half-life, the imaging protocols for thallium-201- and technetium-99m-labeled compounds are somewhat different.

Imaging with thallium-201 and imaging with technetium-99m sestamibi have similar sensitivity (approximately 88%) and specificity (approximately 62%) for detecting CAD (20). Thus, in comparison to stress echocardiography, SPECT imaging (with either thallium or tech-99) has a similar sensitivity but a lower specificity. The reduced specificity of SPECT imaging versus stress echocardiography is related to a higher frequency of false-positive tests with SPECT imaging.

Cardiac performance (i.e., hemodynamic functions) can be assessed with radionuclide techniques using either of two approaches. The first, called first-pass radionuclide angiography, involves analysis of the "first pass" of a radionuclide bolus delivered through the central circula-tion to the heart. The second, more widely applied method involves analysis of the radionuclide following equilibrium, which allows repeat imaging over several hours. This technique is called equilibrium radionuclide angiography or multiple-gated blood pool imaging, and entails the imaging of technetium-99 that is attached to albumin or red blood cells and uniformly distributed throughout the blood volume. These techniques can be used to calculate ejection fraction and assess the right and left ventricles, diastolic and systolic function, regional and global ventricular performance, and ventricular volumes. These techniques were widely used in the 1980s, but continuous improvement of echo-cardiographic technologies has greatly diminished the use of the first-pass or multiple-gated blood pool imaging approaches for evaluating cardiac function.

Positron Emission Tomography

Positron emission tomography scanning, once viewed as primarily a research imaging modality, is becoming an increasingly valuable technique for evaluating CAD. Positron emission tomography perfusion imaging studies are recommended for the identification of myocardial viability (i.e., myocardial tissue that could resume function with improved perfusion secondary to revas-cularization) in patients with established CAD and for the noninvasive diagnosis of CAD (21). Myocardial blood flow and myocardial viability can be assessed with PET through infusion of [^{18}F]-deoxyglucose and/or

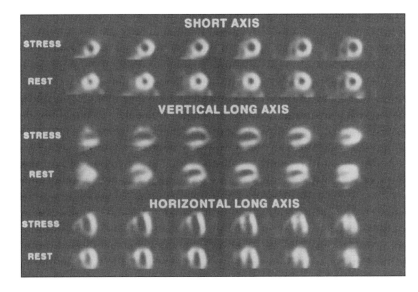

Figure 3.7   SPECT perfusion imaging. Notice differences in images obtained at rest and after stress (i.e.,exercise test) in short axis, vertical long axis, and horizontal long axis views. Dark areas on the stress images that become bright on the rest images indicate the presence of reversible myocardial ischemia.

Reprinted, by permission, from D. Schmidt, S.C. Port, and R.A. Gal, 1995, Nuclear cardiology and echocardiography: Noninvasive tests for diagnosing CAD. In *Heart disease and rehabilitation,* edited by Pollock and Schmidt (Champaign: Human Kinetics), 87.

[^{13}N]-ammonia. These "tracers" provide an index of myocardial cell metabolism and thus cell viability. To date, the initial capital cost of approximately $1 million and the cost of maintaining PET technology have limited its availability. In the future, PET imaging may become more common as the clinical indications for this technique increase and the price of the technology declines.

Newer Noninvasive Cardiac Imaging Techniques

Two newer procedures, electron beam computed tomography (EBCT) (also called cine or ultrafast CT) and magnetic resonance imaging, are becoming more and more available and acceptable for use in the diagnosis of CAD (22). The EBCT has gained a great deal of attention for its reported ability to determine the **patency** (i.e., remaining open) of coronary artery bypass grafts and to detect the presence of coronary artery calcium (23). The EBCT scans reveal the presence of calcium in the coronary arteries. The presence of coronary artery calcium appears to be highly related to the degree of coronary stenosis and future risk for cardiac events. Because of ease of measurement, high sensitivity and specificity for CAD, and relatively low cost (≈$400), EBCT is becoming more widely used and accepted as a diagnostic technique for CAD (24).

Invasive Diagnostic Procedures

In contrast to the diagnostic procedures already described, in which cardiac images are obtained from devices located outside the heart, the techniques discussed next are considered invasive since the measurements are made directly within structures of the heart. Coronary angiography (also referred to arteriography) is the imaging method of choice to establish the presence or absence of CAD and to provide the most reliable information for making critical decisions about the need for medical therapy, angioplasty, or bypass surgery (catheter-based interventions for CAD are discussed in chapter 4). First performed in 1959, coronary angiography is now one of the most widely performed and accurate tests in cardiovascular medicine. More than 1 million coronary angiograms are performed every year in the United States (1) (see figure 1.5).

Catheterization, the technique used to obtain angiograms of the coronary arteries, is generally accomplished through the femoral artery (as depicted in figure 3.8), although brachial or radial artery access is occasionally utilized. After the artery is punctured with a small needle, a guide wire is passed through the needle to the femoral artery. The needle over the guide wire is removed, and a sheath and its dilator are advanced into the vessel. Once the sheath is positioned correctly in the artery, the guide wire and dilator are quickly removed. The guide wire is then loaded into a Judkins coronary catheter, and both are inserted through the femoral sheath. The guide wire is advanced from the femoral sheath into the abdominal aorta under fluoroscopic (X ray) guidance, and both the guide wire and catheter are advanced to the ascending aorta. Finally the catheter is advanced to the ostia (openings in the aorta just superior to the aortic valve) for the two coronary arteries (right and left main coronary arteries). Once the catheter is in place, a few milliliters of a radiographic contrast agent is injected through the catheter into the coronary arteries. While the injection is in progress, cineangiographic equipment is used to visualize and record images of the contrast medium in the coronary arteries. The contrast agent is used to visualize narrowings (i.e., coronary artery lesions) (figure 3.8). Although the industry standard for recording and storing coronary angiograms has been 35-mm cinefilm, digital and optical disc recording are becoming more common. Because of the positioning of the heart, the coronary circulation is imaged in angular views called left anterior oblique and right anterior oblique. These two views allow for optimal visualization of the coronary circulation described in chapter 2.

Recent technologic advances now allow for direct internal visualization of the lumen of the coronary arteries through ultrasonic transducers placed at the tip of the coronary catheter (referred to as intracoronary ultrasound). The transducer provides a cross-sectional picture of the artery and produces excellent images of the arterial wall. These images can be used to describe the characteristics of the coronary lesion and changes after coronary interventions such as angioplasty (discussed in chapter 4).

In addition to coronary angiograms, left ventriculograms (often called LV grams) are routinely obtained during a cardiac catheterization. These images are captured during injection of a larger amount (40-50 ml) of contrast medium through a catheter that has been advanced into the left ventricle. The left ventriculogram is used to assess systolic and diastolic wall motion, allowing estimation of the ejection fraction. Additionally, this technique is used to identify hypokinetic (decreased movement), akinetic (no movement), dyskinetic (small paradoxical "outward" movement during contraction), or aneurysmal (movement in the opposite direction)

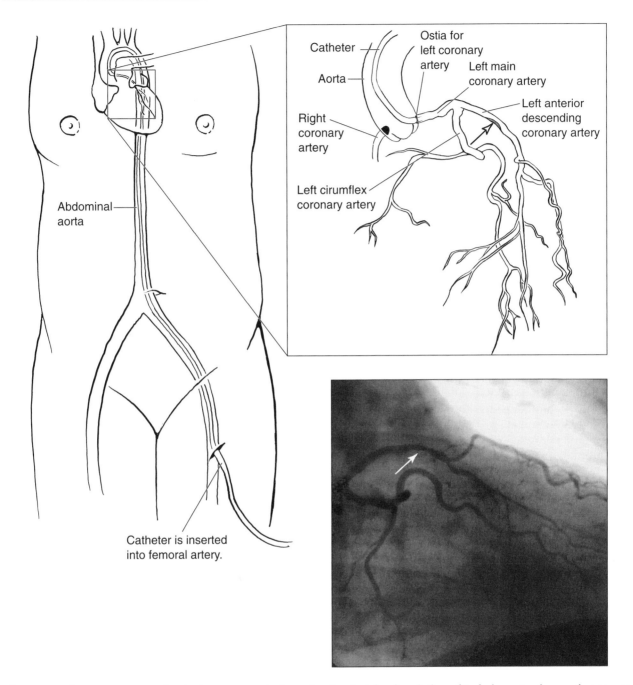

Figure 3.8 Percutaneous transluminal coronary arteriography. See text for description of technique. Angiogram image was obtained from 50-year-old male with recent history of chest discomfort. Angiogram revealed a 40% lesion in the left anterior descending artery (see arrow) and minor irregularities in circumflex coronary artery. This angiogram was obtained from the individual described in Case Study 2.

myocardial segments that can result from myocardial ischemia or infarction (figure 3.9).

The process of obtaining coronary angiograms, left ventriculograms, or intracoronary ultrasounds is commonly called a left heart catheterization, since the information is obtained by an arterial approach into the left side of the heart (i.e., left ventricle and coronary arteries). In contrast, a right heart catheterization is performed

with venous access (usually the femoral vein) to the right side of the heart. This technique allows measurement of pressures within the heart (e.g., pulmonary artery, right atrium, right ventricle, and pulmonary capillary "wedge" pressure, which is an indirect measure of left ventricular filling pressure), as well as pressure gradients across the pulmonic semilunar and atrioventricular valves. Blood sampled at various places in the

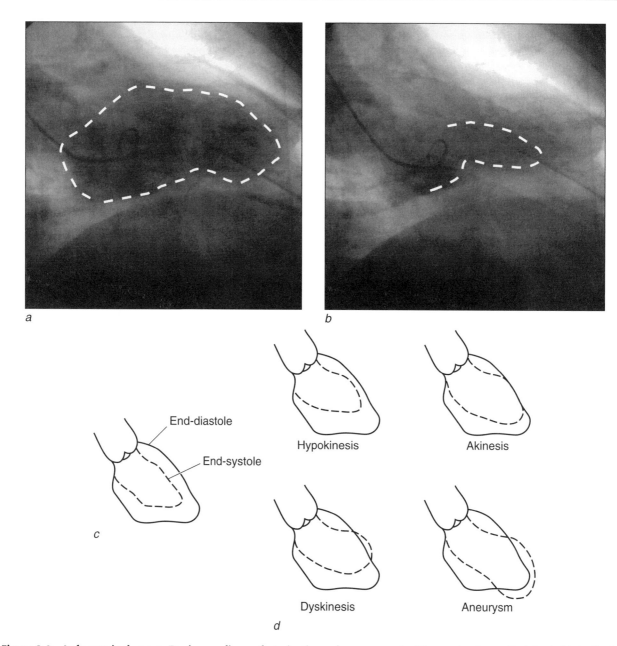

Figure 3.9 Left ventriculogram. During cardiac catheterization, a large amount of the contrast agent is injected into the left ventricle. Images are obtained at *(a)* end-diastolic (after maximal filling) and *(b)* end-systolic dimension (after complete contraction). This technique can be used to estimate ejection fraction (EF% = [EDV – ESV]/EDV × 100), where EDV = end-diastolic volume (ml) and ESV = end-systolic volume (ml). This left ventriculogram was obtained during cardiac catheterization of Case Study 2 presented at the end of this chapter. Drawn figures indicate the position of left ventricle walls at end systole (dotted line) and end diastole (solid line) in a *(c)* "normal" heart, and in *(d)* hearts demonstrating hypokinesis (reduced contraction of one area), akinesis (no contraction of one area), dyskinesis (small paradoxical "outward" movement during contraction), and aneurysm (significant outward "bulging" during contraction). These patterns may be observed after myocardial ischemia/infarction.

heart can be removed and analyzed for oxygen saturation—a technique helpful in the identification of shunts that cause mixing of arterial and venous blood within the heart. Finally, the cardiac output can be calculated with several different techniques during the right heart catheterization.

COST ANALYSIS AND APPLICATION OF DIAGNOSTIC TESTS

Relatively few published studies have compared the cost effectiveness of treadmill exercise testing with that of more expensive imaging procedures.

The average costs (in U.S. dollars) for various diagnostic techniques are as follows: exercise ECG—$330; echocardiography—$900; nuclear imaging—$1200; PET—$1800; and coronary angiography—$4800 (19). The Medicare-allowed charges, however, are approximately one-third of these values (25). The lower cost of one test compared to another does not necessarily result in a lower overall cost of patient care, as the costs of additional testing and interventions may be higher with the lower-cost and less accurate tests. Recent studies have assessed the cost effectiveness of diagnostic testing for CAD by comparing no test, routine exercise ECG testing, exercise echocardiography, and exercise SPECT (thallium or sestamibi) in cohorts of individuals of various ages, both men and women, who had chest pain (25). These were the conclusions:

- All available noninvasive diagnostic techniques operate with an acceptable sensitivity and specificity (except exercise ECG testing, which has a lower sensitivity than the others).

- Direct coronary angiography (e.g., skipping all noninvasive tests) is clearly appropriate and cost effective in middle-aged or older males with classic angina (i.e., those with high pretest likelihood).

- In individuals with moderate pretest probability of CAD, stress echo and SPECT are clearly superior to exercise ECG testing with respect to sensitivity and cost effectiveness.

- No specific test is particularly cost effective in individuals with a low pretest probability.

In an attempt to assist clinicians with the difficult decisions of selecting diagnostic tests, the American College of Cardiology/American Heart Association have developed an algorithm for selecting appropriate tests to evaluate patients with suspected CAD (11). Interested readers should refer to this excellent resource.

SUMMARY

The diagnosis of CAD is normally conducted in a stepwise, incremental process that begins with a review of the medical history and findings from a physical examination. If indicated on the basis of the history and physical, patients should then undergo a series of basic laboratory tests, including a 12-lead ECG, and evaluation of cardiac risk factors. If the patient's risk prediction is high or there is continued suspicion of the presence of CAD, a number of diagnostic procedures can be employed to determine the likelihood of CAD. Selection of the appropriate diagnostic procedure, from the vast number available, can be difficult and must take into account the patient's safety and comfort, the diagnostic power of the test, and the cost effectiveness of the procedure. Several organizations, including the American College of Cardiology/American Heart Association (11), have developed algorithms to help the clinician with this important process.

Case Study 1
Primary Prevention: Low Risk

Although this individual has an increased risk for developing CAD in the future (as described in chapter 1), the lack of CAD symptoms presently indicates that there is no need for further diagnostic studies. In fact, if you refer back to the section on Bayes theorem (table 3.5 and figure 3.3), you will see that this 38-year-old male without any symptoms of CAD has a very low pretest likelihood of CAD (calculated at approximately 2-3% from table 3.5). Thus, figure 3.3 indicates that with a low pretest likelihood there is little value in performing a diagnostic ECG stress test. Even if the test were performed and was in fact abnormal (i.e., ST-segment changes on the ECG suggestive of ischemia), it would only increase the posttest likelihood of CAD to less than 10%. The increased cost and risk of more invasive diagnostic tests (nuclear scan, echocardiogram, catheterization) are unwarranted in this low-risk individual. However, as you will learn in chapters 4 and 6, there are other reasons to do an exercise ECG stress test, including prognosis, exercise prescription, and measuring progress. Although no further diagnostic tests were performed on this low-risk individual, refer to chapters 6, 7, and 8 to learn about his other assessments (body composition) and the lifestyle interventions he received.

Case Study 2
Primary Prevention: High Risk

Medical History

A 50-year-old male with no prior cardiac history began developing dyspnea on exertion, having experienced easy fatigability approximately one month earlier. On day of admission to the hospital, the patient had developed chest tightness lasting 10 min that radiated to left arm and jaw; nausea; shortness of breath; and fatigue at work.

Risk Factors for CAD

Individual has known history of type II diabetes mellitus, 20 pack per year history of smoking (stopped 12 years ago), hyperlipidemia, hypertension, sleep apnea, obesity, and family history of premature CAD. See case study in chapter 1 for calculation and discussion of Framingham risk score.

Physical Examination

BP: 132/60 mmHg

Pulse: 67 bpm, regular rhythm

Heart sounds: normal S_1 and S_2, no murmurs

Peripheral pulses: normal, no bruits

Lungs: clear

All other systems: normal

Laboratory Tests

Chest X ray: no evidence of acute cardiopulmonary disease

12-lead ECG: no evidence of acute myocardial infarction

Cardiac enzymes: slight rise in total CK, but negative for rise in MB or troponin

Impression and Further Assessments

Admitted to hospital and given nitroglycerin (IV), aspirin, beta blocker, and oxygen.

Chest discomfort resolved and patient ruled out for MI without ECG or enzyme changes.

Check fasting lipids in A.M.

Given high-risk status, proceed directly to cardiac catheterization in A.M.

The decision to skip other less invasive diagnostic tests (ECG, nuclear, or echo stress testing) was based on the patient's very high pretest likelihood for CAD (see table 3.5, indicating that a 50-year-old man with typical angina has a 90% pretest likelihood). With such a high pretest probability, the result (positive vs. negative) of noninvasive diagnostic studies has little impact on the posttest probability (still between 75% and 95%), which would still warrant a cardiac catheterization.

Diagnostic Studies

Lipid Profile and Blood Tests

Total cholesterol = 243 mg/dl, triglycerides = 152 mg/dl, HDL = 35, LDL = 178 mg/dl, Hemoglobin A_1c = 11.3% (indicates poor blood glucose control)

Cardiac Catheterization

Left ventriculography: normal wall motion (ejection fraction = 60%) (see figure 3.9)

Coronary angiography (arteriogram) (see figure 3.8): shows proximal left anterior descending artery (LAD) = 40% occlusion

Circumflex = minor irregularities throughout

No other coronary artery disease present

Treatment Plan

Since this person has mild and stable coronary artery disease, lifestyle changes and medication are recommended to prevent further progression of CAD. This individual would benefit from participation in a preventive program. Learn more about the specific interventions he received (chapter 4) and see how well they worked (chapters 8 and 10).

Case Study 3
Secondary Prevention: Post-MI and PTCA/Stent

Medical History

A 61-year-old male with no prior cardiac history and generally good health presented to emergency department of local hospital with chest discomfort that awakened him during the night and did not resolve after he took antacids. Admits to having had bilateral arm pain when mowing lawn one week earlier. Also, two days prior to presentation, patient had sudden onset of epigastric pain after dinner that radiated up to sternum, neck, and arms. He had no associated vomiting, nausea, diaphoresis (sweating), or presyncopal symptoms with any of the episodes of chest discomfort.

Risk Factors

Positive for tobacco (30 pack/year but has not smoked for 15 years), hypercholesterolemia, and family history of heart disease. See case study in chapter 1 for calculation and discussion of Framingham risk score.

Physical Examination

BP: 118/62 mmHg

Pulse: 67 bpm, regular rhythm

Heart sounds: normal S_1 and S_2, no murmurs

Peripheral pulses: normal, no bruits

Lungs: clear

All other systems: normal

Laboratory Tests

Chest X ray: no evidence of acute cardiopulmonary disease

Computed tomography (CT) scan: done to rule out dissecting aneurysm of aorta (negative)

12-lead ECG: shows evidence of acute myocardial infarction (abnormal Q waves in leads I and aVL—indicative of anterolateral MI)

Cardiac enzymes: CK = 375, CK-MB = 5.1%, troponin I = 5.3—indicative of acute MI

Impression and Further Assessments

Admit to cardiac care unit since ruling in for acute MI (ECG and enzyme changes).

Begin anticoagulation with heparin and Integrelin (glycoprotein IIb/IIIa inhibitor—see table 4.6).

Start beta blockers.

Continue oxygen, nitroglycerin drip, and aspirin.

Check fasting lipids in A.M.

Plan for complete echocardiogram (M-mode, 2-D, and Doppler) and diagnostic catheterization in several days (sooner if unstable).

Diagnostic Studies

Lipid Profile

Total cholesterol = 186 mg/dl, triglycerides = 98 mg/dl, HDL = 36 mg/dl, LDL = 131 mg/dl, glucose = 136 mg/dl

Echocardiography

Normal LV chamber size, wall thickness, and contractility (ejection fraction = 55%). No segmental wall motion abnormalities.

Cardiac Catheterization

Left ventriculography: normal wall motion (ejection fraction = 60%)

Coronary angiography (arteriogram):

- Left main coronary artery = 20% occlusion
- Distal LAD = 50% occlusion
- 1st diagonal (off LAD) = 80% occlusion
- Distal circumflex = 95% occlusion
- Mid-RCA = 60% occlusion
- Coronary dominance = right (i.e., posterior descending coronary artery supplied by RCA)

Treatment Plan

This individual was to undergo angioplasty and stenting of distal circumflex lesion ("culprit" lesion that caused anterolateral MI). See chapter 4 to obtain results from these interventions. There were no plans to intervene on other smaller lesions (1st diagonal and RCA); these will be managed with lifestyle modifications and medications described in chapter 4. This patient is an obvious candidate for a cardiac rehabilitation program. Later chapters will describe the interventions he received.

GLOSSARY

Bruit: low-frequency, rumbling sound that can be heard (via stethoscope) in an artery where turbulent blood flow is the result of a large atherosclerotic occlusion

Collateralization: adaptive/protective adaptation in which dormant channels connecting coronary arteries can be opened in response to the presence of ischemia

Dyspnea: shortness of breath

False negative: test result in which the test employed (in this case ECG stress test) fails to identify the presence (identifies no ST-segment changes) of disease (CAD) even when the individual has known disease

False positive: test result in which the test employed (in this case ECG stress test) indicates (ST depression) the presence of disease (CAD) when the individual is disease free

Intermittent claudication: a painful condition in lower extremities caused by significant occlusion in blood vessels supplying the legs; symptom associated with peripheral vascular disease (i.e., atherosclerotic occlusion in leg arteries)

Myocardial perfusion: blood supply to the cells of the heart

Patency: the ability of an artery to remain open, most commonly with reference to a bypass graft or native coronary artery after PTCA

Postprandial angina: angina pectoris that occurs after a meal

Regurgitation: a condition in which a heart valve does not close properly and allows blood to leak back into chamber it was ejected from; most commonly occurs with mitral or aortic valves

Reversible myocardial ischemia: temporary or transient lack of oxygen to myocardial tissue, usually the result of atherosclerotic lesions that do not allow an increase in blood flow despite an increased myocardial demand

Stenosis: narrowing of an anatomical structure, including coronary arteries and heart valves; in a heart valve, most commonly occurs in aortic or mitral valves

Unstable angina: unpredictable pattern of angina (when it occurs, how long it lasts); of greater medical concern than "stable" angina, which is predictable in occurrence

Vasodilatory reserve: ability of blood vessel (coronary arteries) to dilate in response to an increase in myocardial demand; in atherosclerotically diseased artery segments, vasodilatory reserve is diminished

REFERENCES

1. American Heart Association. 1998. *Heart and stroke statistical update.* Dallas: American Heart Association.

2. Eaker, E.D., J.H. Chesebro, F.M. Sacks, N.K. Wenger, J.P. Whisnant, and M. Winston. 1994. Special report: Cardiovascular disease in women. *Heart Dis. and Stroke* 3(2):114.

3. Giuliani, E.R., B.J. Gersh, M.D. McGoon, D.L. Hayes, and H.V. Schaft. 1996. *Mayo clinical practice of cardiology.* 3rd ed. St. Louis: Mosby.

4. Maseri, A., F. Crea, C. Kaski, and T. Croke. 1991. Mechanisms of angina pectoris in syndrome X. *J. Am. Coll. Cardiol.* 17:499–506.

5. Braunwald, E., ed. 1997. *Heart disease: A textbook of cardiovascular medicine.* 5th ed. Philadelphia: Saunders.

6. Caplan, L.R. 1991. Diagnosis and Treatment of Ischemic Stroke. *J.A.M.A.* 266:2413-2420.

7. Goldberg, R., J.M. Gore, J.S. Alpert, J.E. Dalen (1975-1984). 1988. Incidence and case fatality rates of acute myocardial infarction. The Worchester Heart Attack Study. *Am. Heart J.* 115:761–767.

8. Kannel, W. 1987. Prevalence and clinical aspects of unrecognized myocardial infarction and sudden unexpected death. *Circulation* 75 (pt. 2):II4–5.

9. Murray, C., and J.S. Alpect. 1994. Diagnosis of acute myocardial infarction. *Curr. Opin. in Cardiol.* 9:465–470.

10. Nichol, G., R. Walls, L. Goldman, S. Pearson, L.H. Hartley, E. Antman, M. Stockman, J.M. Teisch, C.P. Cannon, P.A. Johnson, K.M. Kuntz, and T.H. Lee. 1997. A critical pathway for management of patients with acute chest pain who are at low risk for myocardial ischemia: Recommendations and potential impact. *Ann. Internal Med.* 127:996–1005.

11. American College of Cardiology/American Heart Association, Committee on Exercise Testing. 1997. Guidelines for exercise testing. A report of the American College of Cardiology/American Heart Association Task force on practice guidelines. *J. Am. Coll. Cardiol.* 30 (1):260–315.

12. Patterson, R.E., and S.F. Herowitz. 1989. Importance of epidemiology and biostatistics in deciding clinical strategies for using diagnostic tests: A simplified approach using examples for coronary artery disease. *J. Am. Coll. Cardiol.* 56 (13):1653–1665.

13. Nesto, R.W., and G.J. Kowalchuk. 1987. The ischemic cascade: Temporal sequence of hemodynamic, electrocardiographic, and symptomatic expression of ischemia. *Am. J. Cardiol.* 57:23C–30C.

14. Uren, N.G., J.A. Melin, B. De Bruyne,W. Wijns, T. Baudhuin, P.G. Camici 1994. Relationship between myocardial blood flow and severity of coronary stenosis. *N. Eng. J. Med.* 330:1782–1788.

15. Weiner, D.A., T.J. Ryan, C.H. McCabe, B.R. Chaitmen, L.T. Sheffield, J.C. Ferguson, L.D. Fisher, and Tristani, F. 1984. Prognostic importance of a clinical profile and exercise test in medically treated patients with coronary artery disease. *J. Am. Coll. Cardiol.* 3 (3):772–779.

16. Roger, V.L., S.J. Jacobsen, P.A. Pellika, T.D. Miller, K.R. Bailey, B.J. Gersh. 1998. Prognostic value of treadmill exercise testing: A population-based study in Olmsted County Minnesota. *Circulation* 98:2836–284.

17. Mark, D.B., M.A. Hlatky, F.E. Harrell, K.L. Lee, R.M. Califf, and D.B. Bryan. 1987. Exercise treadmill score for predicting prognosis in coronary artery disease. *Ann. Internal Med.* 106 (6):793–800.

18. Morrow, K., C.K. Morris, V.F. Froelicher, A. Hide, D. Hunter, E. Johnson, T. Kawaguchi, K. Lehmann, P.M. Ribisl, and R. Thomas. 1993. Prediction of cardiovascular death in men undergoing noninvasive evaluation for coronary artery disease. *Ann. Internal Med.* 118 (9):684–695.

19. Marwick, T.H., ed. 1996. *Cardiac stress testing and imaging. A clinician's guide.* New York: Churchill Livingstone.

20. Gianrossi, R. Detrano, D. Mulvihill, K. Lehmann, P. Dubach, A. Colmbo, D. McArthur, V. Froelicher-1989. Exercise induced ST depression in the diagnosis of coronary artery disease: A meta analysis. *Circulation* 80:87–98.

21. Demer, L.L., K.L. Gould, R.A. Goldstein, R.L. Kirkeeide, NA Mullani, R.W. Smalling, A. Nishikawa, M.E. Merhige.1989. Assessment of coronary artery disease severity by positron emission tomography: Comparison with quantitative arteriography in 193 patients. *Circulation* 79:825–835.

22. Manning, W.J., W. Li, and R.R. Edelman. 1993. A preliminary report comparing magnetic resonance coronary imaging with conventional angiography. *N. Eng. J. Med.* 328:828–832.

23. Brundage, B.H. 1995. Beyond perfusion with ultra fast computed tomography. *Am. J. Cardiol.* 75:69D–73D.

24. Rumberger, J.A. 1999. Electron beam computed tomography coronary calcium scanning. A review of guidelines for use in asymptomatic persons. *Mayo Clinic Proc.* 74 (3):243–252.

25. Kurtz, R.M. 1999. Cost effectiveness of diagnostic strategies for patients with chest pain. *Ann. Internal Med.* 130:719–728.

CHAPTER 4

Prevention and Treatment of Coronary Artery Disease

BEHAVIORAL OBJECTIVES

- To be able to describe the value of specific risk factor interventions for prevention and rehabilitation of coronary artery disease

- To be able to describe various noninvasive and invasive procedures for the treatment of nonemergent coronary artery disease

As described in chapter 1, mortality (i.e., death) from CAD has been declining over the past 30 years. This downward trend in CAD mortality is continuing, and the decrease has occurred among men and women, blacks and whites, and both middle-aged and older persons. This decline is attributable to advances in both primary and secondary prevention of CAD. It appears that national programs directed at reducing risk factors for CAD have contributed to substantial improvement in awareness, treatment, and control of hypertension and hypercholesterolemia, as well as to reductions in cigarette smoking (1). Data from the National Health and Nutrition Examination Surveys (NHANES I, II, III) (2) for adults 20 to 74 years of age reveal a decline in the prevalence of hypertension from 1975 (39%) to 1994 (23%).

Over this same time period, the prevalence of hypercholesterolemia decreased from 26% to 19%, and cigarette smoking among adults 18 years and older declined from 33% to 25%. These favorable trends have been observed for both sexes and for blacks as well as whites (1). The decline in death rate over the past 25 years for patients hospitalized with acute myocardial infarction (MI) can be attributed to an improved understanding of CAD and the subsequent development of medications and technologies used to treat and manage CAD. This chapter describes the various pharmacologic approaches and interventional or surgical procedures used to manage both acute and chronic CAD. Although there is cause to celebrate the steep reductions in mortality from CAD, a recent large population study (3) showed that from 1987 to 1994 the incidence of MI was unchanged or was slightly increased. The paradoxical trend for MI incidence to remain the same or even to increase while mortality from CAD decreases can be explained by less severe infarctions, likely the result of improved and more rapidly delivered medical treatment (e.g., emergency medical response system, aggressive artery-opening treatments), as well as improved long-term treatment approaches. Although there has been some success in the battle against our nation's number-one killer, greater primary and secondary prevention efforts are needed to further reduce the morbidity and mortality associated with CAD.

DETECTION AND PREVENTION OF CORONARY ARTERY DISEASE IN YOUTH

It is widely accepted that the process of CAD starts in the first decade of life and continues to progress across the life span. Furthermore, it has been shown that children who develop risk factors for CAD early in life are more likely to retain those risk factors in adulthood. Some of the data indicating the early onset of CAD come from the Bogalusa Heart Study (4), designed to monitor CAD risk factors in 14,000 children and young adults for several decades. The findings are based on autopsies performed on 93 young adults (mean age of 20) who died unexpectedly from noncardiac causes (usually trauma). Traditional risk factors (obesity, hypertension, smoking, and hyperlipidemia) were strongly associated with the presence of aortic and coronary artery fatty plaques. Recall from chapter 2 that the earliest arterial evidence for CAD is the development of fatty streaks in the artery. In children or young adults with all four risk factors, 35% had aortic plaques and 11% had coronary artery plaques, whereas only 19% and 1.3% of individuals with one risk factor had aortic and coronary artery plaques, respectively. Another recent study showed that by 30 years of age, 19% of men and 8% of women (5) had atherosclerotic stenosis of at least 40% in the left anterior descending coronary artery.

This investigation indicated strong relationships between the severity of atherosclerosis and obesity, cholesterol level, smoking, and hypertension (5). As with the adult population, our nation's children (ages 6-11) and adolescents (ages 12-17) are more overweight than they have been in the past. The NHANES III (2) reveals that the population of overweight children increased from 7.6% to 13.7% from 1976 to 1994 (definitions of overweight/obesity and methods for determination are presented in chapter 6). During this same time, the percentage of overweight adolescents increased from 5.7% to 11.5%. The two factors thought to be contributing to the increased prevalence of overweight children and adolescents are lack of regular physical activity and a higher caloric intake.

It has also become increasingly clear that early detection and management of hypertension and hyperlipidemia are essential in preventing CAD. In teenagers with hypertension, approximately 20% begin to show evidence of **left ventricular hypertrophy,** a known risk factor for CAD. After the age of 3, a child's blood pressure should be assessed annually using age-, gender-, and height-adjusted guidelines (6). Initial management of persistent hypertension in children should focus on weight loss where indicated, increased physical activity, and improved dietary habits (reduction in sugar, fat, and sodium).

Guidelines for hyperlipidemia screening for children have been developed by the National Heart Lung and Blood Institute's Expert Panel on Blood Cholesterol Levels in Children and Adolescents (7). The first step in screening for hypercholesterolemia in children (ages 2-19) is to determine whether there is a family history of CAD and/or a parent with a total cholesterol of ≥240 mg/dl. The presence of either history indicates the need for blood cholesterol and/or lipoprotein analysis. For children beyond the age of 2 years with borderline hypercholesterolemia (low-density lipoprotein = 110-129 mg/dl), the American Heart Association (AHA) Step I Diet (table 4.1) and other risk factor modifications are indicated. Children in the borderline category who don't respond to lifestyle changes in six months, and those with higher low-density lipoprotein levels (>130 mg/dl), require more aggressive lifestyle modification (e.g., AHA Step II Diet—table 4.1) and further investigation to identify **familial disorders** and/or secondary causes of their hyperlipidemia.

Of equal or greater concern is the increased use of tobacco in our nation's adolescents. It has been determined that nearly 35% of high school students are currently smoking; this rate is the highest it has been in 17 years (5). Clearly, early intervention and improved education about tobacco use and other risk factors for CAD in the younger generation are needed if we are to win the war against CAD.

RISK FACTOR MANAGEMENT FOR ADULTS

While optimal management of risk factors should begin early in life, the recognition and ultimately the impact of these risk factors often do not occur until later on. Subsequently, the majority of prevention and rehabilitation specialists will work with adults in formalized primary or secondary CAD prevention settings. Thus the remainder of this chapter focuses on prevention and treatment of CAD in adults.

The first step in risk factor management is to stratify individuals into high-, medium-, and low-risk subgroups. In general, the patient with diagnosed CAD (e.g., angina, MI, bypass, or percutaneous transluminal coronary angioplasty [PTCA]) is at the highest risk for disability and death and therefore is the patient in whom the presence of untreated risk factors is most deleterious. Other individuals may be at high risk because they have atherosclerotic disease in other arterial systems (cerebrovascular, peripheral vascular), possess a combination of several risk factors, or have an extremely elevated level of a single risk factor. The responsibility of the clinician is to match the appropriate level of risk factor management with the patient's level of risk. Patients at the highest risk for disability and death should receive the most aggressive treatment of their risk factors. Risk stratification can also be used to identify subgroups in whom risk factor management strategies are likely to be cost effective. In general, the higher the underlying risk for an adverse outcome and the more powerful the ability of the intervention to reduce the risk, the greater the opportunity to achieve cost effectiveness (8).

The 27th Bethesda Conference (8), supported by the American College of Cardiology, was convened in September 1994 with the specific goal of generating an approach to managing risk factors in the care of patients at risk for CAD.

Table 4.1
American Heart Association Dietary Therapy

Nutrient	Step I diet	Step II diet
Total fat	<30% of total calories	<20% of total calories
Saturated fat	8–10% of total calories	< 7% of total calories
Polyunsaturated fat	<10% of total calories	Same
Monounsaturated fat	<15% of total calories	Same
Carbohydrates	>55% of total calories	Same
Protein	~ 15 % of total calories	Same
Cholesterol	< 300 mg/day	< 200 mg/day
Total calories	Sufficient to achieve and maintain desirable weight	

Step I diet recommended eating pattern for all healthy Americans aged 2 or older.
Adapted from reference (7).

Although this report represents only one approach to managing risk factors and may exhibit some discrepancy from the guidelines of other professional organizations, it does represent a concise, practical framework for risk factor modification. The objectives of the report were to (1) describe the various cardiovascular risk factors for CAD, (2) provide the evidence supporting the association of these risk factors with CAD, (3) determine the usefulness of their clinical measurement, and (4) describe their responsiveness to interventions (e.g., nonpharmacologic and/or pharmacologic treatments). Since chapter 1 describes each risk factor and the evidence supporting its association with CAD, this section focuses on the effectiveness of specific treatments for each risk factor that is modifiable. As seen in table 4.2, which outlines the value of intervention on specific risk factors, the Bethesda report (8) identifies the following four categories: (1) factors for which interventions have been *proven* to lower CAD risk, (2) factors for which interventions are *likely* to lower CAD risk, (3) factors for which modification *might* lower CAD risk, and (4) factors that *cannot be modified* or for which modification would be *unlikely* to lower CAD risk. Since non-modifiable risk factors are described in chapter 1 and since they do not respond to lifestyle or pharmacologic interventions, the remainder of this section focuses on risk factors in the first three categories, providing the evidence for placement of each risk factor in a particular category.

Category I Risk Factors

The risk factors for which interventions have been proven to lower CAD risk (Bethesda Category I) are cigarette smoking, low-density lipoprotein cholesterol, high fat/high cholesterol diet, hypertension, left ventricular hypertrophy, and elevated thrombogenic factors.

Cigarette Smoking

Smoking cessation reduces the risk of damage to the endothelial layer of the artery and also improves CAD risk factors, particularly high-density lipoprotein (HDL) and low-density lipoprotein (LDL). Smoking cessation does not, however, appear to affect systolic blood pressure, and unfortunately can result in significant increases in diastolic blood pressure. The increase in blood pressure secondary to smoking cessation is most likely associated with weight gain. On a positive note, smoking cessation can produce clinical benefits in a relatively short period of time. In patients with a history of MI, the risk of a subsequent cardiac event declines rapidly after the cessation of smoking. Within three years of an MI, former smokers have approximately the same risk for reinfarction as survivors of MI who never smoked (9). A 1% reduction in smoking prevalence rates (currently 25% of American adults smoke) would theoretically result in 924 fewer heart attacks and 538 fewer strokes per year nationwide and would save $44 million per year in direct medical costs. Smoking cessation, which typically includes a behavioral and possibly a pharmacologic component, should be encouraged in all patients. Treatment options to assist with smoking cessation are expanding; these include a variety of nicotine-replacement therapies and one prescription drug, bupropion (brand name: Zyban). While quit rates are higher with any of these agents alone compared with placebo, a combination of a nicotine-replacement therapy, bupropion, and behavioral counseling appears to be most effective for long-term smoking cessation. Chapter 10 presents further description and discussion of smoking cessation approaches.

Low-Density Lipoprotein Cholesterol

The most conclusive evidence that blood lipids are causally related to the development of CAD comes from several randomized, controlled clinical trials. Both primary and secondary prevention trial data indicate that lowering cholesterol, specifically LDL cholesterol, is associated with a reduced risk of CAD (9). While the total cholesterol, HDL, and triglyceride levels are measured directly in most laboratories, the LDL is generally calculated using the Friedewald equation:

$$\text{LDL (mg/dl)} = \text{total cholesterol} - \text{HDL} - (\text{triglycerides}/5)$$

This formula is not accurate with severe hypertriglyceridemia (greater than 400 mg/dl); thus in patients with this condition, LDL should be determined with a specialized and expensive test called gel electrophoresis.

Although several studies from the 1980s demonstrated positive results with aggressive cholesterol lowering in patients without heart disease, the most definitive primary prevention study to date is the West of Scotland Coronary Prevention Study (commonly referred to as WOSCOPS) (10). In this study, 6595 men without a history of MI and a mean total cholesterol of 272 mg/dl were randomized to receive 40 mg of pravastatin (an HMG-CoA reductase inhibitor with brand name of Pravachol) (see table 4.3 for description of cholesterol-lowering medications) each evening or a placebo (inert pill). The average follow-up period for the subjects was approximately five years.

Table 4.2

Cardiovascular Risk Factors: The Evidence Supporting Their Association With Disease, the Usefulness of Measuring Them, and Their Responsiveness to Intervention

Risk factor	Evidence for association with CVD		Clinical measurement	Response to	
	Epidemiologic	Clinical trials	Useful	Nonpharmacologic therapy	Pharmacologic therapy
Category I (risk factors for which interventions have been proved to lower CVD risk)					
Cigarette smoking	+++	++	+++	+++	++
LDL cholesterol	+++	+++	+++	++	+++
High fat/cholesterol diet	+++	++	++	++	−
Hypertension	+++	+++ (stroke)	+++	+	+++
Left ventricular hypertrophy	+++	+	++	−	++
Thrombogenic factors	+++ (fibrinogen)	+++ (aspirin, warfarin)	+ (fibrinogen)	+	+++ (aspirin, warfarin)
Category II (risk factors for which interventions are likely to lower CVD risk)					
Diabetes mellitus	+++	+	+++	++	+++
Physical activity	+++	++	++	++	−
HDL cholesterol	+++	+	+++	++	+
Triglycerides: small, dense LDL	++	++	+++	++	+++
Obesity	+++	−	+++	++	+
Postmenopausal status (women)	+++	−	+++	−	+++
Category III (risk factors associated with increased CVD risk that, if modified, might lower risk)					
Psychosocial factors	++	+	+++	+	−
Lipoprotein(a)	+	−	+	−	+
Homocysteine	++	−	+	++	++
Oxidative stress	+	−	+	+	++
No alcohol consumption	+++	−	++	++	−
Category IV (risk factors associated with increased CVD risk, but which cannot be modified)					
Age	+++	−	+++	−	−
Male gender	+++	−	+++	−	−
Low socioeconomic status	+++	−	+++	−	−
Family history of early-onset CVD	+++	−	+++	−	−

CVD= cardiovascular disease; HDL = high-density lipoprotein; LDL = low-density lipoprotein; + = weak, somewhat consistent evidence; ++ = moderately strong, rather consistent evidence; +++ = very strong, consistent evidence; − = evidence poor or nonexistent.

Reprinted with permission from the American College of Cardiology (*Journal of the American College of Cardiology*, 1996, Vol 27 No 5, pp 962).

Pravastatin lowered LDL cholesterol levels by an average of 25%. The relative risk of coronary events (death or nonfatal MI) was reduced by 31% in the group using pravastatin. The reduction in risk became apparent after six months of treatment and continued to improve during the five years of the study. These findings were supported in the Air Force Texas Coronary Atherosclerosis Prevention Study (known as AFCAPS/TEXCAPS) (11), which showed that individuals on 20 to 40 mg of lovastatin (another HMG-CoA reductase inhibitor with brand name of Mevacor—see table

4.3) had a 40% lower incidence of MI, a 32% lower incidence of angina, and required coronary revascularization (coronary artery bypass graft or PTCA) 25% less often than subjects on a placebo. Importantly, these benefits were observed in subgroups of women, patients over 55 years of age, individuals who smoked, and those who were hypertensive or diabetic.

The National Cholesterol Education Program (NCEP) (7) recently updated its recommendations for individuals without known CAD. A brief review of the recommendations for primary prevention patients is provided. The basic principle of prevention is that the intensity of risk reduction therapy must be adjusted to a person's absolute risk. Risk assessment requires measurement of LDL cholesterol as part of lipoprotein analysis and identification of accompanying risk factors. In all adults age 20 years or older, a fasting lipoprotein profile (total cholesterol, LDL, HDL, and triglyceride) should be obtained once every 5 years. If the values are obtained under non-fasting conditions, only the values for the total cholesterol and HDL are usable. If this occurs, a total cholesterol of >200 mg/dl or HDL < 40 mg/dl warrants a full fasting lipoprotein profile to determine appropriate management based on LDL level. Specific recommendations from the NCEP for individuals without known CAD are as follows:

• Individuals with 0-1 major risk for CAD have an LDL goal of < 160 mg/dl. These low-risk individuals should initiate therapeutic lifestyle changes when LDL is > 160 mg/dl and drug therapy when LDL levels exceed 190 mg/dl.

• Persons with 2+ major risk factors for CAD and a 10-year risk for developing CAD of < 20% (determined from Framingham charts described in chapter 1) have an LDL goal of < 130 mg/dl. Those with a < 10% 10-year risk should initiate therapeutic lifestyle changes when LDL exceeds 130 and drug therapy when LDL exceeds 160 mg/dl. Individuals with a 10-20% 10-year risk should initiate therapeutic lifestyle changes and drug therapy when LDL levels exceed 130 mg/dl.

• Persons with 2+ major risk factors for CAD and a 10-year risk for developing CAD of >20%, as well as those with diabetes or metabolic syn-

Table 4.3
Common Antilipemic Agents by Class

Generic name	Brand name	Mechanism and benefit
Nicotinic acid		
Niacin	Nicobid Niaspan Slo-Niacin	Inhibit lipolysis of adipose tissue and inhibit secretion of lipoproteins from liver. Effectively lower triglycerides, LDL, and raise HDL.
Bile-acid sequestrants (resins)		
Cholestyramine Colestipol	Questran Cholybar Prevalite Colestid	Bind with bile salts in intestines. Effectively lower LDL. Slight increase in HDL.
Fibric-acid derivatives (fibrates)		
Clofibrate Gemfibrozil Fenofibrate	Atromod-S Lopid Tricor	Decrease VLDL synthesis and increase lipoprotein lipase. Effectively lower triglycerides and increase HDL.
HMG-CoA reductase inhibitors (statins)		
Atorvastatin Cerivastatin Fluvastatin Lovastatin Pravastatin Simvastatin Rosuvastatin	Lipitor Baycol* Lescol Mevacor Pravachol Zocor Crestor	Inhibit HMG-CoA reductase, the rate-limiting step in cholesterol production. Increase LDL receptor activity. Effectively lower LDL. Moderate lowering of triglyceride and increase of HDL.

*FDA removed Baycol from the market in August, 2001.

HDL = high-density lipoprotein; LDL = low-density lipoprotein; VLDL = very low-density lipoprotein; HMG-CoA = hepatic hydroxymethylglutaryl coenzyme A.

drome X (described in chapter 1), should be treated as aggressively as individuals with known CAD, thus LDL should be < 100 mg/dl. In these high-risk individuals, LDL levels greater than 100 mg/dl should be managed with therapeutic lifestyle changes, and if LDL exceeds 130 mg/dl, drug therapy is warranted.

The therapeutic lifestyle changes (TLC) strongly promoted by the NCEP include increasing physical activity (approximately 200 kcal/day), weight loss, and the following dietary changes:

- Saturated fat: < 7% of total calories

- Polyunsaturated fat: Up to 10% of total calories

- Monounsaturated fat: Up to 20% of total calories

- Total fat: 25-35% of total calories

- Carbohydrate: 50-60% of total calories

- Fiber: 20-30 g/day

- Protein: Approximately 15% of total calories

- Cholesterol: < 200 mg/day

- Increase consumption of plant stanols/sterols (2 g/day) and soluble fiber (10-25 g/day)

The dietary recommendations of the NCEP are generally consistent with those of the American Heart Association (AHA) with one exception. The NCEP allowance for total fat is slightly higher and is allowed to range from 25-35% of total calories, provided saturated and trans fatty acids are kept low. A higher intake of total fat, mostly in the form of unsaturated fat, can help reduce trigylcerides and raise HDL in persons with the metabolic syndrome X. Both the NCEP and AHA (see table 4.1) recommendations are provided for comparative purposes and because many health care providers are already familiar with the AHA recommendations. According to the AHA, individuals with an elevated LDL should initially follow the Step I diet. If LDL remains elevated despite adherence to the Step I Diet for three months, the Step II Diet should be implemented. In individuals consuming a typical "Western" diet, instituting the AHA Step I Diet generally results in a total cholesterol decrease of 5% to 7%, whereas the Step II Diet should lower total cholesterol by another 5% to 13% (9). Continued elevation of LDL above target levels warrants further clinical examination (i.e., history, physical, lab tests) to screen for secondary causes of dyslipidemia and/or familial disorders. Ultimately, failure to attain the lipid

goals described by NCEP through lifestyle modification should result in initiation of pharmacotherapy.

More than 25 studies to date have evaluated the effects of cholesterol-lowering agents on mortality, morbidity, and progression of CAD in patients with existing CAD. While essentially all studies have shown positive results with cholesterol-lowering medications, one of the most conclusive secondary prevention trials is the Scandinavian Simvastatin Survival Study (known as 4S) (12). This multicenter trial randomized 4444 men and women, aged 35 to 60, with a history of angina or MI and mild hypercholesterolemia to receive 20 to 40 mg of simvastatin (another HMG-CoA reductase inhibitor with brand name of Zocor) or placebo. Simvastatin therapy decreased total cholesterol by 25%, LDL cholesterol by 35%, and triglycerides by 10%. High-density lipoprotein cholesterol was also increased by 8% on simvastatin therapy. Total (i.e., all-cause) mortality was significantly decreased by 30% in the patients treated with simvastatin. The incidence of major coronary events (death and MI) was reduced by 34% in the simvastatin group.

An algorithm for assessing and treating patients with existing CAD, based on LDL levels, has been developed by NCEP (7). In short, in patients with known CAD, an LDL of <100 mg/dl is the goal. Further, after the patient has attained the goal, the NCEP recommends a full fasting lipoprotein analysis at least once every year in individuals with known CAD. Total cholesterol, HDL, and triglyceride goals for secondary prevention are generally similar to those for primary prevention of CAD and were defined in chapter 1. Similar to what occurs with the primary prevention approach, an inability of patients with known CAD to reach the LDL goal through lifestyle behavior changes (diet, exercise, weight loss) should provoke a clinical examination (history, physical exam, blood tests) to identify potential causes of secondary dyslipidemia and/or familial disorders. Ultimately an LDL of >100 mg/dl in a patient with known CAD or risk equivalents (diabetes, metabolic syndrome X, or even a >20% 10-year risk for CAD event) should warrant pharmacologic therapy with an appropriate agent (table 4.3).

Five different classes of medications have been shown to have positive effects on one or more of the lipids. Table 4.3 lists the four most commonly used classes: nicotinic acid (niacin), bile-acid sequestrants (resins), fibric-acid derivatives (fibrates), and HMG-CoA reductase inhibitors (statins). Regardless of the class of medication used, response to therapy should be assessed six to eight weeks after initiation. At the same time, **liver function enzymes** (LDH, SGOT, SGPT) should be assessed through simple blood tests to determine adverse reactions to the medication. If a single medication fails to lower LDL adequately, it is advisable to consider increasing dosage or combining with a second agent. However, it is essential to recognize that the potential for side effects and drug interactions increases with combination therapy (9). In addition to liver dysfunction, potential side effects of cholesterol medications—although fairly uncommon (e.g., <3%)—include **myalgia** (muscle soreness), gastrointestinal problems, and rash.

Despite the recommendations of the NCEP (7) for preventive screening of dyslipidemias, it is not uncommon for patients to have their lipid profile assessed for the very first time when they present to the hospital or physician's office for diagnosis and treatment of their acute cardiac event (i.e., with their heart attack). Often, the lipids obtained at this time will appear to be at desirable levels, suggesting that the individual does not have a dyslipidemia. However, it is now recognized that some of the lipid and/or lipoprotein levels can be suppressed by as much as 40% for as long as 8 to 12 weeks after hospitalization for MI or heart surgery. Although the reason is not clear, it is hypothesized that elevations of stress hormones at the time of an acute coronary or medical event cause perturbations of the lipid profile (9). Consequently, the NCEP (7) now recommends repeating the lipid profile, or waiting and evaluating the lipid profile at least eight weeks after the acute event. Many clinicians believe that if a patient has a LDL greater than 130 mg/dl during hospitalization, drug therapy should be initiated before discharge. If the LDL level is this high during the acute event, it is unlikely that lifestyle changes will be sufficient to reach target levels after the "rebound" in lipids has occurred.

High Fat, High Cholesterol Diet

A diet high in saturated fats and/or cholesterol appears to increase the risk for developing CAD through its impact on other CAD risk factors including hyperlipidemia, hypertension, obesity, and possibly blood coagulation state. As already described, a low fat diet (AHA Step I or II) is the first step of the recommended therapy for primary and secondary prevention of CAD. In controlled settings like hospital metabolic wards, dietary modification has been shown to reduce cholesterol levels by 10% to 15%. However, dietary counseling in subjects living in community settings is apparently not nearly as effective. A **meta-analysis** showed that in community settings, di-

etary modification lowered total cholesterol by only 3% to 6%, depending on the intensity of the diet. Furthermore, a year-long, randomized, controlled trial of 197 middle-aged men and 180 postmenopausal women with moderately elevated LDL levels and low HDL levels showed that subjects randomized to a low fat diet alone had only modest reductions in LDL (8%), which would not have brought the subjects to the LDL goal. However, subjects randomized to a group that performed a combined diet and exercise program (equivalent of 10 miles [16 km] of walking or jogging per week) had a greater decrease in LDL (17%), which allowed them to reach the LDL goal without the use of medications (13).

Results from the Lyon Diet Heart Study (14) indicated that subjects with a prior MI who consumed a "Mediterranean"-type diet (i.e., high in fruits, vegetables, fish, grains, and olive oil) were less likely to experience secondary cardiovascular complications during 46 months of follow-up compared with controls on a "Western"-type diet that was relatively low in saturated fat and cholesterol. Only 26 of 219 (11%) subjects who consumed the Mediterranean diet experienced a major cardiac event compared to 83 of the 204 (40%) individuals consuming the Western diet during the four years of follow-up (figure 4.1).

New evidence suggests that the intake of trans fat may also increase the risk for CAD. Trans fats are unsaturated fats that are produced when polyunsaturated vegetable fats are artificially hydrogenated to make them more solid at room temperature. This process is commonly used to change margarine from a liquid to a more solid (i.e., "stick") form. It is estimated that trans fats constitute about 5% to 10% of the fat in the diet of

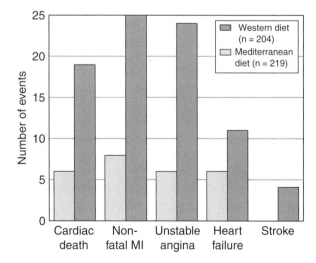

Figure 4.1   Lyon Heart Study results. Comparison of cardiovascular events in individuals consuming a "Mediterranean" diet versus those consuming a "Western" diet.

Americans. The concern over ingesting trans fat comes from the 121,700 female nurses followed in the Nurses' Health Study conducted at Harvard (15). This study showed that individuals in the highest quintile (i.e., upper 20%) of trans fat consumption had a 53% higher risk for CAD than those in the lowest quintile (lowest 20%). As expected, the intake of regular polyunsaturated and vegetable fats was associated with a significantly lower risk for CAD. After dietary and nondietary factors were controlled, neither dietary cholesterol nor total fat intake was associated with an increased risk for CAD. The findings of this study suggest that replacing saturated and trans fats with mono- and polyunsaturated fats in the diet does lower the risk for CAD (15).

Hypertension

The sixth report of the Joint National Committee on Prevention, Detection, Evaluation, and Treatment of High Blood Pressure (JNC VI) (16) gives health care providers a comprehensive overview of contemporary approaches to prevention and early identification of hypertension, as well as to risk stratification and treatment. Hypertensive individuals should be stratified into one of three groups based on the presence or absence of target organ disease, as well as major lifestyle and genetic risk factors (table 4.4). Furthermore, the JNC VI makes clear recommendations for when lifestyle modification versus drug therapy is indicated, including weight loss, regular exercise, and dietary modifications (table 4.4). This recent report (16) places increased emphasis on preventing the progression from high-normal blood pressure to definite hypertension. It has been estimated that a 2-mmHg downward shift in the entire population's distribution of systolic blood pressure would reduce the annual mortality from stroke and CAD by 6% and 4%, respectively.

The variety of pharmacologic agents commonly used to treat hypertension are listed in table 4.5. The JNC VI continues to recommend diuretics and/or beta blockers as the first line of pharmacologic treatment for individuals with hypertension. However, if these agents are not effective at reaching blood pressure goals, the JNC VI recommends substituting another antihypertensive or continuing to add other agents from different classes until target blood pressure is reached. Analysis of 17 randomized trials of hypertension treatment (total of 47,000 patients) indicated that on average, the pharmacologically treated hypertensive patients had lower systolic and diastolic blood pressures (by 13 mmHg and 6 mmHg, respectively) than patients with nontreated hypertension. This degree of blood pressure reduction produced approximately 38% fewer strokes but only a 16% reduction in the incidence of CAD (8). The differential effect of antihypertensive therapy on cerebrovascular compared to cardiovascular disease incidence is not well understood. While hypertension is essentially symptomless, many of the drugs used for treatment of the condition have undesirable side effects and subsequent poor compliance. Furthermore, the cost of these medications can be quite high, particularly in relation to perceived benefit, resulting in a decrease in compliance. Consequently, educating and informing patients about these

Table 4.4
JNC VI Risk Stratification and Treatment of Hypertension

Stage of hypertension (mmHg)	Risk group A	Risk group B	Risk group C
High normal (130-139/85-89)	LM	LM	DT ++
Stage 1 (140-159/90-99)	LM (up to 12 mo.)	LM (up to 6 mo.)+	DT
Stages 2 and 3 (≥160/≥100)	DT	DT	DT

LM = lifestyle modification (exercise, weight loss, dietary changes); DT = drug therapy (see table 4.5 for commonly used anti-hypertensives); + = for patients with multiple risk factors, clinicians should consider drugs as initial therapy plus lifestyle modification; ++ = for those with heart failure, renal insufficiency, or diabetes

Risk Group A = no risk factors and no target organ disease or clinical cardiovascular disease.
Risk Group B = at least 1 risk factor, not including diabetes, and no target organ or cardiovascular disease.
Risk Group C = target organ or clinical cardiovascular disease and/or diabetes, with or without other risk factors.

Example: Patient with diabetes and blood pressure of 142/92 mmHg plus left ventricular hypertrophy should be classified as Stage 1 with target organ disease (left ventricular hypertrophy) and with another major risk factor (diabetes). This patient would be classified as Stage 1, Risk Group C and recommended for immediate initiation of pharmacologic treatment.

Adapted from reference # 16.

Table 4.5

Common Antihypertensive Agents by Class

Generic name	Brand name	Mechanism and benefit
Angiotensin-converting enzyme inhibitors (ACE)		
Benazepril	Lotensin	Prevents conversion of angiotensin I to angiotensin II, which is a powerful vasoconstrictor. Thus lowers blood pressure through peripheral vasodilation. Reduced afterload also beneficial post-MI and in CHF.
Captopril	Capoten	
Enalapril	Vasotec	
Fosinopril	Monopril	
Lisinopril	Zestril, Prinivil	
Quinapril	Accupril	
Ramipril	Altace	
Combination: ACE + diuretic		
Captopril and Hydrochlorothiazide (HCTZ)	Capozide	Combination of vasodilation and diuretic effectively lower blood pressure and afterload.
Enalapril and HCTZ	Vaseretic	
Losinopril and HCTZ	Prinzide, Zestoretic	
Angiotensin II receptor blockers (ARBs)		
Irbesartan	Avapro	Similar vasodilatory response to ACE but works by direct antagonism of angiotensin II receptor (vs. inhibition of converting enzyme).
Losartan	Cozaar	
Valsartan	Diovan	
Losartan + HCTZ	Hyzaar	
Candasartan	Atacand	
Beta adrenergic antagonists (beta blockers)		
Atenolol	Tenormin	Competitively binds with beta 1 receptors on myocardium and prevents action of catecholamines, which results in decreased heart rate and contractility (lower myocardial oxygen demand). Also indicated post-MI and in CHF.
Bisoprolol	Zebeta	
Esmolol	Brevibloc	
Metoprolol	Lopressor, Toprol	
Nadolol	Corgard	
Pindolol	Visken	
Propranolol	Inderal	
Sotolol	Betapace	
Timolol	Blocadren	
Combination: Beta blocker + diuretic		
Propranolol	Inderide	Similar effects as beta blocker plus diuretic effect. Effectively used to reduce blood pressure.
Metoprolol	Lopressor HCTZ	
Atenolol	Tenoretic	
Timolol	Timolide	
Nadolol	Corzide	
Alpha adrenergic antagonists (alpha blockers)		
Doxazosin	Cardura	Competitively blocks vascular alpha 1 receptors, resulting in peripheral arterial dilation.
Prazosin	Minipress	
Terazosin	Hytrin	
Combination: Beta blocker + alpha adrenergic blocker		
Carvedilol	Coreg	In addition to decrease in myocardial demand, inhibition of alpha 1 receptor in peripheral vasculature results in significant vasodilation and afterload reduction. Effectively used to lower blood pressure and in CHF (Coreg).
Labetalol	Normodyne	
	Trandate	
Calcium channel antagonists (calcium blockers)		
Amlodipine	Norvasc	Inhibits the entry of calcium into vascular smooth muscle cells. Results in peripheral vascular
Diltiazem	Cardizem, Dilacor	

Calcium channel antagonists (calcium blockers)		
Felodipine	Plendil	dilation and afterload reduction. Verapamil and
Isradipine	DynaCirc	Diltiazem have antiarrhythmic effect.
Nicardipine	Cardene	
Nifedipine	Adalat, Procardia	
Verapamil	Calan, Isoptin	

Diuretics		
Thiazides		Effects include decreased vascular volume,
Hydrochlorothiazide (HCTZ)	HydroDiuril, Esidrex	decreased sodium balance, and arteriolar
"Loop" diuretic		dilation, resulting in a decrease in peripheral
Bumetanide	Bumex	vascular resistance.
Furosemide	Lasix	
Potassium-sparing		
Spironolactone	Aldactone	

Centrally acting agents		
Clonidine	Catapres	Inhibits or modulates sympathetic outflow from
Guanfacine	Tenex	the central nervous system. Lower blood pres-
Methyldopa	Aldomet	sure is achieved through mild reduction in
Reserpine	Serpasil	heart rate, cardiac output, and a decrease in
		peripheral vascular resistance.

Peripheral vasodilators		
Hydralazine	Apresoline	Arteriole vasodilation lowers blood pressure.
Minoxidil	Loniten	

problems are essential for long-term compliance to antihypertensive medications.

Left Ventricular Hypertrophy

As mentioned in chapter 1, left ventricular hypertrophy has been identified as a risk factor for CAD. It is detected in an electrocardiogram test. Since left ventricular hypertrophy is usually associated with long-standing hypertension, therapy should be directed at lowering blood pressure as already described.

Elevated Thrombogenic Factors

As discussed in chapter 2, plaque rupturing along with the subsequent formation of an intracoronary **thrombus** (i.e., blood clot) is generally the final event that leads to an acute MI. Consequently, it would seem logical that any compound that functions as an **anticoagulant** would decrease the risk for an MI. Therefore the value of aspirin in primary prevention has been tested in two randomized trials, the U.S. Physicians' Health Study and the British Doctors' Trial (8). The American trial included 22,000 male physicians, 40 to 84 years old, assigned to receive aspirin (325 mg every other day) or placebo for five years. There was a 44% reduction in the incidence of MI, limited to those over 50 years of age. However, there was no difference in the incidence of

CAD deaths between the aspirin and placebo groups. In the aspirin-treated group, the risks of hemorrhagic stroke (cerebral bleeding) and gastrointestinal bleeding were slightly increased compared to the risks in the placebo treatment group. In the British trial of 5000 male physicians, 50 to 78 years old, two-thirds were randomly assigned to take aspirin (500 mg per day), and one-third were instructed to avoid it (no actual placebo was used). At six years, while there was no difference in MI or CAD deaths, the aspirin group showed a slight increase in strokes. Because the prevalence of CAD events was quite low among participants in these trials, the absolute risk reduction was quite small. Therefore, the conclusion of the Bethesda conference (8) was that the use of aspirin for primary prevention of CAD events in a healthy population is not recommended. However, men (and probably women) over the age of 50 who possess CAD risk factors should be considered for aspirin therapy. Because of an increased risk for hemorrhagic stroke, aspirin should be used cautiously, if at all, in patients with poorly controlled hypertension.

In contrast, the Bethesda report (8) indicates that the use of aspirin (or other more potent anticoagulants) for secondary prevention in both survivors of myocardial infarction and patients with stable CAD clearly provides protection against death and

Table 4.6
Common Blood Modifying Agents by Class

Generic name	Brand name	Mechanism and benefit
Anticoagulants		
Heparin sodium	Heparin	Inhibits reactions that lead to clotting of blood and the formation of fibrin clots.
Warfarin	Coumadin	Inhibits the synthesis of vitamin K-dependent clotting factors.
Antiplatelet agents		
Acetylsalicylic acid (Aspirin)	Ecotrin Excedrin	Inhibits cyclooxygenase and the conversion of arachidonic acid to Thomboxane A2, a powerful platelet aggregating agent and vasoconstrictor.
Clopidogrel Dipyridamole Ticlopidine	Plavix Persantine Ticlid	Inhibits platelet aggregation by inhibiting ADP stimulation.
Abciximab Eptifibatide Tirofiban	ReoPro Integrelin Aggrastat	Binds with platelet glycoprotein IIb/IIIa receptor, which prevents binding of fibrinogen and adhesive molecules to activated platelets.
Hemorrheologic agents		
Pentoxifylline	Trental	Decreases blood viscosity, which allows for improved blood flow and tissue oxygenation in peripheral vascular disease.
Thrombolytic agents ("clot-busters")		
Tissue Plasminogen Activators (tPA)	Activase Retavase	Binds to fibrin and converts plasminogen to plasmin, which degrades clots.
Streptokinase	Eminase Urokinase	Similar to tPA, converts plasminogen to plasmin.

reinfarction. The advantage of aspirin over other anticoagulants (blood modifiers are listed in table 4.6) is equal effectiveness with lower cost, ease of administration, and less need for monitoring. Thus for post-MI patients, aspirin is still the preferred long-term anticoagulation therapy (8). A meta-analysis of 18,000 patients with known CAD revealed that a medium dose (80-325 mg per day = "baby" aspirin-regular aspirin, respectively) reduced cardiovascular mortality by 13%, nonfatal reinfarction by 31%, and nonfatal stroke by 42% (8).

Category II Risk Factors

The following are risk factors for which interventions are likely to lower CAD risk (Bethesda Category II): diabetes, physical inactivity, low HDL levels, high triglyceride levels, obesity, and postmenopausal status.

Presence of Diabetes

The relationship between fasting blood glucose levels (i.e., **glycemic control**) and prevention of diabetic complications remains controversial. The Diabetes Control and Complications Trial addressed the role of "tight" glycemic control in preventing complications of diabetes by analyzing 1441 patients with insulin-dependent diabetes mellitus, aged 13 to 39 years, who were randomized to receive "intensive" insulin therapy or "conventional" insulin treatment. The intensive therapy comprised administration of insulin by an external insulin pump three or more times a day as indicated by frequent blood glucose monitoring. Conventional therapy consisted of one to two daily injections of insulin. After a mean of 6.5 years, intensive therapy significantly reduced the risk for retinopathy (deterioration of retina in the eye) and **peripheral neuropathy** (deterioration of nerves to hands and feet). Intensive therapy also resulted in a 34% reduction of LDL and a 41% reduction of major cardiovascular complications (9). On the basis of the known adverse effects of prolonged **hyperglycemia,** it is likely that a benefit for CAD risk reduction will result from improved glucose control, but convincing clinical trial data are lacking at the present time.

As described earlier, the NCEP (7) recommends managing elevated LDL cholesterol levels as aggressively in diabetics as in patients with known CAD.

Physical Inactivity

As thoroughly discussed in chapter 1, low levels of physical activity are associated with an increased risk for CAD. One observational study has shown that exercise-induced physical fitness in healthy and diseased subjects is associated with a 44% reduction in mortality. The optimal intensity and duration of exercise to produce CAD risk reduction have not been clearly established, but most guidelines recommend expending at least 1000 kcal per week. In an eight-year follow-up of more than 10,000 Harvard alumni, the self-reported initiation of moderately vigorous sport activity (4.5 METs or higher) was associated with a 41% reduction in CAD mortality and a 23% reduction in all-cause mortality (17). For more information on the risks of physical inactivity, refer back to chapter 1.

Low High-Density Lipoprotein Levels

An HDL cholesterol level of less than 40 mg/dl now is considered low by the NCEP (7) and constitutes a negative risk factor for CAD. Some other professional organizations may have not yet updated their guidelines, hence <35 mg/dl may still be the threshold level in many documents. The primary therapy for low HDL cholesterol is lifestyle modification, emphasizing diet, regular exercise, smoking cessation, and weight reduction as appropriate. According to the NCEP, increasing HDL cholesterol levels is a lesser priority for lipid-lowering therapy than LDL cholesterol reduction. Beyond the described lifestyle changes, nicotinic acid (niacin) and estrogen (for postmenopausal women) are the most commonly used pharmacotherapies. High-density lipoprotein can also be increased through use of a fibric acid derivative (such as gemfibrozil or Lopid) or certain HMG-CoA reductase inhibitors, particularly atorvastatin (Lipitor) (refer to table 4.3 for lipid-lowering agents). The incremental benefit and cost effectiveness of increasing HDL cholesterol in patients who have normal LDL cholesterol levels has not been established (8). Because many lipid-active agents and lifestyle changes affect multiple lipids simultaneously, it has been difficult to demonstrate that increasing HDL cholesterol independently lowers CAD risk. The NCEP (7) does not yet recommend introducing a drug solely for the purpose of increasing HDL in individuals otherwise at low risk for CAD. However, if drug therapy is indicated to lower LDL cholesterol, a secondary goal of increasing HDL could affect the selection of the agent. But it is important to note that the NCEP does recommend consideration of nicotinic acid to increase HDL in patients with CAD even if their LDL cholesterol is below the initiation level for drug therapy (9). It appears that up to 30% of patients with known CAD have a low HDL as their primary lipid abnormality (i.e., total cholesterol and LDL are normal) and are at substantial risk for CAD events. A recent Veterans Affairs study (18) investigated the effect of gemfibrozil (see table 4.3) in men with proven CAD and low HDL (<40 ml/dl) but relatively normal LDL (<140 mg/dl) levels. On average, treatment lasted five years and was associated with a 22% relative risk reduction in cardiac events (defined as MI and death due to CAD). These effects were achieved with a mean reduction in cholesterol (4%) and triglycerides (31%) and a 6% increase in HDL. Treatment with gemfibrozil had no effect on LDL in these patients.

High Triglyceride Levels

Elevated triglycerides are associated with multiple metabolic abnormalities, including low HDL, small dense LDL (known as LDL subclass B), insulin resistance, abdominal obesity, and a subsequent risk for CAD. As in hypercholesterolemia, treatment of triglycerides is influenced by the degree of CAD risk. In patients with known CAD, a strong family history of premature CAD, or diabetes, elevated triglycerides should now be reduced to below 150 mg/dl to decrease CAD risk. The primary treatment for hypertriglyceridemia is lifestyle modification, which should include weight control; a diet low in saturated fat, cholesterol, and sugar; regular exercise; smoking cessation; and alcohol restriction (9). The NCEP guidelines (7) recommend consideration of drug therapy in patients with borderline-high triglycerides and known CAD, a strong family history, a high total cholesterol, or low HDL cholesterol. Suggested pharmacologic agents include fibric acid derivatives or nicotinic acid (see table 4.3).

Obesity

No study has specifically examined the effect of weight loss on CAD events. However, the role of weight reduction in the treatment of hypertension, dyslipidemia, and diabetes makes it an obvious choice for a primary or secondary prevention. Without question the optimal method to lose body weight, particularly body fat, is moderate caloric restriction in conjunction with increased physical activity (8). Regular exercise training and/or physical activity has been shown to be effective for initial weight loss, but is also the most effective approach for maintaining weight loss. It does appear, however, that keeping weight off requires an hour a day of physical activity. This conclusion was drawn from the National Weight Control Registry of 2500 individuals who lost an average of 60 lb (27 kg) and kept it off for more than one year. Those who successfully kept the weight off walked on average 10 miles (16 km) per week in addition to other aerobic activities, weightlifting, and sport-type activities. In addition to their physical activity habits, individuals who successfully kept their weight down reported watching their diet carefully. Although many may view an hour of exercise negatively and see it as too much of a commitment, it is now generally accepted that not all of the exercise has to be done at one time. It appears that several shorter bouts of activity during the course of the day are as effective as one longer period of exercise for maintaining weight loss.

Unfortunately, many individuals, seeking a quicker and easier success, have used a variety of dieting aids, including prescription drugs, to lose weight. In 1997, fenfluramine and phentermine (brand names Pondimin and Redux, respectively) were removed from the market by the FDA because of their reported damage to heart valves (19). A new weight-reducing drug, Orlistat (tetrahydrolipstatin), which works by blocking pancreatic lipase and reducing fat absorption, has been found to be more effective than a low calorie diet alone for losing weight. After one year of treatment, weight loss was substantially greater with Orlistat than placebo (10.2% vs. 6.1%, respectively). In the second year, patients on Orlistat gained less weight back than those on placebo. Moreover, the Orlistat group had significant reductions in blood lipids, blood glucose, and blood pressure. The most common side effect was gastrointestinal distress. Although larger and longer-term safety studies are needed, Orlistat may become the first nondietary suppressant to be useful for pharmacologic treatment of obesity (19). Another drug, Meridia (sibutramine), works by blocking the reuptake of specific neurohormones (serotonin and noradrenalin), which are known to mediate appetite. In essence, use of this drug appears to work by enhancing satiety (i.e., feeling of fullness or satisfaction) and thus reducing food intake. Clinical trials in patients who are obese have confirmed the long-term efficacy and safety of Meridia as a weight-reducing drug (20). However, the impact of pharmacologically induced weight loss on risk factors, and ultimately on risk for CAD events, is unknown.

Postmenopausal Status

Because of the marked difference in the prevalence of CAD between men and women of the same age, estrogens have long been thought to protect against CAD. It has been hypothesized that estrogen-induced changes in blood lipids including lipoprotein(a), fibrinogen, and endothelial function, as well as an antioxidant effect, provide the protection against developing CAD. A large body of evidence supports the use of estrogen in postmenopausal women to prevent the development of CAD. One study showed that after nine years, estrogen users had a 64% lower incidence of CAD mortality than nonusers. Statistically adjusting for other risk factors, including blood pressure, smoking, and lipids, did not diminish the protective effect of estrogen.

In contrast to these positive findings, the Heart and Estrogen Replacement Study (called HERS) (21) failed to detect a reduction in mortality or recurrent MI with estrogen use in women who had documented CAD. In fact, there was a significantly greater risk of thromboembolic events in the estrogen-treated group during the first year. Thus, the use of estrogen for primary prevention appears warranted, while use in secondary prevention is questionable at this time. The differential effect of estrogen in primary versus secondary prevention is not well understood.

Category III Risk Factors

The following factors associated with increased CAD risk are those for which modification might lower risk (Bethesda Category III): psychosocial factors, lipoprotein(a), homocysteine, oxidative stress, and alcohol consumption.

Psychosocial Factors

A number of clinical trials, as well as several meta-analyses, demonstrate that psychosocial stress interventions can reduce cardiac events (death) in individuals with CAD. A recent study from Duke University (22) examined the extent to which either exercise training or stress management techniques could reduce exercise-induced myocardial ischemia and favorably modify clinical outcomes. One hundred and seven patients with known CAD were randomly assigned to a four-month program of exercise (three times per week) or to stress management training. Behavior training consisted of sixteen 90-min group sessions, muscle relaxation techniques, and biofeedback instruction. Compared to the exercise group, the stress management group had a significantly reduced risk of cardiac events and less myocardial ischemia over three years of follow-up. Because psychosocial distress is treatable and because it impacts quality of life, the identification and treatment of anxiety, depression, and hostility should be incorporated into primary and secondary prevention programs. Chapter 10 includes further discussion on psychosocial screening and interventions in preventive and rehabilitative programs.

Lipoprotein(a)

The level of lipoprotein(a) (Lp[a]) in the blood appears to be determined principally by genetics; thus treatment is problematic and controversial (8). Medications have little effect on Lp(a), although recent evidence suggests that niacin and postmenopausal estrogen replacement may have some benefit. Although lowering Lp(a) is theoretically appealing, the impact on recurrent cardiac events has not been studied. Since Lp(a) measurements are not widely available and the clinical significance of lowering Lp(a) is unknown, the NCEP (7) does not recommend the routine measurement of this lipoprotein at this time.

Homocysteine

Although elevated plasma homocysteine levels have been associated with risk of CAD, the benefits of treatment, in terms of CAD risk, are not clear. We know that homocysteine levels can be reduced through increased consumption of foods high in folic acid as well as vitamins B_6 and B_{12}. Clinicians commonly recommend ≥ 0.4 mg per day of folate, ≥ 2 mg and 1.6 mg per day of vitamin B_6 for men and women, respectively, and >0.002 mg per day of vitamin B_{12} to reduce homocysteine levels (23).

Oxidative Stress

As discussed in chapter 2, oxidative modification of LDL appears to be a significant aspect of the atherosclerotic process. Thus, it is reasoned that prevention of such oxidation may prevent CAD. Although the observational studies are promising, there is no conclusive clinical trial evidence that use of antioxidants reduces clinical CAD events. In preliminary findings from a primary prevention trial of beta-carotene and vitamin E in Finnish smokers, overall mortality did not differ significantly between the vitamin E and control groups (24). Furthermore, beta-carotene and vitamin E failed to limit the progression of CAD, angina, or MI among men with established CAD. The low dose of vitamin E (50 mg per day) may

have contributed to the negative findings of these studies. Clinicians commonly recommend 400 IU of vitamin E for high-risk or secondary prevention patients. Moreover, the Heart Outcomes Prevention Evaluation (HOPE) study (25) showed that in patients at high risk for CAD, 400 mg of vitamin E for 4.5 years had no apparent effect on cardiovascular disease outcome. Because supportive evidence is lacking, the NCEP at this time does not recommend the use of antioxidants for primary or secondary prevention of CAD.

Alcohol Consumption

A strong positive relationship between moderate alcohol consumption and reduced risk for CAD has been observed. The exact mechanism responsible for the "cardioprotective" effect of alcohol consumption is not well understood; but beneficial effects on HDL cholesterol, vascular reactivity, and hemostatic factors (e.g., blood clotting) have been identified. Although the mechanism may be different, there does not appear to an advantage to drinking wine versus beer versus other alcoholic beverages, since moderate consumption of each is associated with a similar reduction in CAD mortality. Furthermore, grape juice might offer the same "cardioprotection" as red wine, since both have been shown to inhibit platelets in vivo (26). However, excessive alcohol consumption is associated with an increased risk for cardiovascular disease mortality, secondary to **cardiomyopathy,** arrhythmias, or hypertension. Because of the potential noncardiac risks involved with alcohol use (impaired driving, abuse, etc.) and the lack of data from experimental studies, the use of alcoholic beverages as a "treatment" to reduce the risk of CAD is not recommended. However, moderate alcohol consumption (one to two drinks per day) does not have to be curtailed and may be beneficial in the prevention and treatment of CAD (26).

RISK FACTOR REDUCTION AND REGRESSION OF CORONARY ARTERY DISEASE

As introduced in chapter 1, several studies in the mid-1980s produced the first angiographic evidence in humans that aggressive risk factor intervention, particularly with respect to dyslipidemia, not only stops or delays the progression of CAD but may also result in a reduction of the coronary artery lesion size (commonly referred to as reversal or regression). These early studies relied primarily on the cholesterol-lowering agents available at the time (i.e., bile-acid binding resins and/or nicotinic acid) to successfully lower blood lipids and reverse lesions in native coronary arteries as well as in coronary artery vein grafts. Since then nearly a dozen trials have demonstrated that various cholesterol-lowering agents (most recently the HMG-CoA reductase inhibitors or "statins") significantly reduce progression and often induce regression of CAD lesions, as well as reducing morbidity (MI, coronary artery bypass graft) and mortality associated with CAD.

In the early 1990s, Dr. Dean Ornish was the first to report that lifestyle modifications alone (i.e., no drug therapy) can also effectively decrease progression and evoke regression of coronary lesions in individuals with known CAD. The Lifestyle Heart Trial (27) was a randomized, case-controlled study that followed 35 subjects for a total of five years to determine the effects of comprehensive lifestyle changes on the coronary atherosclerotic progress. Twenty of the subjects received an intensive lifestyle modification program that included a 10% fat (i.e., vegetarian) diet, aerobic exercise, stress management, smoking cessation, and group psychosocial support. The control group followed an AHA Step II Diet and performed regular aerobic exercise. As evidenced by coronary angiograms, the intervention group exhibited an overall regression of coronary atherosclerosis, while the lesions in the control group continued to progress. The average percentage diameter stenosis had decreased by 3.1% by the fifth year in the intervention group, but had in-

creased by 11.8% by the fifth year in the control group. As expected, the change in artery stenosis was found to have a profound impact on myocardial perfusion, such that patients demonstrating regression experienced a decrease in the size and severity of myocardial perfusion abnormalities on a dipyridamole stress test. Most importantly, the rate of cardiac events (MI, hospitalization for procedures) was significantly higher in the control group (45 events in 20 subjects) than in the intervention group (25 events in 28 patients) over the five-year study. Although often criticized for patient selection bias, the Lifestyle Heart Trial has demonstrated that highly motivated subjects following a strict lifestyle change are able to decrease plasma lipid levels, reverse coronary artery lesions, and decrease CAD events and symptoms (27). Figure 4.2 shows coronary angiograms of a patient before and after five years of participation in the intervention group. Notice the clear evidence of CAD regression (60% decreased to 20%) in the left anterior descending coronary artery.

Whereas the Lifestyle Heart Trial used aggressive dietary modification and a comprehensive stress management program to successfully reverse CAD lesions, the Heidelberg Heart Study (28) demonstrated that similar coronary artery benefits can be obtained with vigorous exercise and a low fat diet. Shuler et al. (28) assigned male patients with known CAD to 12 months of either a vigorous exercise program (consisting of 30 min of daily cycle ergometry at home and two group exercise sessions of 1 h per week) and a low fat

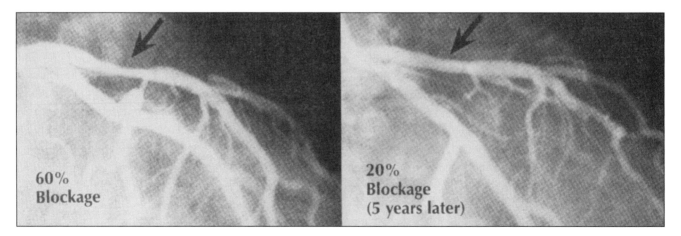

Figure 4.2 Coronary angiogram from intervention group participant in Lifestyle Heart Trial. Image on left represents angiogram for one individual obtained at entry to study; notice 60% lesion in the left anterior descending coronary artery. The image on the right represents an angiogram obtained five years later. Clearly, the percentage of occlusion in the same artery segment is much lower (now 20%).

Image used with permission of Dr. Dean Ornish, Principle Investigator, Lifestyle Heart Trial.

diet (AHA Phase II) or to the "usual care" of their personal physician. In addition to dramatic improvements in blood lipids (LDL and total cholesterol decreased by 12%), the patients in the treatment group were more likely to experience favorable changes in their coronary lesions (7 of 18 patients had clear regression of their CAD) than the patients in the usual-care group (only 1 of 18 patients in this group demonstrated regression of CAD). The positive anatomical changes observed in the intervention group resulted in improved myocardial perfusion (i.e., improved coronary blood flow), whereas patients in the usual-care group tended to have decreased myocardial perfusion. In a follow-up to this study, the same group of investigators (29) reported that cardiac patients who exceeded 2200 kcal of physical activity per week had some regression of their CAD lesions. The authors characterized this amount of activity as approximately 5 to 6 h per week of physical activity. Cardiac patients who reported less than 1000 kcal per week of physical activity exhibited progression of their CAD lesions. Patients reporting an average of 1500 kcal per week of physical activity showed no progression of CAD. The results of these two studies led the authors to conclude that CAD patients willing to devote time and effort to a physical exercise program that exceeds 1500 kcal per week, along with a low fat diet, may experience a decrease in CAD progression or regression and/or an improvement in myocardial perfusion.

Although aggressive dietary modification and vigorous exercise appear to limit progression or induce regression of CAD lesions and to reduce fatal and nonfatal coronary events, it appears that more moderate multifactorial risk reduction programs (i.e., "standard" cardiac rehabilitation programs) can achieve similar positive results. Two meta-analyses (30, 31) of multifactorial cardiac rehabilitation programs revealed a 26% lower mortality rate in patients who combined multifactorial risk factor counseling with regular exercise—a combination promoted in most cardiac rehabilitation programs—than in those who exercised only.

Of the investigations performed to date, the Stanford Coronary Risk Intervention Project (SCRIP) (32) has perhaps the greatest practical significance. This project used aggressive modification of multiple risk factors through lifestyle intervention and medications in a physician-supervised, nurse-managed model. Three hundred men and women with CAD were randomly assigned to usual care (i.e., care through personal

primary physician) or the multifactor risk reduction program for four years. Patients assigned to the risk reduction program received individualized programs for exercise, low fat/cholesterol diet, smoking cessation, weight loss, and medications to improve lipid profiles. In contrast to the usual-care group, the risk reduction group demonstrated significant improvement in modifiable CAD risk factors including blood pressure, blood lipids, and blood glucose. Consequently, progression of atherosclerosis in the risk reduction group was 47% less than for the usual-care group (figure 4.3). In addition, there were 25 hospitalizations for cardiac events in the risk reduction group compared with 44 in the usual-care group. During the last three years of the study, the hospitalization rate was significantly greater in the usual-care versus the intervention group (35 vs. 8, respectively). It is difficult to determine from this investigation which specific intervention (e.g., medications, exercise, diet) was most effective at reducing CAD risk, but clearly a multifactorial approach to modifying known risk factors for CAD has a dramatic impact on the progression or regression of CAD.

On the basis of the existing body of knowledge about the impact of risk factor modification on CAD progression or regression, the American Heart Association and the American College of Cardiology have produced helpful and simple guidelines for managing patients with stable CAD (i.e., secondary prevention) (33). These guidelines can be summarized as the "ABCDES of Secondary Prevention" (table 4.7).

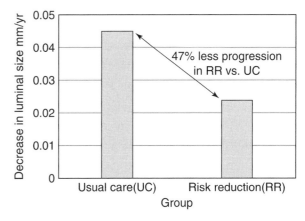

Figure 4.3 Angiographic results from the Stanford Coronary Risk Intervention Program (SCRIP). Graph reveals that participants in the risk reduction group had less decrease in luminal size (47% decrease) than the usual-care group, indicating less CAD progression in the former.

Table 4.7
ABCDES of Secondary Prevention

Anti-platelet/**A**nti-coagulant/**A**nti-anginal drugs/**A**CE inhibitors post-MI
Blood pressure control/**B**eta blockers/**B** vitamins
Cholesterol management/**C**igarette smoking cessation
Diet/**D**iabetes management
Exercise/**E**ducation of the patient/**E**strogen
Social support/**S**tress management

SURGICAL AND INTERVENTIONAL PROCEDURES FOR CORONARY ARTERY DISEASE

There is now little doubt that aggressive management of CAD risk factors can alter the course of CAD progression (i.e., limit progression and evoke regression) in the majority of patients; however, this approach requires time (months to years) and can be used only in the nonemergent treatment of stable CAD. Most studies demonstrating CAD regression through lifestyle and/or pharmacologic intervention, as described earlier, have lasted for one year or longer. Clearly, more rapidly applied treatments are necessary for those with unremitting symptoms, inability to tolerate the necessary pharmacotherapy, lack of motivation to comply, or the presence of certain clinical characteristics associated with poor survival. The two most commonly used revascularization procedures are coronary artery bypass graft (CABG) surgery and percutaneous transluminal coronary intervention (PTCI), which now includes a variety of devices and techniques (i.e., angioplasty, atherectomy, laser treatment, intracoronary stents). Either revascularization procedure is performed after a diagnostic coronary catheterization (described in chapter 3) has revealed the presence of one or more significant coronary lesions.

Coronary Artery Bypass Graft Surgery

Coronary artery bypass graft surgery, first used in the 1960s, continues to be one of the most frequently performed operations nationally. The more than 600,000 surgeries performed each year in the United States (9) result in an annual expenditure of $50 billion. Although the use of invasive cardiac procedures is the subject of constant scrutiny, a recent investigation determined that only 4% of CABG procedures were performed

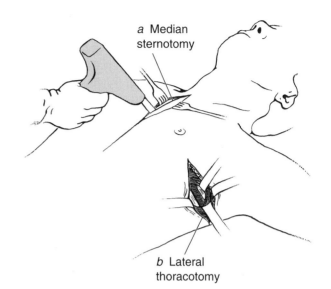

Figure 4.4   **Surgical approaches for coronary artery bypass graft surgery: *(a)* the median sternotomy approach of splitting and separating the sternum (breast bone) to access the heart; *(b)* the lateral thoracotomy approach used for the minimally invasive bypass procedure.**

inappropriately on patients who could have been managed medically (i.e., medications and lifestyle modification) or with other interventions (9). The most commonly used surgical technique to perform CABG involves a median sternotomy (i.e., sawing through the breast bone) (figure 4.4) and opening of the pericardium. By means of cross-clamping the aorta and cannulating the vena cava, blood is rerouted away from the heart and lungs to a cardiopulmonary bypass pump device. This device provides **extracorporeal circulation** to supply blood to other parts of the body during the surgery. Infusion of a cold **cardioplegic solution** into the heart causes the heart to cease contracting, which in turn significantly reduces its metabolic activity. Consequently, the heart is able to survive for several hours without blood supply. The vessels used to "bypass" the occluded coronary arteries are vein grafts, most commonly extracted from the leg (saphenous vein), or internal mammary arteries (also known as internal thoracic arteries) (figure 4.5). The two internal mammary arteries available for CABG surgery are the left and right internal mammary arteries. It is now recognized that atherosclerosis occurs more rapidly in vein grafts than in internal mammary arteries. Consequently, patency (i.e., remaining open) rate at 10 to 12 years is approximately 50% for saphenous vein grafts compared to 90% for internal mammary grafts (9). Thus, most surgeons believe that whenever technically feasible, internal mammary grafts should be used in place of

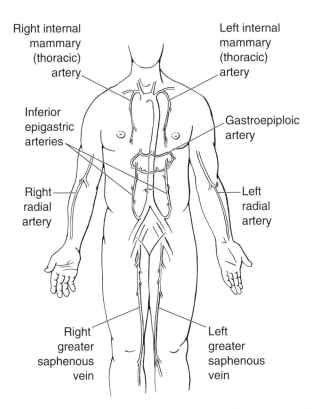

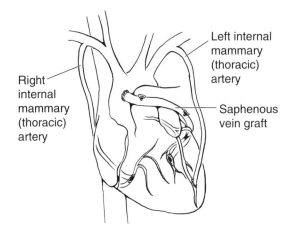

Figure 4.6 Coronary artery bypass graft surgery. Three-vessel (often called triple) bypass using right internal mammary artery (RIMA), left internal mammary artery (LIMA), and a saphenous vein graft to bypass occlusions in the right coronary artery, the left anterior descending coronary artery, and the circumflex coronary artery, respectively.

Figure 4.5 Arterial and venous grafts used for myocardial revascularization procedures.

vein grafts. The superiority of artery grafts over vein grafts for CABG surgery has resulted in identification and subsequent use of other arteries. The gastroepiploic and inferior epigastric arteries in the abdomen can be rerouted to bypass the right coronary artery, and radial arteries from either forearm can be used to bypass coronary lesions (figure 4.5). Despite the availability of several artery grafts, vein grafts may be needed when multiple grafts are necessary, when graft length is an issue (e.g., posterior descending artery bypass), and if CAD progression requires a second CABG. Figure 4.6 depicts a common three-vessel CABG, in which the right and left internal mammary (thoracic) arteries are used to bypass lesions in the right coronary artery and left anterior descending coronary artery, respectively, and a saphenous vein graft is used to bypass a circumflex coronary artery lesion.

Renewed interest in CABG surgery without the use of the cardiopulmonary bypass pump has been stimulated by the desire to avoid blood transfusions, reduce costs, and avoid the negative consequences (e.g., blood clots and microemboli that can affect brain function) of the bypass machine (9). Since 1995, use of the minimally invasive coronary artery bypass (MIDCAB) procedure, performed on a beating

heart through a small thoracotomy (also called port access or keyhole incision) on the lateral aspect of the chest (see figure 4.4), has been increasing. While revascularization of most of the coronary arteries can be performed through the minimally invasive approach, it is most easily and commonly used on the anterior arteries, particularly the left anterior descending. Generally the LIMA is the graft used for the minimally invasive bypass procedures, thus eliminating trauma to the lower extremity associated with harvesting the saphenous vein. Because of reduced trauma and complications, MIDCAB can decrease the length of hospital stay and the overall costs, in selected patients with single-vessel disease, by 40% compared to standard CABG. There is no question that the use of minimally invasive bypass surgery on the beating heart will continue to increase over time.

Percutaneous Transluminal Coronary Interventions

Since the introduction of coronary balloon angioplasty into clinical practice in 1977, improvements in equipment design and operator experience have permitted application of this procedure to the treatment of a broad spectrum of CAD conditions. The more than 400,000 revascularization procedures carried out each year with balloon angioplasty or related devices in the United States now approach the number of CABG surgeries performed in this country.

Following local anesthesia, access to the coronary vessels is obtained through the femoral artery or, less frequently, the brachial artery, in a method similar to that described (in chapter 3) for coronary angiography. A steerable coronary guide wire is advanced through the guide catheter into the coronary vessel and manipulated under fluoroscopic (X ray) guidance across the coronary stenosis. A balloon angioplasty catheter of suitable inflated diameter (usually ≤110% of the estimated normal vessel diameter) is advanced across the guide wire to the stenosis and inflated over a period of seconds to minutes (figure 4.7). Some evidence indicates that outcomes (e.g., increase in lumen size, rate of **restenosis**) may be improved by prolonging inflation time, although the duration of inflation is usually limited by the development of ischemia signs and symptoms associated with the disruption of coronary blood flow. Inadequate improvement in the degree of stenosis may be treated with repeat inflations, a larger balloon, or a different revascularization device.

The mechanisms by which angioplasty improves vessel luminal diameter are somewhat complicated and may depend largely on the characteristics of the lesion itself. For example, softer coronary artery lesions rich in foam cells may be compressible, whereas dense, calcified lesions may fracture to create channels to improve blood flow. In any case, this procedure is highly successful for improving coronary artery blood flow. A large registry of angioplasty data from sites around the United States reveals that approximately 95% of angioplasty procedures result in a

≥20% improvement in luminal stenosis. Figure 4.8 demonstrates the effectiveness of PTCA in a patient with significant coronary occlusion. The rates of death and MI during angioplasty are 1.0% and 4.3%, respectively. As many as 5.0% of patients undergoing angioplasty will experience a complication requiring emergent CABG surgery. Consequently, centers performing angioplasty procedures must have on-site cardiac surgical facilities. The single most important complication associated with angioplasty is abrupt vessel closure, characterized as sudden occlusion of the target or adjacent segments during or shortly after completion of the procedure. The reported incidence of abrupt closure ranges from 4.2% to 8.3% and is typically caused by the dissection of the intimal layer or thrombus formation inside the artery that is obstructing the artery, or by coronary artery vasoconstriction.

A number of preventive pharmacologic measures may limit the occurrence of abrupt vessel closure during angioplasty. In the past, aspirin and/or intravenous infusion of heparin (a potent anticoagulant) was administered before, during, and after the coronary intervention (angioplasty, atherectomy) for three to seven days because this reduced the risk of vessel occlusion and thrombus formation. Several new platelet glycoprotein IIb/IIIa receptor inhibitors (see table 4.6) that work by inhibiting platelet aggregation (i.e., prevent clumping) have been developed and show superiority to conventional therapy. Recent studies indicate that platelet glycoprotein IIb/IIIa re-

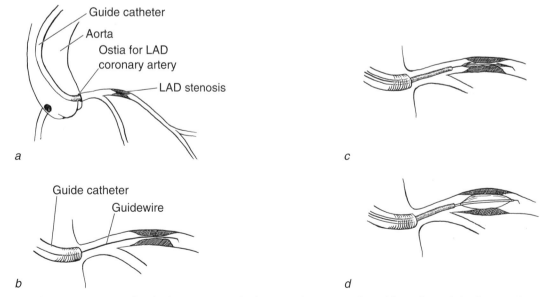

Figure 4.7 Percutaneous transluminal coronary angioplasty (PTCA). Once the guide catheter is in the opening (ostia) of the coronary artery (in this example the left anterior descending coronary artery) *(a)*, the guide wire is passed across the obstruction (lesion) *(b)*. The balloon catheter is then advanced over the guide wire until in position at the lesion *(c)*. The balloon is inflated to dilate the artery segment *(d)*, and then it is deflated and retracted.

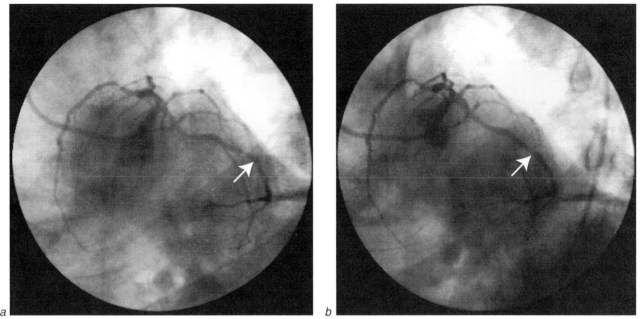

a   *b*

Figure 4.8   Results of successful angioplasty (PTCA). *(a)* A 95% stenosis of distal circumflex coronary artery prior to treatment. *(b)* The same artery segment after balloon inflation and stent placement. The final stenosis after intervention was 0%. Note that this is the actual catheterization of Case Study 3 presented throughout the book. The sections on Case Study 3 in chapters 3 and 4 present details on this catheterization.

ceptor blockers can decrease the risk of complications due to clot formation by 50% to 60%. A variety of other pharmacotherapies to prevent abrupt vessel closure are under investigation, including combining glycoprotein IIb/IIIa receptor blockers with low molecular weight heparins (see table 4.6).

If abrupt closure occurs, initial management typically consists of repeated and prolonged balloon dilation to induce adhesion (i.e., "tack-up") of the dissected intimal layer to the arterial wall or compression of the intraluminal thrombus. A number of new devices, most prominently intracoronary stents that act as "scaffolds" at the angioplasty site, also hold promise for reducing abrupt closure.

Among patients who have undergone initially successful angioplasty, outcomes over the first three to six months are influenced primarily by the development of recurrent stenoses at the treated site (referred to as restenosis), while events over the longer term appear to depend on conventional progression of atherosclerotic disease. The incidence of restenosis has remained largely unchanged since the introduction of angioplasty, with reported rates ranging from 30% to 50%. The risk of restenosis, traditionally defined as an artery obstruction of >50% at follow-up angiography, is greatest during the initial three to six months following the procedure. The most common clinical manifestation of restenosis is recur-

rence of anginal pain. Typically, patients presenting with angina more than six months after the procedure more frequently have progression of CAD in other vessels as opposed to restenosis at the angioplasty site. The pathogenesis of restenosis is complex and likely multifactorial; thus, methods for diminishing or preventing this complication have so far been largely unsuccessful. However, glycoprotein IIb/IIIa receptor blockers and/or intracoronary stenting appear to be capable of reducing the risk of restenosis after successful angioplasty or atherectomy.

Intracoronary Stents

Intracoronary stents may be used to support and maintain an open lumen after successful angioplasty to a native coronary artery or vein or to an artery bypass graft. There has been broad observational experience with the use of stents as a means of treating abrupt closure, and two randomized clinical trials have demonstrated efficacy in reducing the incidence of restenosis. The restenosis rates at seven to eight months postprocedure for stents combined with angioplasty, compared to those for angioplasty alone, were 22% versus 32% and 31% versus 42% in the two studies, respectively (9). Stents currently in clinical use are composed of various metals that have been demonstrated to possess adequate strength but to be biocompatible without degradation. The major disadvantage of metallic stents is the risk for blood clot formation due to interaction between the blood cells and the structure. Thus, stents have been designed with various mesh or coil configurations to minimize the surface area of exposed metal (figure 4.9). Nevertheless, anticoagulation therapy with aspirin, heparin, warfarin (Coumadin), dipyridamole (Persantine), and/or newer agents such as clopidrogrel (Plavix) or ticlopidine (Ticlid), is generally required with a stent (table 4.6). The use of biodegradable stents that would eliminate the need for anticoagulants is currently under investigation.

Radiation Therapy

In a novel approach to reduce restenosis, called **brachytherapy,** radiation is delivered to coronary arteries either by a catheter-based system or by the placement of a radioactive "seed" or stent at the site of the lesion. Both beta and gamma radiation have been used as a source to attempt to reduce smooth muscle proliferation (a significant part of the atherosclerotic process). A study in humans (34) suggests that patients who received catheter-based radiation therapy showed a marked reduction in restenosis (17% vs. 54%) at six months and three years (33% vs. 63%) compared to patients who didn't receive brachytherapy. Furthermore, the combined end point of death, MI, or need for revascularization was significantly lower in the treated versus the nontreated group (23% vs. 55%). However, many issues still need to be addressed with brachytherapy, including optimal radiation dose and source, long-term vascular effects of ra-

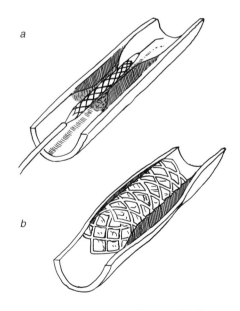

Figure 4.9   Coronary stents. Inflation of balloon catheter allows for expansion and placement of stent. Balloon is deflated and retracted while stent remains embedded in artery wall.

diation, and risk to administrators (i.e., catheterization lab personnel). Some of these questions will be answered in the near future through studies currently being performed.

Coronary Atherectomy

Over the last 10 years, interventional cardiologists have witnessed the development of a variety of devices to remove atheromatous (hence the name atherectomy) material from the coronary arteries. Three atherectomy devices have been approved for clinical use. Two of these, the directional and extraction atherectomy catheters, operate on the principle of physically cutting the stenosis using a spinning blade; the third, rotational atherectomy, abrades and pulverizes the lesion. The directional coronary atherectomy catheter consists of a metal cylinder at its distal end, which houses a rotating cup-shaped blade (figure 4.10). One side of the housing contains a window with a balloon attached to the housing opposite the window. A flexible nose cone at the distal tip of the housing serves as a collecting chamber for excised tissue. Once in place over the coronary stenosis, the balloon is inflated to low pressure, pressing the window against the lesion and invaginating the atherosclerotic plaque into the cutting chamber. The cutter inside the housing is slowly pushed forward as it spins at 2000 rpm (analogous to a deli meat slicer). The excised tissue is pushed forward into the nose cone. A number of cuts are usually performed to reduce the lesion size. Many patients also receive adjunctive balloon angioplasty following atherectomy to achieve the optimal angiographic result. Observational registry experience has demonstrated directional atherectomy to be effective and safe for treating a variety of coronary lesions, with an overall procedural success rate of 85%, increasing to 92% with adjunctive angioplasty (9). Rates of in-hospital death, MI, and emergent CABG were similar to those associated with PTCA (0.5%, 0.9%, and 4.0%, respectively). Furthermore, the restenosis rate after directional coronary atherectomy, to either native coronary arteries or bypass grafts, does not appear to be different from that reported for angioplasty.

The rotational atherectomy catheter (Rotablator) uses a rapidly spinning abrasive tip to grind or "polish" the internal lumen. The distal end of the catheter consists of an elliptical burr coated with tiny diamond chips that rotates at 170,000 to 200,000 rpm while slowly advancing through the atherosclerotic plaque (see figure 4.10). Rotational atherectomy produces particles that typically pass downstream without obstruction of the microcirculation. This technique has been particularly useful for lesions that appear to be heavily calcified and inelastic (i.e., nondilatable with balloon). Adjunctive balloon

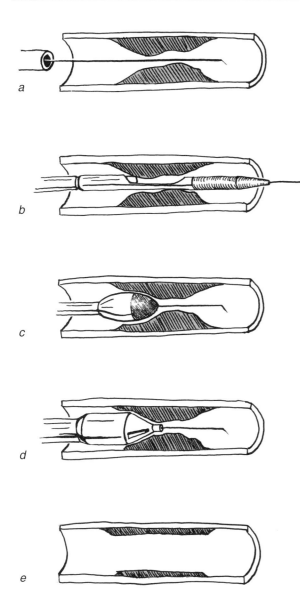

Figure 4.10   Coronary atherectomy. *(a)* Positioning of the catheter guide wire across the lesion. *(b)* Directional atherectomy catheter positioned at coronary lesion. Blade moves back and forth to reduce size of lesion. Atheromatous material that is removed is collected in nose cone of the device. *(c)* Rotational atherectomy catheter spins rapidly to decrease the size of the coronary lesion. Tiny particles remain in the blood. *(d)* Transluminal extraction catheter has spinning metal blades in the nose of the device that suck atheromatous material into the catheter. This device is particularly useful for removal of clots and soft lesions commonly found in vein bypass grafts. *(e)* Often after any of the atherectomy procedures, a balloon catheter inflation (and stent) will be the final step to achieve optimal results (i.e., least amount of stenosis).

angioplasty is almost always required to increase the luminal area, since the burr is relatively small. A multicenter registry of 709 patients who underwent rotational atherectomy indicates high procedural success (95%) and low rates of death (0.9%), MI (5.2%), and emergency CABG (1.7%); all these rates are similar to those for angioplasty. A restenosis rate of 37% was documented in patients six months after rotational atherectomy.

The transluminal extraction catheter, designed to excise and extract atherosclerotic material, has been applied primarily to degenerating saphenous vein grafts and thrombus-containing lesions. It consists of a flexible hollow tube, the distal end of which comprises two blades. Once activated the tube spins at 750 rpm, cutting through the plaque and thrombus with rotating blades. The resultant debris is aspirated by the catheter into an external vacuum bottle (see figure 4.10). A multicenter registry reports an 88% procedural success rate, with major complications occurring in 5.7% of patients. The risk of death, MI, emergent CABG, and vessel perforation after transluminal extraction was 2.2%, 1.3%, 2.3%, and 1%, respectively. Restenosis rates after transluminal extraction range from 45% to 51% in native coronary arteries and 46% to 53% in vein grafts (9).

Other Catheter-Based Interventional Devices

Other new catheter devices have been developed that have mechanisms similar to those of atherectomy catheters or stents. However, instead of mechanical excision of the atherosclerotic material, thermal, photochemical, or acoustic energy is used to ablate coronary lesions. Although several types of ablative techniques are currently under investigation (thermal balloon angioplasty and therapeutic ultrasound), only the excimer laser has been approved by the FDA for coronary revascularization. Laser angioplasty devices directly ablate atherosclerotic lesions by melting or vaporizing tissue. The excimer coronary laser system transmits high-intensity, short-duration pulses of ultraviolet light through a fiber optic bundle catheter to the coronary stenosis, where laser energy is absorbed with the proteins of the plaque. In more than 3500 patients undergoing excimer laser coronary angioplasty, procedural success, defined by increased lumen size, was near 90%; however, adjunctive angioplasty was required in up to 95% of cases to improve the lumen size. Although rates of in-hospital death, MI, and emergent bypass surgery were similar to those observed with balloon angioplasty, coronary dissection and perforation were higher with the laser. Angiographic restenosis occurred in 46% of patients following successful excimer laser angioplasty; this rate, as described earlier, is higher than the 30-40% rate of restenosis observed with angioplasty alone. Clearly, improvement in laser technology is necessary before the use of this type of intervention becomes more common.

While these catheter-based interventional procedures are used extensively for the treatment of "stable" CAD, their use for acute MI is also increasing. It is often said that during an acute MI, "time equals muscle." In other words, the sooner blood flow can be restored to the myocardial tissue, the less chance there is for damage (necrosis) of the tissue. The other approach to rapidly improving blood flow through an occluded coronary artery during an acute coronary event is administration of thrombolytic drugs (see table 4.6). Thrombolytic agents (often called "clot-busters") such as streptokinase or tissue plasminogen activator are injected into the bloodstream to break up the thrombus (blood clot) that has formed in response to the rupture of a coronary lesion.

Novel Emerging Therapies for Severe Coronary Artery Disease

Because of an unacceptably high operative mortality rate, a significant number of patients with severe CAD are not good candidates for the surgical and interventional procedures we have reviewed. Consequently, several alternative therapies to improve myocardial blood flow and reduce anginal symptoms in patients with severe CAD are currently being investigated. One such approach involves the injection of growth factors—vascular endothelial growth factor or fibroblast growth factor (FGF-1). Initial studies indicated that these growth factors were able to stimulate new artery formation in the lower leg. Current studies are under way to determine whether the formation of new coronary arteries (referred to as **angiogenesis**) is possible. In a preliminary study (35), 20 of 40 patients who underwent CABG for multivessel coronary disease also received an injection of FGF-1 into the myocardium during the surgery (figure 4.11). The 20 subjects in the control group underwent a similar procedure but received an injection of heat-denatured (thus ineffective) FGF-1. After 12 weeks, coronary angiography revealed the presence of a capillary network sprouting out from the LAD coronary

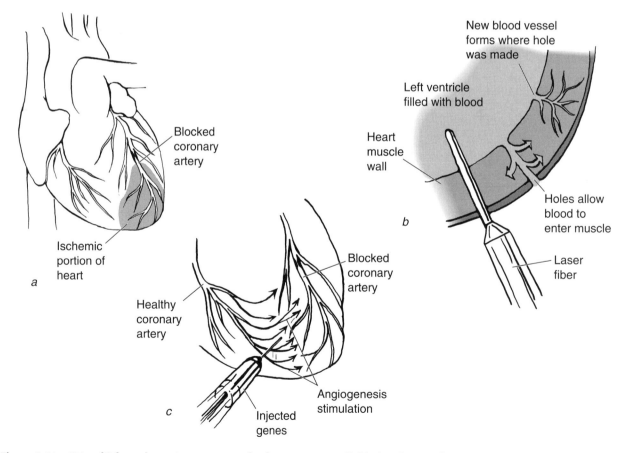

Figure 4.11 "Novel" therapies to treat severe and refractory myocardial ischemia. *(a)* A heart with severe ischemia to an area of the left ventricle (gray area) due to a significant occlusion of the left anterior descending coronary artery. *(b)* The process of transmyocardial revascularization (TMR) in which small holes are made through the myocardium by a laser applied to the heart surface. *(c)* Gene therapy delivered directly to the myocardium (also done via catheter in coronary artery) to provide growth factors to stimulate angiogenesis.

artery into the myocardium in all 20 patients who had received active FGF-1. The control group showed no evidence of new vessel formation. Research is currently being conducted to determine whether the growth of new vessels actually reduces symptoms (angina), improves exercise capacity, or reduces the need for surgical interventions. At least one company has developed a catheter-based delivery system for the growth factor, potentially eliminating the need for injection during a more invasive heart surgery.

A promising novel approach for reducing myocardial ischemia involves creating small channels in the myocardium with a laser. The technique, called transmyocardial revascularization (TMR), entails applying a carbon dioxide or holmium laser directly to the beating heart to make ten to fifty 1-mm channels (figure 4.11). These channels presumably allow oxygen-rich blood from the left ventricle to perfuse the myocardial cell, reducing the ischemia caused by occluded coronary arteries. A recent multicenter U.S. trial (36) randomly assigned 275 patients with severe, refractory angina pectoris to a treatment group (TMR and anti-anginal medications) or a control group (just medications). After one year, 76% of the treatment group had an improvement in angina symptoms, compared with only 32% in the control group. Of the patients having the TMR procedure, 54% had no cardiac events during this period, and 61% had no hospitalization for heart problems. In contrast, only 31% of the control group made it through the year without heart problems, and only 33% were able to stay out of the hospital. While the results of this study and others using TMR are encouraging, the long-term effects are yet to be determined and the procedure is still considered experimental.

SUMMARY

To further reduce the morbidity and mortality associated with CAD, more time and effort must focus on primary prevention, particularly in children and young adults, when lifestyle habits are being formed and when the CAD process begins. Risk factors for CAD should be assessed early in life and on a regular basis across the life span. The presence of one or more risk factors should initially be treated with appropriate lifestyle modification and, when warranted, with medications. Secondary prevention should also initially focus on aggressive risk factor management with appropriate lifestyle changes, medical therapy, or both. There is no question that control of risk factors through lifestyle changes, medication, or both can prevent and reverse CAD. The disadvantage to this approach is time—thus there will always be a need for more rapid, often emergent, treatment of CAD. In fact, these surgical and interventional approaches are a primary reason for recent trends showing a reduction in cardiovascular deaths. A variety of established interventional and surgical techniques are commonly used, and a number of novel therapies are under investigation.

Case Study 1
Primary Prevention: Low Risk

Interventions and Referral

As described in chapter 3, this individual was referred to the primary prevention program at Ball State University to modify risk factors for CAD (hypertension and hyperlipidemia). If lifestyle modifications are ineffective after 6 to 12 months, medications may be warranted for treatment of hypertension and/or hyperlipidemia. Chapter 8 will describe the changes made by this individual through his participation in the Primary Prevention (Adult Fitness) Program at Ball State University.

Case Study 2
Primary Prevention: High Risk

Interventions

With the presence of only minimal CAD (40% in LAD), no catheterization-based interventions were employed. Patient was discharged on the following medications:

Insulin

Potassium 20 meq once a day (qd)

Lasix 80 mg qd

Aspirin 325 mg qd

Nitroglycerin (sublingual) as needed for angina

Atenolol 25 mg qd

Lipitor 20 mg gd

Referral

Met with cardiac wellness coordinator and was referred to cardiac rehabilitation program with the primary objective of limiting progression of CAD by aggressively managing CAD risk factors. Chapters 8 and 10 will describe the significant changes this individual made in his lifestyle.

Case Study 3
Secondary Prevention: Post-MI and PTCA/Stent

Interventions

Patient underwent angioplasty and stent placement to a 95% stenosis in the distal circumflex coronary artery (see figure 4.9). Three separate inflations of the balloon were performed for a total of 109 s. Post-intervention stenosis was 0% (refer to figure 4.8 *a* and *b*). Patient was given ReoPro, Plavix, and aspirin. Patient was discharged the next day on the following medications:

Aspirin 325 mg qd

Lipitor 10 mg qd

Atenolol 50 mg qd

Vitamin E 400 IU qd

Nitroglycerin sublingual as needed

Plavix 75 mg qd for four weeks

Referral

Met with cardiac wellness coordinator and was referred to cardiac rehabilitation program to reduce risk for future cardiac events by aggressively managing risk factors. Chapters 8 and 10 document the changes this individual made in his lifestyle.

GLOSSARY

Angiogenesis: the growth of new blood vessels, such as those in the heart

Anticoagulant: a substance (usually a medication) that inhibits the body's natural blood clotting response

Brachytherapy: the emerging use of radiation to prevent smooth muscle cell growth in blood vessels (particularly coronary arteries after percutaneous transluminal coronary angioplasty)

Cardiomyopathy: failure of the myocardium to contract adequately; can be caused by a variety of pathologies including myocardial ischemia and infections and is generally associated with congestive heart failure

Cardioplegic solution: a solution poured on the heart during a coronary artery bypass graft procedure to arrest the heart, making the procedure easier and decreasing the metabolic needs of the heart tissue

Extracorporeal circulation: condition in which circulation and oxygenation of blood are supported by a machine, as in coronary artery bypass graft surgery when heart and lung function is temporarily arrested

Familial disorders: a variety of genetic disorders that cause abnormal blood lipid profiles

Glycemic control: the ability to keep blood glucose in the normal range, which can be difficult for persons with diabetes (particularly those requiring insulin)

Hyperglycemia: high blood glucose levels

Left ventricular hypertrophy: a thickening of the wall of the left ventricle (which can reduce left ventricle cavity size) due to abnormal underlying pathology, most commonly hypertension

Liver function enzymes: liver proteins; elevated levels in the blood reflect potential liver damage; need to measure in individuals using most cholesterol-lowering medications because of their potential to damage the liver

Meta-analysis: a statistical method in which results of numerous studies are combined to draw conclusion

Myalgia: a painful condition of generalized muscle inflammation that is occasionally caused by the cholesterol-lowering "statins medications" (2-3% of users)

Myocardial perfusion abnormalities: conditions reflective of myocardial ischemia that can be observed on nuclear stress test results

Peripheral neuropathy: deterioration of nerve function to the hands and/or feet, often seen in individuals with poorly controlled diabetes

Restenosis: a partial or complete reocclusion of an artery that had been opened through an interventional procedure such as percutaneous transluminal coronary angioplasty

Thrombus: a blood clot that forms in a coronary artery in response to plaque disruption, often leading to myocardial infarction

REFERENCES

1. Levy, D., and T.J. Thom. 1998. Death rates from coronary disease—progress and a puzzling paradox. *N. Eng. J. Med.* 339 (13):915–917.

2. Troiano, R.P., K.M. Flegal, R.J. Kuczmarski, S.M. Campbell, and C.L. Johnson. 1995. Overweight prevalence and trends for children and adolescents. NHANES II. *Arch. Ped. Adolescent Med.* 149:1085–1091.

3. Rosamond, W.D., L.E. Chambless, A.R. Folsom, L.S. Cooper, D.E. Conwill, L. Clegg, C. Wang, and G. Heiss. 1998. Trends in the incidence of myocardial infarction and in mortality due to coronary heart disease, 1987-1994. *New Eng. J. Med.* 339 (13):861–867.

4. Berenson, G.S. 1998. Association between multiple cardiovascular risk factors and atherosclerosis in children and young adults. *New Eng. J. Med.* 338 (23):1650–1656.

5. H.C. McGill, et al. 2000. Prevalence of advanced atherosclerotic plaque high among young people in US. *Circulation* 103:374–379.

6. Update on the 1987 task force report on high blood pressure in children and adolescents. A working group report from the national high blood pressure education program 1996. *Pediatrics* 98: 649-658.

7. Executive Summary of the third report of the national cholesterol education program (NCEP). Expert Panel on Detection, Evaluation, and Treatment of High Blood Cholesterol in Adults (Adult Treatment Panel III). 2001. *J.A.M.A.* 285: (19) 2486-2497.

8. Pearson T.A., and V. Fuster. 1996. 27th Bethesda Conference: Matching the intensity of risk factor management with the hazard for coronary disease events. *J. Am. Coll. Cardiol.* 25 (5):957–1047.

9. Braunwald, E., ed. 1997. *Heart disease: A textbook of cardiovascular medicine.* Philadelphia: Saunders.

10. Shepherd, J., S.M. Cobbe, I. Ford, C.G. Isles, A.R. Lorimer, P.W. MacFarlane, J.H. Mckillop, C.J. Packard. 1995. Prevention of coronary heart disease with Provastatin in men with hypercholesterolemia: West of Scotland Coronary Primary Prevention Study Group. *New Eng. J. Med.* 333:1301–1307.

11. Downs, J.R., M. Clearfield, S. Weis, E. Whitney, D.R. Shapiro, P.A. Beere, A. Langendorfer, E.A. Stein. W. Kruyer, A.M. Gotto. 1998. Primary prevention of acute coronary events with Lovastatin in men and women with average cholesterol levels. Results of AFCAPS/TCXCAPS. *J.A.M.A.* 279:1615–1622.

12. Scandinavian Simvastatin Survival Group. 1994. Randomized trial of cholesterol lowering in 4,444 patients with coronary heart disease: The Scandinavian Simvastatin Survival study (45). *Lancet* 344:1383–1389.

13. Stephanick, M.J. 1998. Effects of diet and exercise in men and postmenopausal women with low levels of HDL cholesterol and high levels of LDL cholesterol. *New Eng. J. Med.* 339 (1):12–20.

14. deLongeril, M., P. Salen, J.L. Martin, I Monjaud, N. Delaye, N. Mamella. 1999. Mediterranean diet, traditional risk factors, and rate of cardiovascular complications after myocardial infarction. Final report of the Lyon Heart Study. *Circulation* 99:779–785.

15. Hu, F.B., M.J. Stampfer, JE Manson, E. Rimm, G.A. Colditz, B.A. Rosner, C.H. Hennekens, W.C. Willett. 1997. Dietary fat intake and the risk of coronary heart disease in women. *New Eng. J. Med.* 337:1491–1499.

16. The sixth report of the Joint National Committee on Prevention, Detection, Evaluation, and Treatment of High Blood Pressure. 1997. *Arch. Int. Med.* 157:2413–2446.

17. Paffenbarger, R.S., R.T. Hyde, A.L. Wing, I.M. Lee, D.L. Jung, J.B. Kambert. 1993. The association of changes in physical-activity levels and other lifestyle characteristics with mortality among men. *New Eng. J. Med.* 328:538–543.

18. Rubins, H.B., S.J. Robbins, D. Collins, C.L. Fye, J.W. Anderson, M.D. Elam, F.H. Faas, E. Linares, E.J. Shaeffer, G. Schectman, T. Wilt, J. Wittes. 1999. Gemfibrozil for CAD in men with low levels of HDL cholesterol. *New Eng. J. Med.* 341:410–418.

19. National Task Force on the Prevention and Treatment of Obesity. 1996. Long-term pharmacotherapy in the management of obesity. *J.A.M.A.* 276: 1907-1915.

20. Heal, D.J., S. Aspley, M.R. Prow, H.C. Jackson, K.F. Martin, and S.C. Cheetham. 1998. Sibutramine: A novel anti-obesity drug. A review of the pharmacological evidence to differentiate it from d-amphetamine and d-fenfluramine. *Int. J. Obesity* 22 (suppl. 1):518–528.

21. Hully, S., D. Grady, T. Bush, C. Fubert, D. Herrington, B. Riggs, and E. Vittinghoff. 1998. Randomized trial of estrogen plus progestin for secondary prevention of coronary heart disease in postmenopausal women. *J.A.M.A.* 280:605–613.

22. Blumenthal, J.A.,W. Jinag, M.A. Babyak, D.S. Krantz, D.J. Frid, R.E. Coleman, R. Waugh, M. Hansen, M. Applebaum, C. O'Conner, J.J. Morris. 1997. Stress management and exercise training in cardiac patients with myocardial ischemia. Effects on prognosis and evaluation of mechanisms. *Arch. Int. Med.* 157:2213–2223.

23. Rimm E.B., W.C. Willett, F.B. Hu,L. Sampson, GA Colditz, J.E. Manson, C. Hennekens, M. Stampfer,. 1998. Folate and Vitamin B_6 from diet and supplements in relation to risk of coronary heart disease among women *J.A.M.A.* 279:359–364.

24. The Alpha-Tocopherol, Beta-Carotene Cancer Prevention Study Group. 1994. The effect of Vitamin E and beta-carotene on the incidence of lung cancer and other cancers in male smokers. 1994. *New Eng. J. Med.* 330:1029–1035.

25. Vitamin E supplements and cardiovascular events in high-risk patients. 2000. The Heart Outcomes Prevention Evaluation (HOPE) study investigation. *New Eng. J. Med.* 342 (3):154–160.

26. Gordon, N.F. 1998. *Conceptual basis for coronary artery disease risk factor assessment.* In *ACSM Resource Manual.* ed. J. Reitman. Baltimore: Williams & Wilkins.

27. Ornish, D., L.W. Scherwitz, and J.H. Billings. 1998. Intensive lifestyle changes for reversal of coronary heart disease. *J.A.M.A.* 280:2001–2007.

28. Schuler, G., R. Hambrecht, G. Schlief, J. Niebauer, K. Hauer, J. Neumann, E. Hoberg, A. Drinkman, F. Bacher, M. Grunze. 1992. Regular physical exercise and low fat diet. Effects on progression of coronary artery disease. *Circulation* 86:1–11.

29. Hambrecht, R.J., J. Niebauer, and C. Marburger. 1993. Various intensities of leisure time physical activity in patients with coronary artery disease: Effects on cardiorespiratory fitness and progression of atherosclerotic lesions. *J. Am. Coll. Cardiol.* 22:468–477.

30. O'Conner, G.T., J.E. Buring, S. Yusuf, S.Z. Goldhaber, E.M. Olmstead, R.S. Paffenbarger, and C.H. Hennekens. 1989. An overview of randomized trials of rehabilitation with exercise after myocardial infarction. *Circulation* 80:234–244.

31. Oldridge, N.B., G.H. Guyatt, M.E. Fischer, and A.A. Rimm. 1988. Cardiac rehabilitation after myocardial infarction: Combined experience of randomized clinical trials. *J.A.M.A.* 260:945–950.

32. Haskell, W.L., E.L. Alderman, J.M. Fair, D.J. Maron, S.F. Mackay, R.H. Superko, P.T. Williams, I.M. Johnstone, M.A. Champagne, R.M. Krauss. 1994. Effects of intensive multiple risk factors reduction on coronary atherosclerosis and clinical cardiac events in men and women with coronary artery disease. The Stanford Coronary Risk Intervention Project (SCRIP). *Circulation* 89:975–990.

33. Smith, S.C., S.N. Blair, M.H. Criqui, G.F. Fletcher, B. Gersh, A.M. Gotto, K.L. Gould, P. Greenland, S.M. Grundy. 1995. Preventing heart attacks and death in patients with coronary disease. *Circulation* 92:2–4.

34. Malhotra, S., and P.S. Teirstien. 2000. The SCRIPPs Trial—catheter-based radiotherapy to inhibit coronary restenosis. *J. Invasive Cardiol.* 12 (6):330–332.

35. Schumacher, B., T. Stegmann, P. Pecher. 1998. Induction of neoangiogenesis in ischemic myocardium by human growth factors: First clinical results of a new treatment of coronary heart disease. *Circulation* 97:645–650.

36. Allen, K.B., R.D. Dowling, T.L. Fudge, P. Schoettle, S.L. Selinger, D.M. Gangahar, W.W. Angell, M.R. Petracek, C.J. Shaar, and W.W. O'Neill. 2000. Comparison of transmyocardial revascularization with medical therapy in patients with refractory angina. *New Eng. J. Med.* 341 :1029–1036.

PART II

Practical Applications to Coronary Artery Disease Prevention and Rehabilitation

CHAPTER 5

Electrocardiography

BEHAVIORAL OBJECTIVES

- To be able to describe basic electrophysiological events that occur at the cardiac cell membrane
- To be able to describe the basic lead systems used to record resting and exercise electrocardiograms
- To be able to differentiate between normal and abnormal resting electrocardiograms
- To be able to describe a systematic approach to interpreting electrocardiogram recordings

An **electrocardiogram** (ECG) is a graphic recording of the electrical currents that move through the heart during the cardiac cycle. Exercise professionals working in the clinical setting should possess the knowledge to differentiate normal versus abnormal ECG tracings at rest and during exercise. This chapter begins with a section on general principles underlying the recording of the surface ECG and then describes both normal and abnormal patterns in the resting ECG. The focus is on a systematic approach to the interpretation of ECGs.

Although an ECG is considered a medical test most often interpreted by licensed physicians, other health care professionals—exercise physiologists included—routinely encounter ECGs in the clinical setting and need to possess the technical skills necessary to record various types of ECGs, as well as fundamental ECG interpretative skills. Exercise professionals typically encounter two basic forms of ECGs—a 12-lead ECG (figure 5.1) and a single-lead rhythm strip (figure 5.2). Both resting and exercise 12-lead ECGs are used as part of the screening process prior to a patient's participation in a structured exercise program, whereas single-lead rhythm strips are more commonly used to monitor a patient's ECG during exercise training sessions.

ELECTROCARDIOGRAM FUNDAMENTALS

Although we record the electrical forces moving through the heart using **electrodes** attached to the skin surface (often referred to as the surface ECG), the biochemical basis for these electrical forces originates at the level of a cardiac muscle cell membrane. The study of these electrical events is called electrophysiology, and students need a fundamental understanding of cardiac cell electrophysiology so that they can relate what they see on the printed ECG to electrical events occurring within the heart.

Cardiac Electrophysiology and the Surface Electrocardiogram

Cardiac cell membranes are basically electrical conductors designed to stimulate the underlying cell into action. The electrical forces that stimulate the heart muscle cells to contract are conducted throughout the heart by the movement of ions across cardiac cell membranes. An ion is an atom that carries an electrical charge due to the loss or gain of electrons from its nucleus. Ions that carry a positive charge are called cations, and those that carry a negative charge are called anions. With respect to cardiac electrophysiology, sodium (Na^+), potassium (K^+), and calcium (Ca^{++}) are important cations, and chloride (Cl^-) is an important anion. When the cardiac cell is in the resting state (figure 5.3), Na^+, Ca^{++}, and Cl^- are in greater concentration in the extracellular fluid compartment whereas K^+ is in a greater concentration in the intracellular fluid compartment. By movement of these ions across the cell membrane in a sequenced pattern called an action potential, the cell can alter its electrical voltage and thus control its activation.

Movement of these ions across the membrane is accomplished by one of two processes—either diffusion or active transport. These processes are illustrated in figure 5.4. Diffusion is the movement of ions from an area where they are in greater concentration to an area where they are less concentrated. This is often referred to as movement down a concentration gradient. On the other hand, active transport of ions across the cell membrane involves the movement against an ion's concentration gradient (from an area where the ion is less concentrated to an area where it is more concentrated). Diffusion of ions across the membrane occurs through specialized gates often referred to as channels (e.g., Na^+ channels or K^+ channels, etc.). These membrane channels are thought to open (allowing diffusion of the ion to occur) and close (stopping diffusion of the ion) in response to the electrical voltage of the cell membrane. Cardiac cell membranes can alter their permeability (leakiness) to the different ions, allowing one or more to diffuse across the membrane. When ions move across the membrane—by either diffusion or active transport—they carry their net electrical charge with them; and by sequencing the movement of the ions, the cell membrane can alter its electrical voltage. To understand the sequence of ionic movement, we must start with an explanation of the electrical status of the cell membrane at rest.

In the resting state, cardiac muscle cells are referred to as being polarized. This simply means that the interior of the cell—referred to as the intracellular compartment—is electrically more negative than the exterior of the cell, which is referred to as the extracellular compartment. This electrical difference at rest, often referred to as the resting membrane potential (RMP), is extremely important for the optimal functioning of the cardiac cell. How does the cell develop this negative charge on the inside? Two phenomena contribute

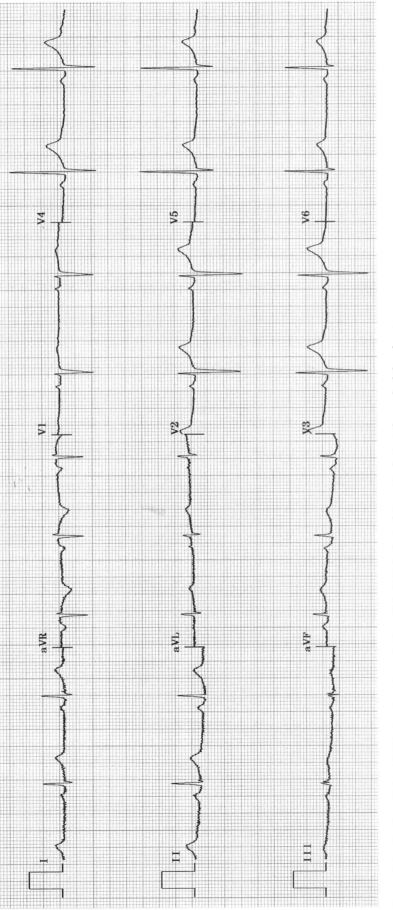

Figure 5.1   Resting 12-lead ECG showing sinus rhythm. This ECG is that of Case Study 1 at the end of the chapter.

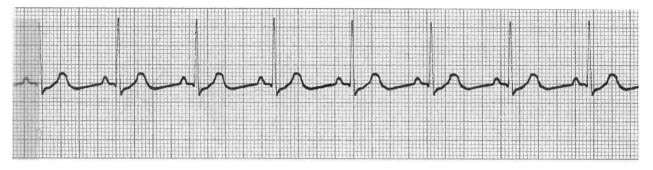

Figure 5.2   Single lead rhythm strip showing normal sinus rhythm.

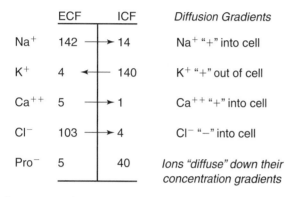

Figure 5.3   Distribution of ions along the cardiac cell membrane and diffusion gradients for movement of ions into and out of the cell.

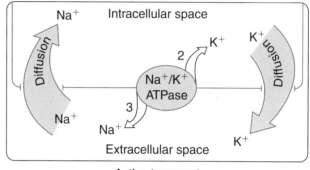

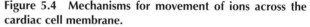

Figure 5.4   Mechanisms for movement of ions across the cardiac cell membrane.

Reprinted, by permission, from Richards et al., *A simple approach of electrocardiography* (Philadelphia: W.B. Saunders), 9, 84.

to the development of the net negative charge at rest. First, a specialized active transport pump (Na^+/K^+ ATPase pump) located along the cardiac cell membrane exchanges three Na^+ ions for two K^+ ions, effecting an unequal trade of positive charges across the membrane. This type of physiological pump is often referred to as an electrogenic pump, because as it extracts more positive charges from the cell than it replaces, it leaves the cell interior electrically negative relative to the exterior compartment. Second, the cardiac cell membrane is selectively permeable to the K^+ ion (not the other ions) in the resting state; this results in some diffusion of K^+ ions down their concentration gradient and out of the cell. When diffusion occurs, the positive charge associated with the K^+ ion also leaves the cell and contributes to a more negative charge on the inside. Collectively, the electrogenic pump and the diffusion of the K^+ ion leave the resting cardiac muscle cell voltage about −90 millivolts (mV). Thus, the membrane is said to be polarized (i.e., negative on the inside and positive on the outside). This sets the stage for the cardiac cell to be stimulated.

The process of depolarization-repolarization along the cardiac cell membrane is referred to as

a **cardiac action potential** (AP). Figure 5.5 shows an AP from a ventricular muscle cell. There are five phases to the AP, with phase 4 designated as the resting, or polarized, stage described previously. The first phase of the AP is referred to as phase 0 (zero) and is primarily the result of diffusion of Na^+ ions into the cell. These Na^+ ions bring their positive charges into the cell, and the membrane voltage very quickly reverses from negative to positive. This process is called **depolarization** of the membrane. Depolarization of the cell membrane stimulates the cardiac muscle cell into action (i.e., contraction), but also creates the need to return the membrane to its resting (i.e., polarized) state. The depolarization phase of the AP coincides with the P wave (in atrial muscle cells) or QRS complex (in ventricular muscle cells) of the surface ECG cardiac cycle.

Following stage 0, the remaining stages of the AP relate to the process of restoring the resting membrane voltage, which is termed **repolarization**. Phase 1 is referred to as early repolarization, during which, as shown in figure 5.5, the membrane voltage begins to recover to a more negative value (moves downward on the graph). This is the result of several changes along the mem-

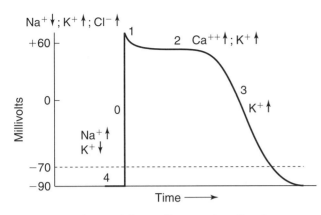

Figure 5.5 Phases of the cardiac muscle cell action potential.

brane. First, the Na$^+$ channels close as the membrane voltage rises over 0 mV, and both the K$^+$ and Cl$^-$ channels begin to open. When K$^+$ and Cl$^-$ begin to diffuse through their respective channels, K$^+$ will carry its positive charge out of the cell and Cl$^-$ will carry its negative charge into the cell. Both processes contribute to a return of the cell interior to a more negative state. The Ca^{++} ion channels along the membrane are also triggered during phase 0, but they are slower to respond than the K$^+$ and Cl$^-$ channels. Because the Ca^{++} channels are slower, diffusion of the Ca^{++} ion begins slightly after onset of K$^+$ and Cl$^-$ diffusion. When the Ca^{++} ions begin to diffuse across the membrane, they carry their positive charge into the cell. This is phase 2 of the AP, or the plateau phase, as the membrane voltage is stabilized (i.e., flat line on the recording of the AP in figure 5.5) for a brief period of time. The membrane is stabilized because the positive Ca^{++} ions diffusing into the cell are offset by the positive K$^+$ ions moving out of the cell. This period of voltage stabilization is very important to normal cardiac cell function because for a brief period of time it actually keeps the membrane from repolarizing. Why is this important? Optimal heart function depends on the chambers being relaxed for a certain period of time between each beat so that the chamber can fill with blood. The plateau phase of the AP briefly keeps the cells from repolarizing so they cannot respond to another stimulus. The plateau phase of the AP in ventricular muscle cells coincides with the ST segment of the surface ECG cardiac cycle.

The last portion of the ventricular muscle cell AP illustrated in figure 5.5 is referred to as rapid repolarization (phase 3). At this point in the AP, Ca^{++} ions are no longer diffusing across the membrane, but K$^+$ ions continue to do so. The positive charges leaving the cell with diffusion of the K$^+$

ion contribute to very quick return of the cell membrane voltage to a more negative state and thus the re-establishment of the RMP (i.e., at -90 mV). At this voltage, the cell is ready to be stimulated again. The rapid repolarization period of the AP in ventricular muscle cells coincides with the T wave of the surface ECG cardiac cycle.

One important feature of the AP within cardiac muscle cells (i.e., atrial and ventricular) is the rather flat slope of phase 4 (see figure 5.5). Under normal conditions, this feature keeps cardiac muscle cells from depolarizing on their own. In contrast, cardiac pacemaker cells (sinoatrial [SA] node and atrioventricular [AV] node) have the capability to initiate a stimulus on their own. This feature within heart nodal cells is referred to as **automaticity,** and is the result of a gradual depolarization of the cell membrane during phase 4 that is termed diastolic depolarization (figure 5.6). You should note that the RMP for the SA nodal cell membrane is less negative than that for muscle cells (–60 mV vs. –90 mV) and that the less negative RMP results in an increased leakiness to both Na$^+$ and Ca^{++} ions. Diffusion of these ions into the cell causes the membrane to gradually depolarize between action potentials and eventually stimulates the nodal cells; this in turn stimulates the right atrium and starts the heartbeat. Under conditions in which the heart is being paced by the SA node (which is most of the time), the heart rate is varied by changes in the cell membrane's permeability to ions, which in turn affect the slope of phase 4 within the nodal cells. The electrical forces in the nodal cells are so small that the electrodes placed on the skin surface cannot sense them, and therefore the surface

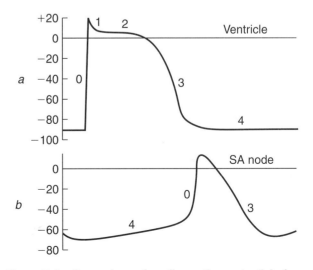

Figure 5.6 Comparison of cardiac action potentials from muscle and pacemaker cells.

ECG does not record SA or AV node electrical forces.

In summary, the surface ECG is a graphic representation of the electrical forces moving through the heart during the cardiac cycle. The biochemical basis for these electrical forces lies in the sequenced movement of ions across the cardiac cell membrane that is known as an action potential. Action potentials are point phenomena, which means that they occur at one point along the membrane. However, the AP at one point stimulates the next adjacent point and thus passes the current along the membrane in this fashion. The electrical current is passed from cell to cell by specialized structures located between the cells called intercalated discs. The electrical force is conducted from cell to cell across the entire myocardium, and this electrical current is sensed by electrodes placed on the skin.

Cardiac Conduction System

The cardiac conduction system is described in detail in chapter 2 (see figure 2.3). We will briefly review it here before discussing the sequence of activation of the heart muscle. The normal heartbeat is initiated by the special collection of nerve cells called the SA (sinoatrial) node, which is located in the upper-posterior portion of the right atrium. As mentioned previously, SA node cells have the characteristic of automaticity, meaning that they can stimulate themselves automatically and then send this electrical impulse out to the right atrium to start the heartbeat. The impulse then travels through the left atrium and down toward the AV node, which serves as a gatekeeper between the upper and lower heart chambers. Once arriving at the AV node, the impulse moves through the bundle of His, and then into two bundle branches that lie on either side of the ventricular septal wall. The impulse moves down the left bundle branch a bit faster than the right bundle branch and therefore stimulates the left side of the septal muscle mass first. The impulse continues down both bundle branches to the Purkinje fibers, which are located along the endocardial surface of both ventricles, and spreads the wave of depolarization along the endocardial surface of both ventricular free walls.

Lead Systems Used to Record the Surface Electrocardiogram

This section presents concepts related to how the ECG is recorded. Recording involves placement of electrodes on the skin surface that conduct the heart's electrical activity from the skin to the ECG machine. The electrodes are placed in specific locations as described further on. Using a combination of two or more of these electrodes, the ECG machine can be used to record 12 unique pictures of the heart's electrical activity through connections referred to as **ECG leads**—hence the 12-lead ECG. We begin by discussing the electrode positions on the body, and then describe how to prepare the individual's skin surface for the electrodes. We next consider the derivation of each of the 12 ECG leads used in the typical recording.

Electrode Landmarks and Skin Preparation

The surface ECG is recorded through placement of electrodes on the skin surface in predetermined locations depending on the type of ECG one needs to record. These electrodes sense the electrical forces moving through atrial and ventricular muscle cells. The standard 12-lead ECG requires 10 electrodes—1 on each limb and 6 across the chest (i.e., precordium) at specified landmarks. For monitoring a single rhythm strip, only three electrodes need be applied to the skin; the landmarks most commonly used are illustrated in figure 5.7. Before the electrodes are applied to the skin surface, the skin should be cleaned with ethyl alcohol that helps to remove skin oil, which can reduce the resistance to electrical flow from the skin to the electrode. For exercise ECGs, the usual procedure is to prepare the skin further by abrading the surface with a very fine sandpaper (or other abrasive pad). This process removes excess dry skin cells and helps to keep the electrode at-

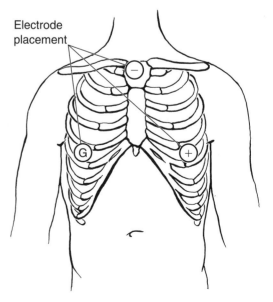

Figure 5.7 Electrode placement for single-lead ECG monitoring. This lead configuration is often used to monitor ECG during exercise training sessions.

tached to the skin during the motion and sweating that occur during exercise testing.

Once the skin surfaces are prepared appropriately, an electrode is attached to each of the four limbs (ankles and wrists), and the precordial electrodes are placed on the chest according to the landmarks identified in box 5.1. For a standard 12-lead ECG, the electrodes attached to the limbs are usually placed on the medial surface of the wrists and ankles. The locations of these electrodes are modified for exercise testing as shown in figure 5.8. This modification of electrode position for exercise was first suggested by Mason and Likar (1) in the 1960s; technicians should ensure that they locate the two leg electrodes below the rib cage, and the two arm electrodes just below the clavicle in the soft space between the anterior deltoid and pectoralis major. Moving the leg electrodes up on the rib cage and/or moving the arm electrodes more medially (i.e., closer to the sternum) may lead to a reduction of motion artifact on the ECG during the exercise test, but it will alter the diagnostic quality of the resting ECG (2). (Describing the various alterations in this modified ECG is beyond the scope of this chapter, and the reader is referred to Mason and Likar for more detail.) For this reason, one should always use a standard ECG (meaning a 12-lead ECG recorded with the limb electrodes placed out on the limbs) as the diagnostic resting ECG prior to exercise testing.

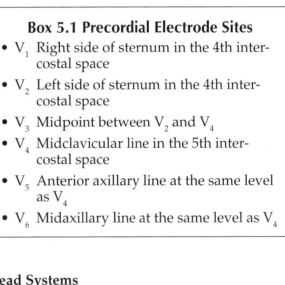

Figure 5.8 Mason-Likar modified ECG electrode placement for 12-lead ECG monitoring. This lead configuration is often used to monitor ECG during exercise testing. Lead V_6 follows the same horizontal level as V_{4-5}, but lies on the midaxillary line.

The precordial chest electrode landmarks are the same for both resting and exercise ECGs and should be located at the landmarks described in box 5.1. The fourth intercostal space is an important landmark for the precordial leads, but some technicians find it difficult to identify. A simple method for finding the fourth intercostal space is to palpate the ridge between the manubrium (triangular-shaped bone above the sternum) and the sternum. You should be able to feel a ridge if you rub your fingers in an up-and-down motion along the top of the sternum. Once you feel the ridge (referred to as the angle of Louis), you'll locate the second intercostal space just below the ridge on each side of the sternum. Count down—palpating with your fingers—two more interspaces, and you have located the fourth intercostal space, where V_{1-2} should be located.

Box 5.1 Precordial Electrode Sites
- V_1 Right side of sternum in the 4th intercostal space
- V_2 Left side of sternum in the 4th intercostal space
- V_3 Midpoint between V_2 and V_4
- V_4 Midclavicular line in the 5th intercostal space
- V_5 Anterior axillary line at the same level as V_4
- V_6 Midaxillary line at the same level as V_4

Lead Systems

The standard 12-lead ECG records the heart's electrical activity in two anatomic planes, the frontal and horizontal planes. As illustrated in figure 5.9, the frontal plane can be described as a plane that runs through the body in such a way that it splits the body into front (anterior) and back (posterior) segments. The horizontal plane can be described as a plane that splits the body into upper (superior) and lower (inferior) segments at heart level. The four limb electrodes are used to derive the ECG leads in the frontal plane, while the horizontal plane is visualized on the ECG by the six precordial electrodes.

Frontal-plane leads
Six of the 12 ECG leads view the heart's electrical forces in the frontal plane. The six frontal-plane leads are further designated as either standard (I, II, and III) (figure 5.10a) or augmented (aVR, aVL,

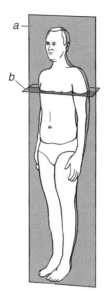

Figure 5.9 Anatomic planes [(a) frontal plane; (b) horizontal plane] derived from the surface electrodes placed on the limbs and chest.

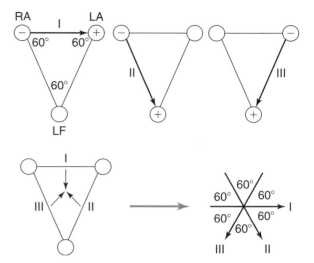

Figure 5.10 (a) Derivation of the three standard ECG leads in the frontal plane. (b) Frontal-plane standard leads forming a triaxial lead system.

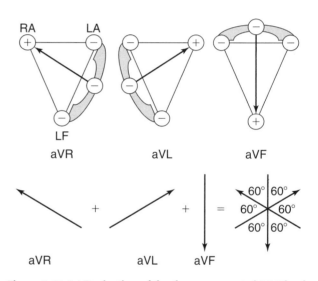

Figure 5.11 (a) Derivation of the three augmented ECG leads in the frontal plane. (b) Frontal-plane augmented leads forming a triaxial lead system.

and aVF) (figure 5.11a). Each lead visualizes the heart's electrical forces from a different location in a 360° circle within the frontal plane of the body. Each standard lead has one positive and one negative electrode. For example, lead I is derived by using the left arm electrode as the positive one and the right arm electrode as the negative one. Standard lead II also uses the right arm as the negative electrode, but uses the left foot as the positive one. And finally, standard lead III uses the left arm as the negative and the left leg as the positive electrode. Varying the location of the positive electrode allows us to view the electrical forces from a different perspective in the frontal plane. As depicted in figure 5.10a, a straight line between the two electrodes, with an arrow pointing to the positive one, serves as the lead axis or geometrical orientation in the frontal plane. This becomes an important feature of each ECG lead as we proceed through the rest of this section and beyond. In addition, the standard leads I, II, and III form an equilateral triangle (three 60° angles), which is known as Einthoven's triangle after the German physician who developed the first ECG in 1903. And finally, as illustrated in figure 5.10b, moving the three standard lead axes inward to where they would hypothetically bisect at heart level transfers the 60° angles to the center of the frontal plane, which results in the end of each lead axis being separated by 60° from the adjacent axes in the 360° frontal-plane circle. This is often referred to as a triaxial (three axes) reference system in the frontal plane.

The other three leads in the frontal plane are referred to as augmented leads, as their voltage

is amplified or augmented by the ECG machine. These leads are illustrated in figure 5.11, a and b. The three augmented leads are derived by using one of the electrodes (i.e., left arm, right arm, or left leg) as the positive electrode and the difference between the other two electrodes as the negative reference point. Conceptually, the negative point for these leads becomes the midpoint between the two other limb electrodes. For example, aVF uses the left leg electrode as the positive one and the midpoint between the two arm electrodes as the negative one (see figure 5.11a), so that the most negative area of the frontal plane for lead aVF is at the head. Ultimately, you will need to think of each lead axis as having a positive and negative end within the frontal plane. As is the case for the three standard leads, the three augmented leads have a 60° relationship within the frontal plane (figure 5.11*b*). When their respective lead axes bisect in the center of the chest over the heart, they too form 60° angles, with the end of each lead axis separated by 60° from the adjacent axes in the 360° frontal-plane circle. This is also an example of a triaxial (three axes) reference system in the frontal plane.

The next conceptual hurdle in understanding the orientation of the six frontal-plane leads is to see them all as a unit within the 360° frontal-plane circle. Figure 5.12 illustrates the combination of the two triaxial lead systems into one hexaxial lead system. In this arrangement, each of the 60° arcs developed by adjacent standard lead axes is bisected by an augmented lead axis, and vice versa. This means that each adjacent lead axis in the frontal-plane arrangement is removed from the next one by only 30°. And finally, so that we can refer to any point in the 360° frontal plane when describing vectors in the next section, the positive end of standard lead I is designated as zero degrees (0°) in the frontal plane, and each of the other lead axes has the degree designation illustrated in figure 5.12. You will note that as you move inferiorly from 0°, the designations are positive numbers (e.g., 30, 60, 90) until you reach 180° on the other side of the frontal plane (lead I's negative end); and as you move superiorly, the designations are negative. We encourage you to study the figures and memorize the lead orientations, as they are very important for understanding several elements of the interpretation of the 12-lead ECG.

Horizontal-plane leads

The other six ECG leads visualize the heart's electrical forces in the horizontal plane (see figure 5.9) and are designated using a capital "V" and a sub-

script number to reflect their position in the horizontal plane (i.e., V_1 through V_6). The six leads in this plane are often referred to as the precordial leads, as their positive electrodes are located at specific landmarks across the precordium. The landmarks are described in box 5.1. The concept of a lead axis for these leads is a bit more abstract because they use one electrode as the positive reference (located at a specified position on the precordium) and the three limb electrodes (RA, LA, and LL) collectively as the negative reference. Using the three limb electrodes as the negative reference—often referred to as the Wilson Central Terminal described by Goldberger and Goldberger (3)—creates a lead axis that extends through the body horizontally, from front to back and side to side (figure 5.13). These six ECG leads provide electrical information about the heart that is clearly unique in relation to the information gathered from the frontal-plane leads. The precordial leads are closer to the heart and generally can produce greater voltages on the recording. Because all the positive electrodes for the six horizontal-plane leads are located within about one-fourth of the horizontal circle of this plane, you will see many similarities in the ECG recording for adjacent leads (e.g., V_3 and V_4, etc.). However, the extreme lead positions in the horizontal plane (i.e., V_1 and V_6) should have distinctly different wave forms that become quite useful in discriminating a normal from an abnormal pattern, which is discussed later in the chapter.

Now that you know the orientation of the 12 conventional ECG leads, we can move on to discuss how we conceptualize the electrical forces that move through the myocardium.

Cardiac Vectors

The electrical forces that move through the heart can be represented by vectors, which are typically symbolized by arrows that denote the direction

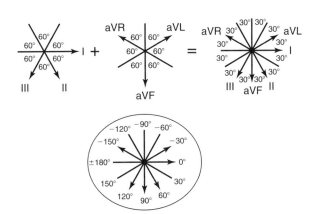

Figure 5.12 The two triaxial lead systems in the frontal-plane combined to form one hexaxial lead system.

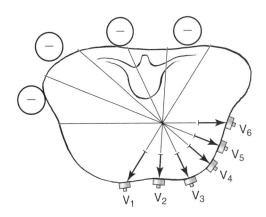

Figure 5.13 ECG lead axes for the six horizontal-plane leads.

(e.g., leftward, rightward, anterior, superior, etc.) and magnitude (i.e., size) of the electrical forces during the cardiac cycle. In a snapshot or still photograph of the electrical forces at any given time during the cardiac cycle, these forces could be summarized by a single vector (i.e., arrow) that would depict the average direction and magnitude of those forces. This would be called an *instantaneous cardiac vector*. However, for understanding the surface ECG, we usually combine or sum the electrical forces for a particular area of the heart muscle (e.g., atrial chambers, ventricular septal wall, etc.) and refer to these as *mean cardiac vectors* representing that portion of the cardiac cycle. A mean cardiac vector for the ventricles is illustrated in figure 5.14. The electrical forces during the cardiac cycle are often subdivided into five mean cardiac vectors—atrial, ventricular septal, major ventricular, posterior-basal, and ventricular repolarization. The vectors are represented on the ECG recording by specific wave forms within the cardiac cycle (figure 5.15). For example, the mean cardiac vector for depolarization of the atrial chambers is represented on the ECG by the P wave of the cardiac cycle. Likewise, repolarization of the ventricles is represented by the T wave. The vector analysis for depolarization of the ventricular muscle mass is multiphasic, which accounts for the fact that most ECG leads contain more than one wave (i.e., some combination of Q, R, and S waves) depicting depolarization of the ventricles. A detailed analysis of the direction and magnitude of each of the five mean cardiac vectors is beyond the scope of this text,

and students can refer to other sources for more details of vector analysis of the cardiac cycle. However, the general principle of vectors is important for understanding the derivation of the ECG wave forms during the cardiac cycle.

An understanding of the cardiac conduction system (described in chapter 2), which regulates the normal sequence of activation of the heart muscle, provides the student with a template for the expected series of electrical vectors throughout the cardiac cycle. When you combine this knowledge with an understanding of the orientation of each ECG lead within the frontal and horizontal planes as just described, you will be ready to begin evaluating the appropriateness of the shape and size of the wave forms on the recorded ECG. In other words, combining information about the direction and magnitude of the mean cardiac vector with knowledge of which ECG lead is being recorded will lead to an understanding of what the ECG wave form should look like. Figure 5.16 illustrates this relationship. However, from a practical point of view, when interpreting an ECG we always start with the ECG recording that has the respective leads labeled (e.g., I, II, III, etc.). Therefore, we typically begin the interpretive process with information about the size and shape of the wave forms and knowledge of which ECG lead we're analyzing. Thus the element from figure 5.16 that's missing in the practical setting when we are interpreting an ECG is knowledge about the direction and magnitude of the mean cardiac vectors. It is this aspect that we use the ECG recording to evaluate.

To put in place the last basic piece of the puzzle to understand how the electrical forces from the heart muscle produce the various waves on the ECG recording, you must comprehend three fun-

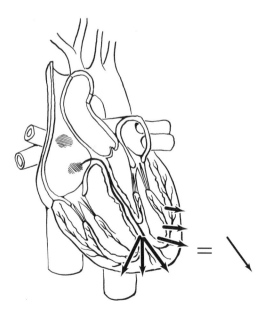

Figure 5.14 The mean cardiac vector represents the sum of all the electrical vectors for a given area of the heart muscle.

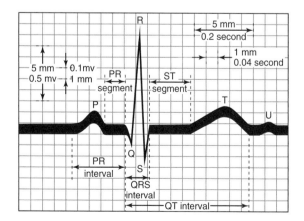

Figure 5.15 ECG cardiac cycle with various waves, complexes, segments, and intervals illustrated on the ECG paper grid.

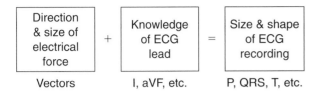

Figure 5.16   Fundamental elements for interpreting the ECG information.

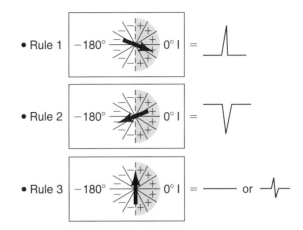

Figure 5.17   Rules for defining the ECG wave form shape based on the direction of the vector relative to the positive end of the ECG lead.

damental rules related to mean cardiac vectors and ECG wave forms. You will most likely need to refer back to the description of the ECG leads in the frontal and horizontal planes when applying these rules. These rules are illustrated in figure 5.17 using standard lead I as the reference lead:

- **Rule 1:** If an electrical force is moving toward the positive electrode in a given lead, the ECG machine will produce a positive or upright deflection on the recording. The more parallel the vector is to the lead axis, the larger the deflection will be.

- **Rule 2:** If an electrical force is moving away from the positive electrode in a given lead, the ECG machine will produce a negative or downward deflection on the recording. Again, the more parallel the vector is to the lead axis, the larger the deflection will be.

- **Rule 3:** The last rule describes the ECG result when the vector is moving perpendicular to the lead axis. In this scenario, the ECG may show one of two results. The machine will produce either a very small deflection or a biphasic deflection. The biphasic wave is the result of the "+" deflection as the force moves toward the electrode, and the "–" deflection is inscribed once the force moves under the electrode and begins the process of moving away from it.

You will note that within the figure, the frontal-plane circle for standard lead I is divided into positive and negative halves or hemispheres (half the 360° circle). The hemisphere containing the positive electrode for lead I (refer to figure 5.12) is designated as positive in the figure because any electrical force moving from the center outward in that half of the circle will produce a positive or upright deflection on the ECG (i.e., rule 1). Now, this electrical force could be a mean cardiac vector for atrial activation or the major activation of the ventricles. In either case, that electrical phase of the cardiac cycle will be viewed as a positive wave on the recording in lead I. If the vector is moving away from the positive electrode for lead

I (middle diagram in figure 5.17), the ECG will record a negative deflection (ECG rule 2). And finally, if the vector is moving in a perpendicular fashion, the ECG may show a flat line (i.e., no electrical force is sensed by the electrode) or a biphasic wave (i.e., Rule 3). Sound simple? Obviously it's not as simple as this, but these basic rules can be applied to aid in the interpretation of the ECG. One final note is that figure 5.17 illustrates these rules using lead I as the frame of reference. However, in the preceding sections we described 12 leads. Each of the 12 leads can be viewed as two hemispheres similar to that shown for lead I in figure 5.17. We can define the hemispheres by using the lead axis that is perpendicular to the reference lead. In figure 5.17, the reference lead is I, and the lead perpendicular to lead I is aVF. Therefore, aVF divides the frontal-plane circle into positive and negative hemispheres with respect to lead I. Likewise, lead I divides the frontal plane into hemispheres with respect to lead aVF. In the latter example, the lower half of the circle would be positive for aVF and the upper half would be negative. The ECG rules listed earlier apply in the same way to any of the leads. By using this concept, you can evaluate the direction of the vectors from the perspective of any of the 12 leads. We will illustrate this concept in the next section when describing the ECG criteria for a sinus pacemaker.

So far we have laid the groundwork for understanding how to interpret an ECG. The following sections describe a systematic approach to ECG interpretation that should give the beginner the tools needed to distinguish between normal and abnormal ECG patterns. It's important to point out that this chapter does not cover all the possible abnormalities that one could encounter in the clinical setting. Readers should consult the ECG textbooks listed at the end of the chapter for more complete coverage. However, we will describe most of the patterns encountered in the clinical setting that would alter our approach to, or interpretation of, exercise testing or training.

SYSTEMATIC APPROACH TO INTERPRETATION

Interpretation of 12-lead ECGs and rhythm strips should follow a systematic process to ensure that important information is not missed. Although various interpretation systems are available, they all stress the importance of reviewing information about the elements listed in box 5.2. The following section provides a template method for reviewing each ECG component that will set the stage for a discussion of abnormal patterns. In short, the student should know the normal criteria and look for them on the ECG recording. If the patterns or intervals do not meet the normal criteria, the final step is to identify the specific problem that caused the pattern to differ from the normal pattern.

Box 5.2 Elements of the Interpretation of the 12-Lead ECG

- Rate and rhythm
- P waves
- PR interval
- QRS complex
- Frontal-plane electrical axis
- Horizontal-plane transition zone
- ST segment
- T waves
- QT interval

Figure 5.15 illustrates several important features of the grid paper used to record ECGs. The units of measure on the vertical axis are millimeters, and the units of measure on the horizontal axis are seconds. Each square millimeter (referred to as a "small" box) represents 0.04 s at the standard speed setting. All ECG paper types have darker bold lines separating every fifth small box on both the vertical and horizontal axes which create larger, 5 mm square boxes. This will serve as a visual reference for several important measurements we will look at later. Electrocardiogram

recordings should be calibrated using a 1-mV electrical force, and this calibration mark should be clearly visible in each channel of the ECG recording (see figure 5.1).

Rate and Rhythm

It is advisable for students to begin an interpretation of an ECG by evaluating the heart rate, pacemaker site, and regularity of the rhythm. One can determine the heart rate in several ways, but should begin visually by locating a QRS complex either on or close to a bold line on the ECG paper and then counting the number of large boxes between adjacent QRS complexes. At the standard paper speed (25 mm/s), there are 300 of these large boxes each minute. Simply take the number of large boxes between beats and divide this into 300 to determine the QRS rate. A more precise heart rate can be calculated by dividing the number of small boxes between adjacent QRS complexes by 1500, as there are 1500 small boxes in each minute at the standard paper speed. The methods just described are most appropriate when the spacing between the cycles is consistent (i.e., regular rhythm). When one notes irregular spacing between cardiac cycles, these methods can be misleading. With irregular rhythms it would be best to count the number of cycles in a defined amount of time—most commonly 6 s—and then multiply this number by the number of like time periods in 1 min (in this instance, 10). Figure 5.18 illustrates the heart rate determination method just discussed. Most clinicians begin by calculating the QRS rate using one of these methods. If there is a 1:1 ratio between the P waves and the QRS complexes, the QRS rate will yield the P-wave rate. However, if the P:QRS ratio is not 1:1, you will need to calculate separate rates for the P waves and QRS complexes.

Next, identify the inherent pacemaker site. As most individuals who present for exercise testing or training will be in a sinus rhythm, we recommend that you look for evidence of a sinus pacemaker first. To identify a sinus pacemaker within a 12-lead ECG, simply look for positive P waves in standard lead II and negative P waves in aVR. As illustrated in figure 5.19, when the SA node serves as the pacemaker, the mean cardiac vector for atrial depolarization will be directed to the left and inferiorly in the frontal plane (i.e., away from its location in the upper, posterior section of the right atrium). According to the basic ECG rules in the previous section, the atrial vector will be moving in the positive hemisphere for lead II and in the negative hemisphere for lead aVR. Thus, the shapes of the P waves will be posi-

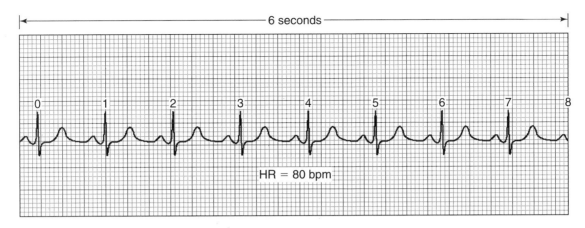

Figure 5.18   Calculating heart rate from ECG rhythm strip. There are 8 cardiac cycles in 6 s, so QRS rate is 80 bpm.

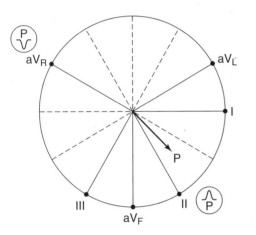

Figure 5.19   Vector for atrial activitation when SA node serves as pacemaker. Based on the vector direction, P waves are always postive in lead II and negative in lead aVR when the sinus node is pacing the heart.

tive in II and negative in aVR when the pacemaker is the SA node. If the tracing meets these criteria, the heart is most likely being paced by the sinus node and the resulting ECG is commonly referred to as a sinus rhythm. Figure 5.1 is an example of a sinus rhythm. There are exceptions to this rule, but it seems to work fairly well as an initial step in the interpretation. If the ECG doesn't meet these criteria for sinus pacemaker, move on to the other steps and evaluate information you may need for identification of the **ectopic** (i.e., outside the SA node) pacemaker site. These criteria for sinus rhythm rely on two ECG leads from a 12-lead ECG. As discussed earlier, many settings in which ECG monitoring is used rely on single rhythm strips rather than 12-lead ECGs. This is the case for monitoring of patients during exercise sessions in a cardiac rehabilitation program. In this situation, one has to know the orientation of the monitoring lead (location of positive and

negative electrodes) in order to evaluate the P-wave information related to pacemaker site. Most programs use a modified lead II for monitoring purposes, and therefore positive P waves on the recording are typically used as evidence of sinus rhythm.

Next, inspect the heart rhythm by measuring the spacing between the cardiac cycles. Cardiac rhythm may be either regular or irregular. If the spacing between cycles varies by no more three small boxes across the ECG, the rhythm is referred to as regular (figure 5.2). If the spacing varies by more than three small boxes, the rhythm is usually referred to as irregular, and this information should be noted.

P Waves and PR Interval

P waves provide important information about the presence of a sinus node pacemaker and the size of the atrial chambers. As previously mentioned, positive P waves in II and negative P waves in aVR usually indicate a sinus node pacemaker; but in addition, P waves should be evaluated for their size and shape in most leads. There are several key points to remember. P waves should be positive in leads I, II, aVF, and V$_{2-6}$ and negative in lead aVR. The other four leads are variable for P-wave direction (i.e., positive or negative). In addition to their direction on the tracing, P waves should be measured for height and width (figure 5.20a). Leads II and V$_1$ are positioned within their respective planes to provide unique information about the size and shape of the P wave. Normal sinus P waves are rarely taller than 2.5 mm and should be less than 0.12 s in duration. P waves that exceed the height criterion may reflect enlargement of the right atrium (figure 5.20b), and P waves that exceed the width criterion may reflect left atrial enlargement (figure 5.20c). Lead V$_1$ (and sometimes V$_2$) often shows a *biphasic* P

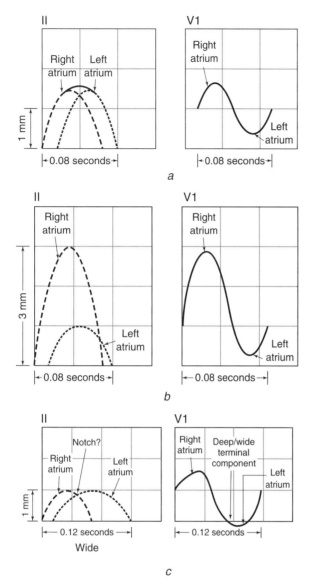

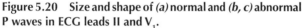

Figure 5.20 Size and shape of *(a)* normal and *(b, c)* abnormal P waves in ECG leads II and V₁.

Reprinted, by permission, from Richards et al., *A simple approach of electrocardiography* (Philadelphia: W.B. Saunders), 9, 84.

wave (figure 5.20, *a-c*), meaning that there are both positive and negative components within the wave. When this is the case, the initial component of the P wave represents the right atrium and should always be positive. The terminal negative component represents the left atrium. An enlargement of the terminal component as illustrated in figure 5.20*c* may suggest the presence of left atrial enlargement. Later in the chapter we will consider these abnormalities in more detail.

The PR interval (PRI) represents the time sequence from the beginning of atrial muscle activation (P wave) to the beginning of ventricular muscle activation (QRS complex). Therefore, the measurement of the PRI begins with the start of the P wave and ends with the start of the QRS

complex (see figure 5.15). This measurement is primarily used to evaluate the function of the AV node. The normal range for the PRI is 0.12 to 0.20 s (three to five small boxes on the ECG grid paper), which means that after leaving the SA node, the electrical impulse should arrive at the ventricles in about one to two tenths of a second. Measure the PRI in several leads, looking for a PRI within the normal range in each lead. If the PRI is within the normal range, next evaluate the consistency of the PRI across the cardiac cycles within a given lead. The PRI should be consistent. If the PRI varies, determine whether it appears to get longer (or shorter) from cycle to cycle. If the PRI is too short (<0.12 s), it may reflect a pre-excitation syndrome. If the PRI is too long (>0.20) or if it varies, it may reflect an AV nodal block. We will return to these abnormalities later.

QRS Complex, Electrical Axis, and Transition Zone

The QRS complex provides important information about the electrical activity of the ventricles. The shape, duration, and consistency of the QRS complex should be evaluated. There are several possible wave forms within the QRS complex (see figure 5.15). Negative deflections at the beginning of the complex (i.e., before an R wave) are labeled Q waves. All positive deflections are labeled R waves. Any negative deflection that follows an R wave is labeled an S wave. Even though we use the term QRS complex to describe the electrical events within the ventricles, a QRS complex does not need to have all three of these wave forms (i.e., Q, R, and S waves). In fact, most do not. Some of the ECG leads may have all three waves, and others will usually have only two of the waves. The QRS shape within a specific ECG lead depends in part on the origin of the stimulus and the sequence of activation.

Start by measuring the duration of the QRS. If you have a 12-lead ECG, we suggest that you measure the duration initially in the right precordial leads (V₁₋₃), as it is usually much easier to determine the beginning and ending of the complex in these leads. However, even if the duration measurement is normal in these leads (≤0.11 s), be sure to make the measurement in several other leads in order to ascertain that the duration is normal in the other lead groups as well. When the QRS complex exceeds the normal limit just identified, the reason may be the presence of bundle branch block, pre-excitation, or a ventricular arrhythmia of some form. We will look more closely at these abnormalities in a later section. Next, evaluate the shape and size of the QRS complex. Look for significant Q waves (a good example can be found later in the chapter with figure 5.46) and voltage criteria for either ventricular enlargement pattern. A significant Q wave is one that exceeds 0.04 s in duration and/or exceeds a depth of approximately one-fourth the size of the R wave that follows it in the cardiac cycle. Significant Q waves may reflect a previous myocardial infarction (MI). After looking for significant Q waves, measure the height of the tallest R wave in the frontal-plane leads. A height of 15 mm or more for this R wave may suggest left ventricular enlargement. In addition, calculate the sum of the S wave in V_2 and the R wave in V_5. A sum that exceeds 35 mm may also suggest left ventricular enlargement. We will return to these topics later in the chapter. For now, make a note of these findings and go to the next step.

The mean cardiac vector for ventricular activation in the frontal plane is referred to as the frontal plane QRS electrical axis. An abnormal QRS axis is associated with several ventricular abnormalities and, as you will see later in the chapter, is often listed as one of the criteria in the differential diagnosis for specific abnormalities (e.g., left axis deviation is associated with left ventricular hypertrophy). Figure 5.21 illustrates the normal range for the electrical axis. A conservative range for the QRS axis is between 0° and +90°

in the frontal plane, although some ECG texts expand this range (up to –30° to +100°). We suggest that the beginning student focus on evaluating whether the axis is between 0° and +90°, as this can be done very quickly and will rule out most ECG abnormalities associated with an abnormal electrical axis (referred to as an axis deviation). To determine whether the electrical axis is within the normal range, simply look at leads I and aVF. If the net QRS voltage is more positive in both leads (i.e., the R wave in either lead is taller than the sum of the Q and/or S waves in the same lead), then the electrical axis for the ventricles is within the normal range (figure 5.21a). If either lead has a net negative QRS, the pattern reflects an axis deviation. The term left axis deviation applies when the net deflection in the QRS in lead I is positive but the net deflection in aVF is negative (figure 5.21b). The term right axis deviation is used when the net deflection in lead I is negative but the QRS in aVF is positive (figure 5.21c). The 12-lead ECG presented later in the chapter (figure 5.43) also illustrates left axis deviation.

The concept behind the frontal-plane electrical axis is also important in the horizontal or transverse plane. However, as the precordial leads are all bunched into one-fourth of the transverse-plane circle (see figure 5.13), the important assessment

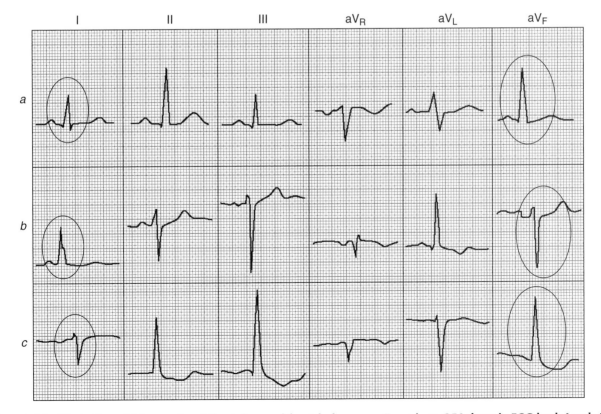

Figure 5.21 Illustration of *(a)* normal and *(b, c)* abnormal frontal-plane axes. Focus is on QRS shape in ECG leads I and aVF.

here is to identify where the QRS complex changes from a more negative complex to one that is more positive. This area is referred to as the transition zone (i.e., where the QRS transitions from negative to positive) and should lie between leads V_3 and V_4. Figure 5.1 illustrates a normal transition zone across the precordial leads. If the transitional QRS occurs in the right precordial leads (e.g., V_{1-2}), the pattern is referred to as an early transition zone; and if it occurs in the left precordial leads (e.g., V_{5-6}), the pattern is referred to as a late transition zone. An early or late transition zone in the precordial leads may be a sign of an abnormality, and this concept too will be revisited throughout the remainder of the chapter.

ST Segment, T Wave, and QT Interval

Following completion of the QRS complex, there are several distinct components of the cardiac cycle related to repolarization of the ventricular muscle mass. The first among these is the ST-segment response (see figure 5.15). The ST-segment component of the cardiac cycle begins with what's referred to as the "j point" (i.e., end of the QRS complex) and ends with the beginning of the T wave. The ST-segment shape must be evaluated at rest, but it is also a very important measurement on the exercise ECG. The ST segment should be isoelectric, meaning it should lie on the same horizontal plane as the T to P segment of the recording as shown in figure 5.22a. The measurement of the ST segment focuses on how far the recording is displaced above or below the isoelectric line. When the ST segment is above the isoelectric line, it is referred to as ST-segment elevation (figure 5.22b); when it's below the isoelectric line, it is referred to as ST-segment depression (figure 5.22c). As the measurement of interest is made on the vertical axis of the ECG paper, the unit of measure for ST-segment responses is millimeters. As with many other ECG measurements, there is a normal range for the ST-segment level on the resting ECG, but the amount of deviation accepted as within normal limits varies and often depends on the shape or contour of the ST segment. For the purposes of this text, a normal range of –0.5 to +1 mm can be used for the resting ECG, and when the measurement deviates beyond this range it should be noted and evaluated further. Beginning ECG students should interpret the ST-segment component cautiously, as certain individuals may have ST-segment displacements on the resting ECG as a normal variant. For example, young males may have as much as 3 to 4 mm of ST-segment elevation in

ST segments

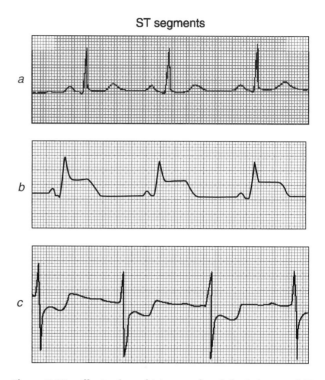

Figure 5.22 Illustration of *(a)* normal and *(b,c)* abnormal ST segment response. Focus is on deviation from the isoelectric line with *b* illustrating elevation and *c* illustrating depression of the ST segment.

the mid-precordial leads (V_{2-4}). Therefore, the interpretation of the ST segment can be more complex than other aspects of the cardiac cycle, and the student is referred to other sources listed at the end of the chapter for a more complete discussion of this topic.

Ventricular repolarization is visualized on the surface ECG as the T wave. The direction, shape, and size of the T waves should be evaluated. T waves generally mirror the direction of the QRS complex within an ECG lead (with the exception of the right precordial leads) and should be asymmetrical in shape (see figure 5.15). A quick rule of thumb for evaluating T waves is that they should be upright (i.e., positive) in leads I, II, aVF, and V_{2-6}; negative in aVR; and variable in the other four leads. T-wave height should be ≤5 mm in the frontal-plane leads and ≤10 mm in the transverse-plane leads. Deviations from these criteria should be noted as abnormal T waves and could be secondary to conduction abnormalities, related to lack of blood flow to the heart muscle (myocardial ischemia), or due to other abnormalities beyond the scope of this chapter. The significance of abnormal T waves will be discussed in more detail later. Evaluate the T waves in figure 5.1 for an example of normal T waves in a 12-lead ECG.

The final measurement of the cardiac cycle is the QT interval (figure 5.15). The QT interval is the time component from the beginning of the QRS complex (either Q wave or R wave) to the end of the T wave and varies as a function of the heart rate response. Various QT interval/heart rate tables are available in most of the recommended resources listed at the end of the chapter, specifically, the ACSM Guidelines (4); these may be used to determine the appropriate QT interval depending on the heart rate response on the ECG. Some ECG authorities advocate the use of a corrected QT interval, which is determined by dividing the QT interval measurement in seconds by the square root of the R-R interval. This measurement should typically not exceed 0.40 on the resting ECG. A visual rule of thumb for evaluating the QT interval on most resting ECGs (heart rates between 60 and 100 bpm) is that it should be less than one-half the preceding R-R interval.

Systematic Interpretation of the 12-Lead ECG

It is always recommended that ECGs be reviewed and interpreted in a systematic fashion to reduce the likelihood of missing important information. Box 5.3 contains a series of interpretation steps modified from the ACSM Guidelines (4). Whether you use this system or another series of steps that covers the same material is not as important as making sure you review all the important elements and then integrate the information to draw an appropriate conclusion about the abnormalities that may exist on the ECG. We provide systematic interpretations of the 12-lead ECGs in the Case Studies at the end of the chapter.

Box 5.3 Systematic Interpretation of the 12-Lead ECG

1. Check for appropriate calibration (1 mV = 10mm) and paper speed (25 mm/s)
2. Calculate heart rate and cardiac rhythm
3. Measure intervals (PR, QRS, QT)
4. Determine the mean QRS axis
5. Look for morphologic abnormalities of the P wave, QRS, ST segments, T waves
6. Compare the present ECG to previous ECGs when available
7. Summarize the abnormal findings

ABNORMAL CARDIAC RHYTHMS

The primary goals of cardiac rhythm interpretation are identification of the origin of the heartbeat (i.e., pacemaker site), calculation of the heart rate (or rates, if the atria and ventricles are not in sync), and the identification of any conduction abnormalities within the AV node. Clinical exercise physiologists should possess the knowledge necessary to identify and differentiate all the cardiac rhythms. Cardiac rhythm interpretation involves a narrower scope of information than is used to interpret a 12-lead ECG. Box 5.4 contains recommended steps for interpretation of cardiac rhythms. Once you've determined the information at each step, compare it with the features for the various arrhythmias presented within the chapter and identify the abnormality.

Box 5.4 Systematic Interpretation of Cardiac Rhythm Strips

1. **Rhythm:**
   Is it regular or irregular?
   If regular, go to next step.
   If irregular, note if there is a *pattern* to the irregular rhythm.

2. **Rate:**
   Calculate the atrial (P wave) and ventricular (QRS) rates.

3. **P waves:**
   Are there sinus P waves present?
   If so, where are they in relation to the QRS (in front or behind)?
   Is there 1:1 ratio for P waves and QRS complexes?

4. **PR interval:**
   Is PRI within the normal range and consistent across the strip?
   If not:
   Is the PRI consistent but too short (<0.12) or too long (>0.20)?
   Does the PRI change (become shorter or longer) across the strip?

5. **QRS complex:**
   Is QRS duration within the normal limit (<0.12)?
   If not, are sinus P waves in front of the QRS?
   Do all the QRS complexes look the same across the strip?

Sinus Rhythms

As reviewed in chapter 2, the sinus node serves as the normal pacemaker of the heart, and individuals presenting for exercise testing or entry into either primary or secondary prevention programs will likely have some form of sinus rhythm on their resting ECG. In addition, the sinus node is usually the underlying pacemaker on a rhythm strip where either **supraventricular** or ventricular ectopic beats, or AV block patterns, are observed. Therefore, it's very important for the exercise program professional to be able to recognize the presence of a sinus pacemaker. The four sinus rhythms are normal sinus rhythm (NSR), sinus **bradycardia,** sinus **tachycardia,** and sinus **arrhythmia.** The features of these cardiac rhythms are presented in boxes 5.5 through 5.8 and illustrated in figure 5.2 and figures 5.23 through 5.25.

Atrial/Junctional Rhythms

Although ectopic rhythms that originate in either the atrial muscle cells or the AV node (AV junction) have different origins, they have many similar features on the ECG and are often presented together. These arrhythmias may represent a contraindication for exercise testing or training, and

---

Box 5.7 Features of Sinus Tachycardia
- **Rhythm:** Regular
- **Rate:** Sinus node rate > 100 bpm
- **P waves:** Sinus P waves
- **PR interval:** Typically between 0.12–0.20 s but may vary according to AV node function
- **QRS complex:** Typically < 0.12 s, but may be prolonged if BBB, pre-excitation, or 3rd AVB are present

Box 5.8 Features of Sinus Arrhythmia
- **Rhythm:** Irregular
- **Rate:** Sinus node rate typically varies between 40–100 bpm
- **P waves:** Sinus P waves
- **PR interval:** Typically between 0.12–0.20 s but may vary according to AV node function
- **QRS complex:** Typically < 0.12 s, but may be prolonged if BBB, pre-excitation, or 3rd AVB are present

Box 5.5 Features of NSR
- **Rhythm:** Regular
- **Rate:** Sinus node rate between 60–100 bpm
- **P waves:** Sinus P waves
- **PR interval:** Typically between 0.12–0.20 s but may vary according to AV node function
- **QRS complex:** Typically < 0.12 s, but may be prolonged if BBB, pre-excitation, or 3rd AVB are present

Box 5.6 Features of Sinus Bradycardia
- **Rhythm:** Usually regular
- **Rate:** Sinus node rate < 60 bpm
- **P waves:** Sinus P waves
- **PR interval:** Typically between 0.12–0.20 s but may vary according to AV node function
- **QRS complex:** Typically < 0.12 s, but may be prolonged if BBB, pre-excitation, or 3rd AVB are present

the exercise professional must be able to recognize them on the resting ECG. In addition, they may occur during an exercise test or session and therefore may represent test or exercise session termination criteria. The most benign form of atrial/junctional arrhythmias is premature beats that have an origin in either location. These are referred to as premature atrial or junctional contractions (i.e., PACs or PJCs) (figure 5.26). They are typically seen in the setting of a sinus pacemaker and generally require no special treatment. However, when either the atrial or the junctional areas establish pacemaker activity, the plot thickens, and it will be necessary to make a decision whether to stop or defer the test or exercise session.

The first step in this process is to recognize the arrhythmia in either the resting or exercise ECG. The atrial arrhythmias in this category are *atrial tachycardia, atrial flutter,* and *atrial fibrillation.* The junctional arrhythmias are *escape junctional rhythm* and *junctional tachycardia.* Again, because of the similarities between atrial and junctional tachycardia, many clinicians use the term supraventricular tachycardia to identify a rhythm strip with the features of either arrhythmia. The features of the various junctional/atrial arrhythmias are presented in boxes 5.9 through 5.13, and example ECG strips are provided in figures 5.26 through 5.30.

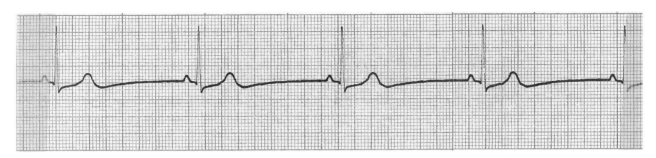

Figure 5.23   Sinus bradycardia. See box 5.6 for features.

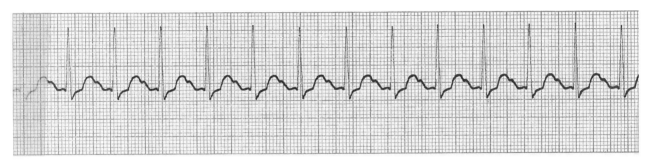

Figure 5.24   Sinus tachycardia. See box 5.7 for features.

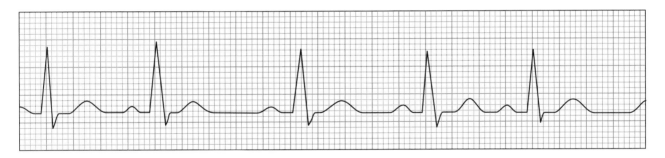

Figure 5.25   Sinus arrhythmia. See box 5.8 for features.

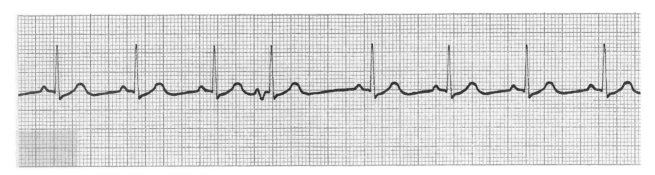

Figure 5.26   Sinus rhythm with premature supraventicular contraction.

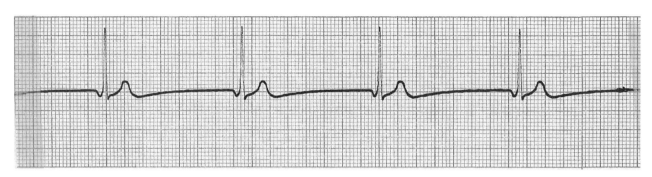

Figure 5.27   Junctional escape rhythm. See box 5.9 for features.

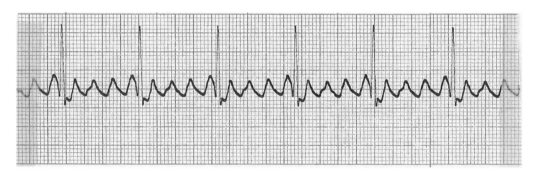

Figure 5.28   Junctional tachycardia. See box 5.10 for features.

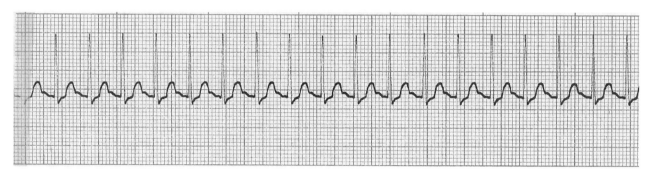

Figure 5.29   Atrial flutter. See box 5.12 for features.

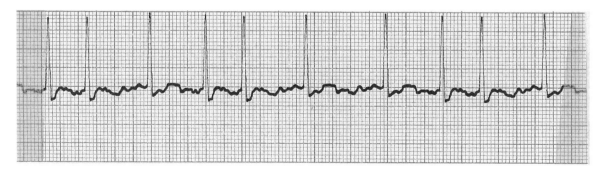

Figure 5.30 Atrial fibrillation. See box 5.13 for features.

Box 5.9 Features of Junctional Escape
- **Rhythm:** Regular
- **Rate:** Usually between 40–60 bpm
- **P waves:** If present, will be inverted; may be in front of, within, or after QRS complex
- **PR interval:** If present, < 0.12 s, consistent
- **QRS complex:** < 0.12 s, unless BBB, pre-excitation, or 3rd AVB are present.

Box 5.10 Features of Junctional Tachycardia
- **Rhythm:** Regular
- **Rate:** Varies between 60–180 bpm; rates of 60–100 referred to as *accelerated junctional rhythm*
- **P waves:** If present, will be inverted; may be in front of, within, or after QRS complex
- **PR interval:** If present, < 0.12 s, consistent
- **QRS complex:** < 0.12 s, unless BBB, pre-excitation, or 3rd AVB are present.

Box 5.11 Features of Atrial Tachycardia
- **Rhythm:** Regular
- **Rate:** Varies between 150–250 bpm
- **P waves:** May be lost in T wave of preceding beat; usually 1:1 ratio (P:QRS) but may be 2:1
- **PR interval:** If measurable usually 0.12–0.20 s, consistent
- **QRS complex:** < 0.12 s, unless BBB, pre-excitation, or 3rd AVB are present.

Box 5.12 Features of Atrial Flutter
- **Rhythm:** Regular
- **Rate:** Atrial ~ 250–350 bpm; ventricular rate varies based on P:QRS ratio (i.e., 3:1, 4:1, etc.)
- **P waves:** Sawtooth pattern between QRS complexes
- **PR interval:** N/A
- **QRS complex:** < 0.12 s, unless BBB, pre-excitation, or 3rd AVB are present.

Box 5.13 Features of Atrial Fibrillation
- **Rhythm:** Grossly irregular
- **Rate:** Atrial > 350 bpm; ventricular rate varies based on AV node function
- **P waves:** No discernable sinus P waves; may see atrial fibrillatory waves between QRS complexes
- **PR interval:** N/A
- **QRS complex:** < 0.12 s, unless BBB, pre-excitation, or 3rd AVB are present.

Ventricular Rhythms

The ventricular arrhythmias are more serious than their supraventricular form (i.e., ventricular tachycardia is more serious than supraventricular tachycardia) and often represent either a contraindication to or termination criteria for exercise testing or training. A common thread for all ventricular arrhythmias is a wide QRS complex. The arrhythmias in this category include premature ventricular contractions (PVCs), ventricular escape, tachycardia, and fibrillation. The most common of these during exercise testing are PVCs. Isolated PVCs may be observed in 30% to 40% of apparently healthy individuals during exercise testing (4). When PVCs are observed on the resting or exercise ECG, they should be classified according to their shape (unifocal vs. multifocal) and frequency (occasional, frequent, bigeminal, trigeminal, couplets, etc.). Unifocal PVCs are those that originate from the same site (i.e., single focus) within the ventricles and therefore look the same on the ECG (figure 5.31a). The term multifocal is used to describe multiple PVCs with more than one shape, as they most likely originate from different locations (i.e., multiple foci) in the ventricles (figure 5.31b). Bigeminal, trigeminal, or quadrigeminal PVCs present in a pattern in which they appear to be grouped with a few sinus beats. The prefix (bi-, tri-, etc.) denotes the number of total beats in the repeating cycle (figure 5.31c). Occasionally, PVCs will occur as consecutive beats. Figure 5.31d illustrates two PVCs in a row, referred to as a couplet.

The ventricles can also give rise to several abnormal pacemakers. Ventricular escape rhythm is a very slow, regular, wide QRS rhythm, whereas ventricular tachycardia and ventricular fibrillation are very rapid rhythms. The features of these arrhythmias are presented in boxes 5.14 through 5.16, and example ECG strips are provided in figures 5.31 through 5.34.

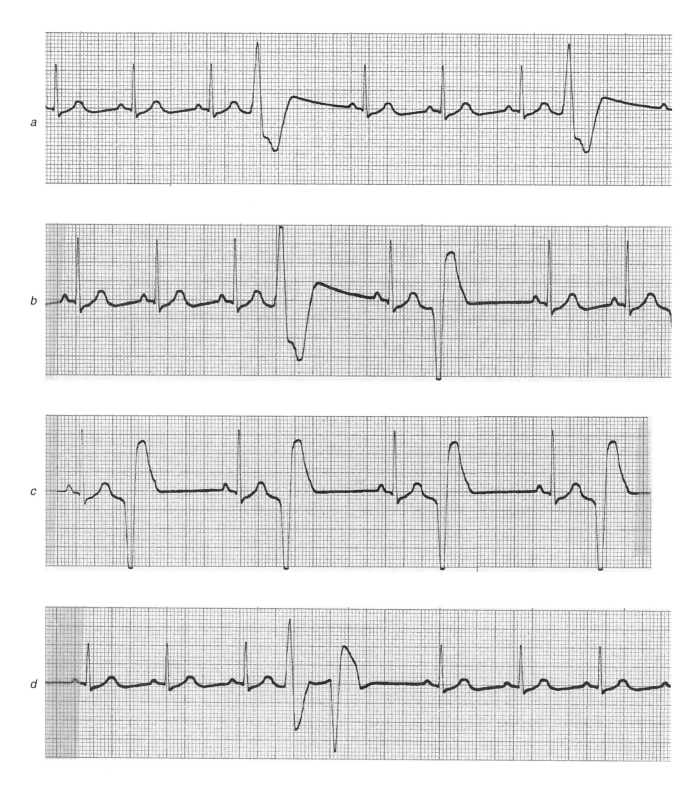

Figure 5.31 Sinus rhythm with premature ventricular contractions (PVCs): *(a)* unifocal *(b)* multifocal; *(c)* bigeminal; *(d)* couplet

Box 5.14 Features of Ventricular Escape

- **Rhythm:** Regular
- **Rate:** Usually between 15–40 bpm
- **P waves:** Absent unless there is 3ʳᵈ AVB
- **PR interval:** N/A
- **QRS complex:** ≥ 0.12 s

Box 5.15 Features of Ventricular Tachycardia

- **Rhythm:** Regular
- **Rate:** Typically 100–250 bpm
- **P waves:** Usually absent
- **PR interval:** N/A
- **QRS complex:** ≥ 0.12 s

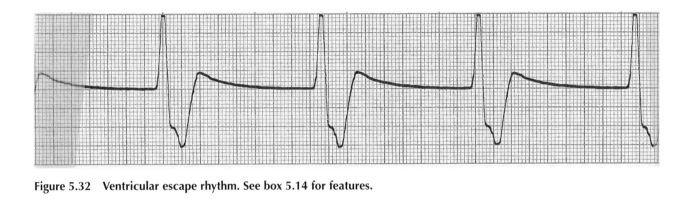

Figure 5.32   Ventricular escape rhythm. See box 5.14 for features.

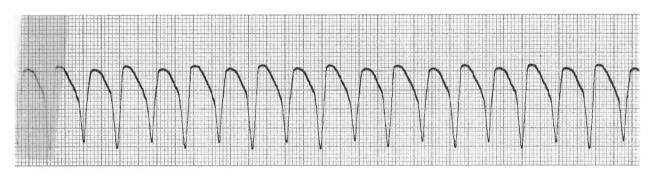

Figure 5.33   Ventricular tachycardia. See box 5.15 for features.

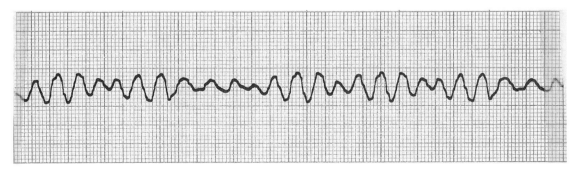

Figure 5.34   Ventricular fibrillation. See box 5.16 for features.

Box 5.16 Features of Ventricular Fibrillation

Totally chaotic with no discernable waves or complexes

Conduction Abnormalities

Conduction abnormalities stem from problems with the electrical conduction system within the heart as reviewed in chapter 2. The most vulnerable areas of the conduction system are the AV node and the bundle branches. The most common problem is a slowing or a complete block of the impulse at some level of the node or bundle branch. The ECG criteria used to identify these abnormalities relate to the timing measurements (i.e., PR interval for the AV node, and QRS duration for the bundle branch blocks). The normal criteria for the PR interval and QRS duration were identified earlier in the chapter.

Atrioventricular Blocks

When an abnormal PR interval is identified on the ECG, it may reflect a conduction abnormality at the AV node (when the PR interval is too long or inconsistent) or a pre-excitation syndrome (when PR interval is too short). These conduction abnormalities may represent a contraindication for exercise testing or training (e.g., high-degree AV block) or may interfere with the interpretation of the exercise test ECG response (e.g., pre-excitation may lead to a false-positive exercise ECG). Therefore, the clinical exercise program professional must be able to identify these conduction abnormalities on the resting ECG and also must be able to recognize them if they show up during the course of an exercise test.

Let's consider the AV blocks first. Four types of AV block patterns are seen on the ECG. The types are referred to by degree (e.g., first, second,

or third degree), with the second-degree form of AV block having two subtypes (I and II). The most benign form is the first-degree AV block, which is not actually a block at all. With first-degree AV block, all the impulses from the sinus node are conducted through the AV node, but the amount of time it takes for the impulse to get through to the ventricles is longer than normal (i.e., PR interval >0.20 s). There is still a 1:1 ratio between sinus P waves and QRS complexes. These features are summarized in box 5.17 and figure 5.35.

Box 5.17 Features of First-Degree AV Block

- **Regularity:** Depends on underlying sinus rhythm

- **Rate:** Varies according to sinus pacemaker (i.e., NSR, bradycardia, tachycardia)

- **P waves:** Sinus; 1:1 ratio with QRS

- **PR interval:** > 0.20 s; consistent

- **QRS complex:** Usually < 0.12 s; may be prolonged if BBB or pre-excitation are present

---

The second-degree AV blocks are more severe and result in some of the impulses from the sinus node not making it through to the ventricles. This results in some P waves appearing on the rhythm strip without a QRS complex following them (i.e., blocked P waves). There are two types of second-degree AV blocks, referred to as types I and II, with the distinguishing feature relating to the PR interval measurement. Type I second-degree AV block (AVB) has a gradually lengthening PR interval across several cardiac cycles until the impulse is finally blocked—which produces a blocked P wave in the ECG. This series of cardiac cycles is typically repeated across the strip with a

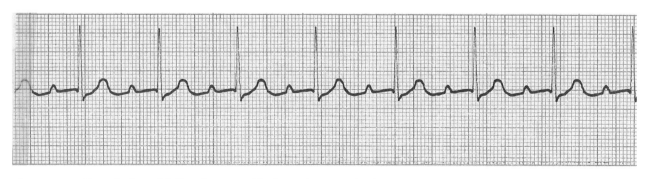

Figure 5.35   Sinus rhythm with first degree AV block. See box 5.17 for features.

Electrocardiography   135

fixed ratio of P waves to QRS complexes. Following the blocked P wave, the next impulse from the sinus node is conducted to the ventricles, and the cycle repeats. The features of type I second-degree AVB are presented in box 5.18 and illustrated in figure 5.36*a*. Type II second-degree AVB is a more severe form of block that results in many more blocked P waves on the rhythm strip. However, when an impulse from the sinus node does get conducted to the ventricles (i.e., QRS follows the P wave), the PR interval measurement is generally consistent across the ECG strip. The features of type II second-degree AVB are presented in box 5.19 and illustrated in figure 5.36*b*.

Box 5.18 Features of Second-Degree AV Block—Type I

- **Regularity:** Depends on underlying sinus rhythm
- **Rate:** Varies according to sinus pacemaker (i.e., NSR, bradycardia, tachycardia)
- **P waves:** Sinus; will have some blocked P waves
- **PR interval:** Gradually lengthening
- **QRS complex:** Usually < 0.12 s; may be prolonged if BBB is present

---

Box 5.19 Features of Second-Degree AV Block—Type II

- **Regularity:** Depends on underlying sinus rhythm
- **Rate:** Varies according to sinus pacemaker (i.e. NSR, bradycardia, tachycardia)
- **P waves:** Sinus; will have increased number of blocked P waves
- **PR interval:** May be within normal range or longer; consistent when present
- **QRS complex:** Usually < 0.12 s; may be prolonged if BBB is present

---

The most severe form of AVB is third-degree or complete heart block. In this form of AVB, none of the impulses that leave the SA node reach the ventricles, which means that the ventricles have to pace themselves. The ECG shows P waves related to the underlying sinus pacemaker, as well as QRS complexes from either an escape junctional or ventricular rhythm. Despite being on the same rhythm strip, the P waves and QRS complexes are not related to each other. With this form of AVB, the PR interval measurement is not consistent, nor does it gradually lengthen as with the second-degree type I form. The PR interval may

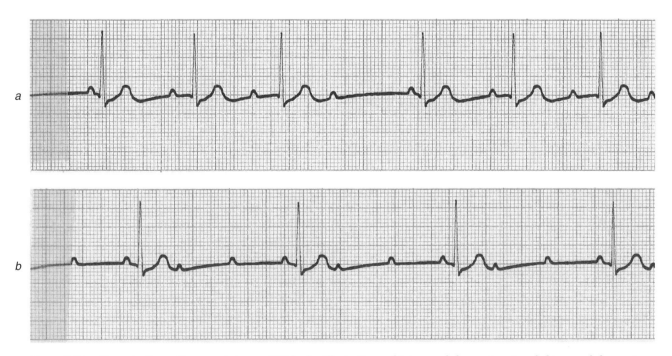

Figure 5.36 Sinus rhythm with second-degree AV blocks. Illustrations of *(a)* second-degree type I and *(b)* second-degree type II. See boxes 5.18 and 5.19 for features.

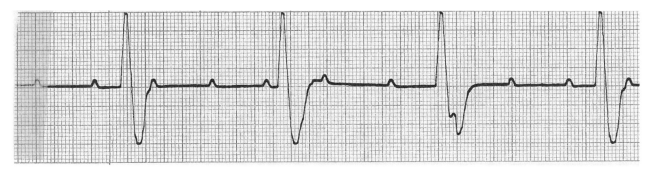

Figure 5.37   Sinus rhythm with third-degree AV block. Note the ventricular escape rhythm. See box 5.20 for features.

even look as though it is getting shorter across the rhythm strip. When this is the case, third-degree AVB is the most likely culprit. When third-degree AVB is identified, the second or escape pacemaker site should be identified and noted. This identification is usually based on the duration of the QRS complexes on the strip. Normal-duration QRS complexes suggest a junctional escape, whereas wide QRS complexes suggest a ventricular escape rhythm. Both junctional and ventricular escape rhythms were discussed earlier, and one of these patterns will be seen on the rhythm strip in the setting of third-degree AVB. The features of third-degree AVB are presented in box 5.20 and illustrated in figure 5.37.

Box 5.20 Features of Third-Degree AV block

- **Regularity:** Depends on underlying sinus rhythm and escape pacemaker location

- **Rate:** Sinus rate may vary (i.e., NSR, bradycardia, tachycardia); escape pacemaker usually at inherent rate

- **P waves:** Sinus; all P waves are blocked

- **PR interval:** Varies

- **QRS complex:** Duration depends on location of escape pacemaker (<0.12 s ~ junctional; ≥0.12 s ~ ventricular)

Pre-Excitation Syndromes

When the PR interval measurement is too short (i.e., <0.12 s), the impulse from the SA node pacemaker is reaching the ventricles sooner than normal, without the normal delay at the AV node. This is referred to as pre-excitation and is the result of an abnormal electrical connection between the atria and ventricles that, in essence, bypasses

the AV node. These specialized conduction fibers are referred to as bypass tracts because they allow the electrical impulse to bypass the normal delay at the AV node; they may be located in either atria or within the AV node itself. The identification of a pre-excitation syndrome begins with the observation of a short PR interval. When you see this, look for evidence of a slurred upstroke (i.e., delta wave) at the beginning of the QRS complex. The delta wave will often cause the QRS complex to exceed the normal duration (≥0.12 s) in several of the leads on the 12-lead ECG. Figure 5.38 illustrates a cardiac cycle with the combination of short PR interval and delta wave, and figure 5.39 illustrates these features on a standard 12-lead ECG. It is important to note that not all pre-excitation syndromes present with each of these features; the reader should refer to texts listed at the end of the chapter for a more complete description of this form of conduction abnormality. However, we should note that individuals with Wolfe-Parkinson-White syndrome

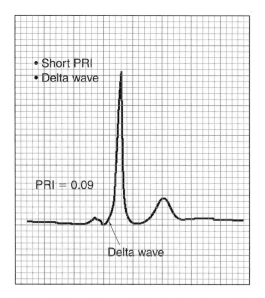

Figure 5.38   ECG cardiac cycle illustrating the result of pre-excitation on the PR interval and QRS complex.

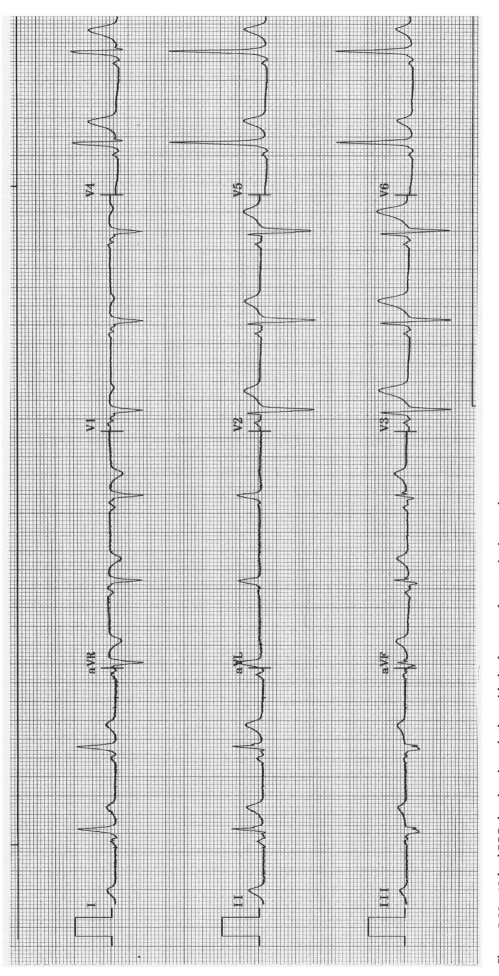

Figure 5.39 12-lead ECG showing sinus rhythm with the features of pre-excitation syndrome.

can often have ST-segment depression during the exercise test, and this may be secondary to the conduction defect, not exercise-induced myocardial ischemia. This pattern is often referred to as a false-positive exercise test. The exercise ECG is referred to as positive because of the presence of ST-segment depression, but because the ST-segment depression does not result from myocardial ischemia, the ST segment change is referred to as a "false-positive" indication of ischemia.

Bundle Branch Block

When a wide QRS is observed in the setting of a sinus pacemaker, it may reflect abnormal conduction (i.e., block) within one of the bundle branches. These abnormalities, referred to as bundle branch blocks (BBB), present some unique challenges to the exercise program professional using ECGs to monitor the heart's electrical function in exercise test or training environments. There are two major bundle branches (i.e., right and left), and either may be blocked. The term right BBB (RBBB) or left BBB (LBBB) is used to describe the pattern observed on the tracing. In addition to widening the QRS complex, each BBB pattern produces significant changes in the shape of the QRS. The changes in the QRS complex with either BBB are related to the abnormal sequence of activation of the two ventricles. The normal sequence of ventricular activation begins along the left side of the interventricular septum and causes the electrical forces to move from the left side of the septal wall to the right side. In the setting of RBBB, this initial electrical force is intact, whereas with LBBB this initial force is altered. The significance of the normal initial forces with RBBB is that the beginning of the QRS complex is also typically normal-looking. It is the late activation of the right ventricle in RBBB that produces the distinguishing feature of this abnormality. The late forces moving through the right ventricle produce a second R wave (the first R wave is the result of the normal activation of the septal wall between the ventricles) in the right precordial leads (i.e., V_{1-2}). A second R wave in a QRS complex is referred to as an R' (pronounced "R prime"), and RBBB typically shows an RSR' in the right precordial leads. The same late forces moving through the right ventricle also often result in a wide S wave in several of the lateral leads (typically I and V_6). The changes in repolarization seen with RBBB (or LBBB) are referred to as *secondary changes* in the ST segment or T waves. The term *secondary* means that the changes are due to the conduction block and are not primary changes that might reflect a lack of blood flow to the heart muscle (more on

this later in the chapter). The secondary ST-T-wave changes with RBBB are usually seen in the right precordial leads. The ECG features of RBBB are summarized in box 5.21, and a 12-lead example is presented in figure 5.40.

Box 5.21 Features of Right Bundle Branch Block
- Sinus rhythm with wide QRS
- RSR' in right precordial leads (V_{1-2})
- May see wide S waves in lateral leads (I or V_6)
- May see secondary ST-T wave changes in right precordial leads

With LBBB, the right ventricle is activated before the left ventricle, and the separation of these forces within the recording of the QRS complex produces a QRS shape distinctly different from that of RBBB. With LBBB, both the initial forces moving across the septal wall and the late forces moving through the left ventricle are oriented leftward. Therefore, a single-phase (i.e., monophasic) QRS shape is typically seen in the lateral leads (I, aVL, V_{5-6}), and the right precordial leads may show a deep QS complex. The secondary ST-T-wave changes with LBBB are typically seen in more leads than with RBBB, and are seen in the lateral leads. The differential diagnosis of right versus left BBB is often confusing for beginning students. Following two steps should help beginners distinguish between RBBB and LBBB. First, when you see a sinus rhythm with a wide QRS, look at the shape of the QRS complex in lead V_1. If V_1 has an RSR' shape, then it's very likely RBBB. If V_1 is all or mostly negative (deep QS complex), it's most likely LBBB. The ECG features of LBBB are summarized in box 5.22, and a 12-lead example is presented in figure 5.41.

Box 5.22 Features of Left Bundle Branch Block
- Sinus rhythm with wide QRS
- "M" shape or monophasic QRS in left precordial leads (V_{5-6}) and leads I and aVL
- May see small R waves or QS complex in V_{1-2}
- Will have secondary ST-T wave changes in most leads

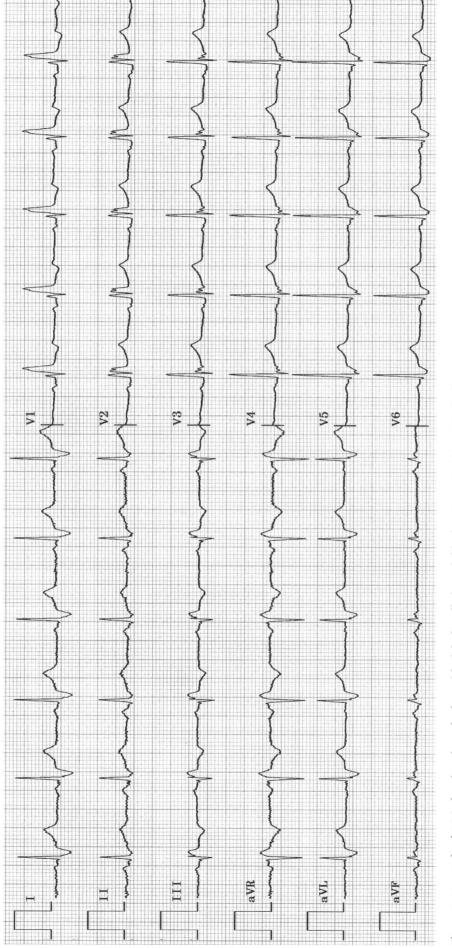

Figure 5.40   12-lead ECG showing sinus rhythm with right bundle branch block pattern. See box 5.21 for features.

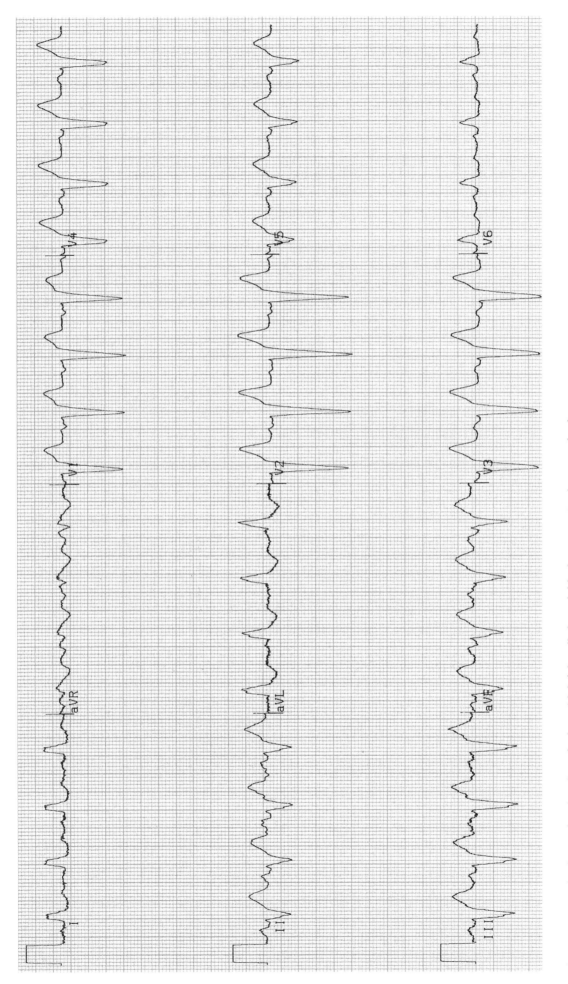

Figure 5.41 12-lead ECG showing sinus rhythm with left bundle branch block pattern. See box 5.22 for features.

CHAMBER ENLARGEMENT

There are numerous cardiovascular disorders that can place an overload on any one of the four heart chambers (hypertension, valvular stenosis, etc.). When cardiac muscle is overloaded, it responds similarly to overloaded skeletal muscle—it increases in size. This leads to an increase in the electrical forces within the affected chamber(s) and will alter the ECG recording. The identification of chamber enlargement on the ECG requires a calibrated tracing (usually 12-lead tracing), with P waves yielding information about atrial size and the QRS complexes yielding information about ventricular size. The clinical exercise professional should be able to recognize the ECG patterns that reflect atrial or ventricular enlargement on the resting 12-lead ECG.

Atrial Enlargement

As mentioned in chapter 2, the heart is normally paced by the SA node, which is located in the superior-posterior portion of the right atrium. As the impulse leaves the SA node it enters the right atrium first, then works its way leftward toward the left atrium and downward toward the AV node. This means that the initial part of the P wave on the ECG strip is the result of the electrical forces moving through the right atrium (see figure 5.20). As the impulse continues leftward it activates the left atrium, and thus the terminal component of the P wave represents the electrical forces of the left atrium. When an enlargement of one or both of the atrial chambers occurs, it affects the shape, height, duration, or mean electrical axis of the P waves on the 12-lead ECG. Earlier in the chapter we noted that P waves should be no more than 2.5 mm tall and no wider than 0.12 s. If either of these criteria is exceeded, one should consider the possibility of atrial enlargement. The changes in P-wave shape associated with right and left atrial enlargement are illustrated in figures 5.20b and c, respectively. An enlargement of the right atrium often increases the size of the P waves in the inferior leads (II, III, and aVF) to ≥2.5 mm tall. If only the right atrium is affected, the duration of the P wave should still be <0.12 s. This increase in height without an increase in duration will produce a P wave that looks peaked. In other words, look for tall, peaked P waves in the inferior leads as evidence of right atrial enlargement (figure 5.20b). The initial component of the biphasic P wave in V_1 may also exceed the height criterion. An enlargement of the left atrium increases the amount of time it takes for the impulse that leaves the SA node to reach the outer edge of the left atrium, and thus increases the duration of the P wave (≥0.12 s). This increase in duration may be seen in several leads, but is usually detectable in leads II and V_1. The increased activation time observed with an enlargement of the left atrium often results in a slight splitting of the right and left atrial forces; this can produce a notch in the P wave in several of the ECG leads. For these reasons, the combination of wide, notched P waves in the inferior or lateral leads is suggestive of left atrial enlargement (figure 5.20c).

By virtue of its location along the right side of the sternum, the precordial lead V_1 provides unique information about the size of both atrial chambers. A biphasic P wave (figure 5.20) is often seen in V_1, with the first component (which should always be positive) representing the right atrium, and the terminal component (which should always be negative) representing the left atrium. This biphasic P wave should meet the normal height and width criteria described earlier. However, a P-wave terminal component (i.e., the second phase) that exceeds 1 mm in width and depth suggests an enlargement of the left atrium. In the setting of left atrial enlargement, the overall P-wave duration in V_1 will usually exceed 0.12 s as well.

Ventricular Enlargement

As is the case with atrial enlargement, any number of pathological conditions may put an overload or strain on the ventricles and ultimately lead to ventricular enlargement. Electrocardiogram criteria used to evaluate ventricular enlargement include a shift in the mean electrical axis of the QRS, increases in size of various wave forms within the QRS, changes in repolarization (ST segments/T waves), and an increase in a measurement referred to as the *intrinsicoid deflection*. Considerable research on ventricular enlargement patterns has resulted in a wide variety of ECG criteria for the determination of enlargement of the right or left ventricle. A full accounting of the various scoring systems is beyond the scope of this text but may be found in the ECG texts listed at the end of the chapter. However, a rather simple way to evaluate the possibility of ventricular enlargement is to use the acronym AVIS. The "A" stands for axis (the mean QRS frontal-plane axis), whereas the "V" stands for voltage (enlargement of the wave forms within the QRS). The "I" represents the intrinsicoid deflection, which is defined as the time interval between the beginning of the QRS complex and the peak of the R wave in that complex (see figure 5.15). Finally, the "S" represents ST-segment/T-wave abnormalities that are often seen with ventricular enlargement. The systematic interpretation of the 12-lead ECG includes an evaluation of all these items, and when you see several of these abnormal elements within the same 12-lead ECG, you should consider right or left ventricular enlargement.

The salient features of right ventricular enlargement based on the AVIS criteria are presented in box 5.23 and illustrated in figure 5.42. Two components of the AVIS criteria provide information related to the direction of the mean electrical forces in the ventricles. When the right ventricular size enlarges to the point where it meets or exceeds the thickness of the left ventricle, the frontal-plane electrical axis and precordial transition zone will be abnormal. Right ventricular enlargement often produces a rightward shift of the frontal-plane electrical axis ($\geq+100°$). In addition, an early transition zone evidenced by an increase in the size of the R wave in the right precordial leads represents a voltage criterion for right ventricular enlargement. The size of the R wave is evaluated relative to the depth of the S wave within the QRS complex in leads V_{1-2}. A ratio of R-wave height to the S-wave height (R/S ratio) in excess of 1.0 in V_{1-2} is a voltage criterion for an enlargement of the right ventricle. An intrinsicoid deflection exceeding 0.035 s and ST-segment depression or T-wave inversion in leads V_{1-2} represent the I and S features of the AVIS acronym with right ventricular enlargement.

Box 5.23 Features of Right Ventricular Hypertrophy
- Right axis deviation
- R/S ratio > 1.0 in V_{1-2}
- Intrinsicoid deflection > 0.035 s in V_{1-2}
- Secondary ST-T wave changes in V_{1-2}

Under normal conditions, the left ventricle is the dominant of the two ventricles with regard to cardiac muscle mass. Therefore, some of the ECG changes associated with an increase in left ventricular mass are simply exaggerations of the normal QRS wave forms. The salient features of left ventricular enlargement based on the AVIS criteria are presented in box 5.24 and illustrated in figure 5.43. Once again, two components of the AVIS criteria provide information related to the direction of the mean electrical forces in the ventricles.

When the left ventricular mass increases above a normal level, the frontal-plane electrical axis will point to the left but will shift in a superior direction. This was referred to earlier in the chapter as left axis deviation ($\geq-30°$). In addition to the shift in the axis, the R-wave height in several of the frontal-plane leads may exceed 15 mm (leads I and aVL are the most sensitive for left ventricular hypertrophy). A commonly used voltage criterion in the precordial leads is a sum of the S wave in V_2 and the height of the R wave in V_5 of ≥35 mm. An intrinsicoid deflection exceeding 0.04 s and ST-segment depression or T-wave inversion in lateral leads V_{5-6} represent the I and S features of the AVIS acronym with left ventricular enlargement.

Box 5.24 Features of Left Ventricular Hypertrophy
- Left axis deviation
- R wave in frontal plane > 15 mm; sum of R wave in V_5 and S wave in V_2 > 35 mm
- Intrinsicoid deflection > 0.04 s in V_{5-6}
- Secondary ST-T wave changes in V_{5-6}

The beginning ECG student should remember that the ECG criteria for ventricular enlargement (right or left) described within this chapter are only suggestive of the presence of an enlarged cardiac muscle mass. An individual could have an enlargement of any of the four heart chambers without having the abnormality visibly apparent on the surface ECG. In addition, there are more sophisticated systems of criteria for the determination of either ventricular hypertrophy pattern. However, when any combination of the criteria in boxes 5.23 or 5.24 is present on the resting ECG, there is a suspicion of chamber enlargement, and this finding may necessitate a more thorough medical evaluation.

MYOCARDIAL ISCHEMIA, INJURY, AND INFARCTION

Entire textbooks have been dedicated to the differential diagnoses of myocardial ischemia, injury, and infarction, so a complete account of this topic is far beyond the scope of this text. Our goal here is to provide the student with some basic ECG signs often caused by either ischemia, acute injury, or infarction. Again, the textbooks listed at

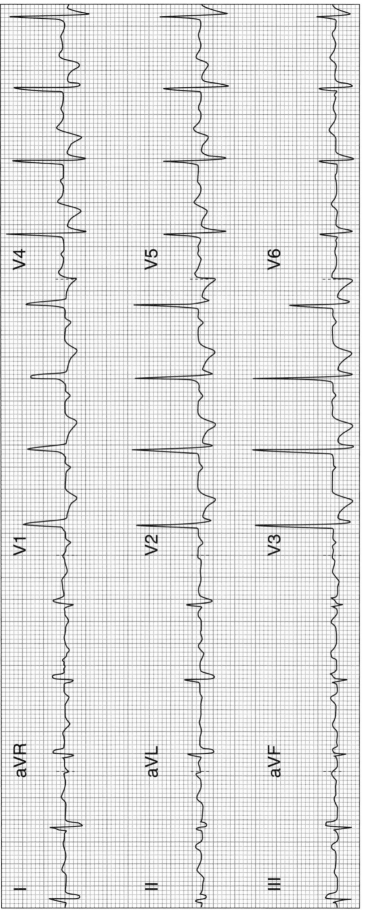

Figure 5.42   12-lead ECG showing features of right ventricular hypertrophy. See box 5.23 for features.

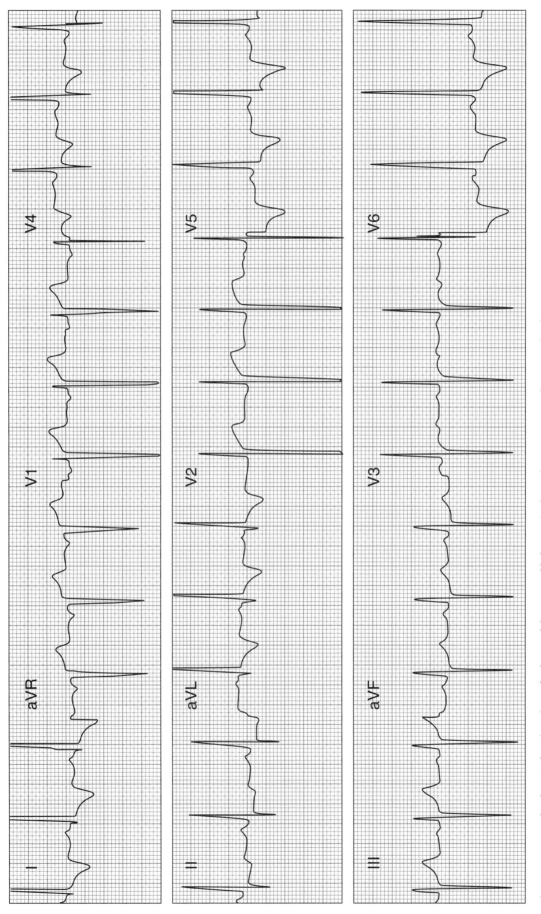

Figure 5.43 12-lead ECG showing sinus rhythm and features of left ventricular enlargement. See box 5.24 for features.

the end of the chapter provide more extensive discussion.

Myocardial ischemia is defined as an inadequate blood flow to cardiac muscle. This creates an imbalance between the myocardial cells' oxygen supply and the demand. This imbalance can occur at rest or can be induced during physical exertion. The most common underlying cause of myocardial ischemia is coronary artery disease. An exercise tolerance test performed for diagnostic reasons is commonly used to elicit an ischemic response within the heart for the purposes of screening for coronary artery disease. Myocardial ischemia may be accompanied by chest pain—often referred to as angina—and may also precipitate life-threatening cardiac arrhythmias and/or an acute MI. However, myocardial ischemia is a reversible process if the oxygen supply-demand relationship is brought back into balance by either a reduction in myocardial oxygen demand (i.e., decrease in workload of the heart) or an increase in oxygen supply. The way in which myocardial ischemia presents on the surface ECG depends, in part, on the amount of muscle mass affected. If the entire thickness of a region of the myocardium is affected (i.e., transmural ischemia), the resting ECG pattern often shows inverted T waves in leads overlying the affected area. However, if only the innermost portion of the muscle mass is affected (i.e., subendocardial ischemia), the ischemia will result in a depression of the ST-segment component of the cardiac cycle. These changes are illustrated in figure 5.44.

Ischemia is the first step in what may be referred to as the ischemic cascade. Figure 5.45 illustrates this concept of progression of ischemia to myocardial injury and ultimately to myocardial infarction. The first two steps of the cascade—ischemia and injury—are thought to be reversible if an adequate amount of oxygen is restored to the myocardial cells. However, once the process of MI results in cell death, those cells are no longer able to function. Each step in the process is associated with significant changes on the ECG that help the physician determine the stage of the cascade and the most appropriate therapeutic approach. The most common ECG pattern associated with myocardial injury is an elevation of the ST segment in ECG leads that overlie the affected region of the myocardium. Examples of the injury pattern are presented in figures 5.45 and 5.46.

When patients who are experiencing an acute ischemic event present to the emergency medical team (e.g., emergency room personnel or paramedics), they have often progressed into the injury stage and may even have progressed to the early stages of MI. Therefore, ECG patterns associated with injury and infarction often overlap on the same ECG tracing. The hallmark ECG change in MI is the development of significant Q waves within the QRS complex. Small Q waves representing the normal electrical forces moving through the ventricular septal wall are seen normally in several of the ECG leads (typically, the lateral or inferior leads). Q waves representing the normal activation of the ventricular septum should be less than 0.04 s in duration (1-mm box) and no deeper than one-fourth the size of the following R wave in the same QRS complex. When Q waves that exceed these criteria are noted on the resting ECG, they are often associated with an MI. Figure 5.47 illustrates the difference between normal and abnormal Q waves.

The proximity of various ECG leads to specific regions of the left ventricle provides the opportunity to localize myocardial ischemia, injury, or infarction patterns on the resting ECG to certain areas of the heart muscle through identification of the ECG lead groups that show the abnormal patterns (e.g., ST-segment changes or significant Q waves). Box 5.25 identifies the various leads with the anatomic regions of the left ventricle that they provide information about (4). For example, if significant Q waves were observed in leads II, III, and aVF on a resting 12-lead ECG, the pattern might reflect a transmural inferior wall MI. Likewise, significant Q waves in the septal and anterior leads (V_{1-4}) would reflect a transmural infarction of the septal and anterior walls of the left ventricle. Figure 5.48 presents an example of such a pattern. However, a cautionary note is in order: when you see significant Q waves in the anterior leads on the resting ECG, you should be sure to measure the duration of the QRS before concluding that this pattern reflects anterior MI. The reason is that LBBB can mimic the anterior MI pattern due to the large Q waves in the anterior leads often seen with this conduction abnormality. The important distinguishing feature is the duration of the QRS. If you see significant Q waves in the anterior leads in combination with a normal QRS duration, you can rule out LBBB as the cause of the Q waves. In such cases, the likely culprit for the Q waves is MI. On the other hand, if you see Q waves in the anterior leads along with a wide QRS (see LBBB criteria in box 5.22), the conduction abnormality may well have caused the Q waves and therefore you cannot make a determination of MI on the ECG evidence alone.

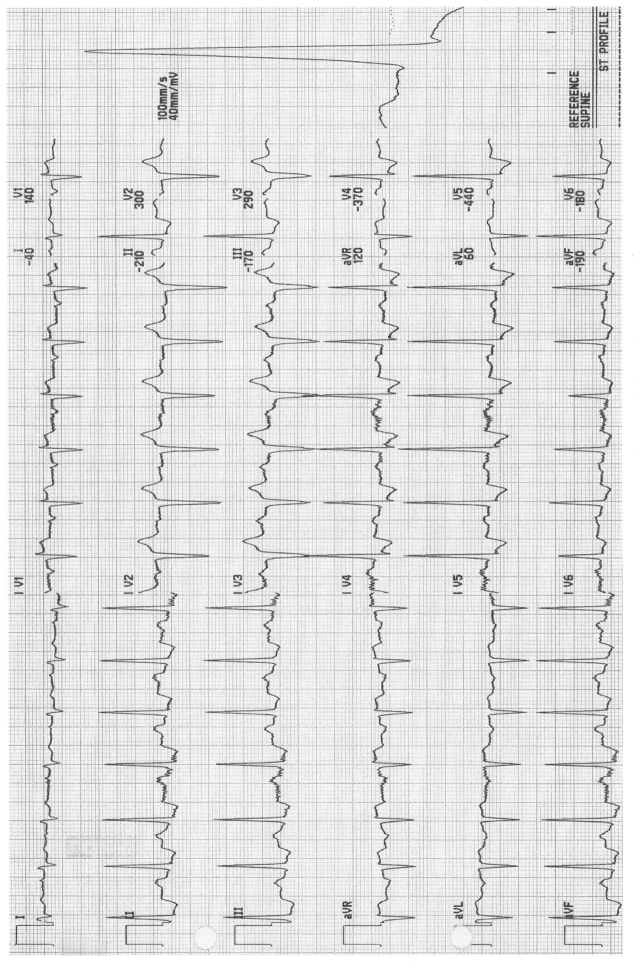

Figure 5.44 12-lead ECG showing sinus rhythm and ST segment / T wave changes associated with myocardial ischemia.

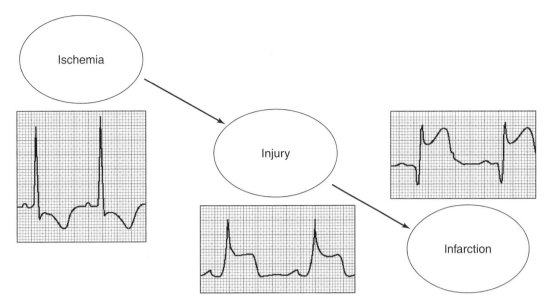

Figure 5.45 Illustration of the ischemic cascade, beginning with myocardial ischemia, progressing next to myocardial injury, and finally to myocardial infarction.

Box 5.25 Localization of Transmural Myocardial Infarction

- V_{1-3} Anteroseptal
- V_{3-4} Localized anterior
- V_{4-6}, I, aVL   Anterolateral
- V_{1-6} Extensive anterior
- I, aVL   High lateral
- II, III, aVF   Inferior
- V_{1-2} True posterior (R/S ratio > 1.0)
- V_1, V_{3R}, V_{4R} Right ventricular

Although highly sophisticated medical technologies are commonly used to determine the extent of myocardial ischemia, the surface ECG remains the major first-line step in the evaluation process. Therefore, clinical exercise program professionals should be able to recognize ECG evidence of acute myocardial ischemia, myocardial injury, and both acute and chronic MI. The interpretation steps suggested within this chapter include inspection of the QRS, ST segment, and T wave to look for evidence of the three I's (i.e., ischemia, injury, and infarction). In conclusion, we concede that the differential diagnosis of myocardial ischemia, injury, and/or infarction is a complex process that is rarely completed without the aid of additional medical information (i.e., signs/symptoms and other diagnostic data), most of which is discussed in chapter 3. Therefore, the ECG should not be interpreted in a vacuum. The clinician will use the ECG findings, along with additional information about the patient, to make a definitive diagnosis of ischemia, injury, or infarction. The information presented here is meant to serve as an introduction to the ECG criteria for these abnormalities, and we certainly encourage the reader to seek more advanced discussions of this topic in the resources listed at the end of the chapter.

SUMMARY

Within this chapter we've presented the basic electrophysiological events occurring at the cardiac cell membrane that are responsible for the transport of the electrical signal through the myocardium. Placing electrodes on the skin surface at specific locations allows the recording of these electrical forces in 12 different leads. Clinical exercise physiologists need to be able to differentiate between normal and abnormal resting and exercise ECG patterns. Within the chapter we present a systematic approach for the interpretation of both 12-lead ECGs and single rhythm strips. It is not possible within one chapter to discuss all the possible ECG patterns that one may encounter in the clinical setting; we have presented a large number of the abnormal patterns, and the information should serve as a solid introduction to ECG interpretation. For more advanced treatments of the topics within this chapter, as well as for discussions of additional ECG patterns, the reader is referred to any of the ECG texts cited at the end of the chapter.

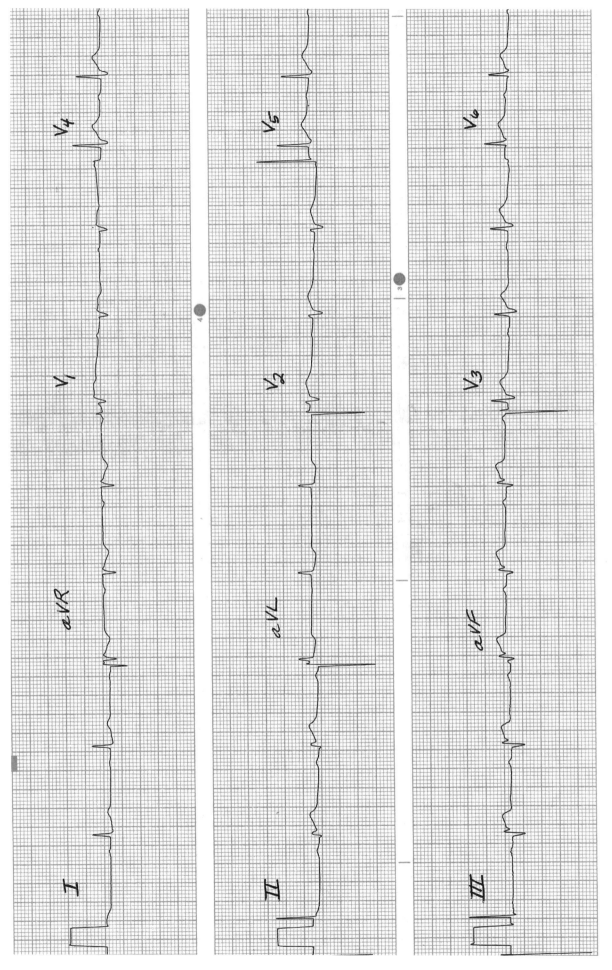
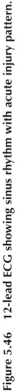

Figure 5.46   12-lead ECG showing sinus rhythm with acute injury pattern.

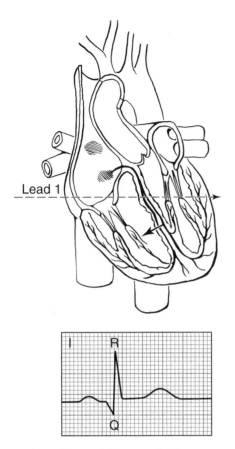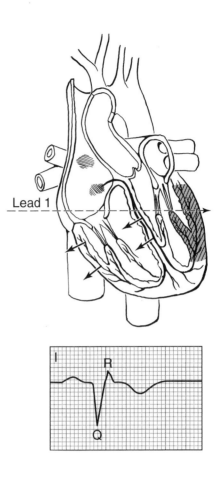

Figure 5.47   Normal vs. abnormal Q wave criteria.

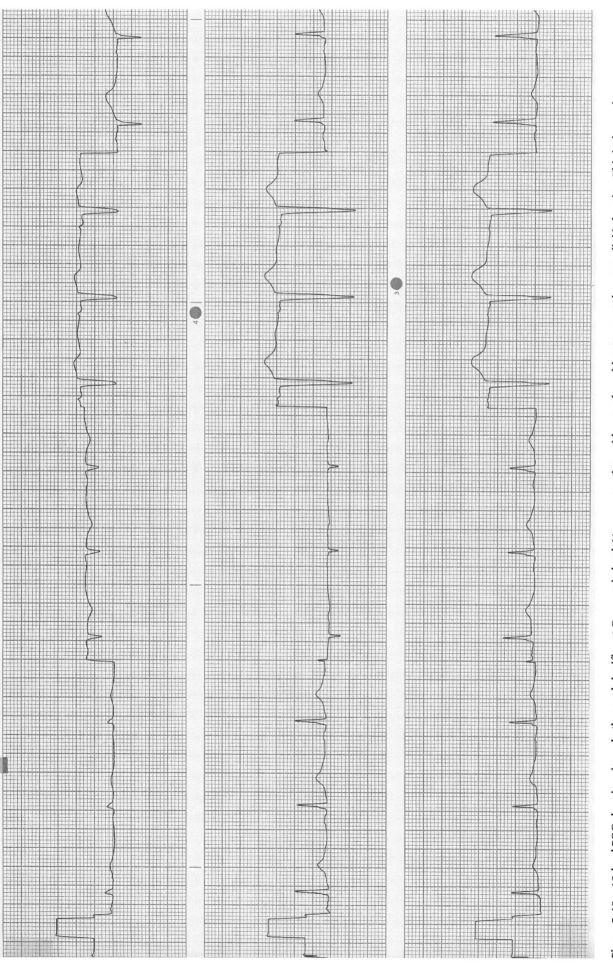

Figure 5.48 12-lead ECG showing sinus rhythm and significant Q waves in leads V$_{1-3}$, representing evidence of an old anteroseptal myocardial infarction. This is the resting ECG for the patient whose data appears in table 7.13.

CASE STUDIES

This section of the chapter presents our interpretation of the resting and exercise 12-lead ECGs for the three case studies. The resting 12-lead for Case 1 was presented earlier as figure 5.1. The 12-lead tracings for Cases 2 and 3 are presented as figures 5.50 and 5.52, respectively. A summary of our interpretations of the resting tracings is provided in table 5.1 for your review. Remember that the exercise ECGs were recorded using the modified electrode placements described earlier in the chapter (see figure 5.8), whereas the resting ECGs were recorded with the limb electrodes in the standard wrist and ankle positions.

Table 5.1
Case Study Resting 12-Lead ECG Interpretations

Element	Case 1 (figure 5.1)	Case 2 (figure 5.50)	Case 3 (figure 5.52)
Heart rate	55	60	57
Rhythm	Normal sinus	Normal sinus	Sinus bradycardia
P waves	< 2 mm < 0.12 s	< 2 mm < 0.12 s	< 2 mm < 0.12 s
PR interval (s)	0.16 Consistent	0.18 Consistent	0.18 Consistent
QRS (s)	0.09 No significant Qs No voltage criteria	0.10 No significant Qs No voltage criteria	0.10 Significant Qs in I and aVL No voltage criteria
Frontal plane axis	+ 50°	+ 30°	- 20°
Transition zone	V_{3-4}	V_{3-4}	V_{2-3}
ST segment	WNL	WNL	WNL
T waves	WNL	WNL	WNL
QT interval (s)	0.38	0.40	0.40
Summary	Sinus bradycardia	NSR	Sinus bradycardia Lateral MI (age indeterminant) Left axis deviation

bpm = beats per minute; WNL = within normal limits; NSR = normal sinus rhythm.

Case Study 1
Primary Prevention: Low Risk

Case 1 had a regular sinus rhythm with a rate of approximately 55 bpm. He had normal-size and -shape P waves, which rules out ECG evidence for atrial enlargement. He had one P wave in front of each QRS. He had a consistent PRI of 0.16 s in lead II, which, when combined with the fact that there is a 1:1 ratio for P waves and QRS complexes, rules out any of the AV block patterns. He had a normal-duration QRS complex (0.09 s) with no evidence of significant Q waves or any voltage criteria (see boxes 5.23 and 5.24). This allows us to rule out BBBs, as well as ECG evidence for old MI or ventricular hypertrophy. His frontal-plane electrical axis was approximately +50°, and his transition zone was at V_4. Both of these measures are within normal ranges. His ST segments and T waves were within normal limits and thus we can rule out ECG evidence for myocardial ischemia/injury. And finally, his QT interval of 0.38 is within the normal range for a sinus rhythm just under 60 bpm. Therefore, our summary interpretation would be sinus bradycardia.

As discussed in earlier chapters, this man completed a maximal exercise test prior to entry into the preventive exercise program at Ball State University for the purpose of measuring his functional capacity. Specifics about the exercise test and his physiological results will be presented and discussed in chapter 6. Here, we present and provide an interpretation of his peak exercise 12-lead ECG, which was recorded at 13 minutes, 20 seconds into the BSU Bruce ramp protocol (figure 5.49). His peak exercise ECG shows sinus tachycardia of approximately 186 beats per minute with no arrhythmias or significant ST-segment changes in any lead groups. His peak exercise response was therefore viewed as normal. As is policy within the Ball State program, the exercise test results were forwarded to the individual's personal physician, who subsequently concurred that the exercise ECG response was normal. Recalling the diagnostic terminology presented in chapter 3, this man's ECG response was "negative" for myocardial ischemia. Based on the normal ECG and the other normal exercise responses discussed in chapter 6, this man was cleared by his personal physician for participation in the exercise program.

Case Study 2
Primary Prevention: High Risk

Case 2 also presented with a regular sinus rhythm of approximately 60 bpm. His resting 12-lead ECG (figure 5.50) also met all the normal criteria within each of the interpretive elements listed in box 5.2. He had normal-size and -shape P waves, which rules out ECG evidence for atrial enlargement. He had one P wave in front of each QRS. He had a consistent PRI of 0.18 s in lead II, which, when combined with the fact that there is a 1:1 ratio for P waves and QRS complexes, rules out any of the AV block patterns. He had a normal duration QRS complex (0.10 s) with no evidence of significant Q waves or any voltage criteria (see boxes 5.23 and 5.24). This allows us to rule out BBBs, as well as ECG evidence for old MI or ventricular hypertrophy. His frontal-plane electrical axis was approximately +30°, and his transition zone was between V_3 and V_4. Both of these measures are within normal ranges. His ST segments and T waves were within normal limits and thus we can rule out ECG evidence for myocardial ischemia/injury. And finally, his QT interval of 0.40 s is within the normal range for a sinus rhythm of 60 bpm. Therefore, our summary interpretation would be normal sinus rhythm.

Case Study 2 completed his maximal exercise test at Wake Forest University. Details about the exercise test and his physiological responses will be presented and discussed in detail in chapter 6. Here we discuss the exercise ECG response which is presented in figure 5.51. His peak exercise ECG shows sinus tachycardia of approximately 103 bpm with no arrhythmias or significant ST-segment changes in any lead groups. His peak exercise response was therefore viewed as normal or negative for exercise-induced myocardial ischemia. However, as was discussed in earlier chapters, this man does have a moderate stenosis in his proximal LAD. Does this mean that the exercise ECG failed to detect the disease (i.e., a false negative exercise ECG)? As you've no doubt come to appreciate by this point in the book, the answer to the question is not a simple yes or no! Let us explain. First, evidence of mild single vessel CAD (i.e., 1 lesion of only 40%) is often undetectable on a 12-lead exercise ECG. Second, the peak HR was only 103 bpm (due to the beta blocker) and therefore the workload on the heart—defined by the peak rate pressure product (RPP)—was not very high at peak exercise. When you combine the mild lesion with the low RPP, it is not hard to imagine why the ECG result was negative. But remember that it was "negative" up to the peak RPP observed during the exercise test (103 bpm × 142 mmHg). Should the man exceed this RPP during the training program, the ECG response could be different. And furthermore, you may recall from the discussion of this man's diagnostic workup in chapter 3 that his exercise test was actually performed after his cardiac catheterization. Therefore, the focus of his exercise test was not to diagnose CAD because the cardiac rehabilitation team at Wake Forest already knew his disease status. Now, we can already hear some of you asking the question, "If you already knew his CAD status, why did he need a diagnostic exercise test?" As will be discussed in chapter 6, exercise tests are often performed for more than just diagnostic reasons. At this point in the discussion it is important to remember that this man presented to the emergency room with chest pain (see Case Study 2 report in chapter 3). In this case, the exercise test would have served to identify an ischemic threshold (if

he had had an ischemic response to exercise), and the test results would have also provided a baseline functional capacity for comparison purposes during follow-up evaluations. As described above, this man did not have an ischemic response during the test up to the RPP achieved during the test (i.e., no ECG changes or symptoms), and he was thus cleared for participation in the exercise program. His fitness assessment and exercise prescription will be discussed in detail in the next two chapters.

Case Study 3
Secondary Prevention

Case 3 presented with a regular sinus rhythm just under 60 bpm (57), so we would interpret his cardiac rhythm as sinus bradycardia. He had normal-size and -shape P waves, which rules out ECG evidence for atrial enlargement (figure 5.52). With one P wave in front of each QRS and a consistent PRI of 0.18 s in lead II, we can again rule out any AV block pattern. He had a normal-duration QRS complex (0.10 s), allowing us to rule out BBB. As you recall from discussions of this man in earlier chapters, he has a history of anterior MI. The significant Q waves in leads I and aVL represent the ECG evidence of the old infarction. These two leads are considered anterior/lateral leads (see box 5.25); but when the Q waves are limited to just I and aVL, the ECG label of lateral MI is typically used. His frontal-plane electrical axis was approximately −20°, which represents left axis deviation; and his transition zone was slightly early between V_2 and V_3. His ST segments and T waves were within normal limits; thus we can rule out any ECG evidence for residual myocardial ischemia/injury following the MI. His QT interval of 0.40 s is within the normal range for a sinus rhythm of 57 bpm. Therefore, our summary interpretation would be sinus bradycardia, with ECG evidence of old lateral MI pattern.

As has been described in earlier chapters, this man is a patient in the Cardiac Rehabilitation Program at Wake Forest University. As with cases 1 and 2, details about the exercise test and his physiological responses will be presented and discussed in detail in chapter 6. Here we present and discuss

his peak exercise ECG response from the treadmill test completed at 3 months into the rehabilitation program (figure 5.53). The 12-lead exercise ECG shows sinus tachycardia of approximately 128 bpm with no arrhythmias. However, you will note the ST-segment depression in leads V_{2-6} at peak exercise. This man did not report any chest pain during or following the test, but did report shortness of breath as the major symptom resulting in test termination. The ST-segment depression in the anterior leads meets the generally accepted criteria for a positive test (i.e., > 1 mm of horizontal or downsloping depression), and therefore this test could be labled a "positive" one. But remember, ST-segment depression during exercise is not 100% accurate as a marker of myocardial ischemia (i.e., test specificity < 100%). The ST changes were noted in the patient's chart but due to the absense of chest pain, and the normal exercise echo he had several months earlier (see discussion in chapter 3), the attending physician interpreted the exercise response as "clinically negative" and cleared him for further participation in the exercise program. As will be discussed in chapter 7, his target training intensity for subsequent training sessions would be set safely below the HR level that produced the ST-segment changes noted during this test. This patient would be monitored by the cardiac rehabilitation staff for any changes in symptoms that might shed light on the ECG change noted on the GXT (graded exercise test). More on his exercise prescription and training responses will be presented in the chapters ahead.

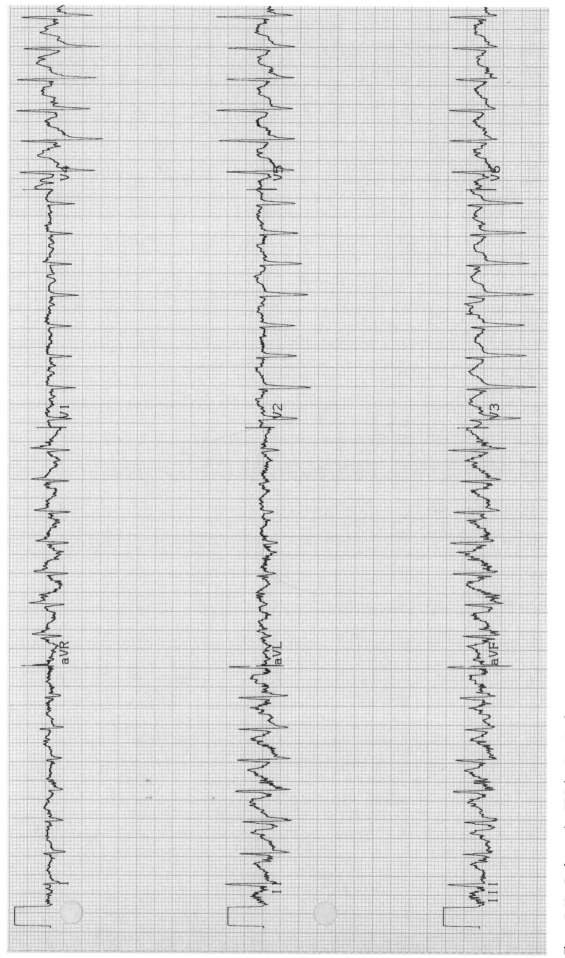

Figure 5.49   Peak exercise ECG for Case Study 1.

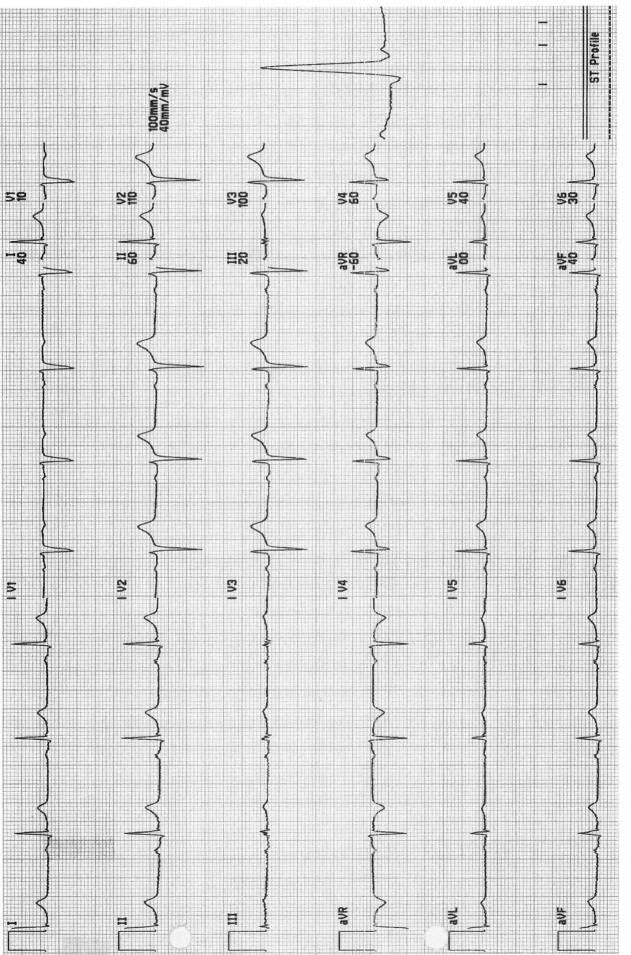

Figure 5.50   Resting 12-lead ECG for Case Study 2. See table 5.1 for interpretation.

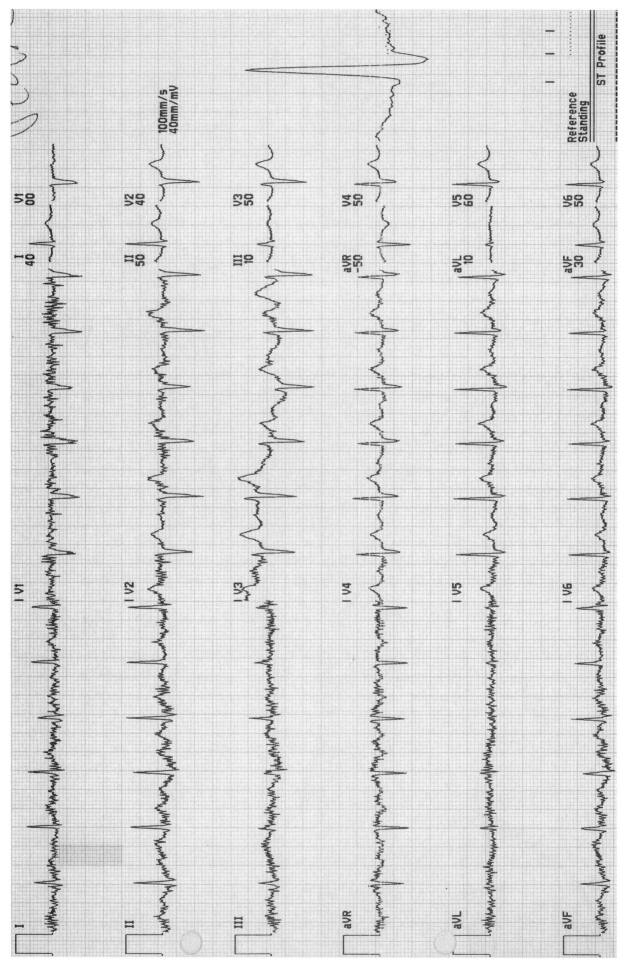

Figure 5.51 Peak exercise ECG for Case Study 2.

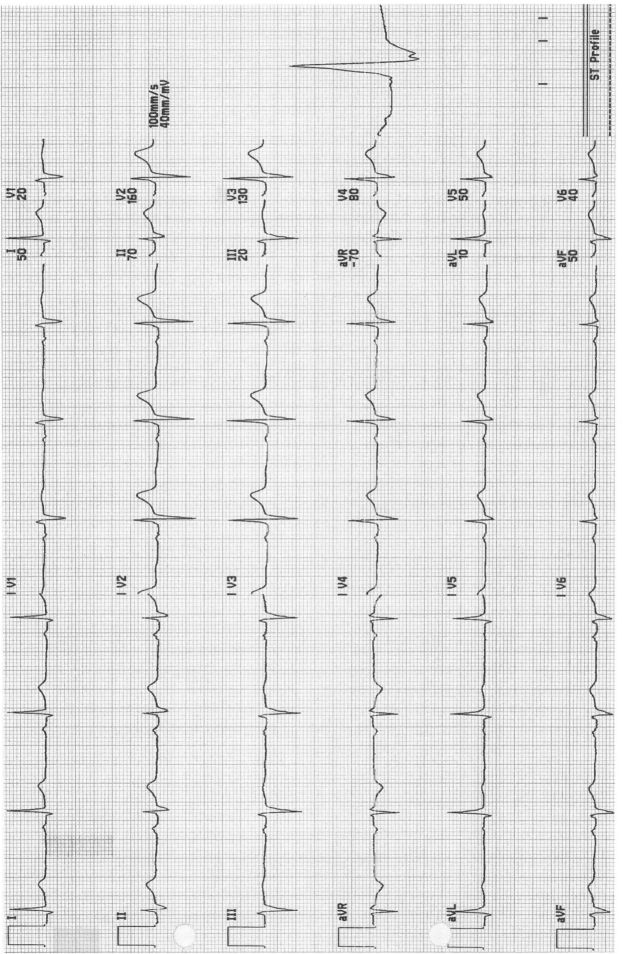

100mm/s
40mm/mV

V1
20

I
50

V2
160

II
70

V3
130

III
20

V4
80

aVR
-70

V5
50

aVL
10

V6
40

aVF
50

I V1

I V2

I V3

I V4

I V5

I V6

I

II

III

aVR

aVL

aVF

ST Profile

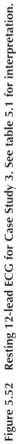

Figure 5.52   Resting 12-lead ECG for Case Study 3. See table 5.1 for interpretation.

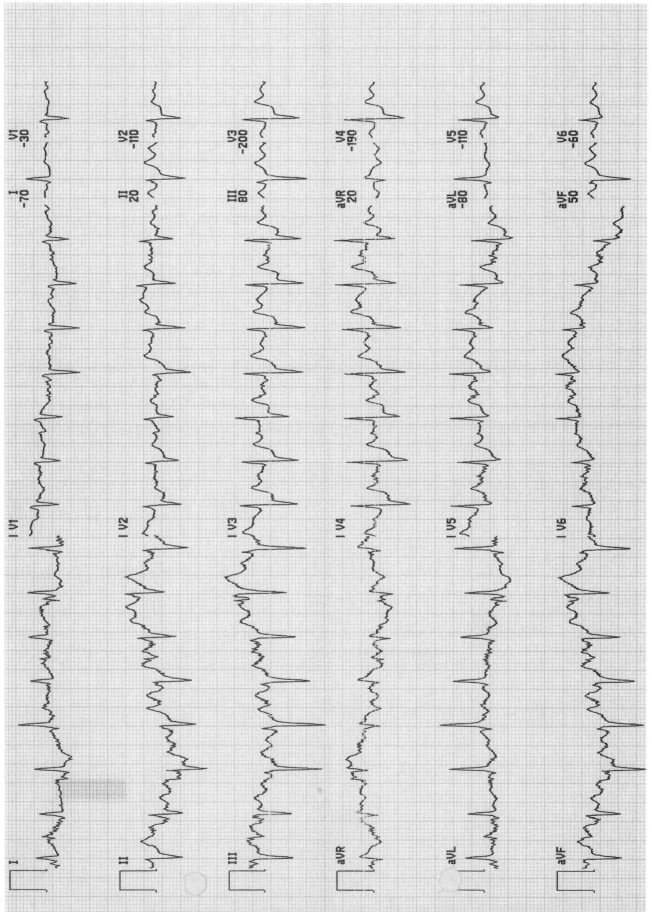

Figure 5.53   Peak exercise ECG for Case Study 3.

GLOSSARY

Arrhythmia: an abnormal heart rhythm produced as the result of a change in the regularity of a sinus rhythm (i.e., sinus arrhythmia) or a change in the pacemaker site (i.e., nonsinus pacemaker)

Automaticity: a characteristic of certain cardiac cells, specifically the ability to initiate stimulus spontaneously without reliance on a signal from outside the heart

Bradycardia: a heart rate slower than the normal inherent rate for a specified pacemaker site (i.e., <60 bpm for the sinus node = sinus bradycardia)

Cardiac action potential: a transient change in membrane permeability that results in movement of ions across the cell membrane, producing a sequenced change in membrane voltage

Depolarization: process of cardiac cell activation that results from the diffusion of cations (usually Na^+) into the cell, changing the voltage on the inside to a more positive value

ECG lead: a combination of two or more electrodes used by the ECG machine to create an electrical field (positive and negative poles) for sensing the heart's electrical forces (i.e., leads I, II and III, etc.)

Ectopic: a stimulus site outside the sinus node, as in ectopic beat or ectopic pacemaker

Electrocardiogram: a graphical representation of the electrical forces within the heart during the cardiac cycle

Electrode: a metal or other composite material that serves as the physical connection between the skin surface and the ECG machine

Repolarization: the process of returning the cardiac cell to its resting charge (i.e., –90 mV for ventricular muscle cells)

Supraventricular: referring to a site above the ventricles (i.e., atrial or junctional)

Tachycardia: a heart rate faster than the normal inherent rate for a specified pacemaker site (i.e., >100 bpm for the sinus node = sinus tachycardia)

REFERENCES

1. Mason, R.E., and I. Likar. 1966. A new system of multiple-lead exercise electrocardiography. *Am. Heart J.* 71:196–205.
2. Gamble, P., H. McManus, D. Jensen, and V.F. Froelicher. 1984. A comparison of the standard 12-lead electrocardiogram to exercise electrode placements. *Chest* 85:616–622.
3. Goldberger, A.L., and E. Goldberger. 1994. *Clinical Electrocardiography.* 5th ed. St. Louis: Mosby.
4. American College of Sports Medicine. *ACSM's Guidelines For Exercise Testing And Prescription.* Franklin, B.F., M.H. Whaley, and E.T. Howley, eds. 2000. 6th ed. Baltimore: Lippincott, Williams & Wilkins, 368.

SUGGESTED READINGS

Dubin, D. 1989. *Rapid Interpretation of EKGs.* 3rd ed. Tampa: Cover.
Wagner, G.S. 2000. *Marriott's Practical Electrocardiography.* 10th ed. Baltimore: Lippincott, Williams & Wilkins.

CHAPTER 6
Physical Fitness Assessment and Interpretation

BEHAVIORAL OBJECTIVES

- To be able to describe the components of physical fitness and how each component of physical fitness is measured

- To be able to contrast indirect and direct measures of cardiorespiratory fitness

- To be able to describe procedures that should be completed prior to and during a maximal exercise test

- To be able to interpret results from maximal exercise testing

Physical fitness is positively associated with quality of life. In this chapter we present standard methodologies for measuring the various components of physical fitness. (Note that at the end of this chapter there are some basic data sheets and ancillary testing forms.) Results from these assessments allow the exercise program professional to individualize exercise prescriptions to meet specific patient needs. Since cardiorespiratory fitness and body composition are components of physical fitness that are related to many diseases, we devote the majority of the chapter to reviewing their measurement.

WHAT IS PHYSICAL FITNESS?

There is no one universally accepted definition of physical fitness; in general, however, physical fitness is thought of as the ability or capacity of the body to exercise. In the early- and mid-1900s, measurement of physical fitness focused mainly on sport-related skills, with test batteries commonly including components such as agility, balance, endurance, power, and reaction time. It wasn't until later in the 20th century that educators, health care professionals, and researchers pushed for measurement of other components of physical fitness that were more directly associated with health and disease prevention. We now recognize two types of physical fitness, termed skill- or sport-related physical fitness and health-related physical fitness. Authors from the Centers for Disease Control and Prevention defined physical fitness as a set of attributes that people have or achieve that relates to the ability to perform physical activity (1). Another definition, which includes the components of health-related physical fitness, is a general state of well-being characterized by the ability to sustain work or the ability to perform occupational, recreational, and daily activities without becoming unduly fatigued. This requires an effective integration of and sufficient capabilities in **cardiorespiratory endurance, muscular strength, muscular endurance, body composition,** and **flexibility** (2). These components of health-related physical fitness are defined in the glossary.

BASIC BODY COMPOSITION MEASUREMENT

Measurement of an individual's body composition has long been considered an important part of a health risk appraisal. This is even more the case since the recent pronouncement of the American Heart Association indicating that obesity is a major risk factor for coronary artery disease (3). Unfortunately, no in vivo methods for measuring total body fat content are available, so clinicians can only estimate body fat percentage. The accuracy of these estimations varies considerably according to the method. All those who perform these measurements should heed a quotation attributed to one of the pioneers in the field of body composition, Dr. A.R. Behnke: "Nothing is measured with greater error than the human body."

Height and Weight Measurements

One of the simplest methods for measuring body composition is to compare measurements of body weight and body height. In part because of its simplicity, this method is often underappreciated.

A variety of approaches have been developed to measure body height or stature. It is common, for example, to measure height from a rod attached to platform weight scales or from a measuring tape affixed to a wall. But because measurements made with these devices are less accurate and precise than with other methods, their use is not recommended. Ideally, height should be measured using a stadiometer. A stadiometer is composed of a vertical board with an attached measurement scale and a movable horizontal headboard. The correct measurement position of the patient is with the heels, buttocks, scapulae, and posterior aspect of the cranium in contact with the vertical board. Patients should remove their shoes and stand with their heels together (feet forming a 60° angle); they are measured while holding their breath after a deep inspiration. The headboard is positioned so that it compresses the hair and touches the most superior point on the head. This measurement should be made to the nearest 0.25 in. (figure 6.1; form A, p. 191). Readers will find more detailed information on measuring stature, as well as recommended adaptations for patients who cannot be positioned correctly, in the excellent chapter on this subject in the *Anthropometric Standardization Reference Manual* (4).

As with stature-measuring devices, there are many different types of scales for measuring body weight, ranging from simple household models to sophisticated electronic instruments. For standardization purposes, a leveled platform and balance-beam scale with movable weights and an adjustment screw is recommended. It has become increasingly common to use electronic scales interfaced to computers to provide imme-

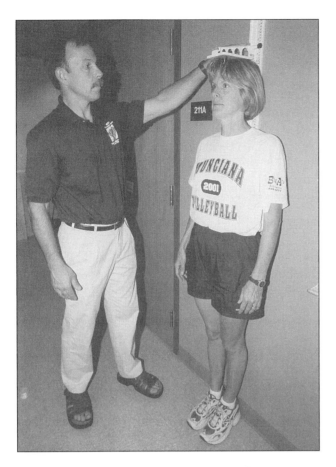

Figure 6.1   A patient is measured with a stadiometer.
Photo Courtesy of Ball State University Photo Services.

diate data storage. With this type of system, weights obtained on the electronic scale should be checked regularly against weights obtained on a balance-beam scale to verify their accuracy. The patient should be measured in standardized clothing (e.g., a hospital gown or shorts and a T-shirt) without shoes and after voiding the bladder; the measurement is taken to the nearest 0.1 kg. Since body weight may fluctuate throughout the day, it is advisable to record the time of day the measurement is taken and to attempt to take serial measures at a similar time of day.

Among the advantages of using height and weight measurements are that they are economical, quick to perform, and easily understood by patients. Also, from a technical standpoint, they can be performed with a high degree of accuracy and precision both within and between technicians (4). The major disadvantage to height and weight measures is that they do not differentiate the types of body tissues (i.e., two people could have the same height and weight yet very different body fat percentages). Although this is often an issue in athletic populations, it is generally less

so in the average adult population, who are typically both overweight and underactive.

Relative Weight and Body Mass Index

Various classification schemes using height and weight measurements are available. Basically, these schemes place patients into one of four general categories: underweight, desirable weight, overweight, or obese.

The relative weight method compares a person's actual weight to a normative weight for that person's height and expresses the result according to the following formula:

$$\text{relative weight (\%)} = \frac{\text{measured weight}}{\text{normative weight}} \times 100$$

One advantage of this system is that it allows clinicians to select the normative weight they believe best suits the patient. Recommended references for normative weights are the 1995 USDA healthy weight table (table 6.1) (5) and the Hamwi formula (6). As table 6.1 shows, a given weight range for each height represents ±13.5% of the midpoint of the range. In other words, for any height, a range of weights is considered within normal limits. The midpoint weight is selected for use in the relative weight formula (e.g., for a person who is 64 in. tall, the midpoint of the weight range of 111-146 is 128.5 lb). The Hamwi formula determines the normative weight as follows:

5 ft = 100 lb [women] +
5 lb for each inch taller than 5 ft
5 ft = 106 lb [men] + 6 lb
for each inch taller than 5 ft

Using this method for the same 64-in.-tall woman would result in a normative weight of 120 lb (i.e., 60 in. = 100 lb + [5 lb/in. × 4 in.]). Assuming this woman weighed 150 lb, calculations of her relative weight would be as follows:

150/126 × 100 = 119% or 150/120 × 100 = 125%

Classification of patients using the relative weight method proceeds according to the values in table 6.2. The principal advantage to the relative weight system is that it has been used for many years by clinicians in practice and thus is well accepted and understood. The obvious disadvantage is that the relative weight will vary depending on which method is used to establish the normative weight. Note the 8.5 pound difference in normative weight between the two methods in our example.

Table 6.1
**1995 USDA Healthy Weight Ranges
for Men and Women**

Height (ft, in; no shoes)	Weight (in pounds; without clothes)
4'10"	91-119
4'11"	94-124
5'0"	97-128
5'1"	101-132
5'2"	104-137
5'3"	107-141
5'4"	111-146
5'5"	114-150
5'6"	118-155
5'7"	121-160
5'8"	125-164
5'9"	129-169
5'10"	132-174
5'11"	136-179
6'0"	140-184
6'1"	144-189
6'2"	148-195
6'3"	152-200
6'4"	156-205
6'5"	160-211
6'6"	164-216

From USDA 1995 Dietary Guidelines for Americans.

Table 6.2
Relative Weight Classifications

Relative weight	Classification
<80%	Severely underweight
80–86.5%	Underweight
86.5–113.5%	Desirable weight
113.5–120%	Overweight
>120%	Obese

The American Heart Association definition of obesity is a relative weight of ≥120%.

Determination of Body Fat Distribution

Including a measure of body fat distribution can give the exercise program professional increased confidence in evaluating the potential health risks of excess body weight in relation to height. Research evidence now suggests that the most serious health risks result when an individual preferentially stores excess fat in the upper half of the body, particularly when the fat is located viscerally (7). This is commonly referred to as upper-body, apple-shaped, android, or central obesity. Although early methods of assessing body fat distribution included measures of both waist and hip circumferences, the Expert Panel on the Identification, Evaluation and Treatment of Overweight and Obesity in Adults now recommends that health risk assessment be made from the waist circumference alone (8). This measurement, which is highly accurate, reliable, as well as quick and easy to perform, may provide the most important information about the patient's health risks associated with body composition. Suggested thresholds for increased risk of developing hyperinsulinemia, hypertension, hypertriglyceridemia, or low high-density lipoprotein are a waist circumference >40 in. (102 cm) for men and >35 in. (88 cm) for women (table 1.5).

Measurement of waist circumference should be made to the nearest 0.1 cm with a non-elastic measuring tape that has metric unit markings and a tension gauge to allow for consistent pressure. From a position at the participant's side, the technician should make the measurement on bare skin (the tape should not compress the skin), at the end of a normal expiration, and at the site location used in many research studies—the narrowest part of the torso (above the umbilicus and below the xiphoid process).

Another classification system that is seeing increased use is the body mass index (BMI). The BMI ($kg \cdot m^{-2}$) is calculated as follows:

$$\frac{body\ weight\ (kilograms)}{height\ (meters\ squared)}$$

The BMI has been employed for a long time as a primary method to describe body composition of individuals in large scale research studies. It has recently gained acceptance in clinical practice primarily because it eliminates the subjectivity of selecting a normative weight for calculation. Classification of patients' weight status using BMI is determined according to the values in table 1.5.

Another recommendation for identifying the site location, just above the uppermost lateral border of the right iliac crest, has been proposed by the National Health and Nutrition Examination Survey (NHANES III) and is shown in figure 6.2.

Summary

For most adult populations, measurements of height, weight, and waist circumference provide data sufficient for an accurate assessment of the patient's health risks associated with body composition. The advantages of performing only a "basic" body composition assessment are that it is easily understood by both clinicians and patients, is reliable and accurate, is quick and easy to perform, and is highly cost effective. Thus, for most patients seen in a clinical exercise program setting, a "basic" body composition assessment is all that is needed. For the few patients about whom the clinician has uncertainties with

regard to health risk status, it is advisable to pursue a more advanced assessment of body composition.

ADVANCED BODY COMPOSITION MEASUREMENT

Knowledge about bone density, total body water, or skeletal muscle mass is of interest and importance to clinicians for certain patients; however, in most clinical exercise programs it is not feasible to measure these components. More commonly, advanced body composition measurement involves a method of estimating body fat percentage. It is important for the student to understand that since an in vivo method to measure total body fat percentage does not exist, all methods are considered indirect. The only direct method for determining body composition is via cadaver analysis, which is an unpopular choice for patients. Indirect methods are based on assumptions about the makeup of various body tissues as determined from cadaver analyses. For example, one assumption underlying body density-based methods is that the average density of all fat-free tissue (within and between individuals) has a value of $1.1 g/cm^3$. This value was derived from cadavers of mostly young- to middle-aged Caucasian men, which makes its application to patients with different characteristics suspect (e.g., since we know that bone density decreases with age, we would expect error in the outcome measure). Doubly indirect methods involve measuring a component of the body—for example, a group of skinfolds or circumference measures—and then establishing a regression (prediction) equation to estimate an indirect method outcome measure (e.g., body density or total body water). It is important to understand that anytime a prediction equation is used to determine a variable (e.g., predicting body fat percentage), the estimated value may not be exactly correct. In other words, the predicted value can differ from the actual value. This difference, sometimes called the prediction error, is commonly quantified by the standard error of estimate (SEE) (figure 6.3). The measurement error with doubly indirect methods is thus even greater than with indirect methods.

We will briefly review indirect and doubly indirect methods of obtaining body fat estimates. Students requiring more thorough information on this topic should refer to some of the references at the end of the chapter that provide more detailed information.

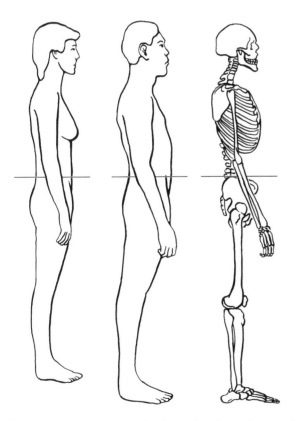

Figure 6.2 Measurement site for waist circumference. Locate site just above uppermost lateral border of the right iliac crest and in line with the midaxillary line. Measurement is taken in the horizontal plane with the measuring tape held parallel to the floor (8).

From the United States Department of Health and Human Services, Public Health Services, 1996.

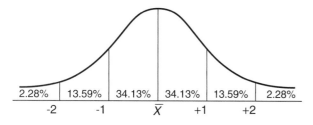

2.28%	13.59%	34.13%	34.13%	13.59%	2.28%
-2	-1	$\overline{X}$	+1	+2	

Figure 6.3 In a bell-shaped curve looking at a "normal" population, two-thirds (68%) of the population have values within ± 1 standard deviation (SD) of the mean value ($\overline{x}$) of the population. (Ninety-five percent are within ± 2 SD and 99% are within ± 3 SD.) The SEE can be viewed as the SD at any given point along a prediction (regression) line.

Criterion Methods of Body Fat Estimation

A number of methods are available that are considered criterion or reference measures of body fat percentage. Although few clinical exercise programs—with the exception of those at academic or research institutions—actually employ a criterion method, the most commonly used procedure is the measurement of body volume by either hydrostatic weighing or air-displacement plethysmography. Body density is determined by the following formula:

body density = body mass (weight)/body volume

The body density value is then used in what is called a two-compartment model that divides the body into fat tissue and fat-free tissue. The most common two-compartment model equation is the Siri equation (9):

$$\text{body fat percentage} = \frac{495}{\text{body density}} - 450$$

Lohman (10) has proposed that the standard error of estimate for predicting body fat percentage from body density is ±2.7%.

Hydrostatic or underwater weighing is usually considered the "gold standard" method for determining body fat percentage, even though it is really an indirect method (i.e., body volume is determined and used to estimate body fat percentage). Hydrostatic weighing requires measurements of body weight (on land), weight while the person is submerged under water, and residual lung volume. These latter two measurements require specialized equipment and instrumentation (body or tank of water with submergible seat connected to a sensitive scale, and a helium or nitrogen gas analyzer) and present some challenges to the patient performing the test. The patient must maximally exhale and must stay under the water long enough to get a stable underwater weight reading; this is difficult for many and beyond the capabilities of some. Because of the patient performance requirements, the specialized equipment needs, and the time required to complete a test (≈30 min per patient), this procedure is seldom used in clinical exercise programs. However, it is important to remember that hydrostatic weighing is the most commonly used criterion measure against which new methods of body composition are compared.

A newer method of measuring body volume was introduced in the 1990s based on the principle of air-displacement plethysmography. Various types of plethysmographs have been experimented with over the past 50 years, yet all suffered from either technological or practical limitations that precluded their widespread use. The development of the BOD POD gave clinicians the opportunity to measure patients' body volume with an air-displacement plethysmograph (figure 6.4) (11).

The measurement of body volume from air-displacement plethysmography is based on Boyle's law, which states that there is an inverse relationship between pressure and volume if temperature is held constant. The BOD POD is a dual-chamber plethysmograph with a volume-perturbing element in the rear chamber. To operate the BOD POD, one establishes the volume of the front chamber when empty and then with a person sitting in it, then calculates body volume by subtraction. This method also requires the determination of thoracic gas volume via instrumentation provided with the BOD POD. The procedure requires the individual to wear only a tight-fitting, unpadded nylon swimsuit. From a practical standpoint, measurements made via the BOD POD overcome many of the limitations imposed by hydrostatic

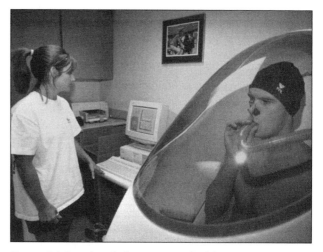

Figure 6.4 A patient being measured with a BOD POD.
Photo Courtesy of Ball State University Photo Services.

weighing and do not take as long (≈10 min per patient). However, more research is needed to establish the validity and reliability of this device.

It is important to recognize that the procedures to measure body volume (and thus density) are considered both reliable and valid. Error comes from estimating percent body fat from body density. As mentioned earlier, the Siri equation is the prediction equation most often used. However, newer equations have recently been developed for populations of different racial groups and are also gender-specific. These equations appear to reduce the error in estimating percent body fat from body density (12).

Doubly Indirect Methods

The two most common and most thoroughly studied doubly indirect methods are measurement of a sum of skinfolds (SF) and bioelectrical impedance analysis (BIA). Two assumptions underlying the sum-of-skinfold method are that ≈50% of the total body fat is located in the subcutaneous adipose depots and that measurement of selected sites is representative of the total body. The ACSM

recommendations for standards for skinfold measurement sites and procedures are provided in table 6.3. The BIA method assumes that fat-free mass contains a constant value of water (≈73%) and that measurements of impedance to a low-level electrical current passed through the body are reflective of the total body water.

A major limitation of both the SF and BIA methods is that the accuracy of the estimate is influenced by the degree of similarity or difference between the patient and the subjects used in the original research that established a prediction equation. Literally hundreds of prediction formulas have been developed to predict body fat percentage. Use of population-specific formulas could theoretically reduce error; however, it is usually deemed impractical to select a different equation for each individual tested. Thus, most clinical exercise programs use generalized equations both for practical reasons and for consistency. The SF and BIA methods have similar standard error of estimates, ranging from approximately 3% to 4% (13) (remember that the standard error of estimate of the indirect densitometry method was estimated to be ±2.7%).

Table 6.3
Standardized Description of Skinfold Sites and Procedures

Skinfold site	Description
Abdominal	Vertical fold; 2 cm to the right side of the umbilicus
Triceps	Vertical fold; on the posterior midline of the upper arm, halfway between the acromion and olecranon processes, with the arm held freely to the side of the body
Biceps	Vertical fold; on the anterior aspect of the arm over the belly of the biceps muscle, 1 cm above the level used to mark the triceps site
Chest/Pectoral	Diagonal fold; one-half the distance between the anterior axillary line and the nipple (men) or one-third of the distance between the anterior axillary line and the nipple (women)
Medial calf	Vertical fold; at the maximum circumference of the calf on the midline of its medial border
Midaxillary	Vertical fold; on the midaxillary line at the level of the xiphoid process of the sternum (an alternate method is a horizontal fold taken at the level of the xiphoid/sternal border in the midaxillary line)
Subscapular	Diagonal fold (at a 45° angle); 1 to 2 cm below the inferior angle of the scapula
Suprailiac	Diagonal fold; in line with the natural angle of the iliac crest taken in the anterior axillary line immediately superior to the iliac crest
Thigh	Vertical fold, on the anterior midline of the thigh, midway between the proximal border of the patella and the inguinal crease (hip)

Procedures

All measurements should be made on the right side of the body

Caliper should be placed 1 cm away from the thumb and finger, perpendicular to the skinfold, and halfway between the crest and the base of the fold

Pinch should be maintained while reading the caliper

Wait 1 to 2 s (and no longer) before reading caliper

Take duplicate measures at each site and retest if duplicate measurements are not within 1 to 2 mm

Rotate through measurement sites or allow time for skin to regain normal texture and thickness

Reprinted, by permission, 2000, *ACSM's Guidelines for Exercise Testing and Prescription*. 6th ed. (Philadelphia: Lippincott, Williams, and Wilkins), 65.

Interpretation of Body Fat Percentage Estimates

There are many different classification schemes or charts that are available to interpret body fat percentage values. Unfortunately, there are no universally accepted standards for what is considered a normal body fat percentage. A simple "rule of thumb" method that we have used is the following: average body fat percentage for college-aged men and women is 15% and 22%, respectively. An allowance of an additional 2% body fat is added for each additional decade of age beginning at age 30 to provide a value for average body fat percentage (e.g., for 30-39-year-old men and women, average values would be 17% and 24% respectively). Note this allowance with age is used to reflect "average" body fat percentage. Ideally, we should not gain body fat as we age. Body fat percentages that are > 5% above the average value would be considered "obese."

Summary

The biggest factor negatively influencing a decision to use advanced body composition methods is the relatively large prediction error (±3-4%) associated with the measurements. However, estimates of body fat percentage may be desirable when the clinician has some doubt about a patient's body composition classification from height/weight and waist circumference measurements.

MUSCULAR STRENGTH AND ENDURANCE AND FLEXIBILITY MEASUREMENT

Before the 1990s, clinical exercise programs were designed to stimulate improvement in or maintenance of desirable levels of cardiorespiratory endurance and body composition, giving little or no attention to the other components of physical fitness. In the 1990s, however, many position papers and guideline statements on the benefits of physical activity and exercise provided recommendations for including training for muscular strength, muscular endurance, and flexibility in all clinical exercise programs (8, 14-17). These recommendations came out of accumulating research demonstrating both the health and the functional benefits associated with these components of physical fitness. Cardiac rehabilitation programs are starting to include measures of muscular strength, muscular endurance, and flexibility to their outcome assessments. Thus, it is important to understand the assessment of these components of physical fitness.

There is no single measure for assessing total body muscular strength (or muscular endurance or flexibility). Since exercise training adaptations are specific to the muscle group (and joint) and energy system utilized (i.e., the principle of specificity), assessment of these three components of physical fitness requires measurement of the muscular strength or endurance of specific muscle groups or the flexibility of specific joints. This requirement to measure multiple muscle groups or joints creates an obstacle to assessing these components of physical fitness. Some programs have attempted to use single measures (e.g., hand-grip strength or sit-and-reach tests) as general markers, but there are no established global measures.

Assessment of Muscular Strength

Many different devices are available to measure muscular strength, including computerized isokinetic systems, strain gauges, cable tensiometers, dynamometers, and free weights. When assessing strength it is important to understand the difference between dynamic and static muscular contractions. Dynamic contractions are those in which the length of the muscle is changing when force is produced. Contractions in which the muscle is shortening are called concentric, whereas those in which the muscle is lengthening are referred to as eccentric contractions. For a specific muscle group, strength can be measured during performance of either a dynamic or a static contraction. It is also important to understand that force-production capabilities vary throughout the range of motion of a muscular contraction and that the pattern of change in this force-production range differs from one muscle group to another.

Thus, the assessment of muscular strength can get quite involved. In some settings, particularly those focusing on treatment or rehabilitation for musculoskeletal problems, the assessment of muscular strength may require multiple measurements with a high level of sophistication. This level of assessment is beyond the scope of this textbook.

Most clinical exercise programs can perform one repetition-maximum (1-RM) tests of a few of the major muscle groups to provide a simple yet effective assessment of a patient's muscular strength. Advantages of the 1-RM assessment are that it is simple to perform; it allows the option of using free weights or resistance-exercise machines; it provides the ability to test multiple muscle groups; and it is practical, since most strength requirements of activities of daily living involve dynamic contractions of a fixed weight (e.g., lifting a bag of groceries). The 1-RM assessment has several disadvantages, though: performing the initial assessment of each muscle group may take 10 min or more; there may be a learning effect, since some skill is involved; and poor technique (e.g., allowing varying contributions of accessory muscle groups) can influence the results. Recommended procedures for a 1-RM assessment are listed in box 6.1. Ideally, one should use a group of exercises that assess the strength of the major muscle groups. The test battery could include all or some of the following exercises: bench press, lat pull-down, arm curl, seated abdominal crunch, seated back extension, leg press, leg extension, leg curl. Although most of these exercises can be done with free weights, resistance-exercise machines are most often preferred for both convenience and safety reasons. Regardless of which modality is used for testing, procedures should be established to standardize the position of the patient (e.g., foot and hand position, seat height) during each lift, as differences could create variability in the results.

Box 6.1 Procedures for a 1-RM Assessment

Provide a thorough explanation, and if necessary, a demonstration of the lifting technique. Emphasize correct posture, isolation of desired muscle group, and correct breathing pattern (e.g., do not hold breath and exhale during contraction).

Have patient perform a warm-up or practice trial of the lift. Select a weight that can be easily lifted and have the patient complete 5-10 repetitions. A good rule of thumb to select an appropriate starting weight for men is to take 33% of body weight for the bench press and 100% of their weight for the leg press (for women, use 25% and 75%, respectively). It should be recognized that with some patients, such as the elderly, much lower weights should be used.

Increase the weight depending on the ease of the previous lifts. If the weight can be lifted more than once, have the client stop and rest for at least one minute, then add additional weight and repeat the lift. This is continued until only one contraction can be completed at a given weight. This value is recorded as the 1-RM. The goal is to reach 1-RM within three to five trials (figure 6.5).

Interpretation of strength testing is hindered by the limited amount of normative data available. Indeed, many programs have to rely on norms they have developed with their clients over the years. Interpreting strength measures is further complicated by the fact that the available norms are specific to the type of equipment used for the assessment. For example, one set of commonly used normative standards for 1-RM measures comprises those established by the Cooper Clinic, which used Universal brand exercise machines for the testing. Applying these norms to individuals tested with free weights or another brand of resistance-training machine would not be appropriate. Although it may be difficult to find an appropriate set of norms to classify strength in a patient, serial measurements over time are still useful for tracking a person's strength.

Assessment of Muscular Endurance

The muscular endurance component of physical fitness has been commonly measured on individuals beginning in their school years with various forms of calisthenics-type exercises including push-ups, pull-ups, and sit-ups. Although widely used, particularly in younger populations, these tests have a number of limitations that bring their validity into question. One major disadvantage is that differences in individuals' limb lengths and body weight affect the results. A number of normative data sets are available for these tests. It is important to follow the specific procedures that were used in the development of the normative set if one decides to evaluate clients using a test of this type.

In part because of the limitations of tests using calisthenics-type exercise, other tests of muscular endurance have been suggested. One of these is the YMCA bench press test, which evaluates the maximal number of lifts of a fixed weight (80 lb [36 kg] for men, 35 lb [16 kg] for women) that an individual can complete (18). Although normative values are available for this test, it is not widely used because for many individuals, particularly those with lower body weights and less absolute chest and arm strength, the test is more a measure of strength than of endurance. Recently some programs have begun using tests that evaluate how many times a patient can lift a given amount of weight. The amount of weight can be set as a percentage of body weight or, ideally, of the patient's 1-RM. To date, no widely accepted set of guidelines has been established for this type of muscular endurance testing. Neiman (19) proposed using 70% of 1-RM for the weight and has suggested an "optimal" standard of 10 to 15 contractions for most people and 20 to 25 for athletes. Until firm guidelines are established, differences in protocols will likely exist between programs. Even though these differences present a limitation to this type of muscular endurance testing, the method's practicality makes it desirable. Additionally, evaluations of patients' test scores over time allow the clinician to easily interpret changes in muscular endurance.

Assessment of Flexibility

Although conceptually flexibility is recognized as an important component of physical fitness, its assessment is not well understood or consistently administered. The most common test of flexibility is the sit-and-reach test; it has been proposed that this indirect technique measures the flexibility of the lower back. Since poor flexibility in the lower back has been proposed as a potential risk factor for low back pain and related disability, which has an extremely high prevalence in adults, the sit-and-reach test has gained widespread use. Unfortunately, no substantive evidence exists to support the proposed relationship. This fact, along with knowledge that limb-length differences affect the results and that hamstring muscle flexibility also greatly influences the results, limits the value of this test as a measure of flexibility.

In clinical settings, measurement of the flexibility of multiple joints is recommended. This can be accomplished with relatively inexpensive equipment that includes a universal goniometer (figure 6.6), a Leighton flexometer, and possibly

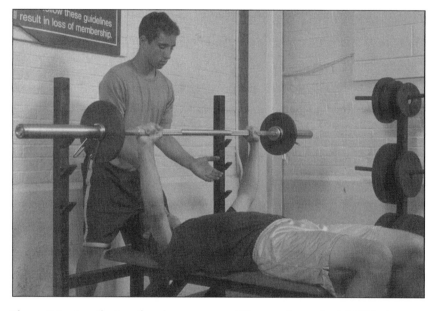

Figure 6.5   A patient performing a one repetition-maximum (weightlifting).

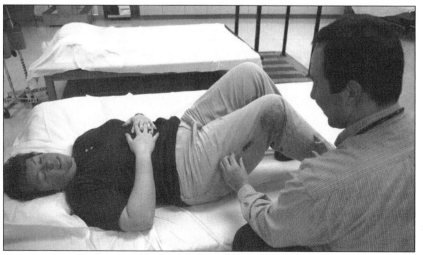

©William Crane

Figure 6.6   Patient being measured with a goniometer.

an inclinometer. Although mechanical operation of the equipment is quite simple, knowledge of and ability to locate anatomical landmarks are necessary for accurate and reliable measurements. Because of the unique landmarks and equipment positioning required for each joint, it is beyond the scope of this text to present flexibility assessment procedures. Maud and Cortez-Cooper (20) provide an excellent review of the methods of multiple-joint flexibility assessment, complete with procedures and normative tables.

Summary

Muscular strength, muscular endurance, and flexibility are now well-accepted components of health-related physical fitness. The specificity principle presents some challenges for assessment of these components, so programs may need to be somewhat creative in developing test batteries. Certainly more research is needed to develop methods and norms for interpreting these components of fitness.

CARDIORESPIRATORY FITNESS

Cardiorespiratory fitness has long been considered the hallmark measure of physical fitness. This is attributable, in large part, to its whole-body nature. The criterion measure of cardiorespiratory fitness, maximal oxygen uptake ($\dot{V}O_2max$), is derived from cardiac output $\times$ arteriovenous oxygen content difference. When we consider the physiological determinants of $\dot{V}O_2max$, which include effective integration of the cardiac, circulatory, respiratory, and muscular systems, it is clear why this measure relates so well to an individual's ability to function. For this reason this component of fitness is sometimes called functional capacity.

As reviewed in chapter 1, cardiorespiratory fitness is also positively related to health and prevention of disease. Additionally, measurement of $\dot{V}O_2max$ is important in various clinical populations for both prognostic and diagnostic reasons. For example, $\dot{V}O_2max$ is on the list of criteria that are evaluated to determine the suitability of a patient for cardiac transplantation. Because of its importance, we devote the remainder of the chapter to the assessment of cardiorespiratory fitness.

Maximal Exercise Testing

$\dot{V}O_2max$ is assessed by measuring pulmonary gas-exchange parameters (minute ventilation and inspired and expired oxygen and carbon dioxide) during a maximal exercise test. Although this procedure is generally considered safe, there are known risks that include major medical complications (serious arrhythmias, myocardial infarction, stroke) and death. Numerous surveys aimed at quantifying the risk of medical complications during exercise testing have yielded values ranging from 0.3 to 8.4 events per 10,000 tests (0.1-0.4%). An exact risk level is difficult to determine since this is influenced by many factors, including patient characteristics, testing protocol and procedures, and skill of test administrators.

As with any type of test, the first consideration should be the rationale for performing the evaluation. There are many indications for exercise testing as summarized in box 6.2. The American College of Cardiology and the American Heart Association have made recommendations for the appropriate use of exercise testing, including a classification scheme (table 6.4) for determining the value of an exercise test (21).

Box 6.2 Indications for Maximal Exercise Testing

To obtain the "true" measure of cardiorespiratory fitness

To use as a diagnostic measure for CAD and to monitor progression of CAD

To use as a prognostic indicator of various diseases

To obtain data for an exercise prescription

To obtain information of relevance to exercise program participation safety

---

Given a sound indication for performing an exercise test, it is necessary to screen patients prior to beginning. Through screening one can risk stratify the patient (low, moderate, or high risk) and thus be able to compare the risks of exercise testing to its benefits. Some conditions, such as unstable angina or an uncontrolled ventricular arrhythmia, pose significant risks for the patient and thus would be considered contraindications to proceeding (box 6.3). The American College of Sports Medicine (ACSM) has developed and regularly updates recommendations for exercise testing and the appropriate pretest screening (12). These guidelines are quite comprehensive. Although some of these recommendations are summarized here, students requiring more detailed information will need to review the appropriate section of the ACSM Guidelines.

Table 6.4
ACC/AHA Classification of Indications for Exercise Testing

Classification	Indication for exercise testing
I	Conditions for which there is evidence and /or general agreement it is useful and effective.
II	Conditions for which there is conflicting evidence about its usefulness/efficacy.
IIa	Weight of evidence/opinion is in favor of usefulness/efficacy.
IIb	Usefulness/efficacy is less well-established by evidence/opinion.
III	Conditions for which there is evidence and/or general agreement it is not useful/effective and in some cases may be harmful.

From (21).

Box 6.3 Contraindications to Exercise Testing (ACSM)

Absolute

A recent significant change in the resting ECG suggesting significant ischemia, recent myocardial infarction (within 2 days), or other acute cardiac event

Unstable angina

Uncontrolled cardiac arrhythmias causing symptoms or hemodynamic compromise

Severe symptomatic aortic stenosis

Uncontrolled symptomatic heart failure

Acute pulmonary embolus or pulmonary infarction

Acute myocarditis or pericarditis

Suspected or known dissecting aneurysm

Acute infections

Relative*

Left main coronary stenosis

Moderate stenotic valvular heart disease

Electrolyte abnormalities (e.g., hypokalemia, hypomagnesemia)

Severe arterial hypertension (i.e., systolic blood pressure of >200 mmHg and/or a diastolic blood pressure of >110 mmHg) at rest

Tachyarrhythmias or bradyarrhythmias

Hypertrophic cardiomyopathy and other forms of outflow tract obstruction

Neuromuscular, musculoskeletal, or rheumatoid disorders that are exacerbated by exercise

High-degree atrioventricular block

Ventricular aneurysm

Uncontrolled metabolic disease (e.g., diabetes, thyrotoxicosis, or myxedema)

Chronic infectious disease (e.g., mononucleosis, hepatitis, AIDS)

---

*Relative contraindications can be superseded if benefits outweigh risks of exercise. In some instances, these individuals can be exercised with caution and/or using low-level end points, especially if they are asymptomatic at rest.

Reproduced with permission. ACC/AHA Guidelines for Exercise Testing. *J Am Coll Cardiol* 1996;30:260-315. Copyright 1997 by the American College of Cardiology and American Heart Association, Inc.

The minimal level of screening for risk stratification of a patient requires information on present health status; known risk factors; and signs or symptoms of cardiovascular, pulmonary, or metabolic disease. Much of this information can come from a good medical history review (questionnaire) and some basic clinical measurements. Table 6.5 provides a summary of the risk factor and sign and symptom lists as well as the recommended risk stratification classifications as proposed by ACSM. We developed a basic questionnaire that clinicians can use to quickly and easily obtain an initial risk stratification according to the ACSM recommendations (see form B, page 192). Note that most or all of the information required for the risk stratification can be obtained directly from the patients' responses on this questionnaire. Some patients may respond with "unknown" to the questions about blood pressure, obesity, cholesterol, and glucose measurements. However, exercise program staff can typically obtain this information by performing a standard resting blood pressure assessment; taking measurements of height, weight, and waist

Table 6.5
ACSM Risk Stratification Recommendations

Risk Category	Initial risk stratification criteria
Low risk	Younger individuals who are asymptomatic and ≤1 risk factor
Moderate risk	Older individuals or those with ≥2 risk factors
High risk	Individuals with ≥1 sign/symptom or have known cardiovascular, pulmonary disease, or metabolic disease

Age criteria:	Younger = <45 years (men) or <55 years (women) Older = ≥45 years (men) or ≥55 years (women)
Risk factor list*:	Cigarette smoker; family history; hypercholesterolemia; hypertension; impaired fasting glucose; obesity; sedentary lifestyle; high HDL-cholesterol (negative risk factor)
Sign/symptom list:	Pain, discomfort (or other angina equivalent) in the chest, neck, jaw, arms, or other areas that may be due to ischemia; dizziness or syncope; orthopnea or paroxysmal nocturnal dyspnea; ankle edema; palpitations or tachycardia; intermittent claudication; known heart murmur; unusual fatigue or shortness of breath

*Thresholds for each risk factor are presented in the ACSM Guidelines for Exercise Testing and Prescription (12).

Reprinted, by permission, 2000, *ACSM's Guidelines for Exercise Testing and Prescription*. 6th ed. (Philadelphia: Lippincott, Williams, and Wilkins), 26.

circumference; and collecting a fasting blood sample.

Given the initial risk stratification, the ACSM has specific recommendations for further evaluation. All high-risk patients should have a current medical exam and a maximal exercise test. This same recommendation applies to moderate-risk patients beginning (or increasing to) a vigorous-intensity exercise program.

Pretesting Procedures

The patient should receive, preferably in written form, a set of pretest instructions to follow in preparation for the exercise test (see form C, p. 193). These include being well rested (adequate amount of sleep and no unusual exertion within 24 h of the test), limiting food intake to no more than a small snack (e.g., piece of fruit) and ingesting no caffeine or alcohol for 3 h prior to the test, continuing to take all medication as regularly scheduled unless told specifically otherwise by the physician conducting the test, and wearing loose-fitting (preferably athletic) clothing and some type of exercise footwear. A number of preliminary steps precede the start of an exercise test. The first is administration of an informed consent, which is necessary for both legal and ethical reasons. Much more than a form that you require a patient to sign, an informed consent is a process to be completed with the patient. The essential elements of the process are to provide an adequate explanation of the testing procedures, including what will be required of the patient; describe the risks and the benefits of the test; and explain that the patient is able to withdraw consent at any time (i.e., can stop the test at any time). In the description of risks it is advisable to explain that procedures are

designed to minimize risks wherever possible. Many generic templates for informed consent forms are available in various sources (including the ACSM Guidelines). Since the testing procedures vary from site to site, it is important to customize an informed consent form to the specifics of each site (see form D, p. 194). The actual administration of the informed consent requires the patient to read the form, have the opportunity to ask any questions for clarification purposes, and then sign the form in the presence of a witness.

The patient should then be prepared for any monitoring to be conducted during the test. Preparation includes selecting the appropriate size blood pressure cuff (length of bladder should be ≥80% of the circumference of the arm), explaining appropriate responses for any perceptual scales (ratings of dyspnea, chest discomfort, and perceived exertion), and applying ECG electrodes. We have found it helpful to read standardized instructions to all patients explaining use of the perceptual scales (table 6.6). This assures that the essential information is covered and that the data are useful for potential research applications.

Because of the importance of the ECG for both safety (monitoring during the test) and potential diagnosis (posttest interpretation), a high-quality tracing is essential. This requires preparation of the skin to lower the resistance to the conduction of the electrical signal. The locations of the electrodes (shown in figure 5.8) for the limb leads are modified for the exercise test to reduce artifact (figure 6.7). Specifically, these electrodes are placed on the torso, with the ankle sites placed just below the rib cage at the midclavicular line and the wrist sites just below the right and left clavicle in the infraclavicular fossa. It is important not to use

Table 6.6
Useful Perceptual Rating Scales During Exercise Testing

5-grade angina scale	5-grade dyspnea scale	10-grade angina/dyspnea scale	
0 No Angina	0 No dyspnea	0	Nothing
		0.5	Very, very slight
1 Light, barely noticeable	1 Mild, noticeable	1	Very slight
2 Moderate, bothersome	2 Mild, some difficulty	2	Slight
3 Severe, very uncomfortable	3 Moderate difficulty, but can continue	3	Moderate
4 Most pain ever experienced	4 Severe difficulty, cannot continue	4	Somewhat severe
		5	Severe
		6	
		7	Very severe
		8	
		9	
		10	Very, very severe
			Maximal

From (14).

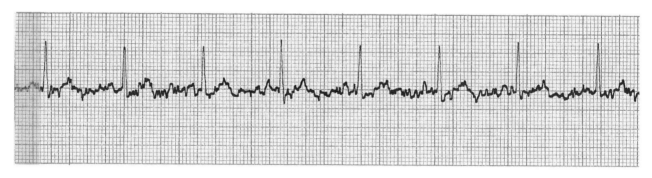

Figure 6.7   Picture of artifact on ECG from poor preparation.

these modified leads for a diagnostic resting ECG, as changes in the electrical axis and amplitude of the wave forms have been shown to occur when compared to the tracings obtained with the standard limb lead placement. Once the ECG sites are identified (site area should be shaved if necessary and marked with a felt-tip pen), the preparation consists of cleansing the skin with an alcohol-soaked gauze pad, then rubbing with an abrasive pad. The electrodes are then carefully placed on the skin; care should be taken to make sure that they adhere completely (figure 6.8).

Mode of Exercise

The first decision to be made concerning exercise testing is what mode to use. The two most com-mon modes are treadmill and cycle; but depending on the patient characteristics, the purpose of the test, and the equipment available, other modes such as arm, combined arm and leg, stepping, and recumbent cycling can be used. Historically, the majority of clinics in the United States (a 1980 survey reported 71%, and a 2000 survey reported 78%) performed treadmill testing, whereas cycle testing was more common elsewhere (22, 23). Today most clinics with the resources and space have both the treadmill and cycle available, and in some cases other modes. Treadmill and cycle testing both have advantages and disadvantages (box 6.4). The treadmill is the ideal mode for exercise testing principally because walking is the most common activity for the majority of individuals. Additionally,

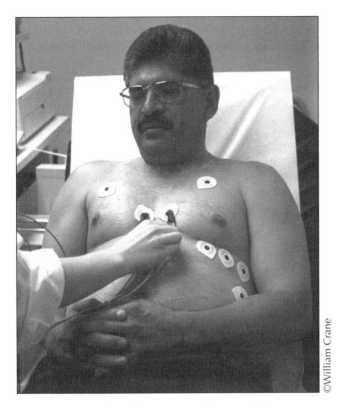

©William Crane

Figure 6.8   A patient being prepared for an ECG.

Box 6.4 Factors to Consider in Exercise Test Mode Selection

Treadmill: Advantages

Is a more common activity

Provides "true" maximal physiological responses

Has a greater potential for detecting ST segment changes and/or angina

Can manipulate rate of work by both speed and grade change

Treadmill: Disadvantages

Is more expensive and requires more space

Is generally noisier (issue for BP measures)

Has potential risk of injury if patient slips

Has potential for more ECG artifact

High elevations may cause local calf muscle fatigue, which may result in less than maximal effort

Cycle: Advantages

Is less expensive and requires less space

Is generally quieter

Generally involves no injury risk

Eliminates body weight as a work determinant

Cycle: Disadvantages

Is a less common activity

Generally will use a fixed pedal rate on mechanically-braked ergometers and thus can only manipulate pedal resistance

Local fatigue of leg muscles may result in less than maximal cardiovascular stress

treadmill tests have been shown to provide the highest $\dot{V}O_2$max values. Cycle testing is preferable for patients who have an orthopedic limitation that hinders their ability to ambulate. Additionally, in some populations (e.g., among individuals who are elderly) for whom maintaining balance on the treadmill belt is an issue (and thus increases patient anxiety), cycle testing is preferable. Arm testing is required for persons with a disability that prohibits adequate amounts of work with the legs, as well as for some patients whose occupation requires repetitive lifting with the arms. When there is concern that a patient will not be able to produce the required maximal exercise effort, pharmacological tests (as discussed in chapter 3) are commonly used for diagnostic purposes.

Protocol Selection

Once the mode has been determined, it is necessary to select a specific protocol. A protocol for an exercise test defines the rate of work increases that will be required of the patient. Although many protocols are available, all can be categorized on the basis of several characteristics: submaximal versus maximal, discontinuous versus continuous, and incremental versus ramp. Selecting a particular protocol for an exercise test requires consideration of a variety of factors, with the most important one being the purpose of conducting the test. The purpose of the test could range from an estimation of $\dot{V}O_2$max in a young, low-risk participant in a community health/fitness program to diagnosis of a middle-aged, high-risk patient in a clinical exercise program. For the $\dot{V}O_2$max estimation one could use a submaximal protocol and pulse rate monitoring; the diagnosis would require a graded maximal protocol with monitoring of a number of different variables (e.g., heart rate, blood pressure, ECG, signs and symptoms). Even though the exercise test may have one primary purpose, in most clinical programs (both primary and secondary prevention) it is desirable to maximize the amount of data from the test for multiple uses (e.g., fitness assessment, exercise prescription, diagnosis and/or prognosis).

The protocol selected should include a short warm-up period (1-2 min) at a low intensity (2-3 METs) and should allow the patient to reach maximal physiological effort in no less than 6 min or more than 15 min (with an ideal test time range of 8-12 min). It has been shown that test durations <6 min or >15 min may not result in maximal responses for some physiological measures, including $\dot{V}O_2$max (24). Traditionally, most exercise testing laboratories utilized standardized incremental protocols—an incremental protocol is one that consists of multiple stages (a workload that is set for a fixed period of time). Typically the increase in work rate with each stage is similar, as are stage durations. Most incremental protocols were designed with stage durations of 2 or 3 min so that patients would reach a steady state at each stage. The rate of increase in work rate with each stage is typically between 1 and 3 METs for most incremental protocols.

Treadmill Protocols

One distinguishing characteristic of the incremental type of treadmill protocol is the way in which the work rate is increased. Treadmill protocols are described as either fixed or variable speed. A basic advantage of a fixed-speed protocol is that patients need to adjust their gait only once (from warm-up speed to test speed) during the test. Another desirable feature is that it is possible to select a comfortable walking speed and then maintain it for the entire test. The disadvantage of fixed-speed protocols is that increases in work rate can be obtained only by increasing elevation (which generally constrains the rate of increase); patients capable of performing longer tests face steep treadmill grades (>15%), which may result in local fatigue of the gastrocnemius muscles and thus lead to a premature end of the exercise test.

Many standardized incremental treadmill protocols have been developed. The defining features of these protocols are their starting work rate, the amount of increase in work rate with each stage, whether they are fixed or variable speed, and their stage duration (table 6.7). The two most commonly used incremental protocols are the Bruce and the Balke. A survey of exercise testing clinics in 1980 showed that 67% used the Bruce protocol and 10% used the Balke protocol (23). A recent survey of Veterans Affairs Medical Centers indicated that these facilities used the Bruce protocol, or a modification thereof, in 82% of the exer-

cise tests performed on treadmills (22). Certainly, familiarity with a procedure, both within a clinic and for communications among clinicians, would be a primary reason for utilizing the Bruce or Balke protocol. Another benefit is the large body of knowledge relating to individuals' physiological responses during exercise testing with these procedures. Especially important is the knowledge of the metabolic requirements at both submaximal and maximal levels.

The defining characteristics of the Bruce protocol are outlined in table 6.8. Among criticisms of the Bruce protocol have been the relatively high beginning work rate, the large work rate increments, and the variable speed. The original work rate requirements limited the use of this protocol in populations with relatively low functional capacity (e.g., <7 METs), as test times were too short. This limitation has been overcome through a modification of the Bruce protocol—the addition of a preliminary stage or two (stages 0 and 0.5).

Table 6.7
Features of the Bruce and Balke Protocols

Feature	Bruce	Balke (original)	Balke (modified)
Speed (mph)	Variable 1.7–6.0	Fixed 3.3	Fixed 3.0
First stage (METs)	4.5	3.3	3
Stage duration (min)	3	1	2
Work rate Δ (per stage)	2.5–3 METs	0.5 METs	1 MET

Table 6.8
Characteristics of the Bruce Protocol

Stage/time (min)		Speed (mph)	Grade (%)	Intensity (METs)
0		1.7	0	2
0.5		1.7	5	3
1	0–3	1.7	10	4.5
2	3–6	2.5	12	7
3	6–9	3.4	14	10
4	9–12	4.2	16	13
5	12–15	5.0	18	16
6	15–18	5.5	20	19
7	18–21	6.0	22	21

The variable-speed element of the protocol requires an individual to make numerous gait adjustments and may lead to a transition from a walk to a run for those who continue past 9 min on the test. This transition typically occurs during stage 4 and may lead to premature test termination for some individuals who struggle to find a comfortable gait. Certainly, monitoring of both ECG and blood pressure becomes much more problematic when a patient begins to run (figure 6.9). Despite these limitations, many clinicians still prefer to use the Bruce protocol for a majority of their patients because of its familiarity and the reasonably short test times (<10 min).

The defining characteristics of the Balke protocol are highlighted in table 6.7. Criticisms of the original protocol were that the speed was uncomfortable for many patients, that the stages were too short, and that for many patients with average or above-average functional capacities the test duration would be quite long. Modifications have been made to the original Balke protocol in order to address the first two criticisms. Although many different modifications exist, the most common one reduces the speed to 3 mph (4.8 km/h) and uses increments of 2.5% grade (1 MET) every 2 min. Other modifications have used even slower fixed speeds (e.g., 2 mph [3.2 km/h]) for populations with lower functional capacities.

Cycle and Ramp Protocols

For cycle testing there has been less standardization of protocols, in large part because of the differing nature of the work requirements between individuals. For treadmill tests, the increments per stage are equal with regard to the relative units of METs for all individuals, since the resistance component of the work is determined by the body weight. For cycle exercise, the resistance component of the work is determined by the external load placed on the pedals. This type of resistance results in an equal absolute energy requirement between individuals; however, the relative energy expenditure (METs) varies with body weight (table 6.9). This results in potentially drastic differences in relative energy expenditure requirements between individuals using the same cycle exercise test protocol. Thus, determination of an appropriate protocol for cycling requires setting both a reasonable initial load and a rate of increment based on an estimation of the individual's maximal absolute functional capacity. The work rate for cycling is dependent on both the load on the pedals and the frequency of pedaling (rpm). With mechanically loaded (braked)

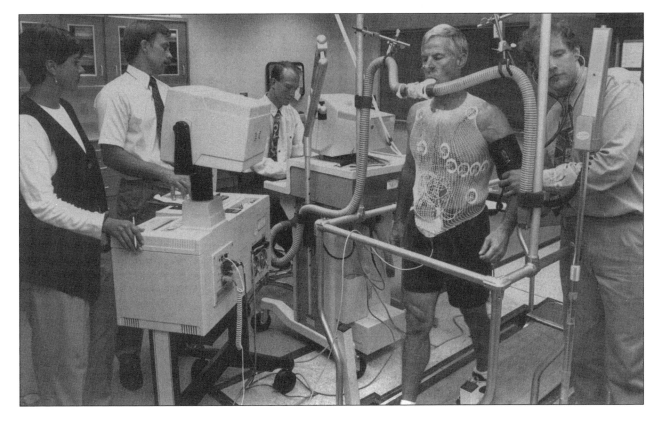

Figure 6.9   A patient performs a maximal exercise test.
Photo Courtesy of Ball State University Photo Services.

Table 6.9

Differences in Absolute and Relative Energy Requirements at a Fixed Work Rate

	Person A	Person B
Work rate	100W	100W
Body weight	100kg	50 kg
"Absolute" $\dot{V}O_2$ (ml/min)	1780	1430
"Relative" $\dot{V}O_2$ (ml/kg/min)	17.8	28.6

ergometers, the resistance on the pedal remains fixed and thus the work rate will vary with pedal speed. This requires maintenance of a fixed speed (usually 50 rpm) during the test to keep work rates standardized. Electrically loaded cycles, on the other hand, adjust the load on the pedal according to the pedal frequency in order to maintain a constant work rate. A typical incremental type of cycle protocol starts at an initial work rate of between 25 and 100 W with stage increases of either 25 or 50 W every 2 or 3 min. Electrically loaded cycles allow for even smaller initial loads and smaller stage increases than the 25-W minimum obtained with mechanically loaded cycles. Another feature of the electrically loaded cycles is a means to make small changes in the work rate more rapidly during the test. This has led to the development of ramp-style protocols. Although conceptually, ramp protocols are thought to provide consistent and continuous increases in work rate over time, in reality they deliver small increases in work rate over very short time increments (5-20 s). When they were first proposed, many believed that ramp protocols would provide better data, both for interpretation of gas-exchange kinetics measures (e.g., measures used for ventilatory threshold detection) and for translation to exercise prescription, than incremental protocols did. Although these purported benefits of ramp protocols have not been evaluated adequately in research studies, other advantages of ramp protocols have been established. Two documented advantages are an improved ability to predict maximal oxygen uptake from exercise test time and a stronger relationship between exercise test time at ischemia and ambulatory ischemia. The latter finding suggests that ramp-type protocols would also better serve to document the efficacy of interventions for ischemia.

Originally, the use of ramp protocols was limited to tests performed with an electrically loaded

cycle. However, in the late 1980s, technology emerged that allowed programming of treadmill controllers to deliver ramp protocols. Two variations of ramp treadmill protocols are currently being used—individualized ramp protocols and standardized ramp protocols.

An individualized ramp protocol is designed to have the patient reach maximum effort in an ideal test time of between 8 and 12 min. This approach requires knowledge of the patient's expected maximal work rate, which is ideally obtained from a previous, recent exercise test. However, for those who do not have recent exercise test data, an estimation of their predicted $\dot{V}O_2$max must be derived from their demographic characteristics. (The relatively large errors in predicted $\dot{V}O_2$max can be a major limitation to the use of individualized protocols.) Another feature of an individualized ramp protocol is that one can select any speed, which is ideal for customizing to a patient's comfort level. The desired speed and the expected $\dot{V}O_2$max information are then used to determine the peak grade from the ACSM metabolic equation for walking.[1] The time and rate of change in work rate from the beginning to the estimated end of the test can be derived in the same way; however, many exercise testing systems now offer computerized methods that will develop a ramp rate. Dr. Jonathan Myers and colleagues have demonstrated the usefulness of individualized ramp protocols (25-27). If $\dot{V}O_2$max is not measured, it can be predicted from peak speed and grade using the ACSM metabolic equations.

Standardized ramp protocols use the same speed and grade increments for all patients, allowing for data comparisons between patients at equivalent test times (see figure 6.10). The one major limitation to standardized ramp protocols, as with incremental protocols, is that one specific protocol is not suited to all populations. The BSU [Ball State University]/Bruce ramp protocol (table 6.10) was designed to have characteristics similar to those of the incremental Bruce protocol (28)—specifically, identical work rate requirements at each 3-min period throughout the test. This protocol was conceptualized to allow clinics that have traditionally used the Bruce protocol, yet wish to obtain the advantages offered by a ramp-style protocol, to make the transition. A nice benefit of the BSU/Bruce ramp protocol is that patients can typically walk longer prior to needing to jog ($\approx$11 min) than if they were using the Bruce protocol (9 min). Clinics that do not mea-

---

1 $\dot{V}O_2$ (ml·kg^{-1}·min^{-1}) = (speed [m·min^{-1}] • 0.1) + (speed [m·min^{-1}] • grade [frac.] • 1.8) + 3.5

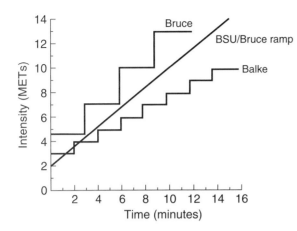

Figure 6.10 Diagrammatic representation of the increase in metabolic requirements using incremental (standard Bruce and modified Balke) and ramp (standardized BSU/Bruce ramp) treadmill protocols.

sure oxygen uptake can use a validated equation to predict $\dot{V}O_2$max from exercise test time from the BSU/Bruce ramp protocol. This equation, along with published equations for the Bruce and Balke protocols, is presented in table 6.11.

Estimates of Functional Capacity

As discussed earlier, selection of an appropriate test protocol depends in part on having an estimate of the patient's $\dot{V}O_2$max prior to the test. There are a number of approaches to this, but all rely on having descriptive information on the patient. Usually the more that is known about the patient, particularly about factors known to be associated with $\dot{V}O_2$max, the better the prediction. Among the most helpful characteristics are gender, age, activity status, and body composition.

The simplest approach to estimating a patient's $\dot{V}O_2$max is to use a normative table to determine what an "average" value is for a particular gender and age group (table 6.12). For example, using the norms developed from over 4000 people in the Ball State University Adult Physical Fitness research database who met maximal criteria during exercise tests, the average $\dot{V}O_2$max for 50- to 59-year-old women is 26.1 ± 5.8 ml·kg⁻¹·min⁻¹. You might adjust the expected value by adding one standard deviation to the average if, for example, you know that the patient is a regular exerciser. Conversely, you might adjust the expected value by subtracting one standard deviation from the average if you know that the patient is sedentary and obese.

A slightly more scientific approach is to use statistical regression equations to estimate

$\dot{V}O_2$max. A number of studies that developed such equations were published in the 1990s, including two with our data from Ball State and Wake Forest Universities. These studies all used gender, age, a rating of physical activity, and some measure of body composition to predict $\dot{V}O_2$max. The equations developed from Ball State and Wake Forest Universities are provided in table 6.13 and used in the case studies at the end of the chapter.

Of note are the wide range of "average" values in the normative table (6.12; i.e., ±SD) and the relatively large standard error of prediction in the regression equations (tables 6.11 and 6.13), demonstrating that $\dot{V}O_2$max varies widely (even between individuals of similar characteristics) and thus is a difficult variable to predict.

Exercise Testing Procedures

A number of different variables can be monitored during an exercise test. Generally it is considered essential to monitor the patient's ECG, heart rate, blood pressure, signs, and symptoms. Additional helpful information can come from measurements of gas exchange during the test. The following is a brief overview of specific requirements for monitoring each of the variables mentioned. Recommendations as to when each variable should be measured prior to, during, and after the exercise test is provided in table 6.14.

Standardization of the procedures and the timing of the measures are important to allow for accurate interpretation of test data, especially from serial tests on the same patient (form E, p. 195).

The ECG technician should make all the initial settings on the recorder (specific to the manufacturer) and should record a tracing of the ECG as soon as the patient is connected to the ECG system. It is important to review this initial tracing to make sure that the quality of the ECG preparation was good and that the electrodes are picking up a clean signal—basically, to ensure that the recording is free from artifact and that the individual lead recordings do not exhibit excessive wandering from a baseline level. It is also important to ascertain that the electrodes were accurately connected with the lead wires (e.g., limb leads not switched). The ECG should be monitored continuously prior to, during, and after the exercise test. Any deviations from a normal ECG (see chapter 5) should be documented with either an ECG recording or a notation on the exercise test data sheet. This technician also typically records all the data collected according to the time

Table 6.10
Characteristics of the BSU/Bruce Ramp Protocol

Increment	Time	Speed	Grade	Increment	Time	Speed	Grade
1	0:00	1.7	0.0	33	10:40	4.0	15.2
2	0:20	1.7	1.3	34	11:00	4.1	15.4
3	0:40	1.7	2.5	35	11:20	4.2	15.6
4	1:00	1.7	3.7	36	11:40	4.2	16.0
5	1:20	1.7	5.0	37	12:00	4.3	16.2
6	1:40	1.7	6.2	38	12:20	4.4	16.4
7	2:00	1.7	7.5	39	12:40	4.5	16.6
8	2:20	1.7	8.7	40	13:00	4.6	16.8
9	2:40	1.7	10.0	41	13:20	4.7	17.0
10	3:00	1.8	10.2	42	13:40	4.8	17.2
11	3:20	1.9	10.2	43	14:00	4.9	17.4
12	3:40	2.0	10.5	44	14:20	5.0	17.6
13	4:00	2.1	10.7	45	14:40	5.0	18.0
14	4:20	2.2	10.9	46	15:00	5.1	18.0
15	4:40	2.3	11.2	47	15:20	5.1	18.5
16	5:00	2.4	11.2	48	15:40	5.2	18.5
17	5:20	2.5	11.6	49	16:00	5.2	19.0
18	5:40	2.5	12.0	50	16:20	5.3	19.0
19	6:00	2.6	12.2	51	16:40	5.3	19.5
20	6:20	2.7	12.4	52	17.00	5.4	19.5
21	6:40	2.8	12.7	53	17:20	5.4	20.0
22	7:00	2.9	12.9	54	17:40	5.5	20.0
23	7:20	3.0	13.1	55	18:00	5.6	20.0
24	7:40	3.1	13.4	56	18:20	5.6	20.5
25	8:00	3.2	13.6	57	18:40	5.7	20.5
26	8:20	3.3	13.8	58	19:00	5.7	21.0
27	8:40	3.4	14.0	59	19:20	5.8	21.0
28	9:00	3.5	14.2	60	19:40	5.8	21.5
29	9:20	3.6	14.4	61	20:00	5.9	21.5
30	9:40	3.7	14.6	62	20:20	5.9	22.0
31	10:00	3.8	14.8	63	20:40	6.0	22.0
32	10:20	3.9	15.0				

Highlighted increments are at same time, speed, and grade as the standard Bruce protocol.

Reprinted, by permission, from L.A. Kaminsky and M.H. Whaley, 1998, "Evaluation of a new standardized ramp protocol: the BSU/Bruce ramp protocol," *Journal of Cardiopulmonary Rehabilitation* 18:444.

Table 6.11
Regression Equations to Estimate $\dot{V}O_2$max (ml·kg^{-1}·min^{-1}) From Exercise Test Time

Protocol/population studied	Prediction equation
Bruce (29) 200 men and women	$14.8 - 1.379$ (min) $+ 0.451$ (min^2) $- 0.012$ (min^3) ± 3.4
Bruce (handrail support) (30) 128 men	$8.545 + 2.282$ (min) ± 4.92
Balke (original) (31) 51 men	$14.99 + 1.444$ (min)
Balke (modified) (32) 49 women	$5.2 + 0.023$ (sec)
BSU/Bruce Ramp (28) 698 men and women	3.9 (min) $- 7.0 \pm 3.4$

min = test time in minutes; sec = test time in seconds.
Modified Balke used a fixed speed of 3 mph, started at 0% and increased grade 2.5% every 3 minutes.

Table 6.12
Normative Values for $\dot{V}O_2$max (ml·kg^{-1}·min^{-1}) Based on Gender and Age

Age range (sample size [M/W])	Men	Women
20–29 years (264/210)	45.9 ± 10.8	35.2 ± 9.2
30–39 years (705/410)	42.5 ± 9.3	30.9 ± 7.0
40–49 years (866/462)	38.9 ± 9.0	28.6 ± 7.0
50–59 years (593/335)	35.6 ± 8.7	26.1 ± 5.8
60–69 years (231/168)	33.0 ± 7.8	23.1 ± 5.5
70–79 years (41/22)	27.8 ± 6.6	20.7 ± 3.6

Minimal criteria for inclusion of data was an exercise test R value of >1.0.
From Whaley, Kaminsky, and Getchell. Adult Physical Fitness Research Database.

sequence noted in table 6.14. It is important to continually observe the patient for signs of distress and to regularly ask the patient if he or she is experiencing any symptoms. If gas-exchange measurements are being obtained, the patient should be instructed to remove the mouthpiece to report any symptoms or concerns experienced during the exercise test.

It can be difficult to obtain blood pressure measurement during exercise, especially for a novice technician. Use of the auscultatory technique requires good basic skills and ability when performed with a patient at rest. The technique becomes more challenging during exercise, especially with treadmill protocols, which involve extraneous noise from the ergometer and from movement of the patient. An accurate blood pressure measurement requires use of the correct cuff size (length of bladder ≥80% of the circumference of the arm) and is aided by a high-quality stethoscope. It is helpful to palpate the brachial artery and mark the location on the skin for subsequent placement of the stethoscope bell. The bladder should be centered over the brachial artery (note that tubes coming out of the cuff should not get in the way of the placement of the stethoscope bell), with the lower edge of the cuff positioned at least 1 in. [2.5 cm] above the antecubital space. The technician begins the measurement by stabilizing the patient's arm (e.g., by holding the patient's arm between the technician's arm and torso) and placing the bell of the stethoscope lightly over the brachial artery. Then the cuff is rapidly inflated to a pressure that is 20 mmHg higher than the estimated systolic blood pressure. Pressure in the cuff is reduced (rate of 2-3 mmHg/s) until the first Korotkoff sound is heard. The Korotkoff sounds are the actual sounds heard with a stethoscope during a blood pressure reading. This gradual deflation of the cuff pressure is important for obtaining an accurate measurement, as too rapid a reduction can result in significantly lower readings. Once a clear set of sounds is heard, the pressure in the cuff can be dropped more rapidly until the pressure reaches ≈20 mmHg higher than the estimated diastolic blood pressure. Then the deflation rate is reduced to approximately 2 to 3 mmHg/s again until the sounds disappear (fifth Korotkoff phase), which indicates diastolic pressure. Note that sometimes

Table 6.13
Regression Equations to Estimate $\dot{V}O_2max$ (ml·kg^{-1}·min^{-1}) From Patient Characteristics

Source/population	Equation
Ball State APFP/Healthy (no CAD)	$\dot{V}O_2max = 50.55 - 0.324$ (age-yrs) + 5.664 (gender) + 2.157 (PA-BSU) − 0.46 (BMI) SEE = ± 5.60; r = 0.84
Wake Forest CR/CAD Patients	$\dot{V}O_2max = 40.74 - 0.208$ (age-yrs) + 4.283 (gender) + 1.187 (PA-WFU) − 0.406 (BMI) SEE = ±3.86; r = 0.66

Gender: (female = 0; male = 1)
Ball State physical activity habits code scheme:
1 = sedentary lifestyle
2 = sedentary occupation with moderate recreational activity
3 = moderate occupational and recreational activity
4 = heavy occupational with moderate recreational activity
5 = participates regularly in endurance exercise (e.g., ≥3 days per week of walking, running, swimming, cycling, aerobic dancing, etc.)
6 = highly trained (e.g., >20 miles per week of running, cycling, swimming).

From Whaley MH et al. Medicine and Science in Sports and Exercise, 27:85-91, 1995.

Wake Forest Physical activity habits code scheme:
0 = no activity outside the rehabilitation program
1 = 2-3 days of activity outside the rehabilitation program
2 = greater than 3 days of activity outside the rehabilitation program
From Fox, J.L. et al. Journal of Cardiopulmonary Rehabilitation, 19:313, 1999.

Table 6.14
Recommended Monitoring Intervals Associated With Exercise Testing

Variable	Prior to exercise test	During exercise test	After exercise test
ECG	Monitored continuously; recorded supine position and posture of exercise	Monitored continuously; recorded during the last 15 s of each stage (interval protocol) or the last 15 s of each 2 min time period (ramp protocols)	Monitored continuously; recorded immediately post exercise, during the last 15 s of first minute of recovery and then every 2 min thereafter
HR	Monitored continuously; recorded supine position and posture of exercise	Monitored continuously; recorded during the last 5 s of each minute	Monitored continuously; recorded during the last 5 s of each minute
BP	Measured and recorded in supine position and posture of exercise	Measured and recorded during the last 45 s of each stage (interval protocol) or the last 45 s of each 2 min time period (ramp protocols)	Measured and recorded immediately post exercise and then every 2 min thereafter
Signs and symptoms	Monitored continuously; recorded as observed	Monitored continuously; recorded as observed	Monitored continuously; recorded as observed
RPE	Explain scale	Recorded during the last 5 s of each minute	Obtain peak exercise value then not measured in recovery
Gas exchange	Baseline reading to assure proper operational status	Measured continuously	Not needed in recovery

with exercise, sounds can be heard all the way to zero. In these circumstances it is desirable to record the fourth Korotkoff sound (muffling of sound) as the diastolic pressure.

In this era of rapidly evolving technology, it bears mentioning that automated blood pressure measurement devices are available. Because of the challenges in obtaining quality blood pressure measurements during exercise, the potential for use of an automated system is appealing. To date, the majority of the automated systems are designed only for resting measurements. One review paper evaluating the performance of many automated devices indicated that only ≈50% of them had satisfactory accuracy and reliability (33). A few manufacturers are marketing products that can be used during exercise. Validation studies on the performance of these devices are necessary before they obtain widespread acceptance. Users of this technology need to be cautioned to be sure that technicians are appropriately trained, that the data are critically evaluated for reasonableness, and that the system's calibration is regularly checked.

A comprehensive list of both absolute and relative test termination criteria from the ACSM *Guidelines for Exercise Testing and Prescription* (12) is provided in box 6.3. Although terminating the exercise test is ultimately the responsibility of the test supervisor, all technicians should be familiar with indications for stopping an exercise test. Some facilities in certain situations may have specific test end points established prior to the test—for example, if the patient reaches his age-predicted maximal heart rate. However, in most cases, patients are encouraged to give their best effort, and the test is continued—unless specific signs or symptoms are observed—until the patient requests that it be stopped. Note that to perform a maximal effort, most patients require considerable encouragement and feedback from the technicians. Since there is no definitive physiological marker of maximal effort, with the possible exception of a true $\dot{V}O_2$ plateau, the decision to terminate the test relies on the clinical judgment of the test supervisor. Common indicators of maximal effort are discussed in the next section. It has been the authors' practice to enthusiastically encourage patients to produce a maximal effort. One method that we employ is to have patients give a signal (wave their hands in front of them) when they feel they are getting close to maximal effort. At that time we ask patients if they can continue for an additional 20 to 30 s and encourage them to do so. At the end of this time period the patients are asked again if they can continue. Most patients are able to "push" themselves to a higher work

level with this type of encouragement, since they know they are in control of stopping the test.

Box 6.5 ACC/AHA Indications for Terminating Exercise Testing

Absolute Indications

Drop in systolic blood pressure of ≥10 mmHg from baseline blood pressure despite an increase in workload, when accompanied by other evidence of ischemia

Moderate to severe angina

Increasing nervous system symptoms (e.g., ataxia, dizziness, or near syncope)

Signs of poor perfusion (cyanosis or pallor)

Technical difficulties monitoring the ECG or systolic blood pressure

Patient's desire to stop

Sustained ventricular tachycardia

ST elevation (≥1.0 mm) in leads without diagnostic Q-waves (other than V_1 or aVR)

Relative Indications

Drop in systolic blood pressure of ≥10 mmHg from baseline blood pressure despite an increase in workload, in the absence of other evidence of ischemia

ST or QRS changes such as excessive ST depression (>2 mm horizontal or downsloping ST-segment depression) or marked axis shift

Arrhythmias other than sustained ventricular tachycardia, including multifocal premature ventricular contractions, triplets of premature ventricular contractions, supraventricular tachycardia, heart block, or bradyarrhythmias

Fatigue, shortness of breath, wheezing, leg cramps, or claudication

Development of bundle branch block or intraventricular conduction delay that cannot be distinguished from ventricular tachycardia

Increasing chest pain

Hypertensive response*

*Systolic blood pressure of more than 250 mmHg and/or a diastolic blood pressure of more than 115 mmHg.

Reproduced with permission. ACC/AHA Guidelines for Exercise Testing. *J Am Coll Cardiol* 1996;30:260-315. Copyright 1997 by the American College of Cardiology and American Heart Association, Inc.

The posttest recovery period typically has two phases, active and passive. Close observation and monitoring of the patient are important in the recovery period, as it is common for patients to develop symptoms after they have completed the test. In most adult fitness settings and in situations when the test has a major purpose other than diagnosis of an ischemic response, the recovery period begins with a short interval (1-3 min) of low-level exercise (walking ≤ 2 mph [3.2 km/h], cycling <25 W). This is followed by a 3- to 7-min period with the patient in the supine position. In cardiac rehabilitation programs and when the primary purpose of the test is diagnosis of an ischemic response, having the person lie down immediately after the test can improve the sensitivity of the test by increasing the "stress" on the heart. This increased work of the heart is due to the increased venous return that occurs because of the postural change. Most patients prefer a short active posttest period as it speeds their recovery, in part via the metabolism of exercise metabolites (e.g., lactic acid and catecholamines) by the working skeletal muscles. Additionally, many patients benefit from a drink of water immediately after the exercise test, particularly if it included gas-exchange measurements. It is also important for technicians to be aware that occasionally patients become nauseous and/or light-headed during recovery. These patients need to be observed for a prolonged period of time and periodic blood pressure measurements made when hypotension is suspected. It is ideal to have someone transport these patients home when they are ready to leave the testing facility (form F, p. 196).

Interpretation of Exercise Test Results

This section provides a brief overview of interpretation of the results of an exercise test. Students should keep in mind that an exercise test yields a wealth of information and that truly mastering the interpretation of results requires the ability to integrate all of the data.

In its most basic form, interpretation of the results of a test comes down to determining whether the results are normal (sometimes termed "negative") or abnormal (sometimes termed "positive"). Obviously, if a test had to be stopped because the patient showed a sign (e.g., cyanosis or cold, clammy skin) or a symptom (e.g., chest discomfort or wheezing), the test must be considered abnormal and the patient should be referred to her primary care physician. Specific findings on the ECG as discussed in chapter 5, or in the blood pressure response (e.g., elevation in diastolic blood pressure >100 mmHg or systolic

pressure >260 mmHg), would also signify an abnormal test (form G, p. 197).

Given a test with no abnormal findings, the next interpretation decision addresses whether the test produced a maximal effort. The only universally accepted criterion for a true maximal exercise test is a plateau in the $\dot{V}O_2$ response (i.e., no increase in $\dot{V}O_2$ with an increase in work level). Unfortunately, this response is not observed in many patients and may be more difficult to assess with the use of ramp protocols versus incremental protocols. Attainment of age-predicted maximal heart rate is generally considered a poor indicator of maximal effort since the 95% confidence interval ranges from ±20 to 30 bpm (34). Indeed, some patients actually demonstrate what is termed chronotropic incompetence, an abnormally low maximal heart rate, with exercise testing. Subjective ratings from patients are helpful, but not definitive enough to establish whether a maximal effort was obtained. Clinicians consider peak exercise test perceived exertion ratings of ≥18 (on the Borg 6-20 scale) as indicative of a good effort; however, cardiac patients commonly report peak values of only 15 to 17. It is also useful to directly ask patients after the test if they felt as though they could have continued the test any longer. Probably the most commonly used variable for determining maximal effort during tests including gas-exchange measurements is the respiratory exchange ratio ($R = \dot{V}CO_2/\dot{V}O_2$). The most liberally used criterion R for a maximal effort is a value of ≥1.0; a value of ≥1.1 is considered a more conservative indicator. It is known that metabolic measurements made with breath-by-breath technology typically produce higher maximal R values; thus a criterion value of an R ≥1.15 is common in these laboratories.

Although not as much information is available on interpretation of submaximal responses to exercise testing, evaluation of these data is helpful for clinicians. Since the absolute values for heart rate and blood pressure vary between individuals, the best way to evaluate responses is to express a change relative to the change in power output requirements (METs) of the test. Data from our research database of exercise test results suggest the following mean rates of change for submaximal heart rate and blood pressure, respectively: men, 9 ± 2 bpm/MET; women, 11 ± 2 bpm/MET; both genders, 6 ± 3 mmHg/MET. It is important to recognize that these are mean values from men and women who were not taking any medications affecting heart rate or blood pressure, and that responses vary between individuals with different characteristics. The characteristic that most influences these rates of change is cardiorespiratory fitness level. Thus, it is expected that those with higher-than-average cardiorespiratory fitness levels will have lower-than-average submaximal heart rate and blood pressure responses. The opposite, of course, is true for those with lower-than-average cardiorespiratory fitness levels.

Another useful submaximal response to interpret is that of a break point or a threshold in the physiological response to increasing intensity of exercise. Among the various break point responses that have been identified, the most common is the ventilatory threshold (sometimes called the anaerobic threshold), which obviously requires measurement of various gas-exchange parameters during the test. There are many different procedural options for identifying a ventilatory threshold (see Myers [35] for a more complete discussion). Many metabolic measurement systems now offer online computer-derived assessment of the ventilatory threshold using the V-slope technique, which detects a change in the linear response between $\dot{V}CO_2$ and $\dot{V}O_2$ during the test. We have also conducted research with colleagues from Fukoka University in Japan on detection of what is termed the double-product break point (36). The double product, also called the rate-pressure product, is the mathematical product of heart rate times systolic blood pressure. Exercise specialists have long recognized the potential value of these threshold measures in individualizing the exercise prescription for patients. More recently, clinicians have begun to investigate the potential of these measures as diagnostic indicators (figure 6.11).

Recommendations for Frequency of Testing

There are no established guidelines for how often an individual should have an exercise test. In deciding to recommend a current exercise test for a patient, the practitioner again needs to determine what the indication for the test is (box 6.2). We have generally followed a schedule consisting of annual tests for high-risk patients, tests every two years for moderate-risk patients, and tests every four years for low-risk patients participating in our organized exercise programs. Certainly, physicians may recommend testing earlier for selected patients or for patients who develop new symptoms or have a significant change in health status.

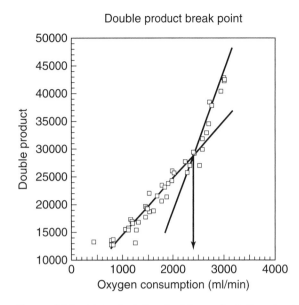

Figure 6.11 Note that the double product (heart rate × systolic blood pressure) rises linearly with increases in oxygen uptake until the break point is reached. This is one of several variables that exhibit this type of relationship with graded exercise testing.

Reprinted from the *American Journal of Cardiology*, Vol 17, P.H. Brubaker et al., "Identification of the anaerobic threshold using double product in patients with CAD", Page 361, Copyright 1997, with permission from Excerpta Medica Inc.

Indirect Methods for Assessing Functional Capacity

In certain circumstances, clinicians may desire an indication of a patient's functional capacity but are not able to justify the time and expense associated with a maximal exercise test. In these situations they consider alternative tests such as a submaximal exercise test or a timed (usually 6 min) walking test.

Submaximal exercise tests are more commonly used in fitness centers dealing with low-risk patients. The physiological basis for most of these tests is the known linear relationship between heart rate and oxygen consumption. The submaximal exercise test most commonly used in fitness centers follows the YMCA protocol. This protocol requires measurements of pulse rate at each of two to four power-output settings on a cycle ergometer and plots of those values against estimates of oxygen consumption at these work rates. A detailed description of the procedures for this test can be found in the ACSM Guidelines (12). The linear relationship between these two variables (heart rate and work rate) is established, and an extrapolation is then made to estimate $\dot{V}O_2$max. Among the assumptions this method relies on are that the linear relationship between heart rate and oxygen consumption holds through maximal levels, that the decline in maximal heart rate is uniform with age, that the mechanical efficiency is the same for all individuals, that submaximal heart rates are reliable at fixed work rates, and that maximal oxygen uptake can be predicted from maximal power-output values on the cycle ergometer. Unfortunately, individuals' responses do not always meet these assumptions, and the result is relatively high prediction errors that have been shown to range from 7% to 27% (37).

In clinical exercise programs, particularly those involving patients with limited functional capacity (such as persons with pulmonary disease or chronic heart failure), a more common method to estimate functional capacity is the 6-min walk test. Beyond its use in estimating functional capacity, this test has shown some promise for its potential clinical utility to evaluate the efficacy of therapeutic agents, provide prognostic data, and predict mortality (38). The test requires patients to ambulate as far as they can over a premeasured course (typically back and forth in a clinic hallway) in a 6-min time period (figure 6.12). Ideally patients are read a set of standardized instructions and are encouraged to produce their best effort. Rest breaks are allowed as needed. Since patients commonly demonstrate a learning effect when performing this test, the recommendation is to perform at least two trials. Additionally, since encouragement has been shown to positively influence the results, it is important to provide a consistent level of encouragement for all tests. Although this test has gained favor as an assessment tool for documenting outcomes in some rehabilitation programs, few studies to date have evaluated the ability of the 6-min walk test to predict peak $\dot{V}O_2$. Those few studies have shown prediction errors ranging from 15% to 27%.

SUMMARY

This chapter focuses on the assessment and interpretation of the five health-related components of physical fitness. These measurements are useful for many purposes, including risk stratification, diagnostic and prognostic evaluations (in which they serve as supplemental information), exercise prescription, and outcome assessments. The clinical exercise physiologist is considered an expert in the assessment and interpretation of physical fitness and thus needs to master these skills and knowledge.

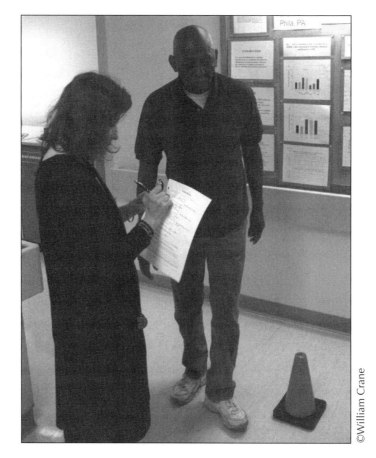

©William Crane

Figure 6.12   An elderly patient performing a 6-min walk test.

Case Study 1
Primary Prevention: Low Risk

Our 38-year-old man completed the routine screening and testing prior to entering the Ball State Adult Physical Fitness Program. Tables 6.15 and 6.16 show the data on his body composition and maximal exercise test results.

A quick review of his basic body composition revealed the following:

- BMI = 91.8 kg / (1.81 m × 1.81 m) = 28.1 kg/m^2
- He would be classified as "overweight" with an "increased disease risk" based on his waist circumference (< 102 cm) (using information from table 1.5).
- An estimate of his body density (using the sum of all 7 sites = 166 mm) can be calculated by the formula found in the ACSM Guidelines text (12):

$$1.112 - 0.00043499(166) + 0.00000055(166)^2 - 0.00028826(38) = 1.044 \text{ g/ml}$$

Then using the Siri equation his body fat is predicted to be: (495/1.044)–450 = 24.1%, which would be considered "obese" (>5% above the rule of thumb average of 17% for a man his age). It is interesting to note that if only three sites were used (chest, abdomen, thigh equation found on form A) his estimated body fat is 20.1%. This points out some of the potential for error when predicting body fat percentage.

His pre-exercise test screening did not reveal any contraindications to testing, nor any limitations for the mode of exercise. To help select a protocol the testing staff obtained a quick estimate of his maximal oxygen uptake (41.7 ml/kg/min or approximately 12 METs) using the non-exercise equation found in table 6.13:

$$\dot{V}O_2\text{max (ml/kg/min)} = 50.55 - (0.324 \times 38 \text{ yrs}) + (5.664 \times 1 \text{ [gender code]}) + 2.157 \times 5 \text{ [PA code]}) - 0.46 \times 28.1 \text{ [BMI]})$$

In the Ball State and Wake Forest programs we prefer ramp style protocols. In this case it was determined that the BSU/Bruce ramp would be a reasonable protocol to provide an exercise test of between 6-15 minutes in duration (table 6.16).

This test was considered a maximal effort, as indicated by the R value of 1.19 exceeding the criterion of 1.0 (or for breath-by-breath measurements, as was used in this test, of 1.15). The maximal heart rate value of 187 bpm actually exceeded his age-predicted value of 182 bpm (220-38), his maximal systolic blood pressure of 186 mmHg was within the expected range (increase of 6 mmHg/MET), and he rated his perceived exertion as 20.

Read on in chapter 7 to learn about the exercise prescription that was developed for our 38-year-old man and then how he progressed with his exercise training in chapter 8.

Table 6.15
Body Composition Data Collection

Weight (kg)	91.9
Height (cm)	181.0
Waist circumference (cm)	95.8
Midaxillary skinfold (mm)	25.5
Chest skinfold (mm)	15.5
Tricep skinfold (mm)	25.5
Subscapular skinfold (mm)	22.0
Suprailiac skinfold (mm)	27.5
Abdominal skinfold (mm)	32.0
Thigh skinfold (mm)	18.0

Table 6.16
Maximal Exercise Testing Data Collection

Mode	Treadmill
Protocol	BSU/Bruce ramp
Test time (min)	13.33
Test work rate	4.6 mph / 16.8%
Measured $\dot{V}O_2$max (ml/kg/min)	45.2
Heart rate (bpm)	187
Blood pressure (mmHg)	186/86
R ($\dot{V}O_2/\dot{V}CO_2$)	1.19
RPE	20
Reason for test termination	Overall fatigue

Case Study 2
Primary Prevention: High Risk

As we learned in chapters 3 and 4, this 50-year-old man has type II diabetes, and a coronary angiography revealed he had a 40% occlusion of the left anterior descending (LAD) coronary artery. He was referred to the Wake Forest University Cardiac Rehabilitation program and performed the routine pre-exercise training battery of tests as summarized in the table 6.17.

A quick review of his basic body composition revealed the following:

- BMI = 163.8 kg / (1.994 m × 1.994 m) = 41.2 kg/m^2
- He would be classified as "obese" (grade III) with an "extremely high disease risk" based on his waist circumference (> 102 cm) (see table 1.5).
- As we learned in the previous chapters he has type II diabetes, hyperlipidemia, and hypertension. All of these along with his abdominal obesity are suggestive of the metabolic syndrome (see chapter 9).

From a clinical perspective, the basic body composition analysis provided all the information that was required. Being a research institution, the staff at Wake Forest University routinely collects advanced body composition data as well. However, it is important to emphasize that this additional information (advanced body composition) is of little value in this patient's case. Collecting this information on patients with higher levels of obesity (grade III in this case) can be problematic as noted by the difficulties in obtaining accurate skinfold measurements (note the value for the chest skinfold of 50+?, suggesting that the technician could not obtain a measurement with confidence).

At Wake Forest University, prior to the exercise testing session, the laboratory staff meets to review the patient's characteristics and select the test mode and protocol. Based on the patient's characteristics the staff opted for a treadmill mode and selected an individualized ramp protocol (see specific characteristics in table 6.18). You will note that at Wake Forest the preferred treadmill time is targeted at 12 minutes with the cardiac patient population.

In interpreting the test results, the first obvious observation is that the maximal heart rate was only 103 bpm. This value is >3 standard deviations lower than his age-predicted maximal heart rate (170 bpm). However, it is important to remember (see case studies in previous chapters) that this patient was taking a beta-blocker medication (atenolol) which will blunt the heart rate response. The other indicators were supportive, yet not entirely conclusive, of a maximal effort. The maximal RPE of 17 is common for cardiac patients, but the R of 1.11 is slightly lower than what is commonly observed for maximal effort when the data is collected (as was this test) with a breath-by-breath metabolic system (R >1.15). Additionally, the blood pressure

Table 6.17
Body Composition Data Collection

Weight (kg)	163.8
Height (cm)	199.4
Waist circumference (cm)	125.0
Midaxillary skinfold (mm)	45.8
Chest skinfold (mm)	50+?
Triceps skinfold (mm)	19.2
Subscapular skinfold (mm)	40.2
Suprailiac skinfold (mm)	33.8
Abdominal skinfold (mm)	42.8
Thigh skinfold (mm)	18.0

Table 6.18
Maximal Exercise Testing Data Collection

Mode	Treadmill
Protocol	Individualized ramp (2.5 mph; programmed to reach 7 METs in 12 min)
Test time (min)	7
Test work rate	2.5 mph / 7%
Measured $\dot{V}O_2$max (ml/kg/min)	16.1
Heart rate (bpm)	103
Blood pressure (mmHg)	136/70
R ($\dot{V}O_2/\dot{V}CO_2$)	1.11
RPE	17
Reason for test termination	Knee pain

response was blunted, which could also be attributable to the beta-blocker and the diuretic (lasix) the patient was taking. You should also note that the reason reported for terminating the test was knee pain. Thus, the interpretation of whether this was a true cardiovascular maximum test is somewhat equivocal. In retrospect, it may have been preferable to use a cycle (non-weight bearing) mode of exercise for this test. Indeed, this patient reported having osteoarthritis secondary to his obesity, which quite possibly limited his performance on this exercise test.

Another aspect of this test to evaluate is the short test time (7 min compared to the target of 12 min). Some of this shorter time possibly could be attributed to stopping the test prematurely. How-ever, we have recently developed a non-exercise equation to predict $\dot{V}O_2$max from the Wake Forest database of cardiac patients (table 6.13). Interestingly, had this equation been available and used, his targeted MET level would have been 5.1 when calculated as follows:

$$\dot{V}O_2\text{max (ml/kg/min)} = 40.74 - (0.208 \times 50 \text{ yrs}) + (4.283 \times 1 \text{ [gender code]}) + (1.187 \times 0 \text{ [PA code]}) - 0.406 \times 41.2 \text{ [BMI]})$$

Being that his measured maximal METs were 4.6 (16.1 / 3.5), this prediction method would have yielded a more reasonable target level than 7 METs for this exercise test. Read on in chapter 7 to see how the exercise prescription for this patient was formulated.

Case Study 3
Secondary Prevention

For this case we are presenting data for both his baseline assessment and his 3-month post-training assessment. As is often the case with cardiac patients, test data is available as part of the diagnostic evaluation or treatment program for the patient in conjunction with a cardiac-related symptom. Review this patient's case information in chapters 3 and 4 for his history. The baseline data for the exercise test is information provided by the patient's physician (body composition data collected at Wake Forest). For this case our approach will be slightly different than that for cases 1 and 2. We will not review all the calculations and interpretations for all the assessments, rather we will highlight some of the interesting measurement issues that arose in these two assessments.

Calculations of BMI gave values of 29.4 kg/m² at baseline and 28.6 kg/m² at 3 months. Waist circumference data was only collected at 3 months. Thus, interpretation at baseline was "overweight" and at 3 months was "overweight" with "increased disease risk." As was the situation in Case Study 2, the need for advanced body composition data for this patient is debatable. One thing to consider if you choose to measure skinfolds is the potential for variability in your measurements. Notice the large change in the measures for the suprailiac (30.0 to 16.2) and thigh sites (12.7 to 25.4) from baseline to 3 months. Measurement error, which is a major concern with skinfold measures, should be suspected here. Interestingly, the sum of 7 skinfolds was essentially the same—156 mm for both assessments—which would suggest that there was no change in percent body fat over the 3 months (table 6.19).

The cardiac rehabilitation staff was provided with results from a stress echocardiogram administered

Table 6.19
Body Composition Data Collection

	Baseline at Wake Forest	Three mo. at Wake Forest
Weight (kg)	101.1	98.2
Height (cm)	185.4	185.4
Waist circumference (cm)	Did not measure	100.5
Midaxillary skinfold (mm)	13.2	16.2
Chest skinfold (mm)	31.0	25.6
Triceps skinfold (mm)	15.4	14.2
Subscapular skinfold (mm)	20.4	25.0
Suprailiac skinfold (mm)	30.0	16.2
Abdominal skinfold (mm)	33.4	33.2
Thigh skinfold (mm)	12.7	25.4

at the local hospital for this patient upon entry to the program. This patient was taking atenolol, which can explain the significantly lower maximal heart rate (age-predicted = 159 bpm). You will note that $\dot{V}O_2$max was estimated and not measured during this test. The estimate could have been generated from either exercise test time (using an equation like those found in table 6.13) if a standardized protocol was used or, more likely in this case, from the maximal treadmill speed and grade using the ACSM metabolic equations. The other point to note here is the limited information that is provided in some standard test summary reports (table 6.20).

For the 3-month test we can see that the testing staff stayed consistent with the mode of exercise as there were no problems associated with treadmill exercise on the baseline test. However, the staff elected to use an individualized ramp protocol (see section in this chapter to review the advantages of ramp protocols) for the test. One of the most revealing findings of this test was the markedly lower $\dot{V}O_2$max of 22.4 ml/kg/min. This is approximately 3 METs lower than the value predicted from this patient's baseline test—and this is after 3 months of exercise training! These results illustrate clearly some of the important interpretation issues exercise program professionals face when they work with predicted versus measured values. To make a more apples-to-apples comparison, we can make an estimate of the $\dot{V}O_2$max based on the final treadmill speed and grade from this second test using the ACSM walking equation:

Table 6.20
Maximal Exercise Testing Data Collection

	Baseline at local hospital	Three mo. at Wake Forest
Mode	Treadmill	Treadmill
Protocol	Modified Bruce	Individualized ramp (3.0 mph; programmed to reach 10 METs in 12 min)
Test time (min)	Not reported	11
Test work rate	Not reported	3.0 mph / 15%
$\dot{V}O_2$max (ml/kg/min)	Estimated 32.6	Measured 22.4
Heart rate (bpm)	136	128
Blood pressure (mmHg)	Not reported	178/84
R ($\dot{V}O_2$/$\dot{V}CO_2$)	Not measured	1.12
RPE	Not reported	17
Reason for test termination	Not reported	Shortness of breath

$$\dot{V}O_2\text{max (ml/kg/min)} = (0.1 \times 80.4) + (1.8 \times 80.4 \times .15) + 3.5 = 33.2 \text{ ml/kg/min}$$

Notice this is quite comparable to the 32.6 ml/kg/min predicted for the test at baseline. Read on in chapters 7 and 8 to see how these test results were used to prepare this patient's exercise prescription and help us to interpret his response to exercise training.

BODY COMPOSITION WORKSHEET

Client Name _____ **Date** _____ **Time** _____ **Technician** _____

Previous Body Comp. Data (BMI; % fat; date) _____ Resistance Exerciser Y / N

<u>Weight History Review</u>

Weight at age 18 _____ lbs   Cyclic Wt Loss <u>Y / N</u>

Recent Wt Loss <u>Y / N</u> if yes, (lbs, time) _____

<u>Visual Impression Record</u>
(circle impressions)

%fat appearance <10 10-15 15-20 20-25 25-30 >30

overall appearance   Lean   Muscular   Average   Fat

Basic Body Comp. Weight (nearest 0.25 lb) _____ lbs. / 2.2046 = _____ kg

Height (nearest 0.25 in) _____ in $\times$ 0.0254 = _____ m

Body Mass Index _____ kg / (____ m $\times$ ____ m) = _____ (kg/m^2)

Waist Circumference (1) _____ (2) _____ (mean) _____ cm

BMI Classification _____ Body Fat Distribution Disease Risk Classification _____

Advanced Body Comp.

Bioelectrical Impedance Analysis

impedance _____

% fat _____

BIA Considerations:

Caffeine (last 3h) <u>Y / N</u>   Void bladder (last 1h) <u>Y / N</u>

Large fluid intake <u>Y / N</u>   Drug (diuretic) concerns <u>Y / N</u>

Alcohol (last 24h) <u>Y / N</u>   Menstruating <u>Y / N</u>

Diet (very-low cal. or low carb) concerns <u>Y / N</u>

Time since last vigorous exercise _____ last meal _____

Skinfolds (mm)

Women

Triceps ____ / ____ / ____   Suprailiac ____ / ____ / ____   Thigh ____ / ____ / ____   Sum _____

Body Density _____ = $1.099421 - 0.0009929 \text{(sum)} + 0.0000023 \text{(sum)}^2 - 0.0001392 \text{(age)}$

Or

Triceps ____ / ____ / ____   Suprailiac ____ / ____ / ____   Abdomen ____ / ____ / ____   Sum _____

Body Density _____ = $1.089733 - 0.0009245 \text{(sum)} + 0.0000025 \text{(sum)}^2 - 0.0000979 \text{(age)}$

Men

Chest ____ / ____ / ____   Abdomen ____ / ____ / ____   Thigh ____ / ____ / ____   Sum _____

Body Density _____ = $1.10938 - 0.0008267 \text{(sum)} + 0.0000016 \text{(sum)}^2 - 0.0002574 \text{(age)}$

Or

Chest ____ / ____ / ____   Triceps ____ / ____ / ____   Subscapular ____ / ____ / ____ Sum _____

Body Density _____ = $1.1125025 - 0.0013125 \text{(sum)} + 0.0000055 \text{(sum)}^2 - 0.000244 \text{(age)}$

Estimate of % fat _____ = (495 / Body Density) - 450

Form A

ACSM Initial Risk Stratification Questionnaire

Please provide accurate information for all requested items. Ask a staff member to assist you if you need clarification of any item.

Name: _____ Phone: _____ Email:_____

Address: _____

Date of Birth: _____ Occupation/phone: _____

Physician name/location/phone number _____/_____

Date/purpose of last physician visit: _____/_____/_____

current body weight:_____ height:_____ waist size:_____

Write a **Y** for all statements that are true, write a **N** for all statements that are false, and write a **U** for all statements that are unknown.

Cardiovascular Risk Factors

_____ You have a first-degree relative who had a heart attack **or** coronary revascularization **or** sudden death before age 55 (father or brother) or age 65 (mother or sister).

_____ You smoke cigarettes **or** you quit smoking cigarettes within the last 6 months.

_____ Your systolic blood pressure is $\geq$ 140 **or** your diastolic blood pressure is $\geq$ 90 mmHg **or** you take blood pressure medication.

_____ Your LDL cholesterol is $\geq$ 130 mg/dL (*if LDL not known*: your total cholesterol is $\geq$ 200 mg/dL) **or** your HDL-cholesterol is < 40 mg/dL **or** you take lipid lowering medication.

_____ Your blood sugar is $\geq$ 110 mg/dL.

_____ You are sedentary (i.e., you get less than 30 minutes/day of moderate intensity physical activity on most days **and** you do not participate in a regular exercise program).

_____ Your HDL-cholesterol is $\geq$ 60 mg/dL.

Symptoms

_____ You experience pain or discomfort in the chest, neck, or arms.

_____ You experience shortness of breath at rest or with mild exertion.

_____ You experience dizziness or have had episodes of blackouts.

_____ You have swelling of the ankles.

_____ You experience shortness of breath with change of posture or while sleeping.

_____ You experience episodes of rapid heart beats or skipped heart beats.

_____ You experience pain or cramping sensations in your legs when walking.

_____ You experience fatigue or shortness of breath with usual activities.

Medical History   ***List all other notable health problems, injuries, or conditions:***

You have or have had: _____

_____ heart murmur _____ heart attack   _____

_____ heart surgery _____ a lung disease _____

_____ a metabolic disease (diabetes, thyroid disorder, kidney or liver disease)

Name and phone number of person to contact in an emergency: _____

List names/doses/frequency of all medications taken (if not taking any medication write NONE): _____

_____

Staff Comments (*explain all Y or U responses*): _____

_____

ACSM Initial Risk Stratification (*circle correct classification*):   Low   *Moderate*   **High**

Recommended Follow-up: _____

Form B

PREVENTATIVE/REHABILITATIVE EXERCISE PROGRAM

Pre-Exercise Testing Instructions

Your exercise test is scheduled for _____ on _____ at _____.
                                     day   date   time

For safety reasons, as well as to allow you to perform to the best of your ability, the following instructions should be followed prior to your exercise test:

1. Come to the laboratory well rested. Get a good night's sleep and avoid any strenuous, vigorous activities the day before your exercise test.

2. You should abstain from food, tobacco, and caffeinated beverages for a minimum of 3 hours and from alcohol for a minimum of 12 hours prior to the exercise test. Water consumption is both allowed and encouraged. (Note: those being tested in the early morning hours may have some clear juice if desired.)

3. If you are presently taking medications please **continue** taking them as scheduled prior to the exercise test unless specifically instructed to do otherwise by your physician.

4. Come dressed in or bring with you exercise attire. Recommended attire includes exercise shoes (ex., running/walking shoes, aerobic shoes, sneakers), white socks, shorts or loose fitting exercise pants, and a loose fitting short sleeve blouse or t-shirt. Women should remove lipstick before the exercise test.

5. Changing and shower facilities are available in the laboratory. However, it should be noted that most participants shower and change at home following the exercise test.

If you have any questions or need to reschedule your appointment, please call _____ at _____ between 8:00 - 5:00, Monday through Friday. If you need to cancel your appointment before 8:00 a.m. on the morning of your scheduled examination, please call the testing laboratory staff at _____.

Form C

PREVENTATIVE/REHABILITATIVE EXERCISE PROGRAM

INFORMED CONSENT
(For Exercise Testing of Low or Moderate Risk Participants)

I, _____, do hereby voluntarily consent to participate in a fitness assessment prior to beginning participation in the preventative exercise program. This assessment will consist of, but is not limited to, a health history questionnaire, resting ECG and blood pressure, blood lipid analysis, pulmonary function measurements, body composition measurements, and a graded exercise test. In obtaining the blood sample there will be a stinging sensation experienced when the needle is inserted. Occasionally, some localized bruising and tenderness appears around the site. If I am over the age of forty-five, or have two or more risk factors (e.g., high blood pressure, smoking, sedentary, etc.) or symptoms of heart problems, it is strongly encouraged that I have a medical examination by my personal physician prior to engaging in the exercise test. It is my understanding that my personal physician can be informed of the results of the fitness testing program in which I am hereby choosing to participate. I also understand that I will be interviewed by a physician or other persons prior to my undergoing the exercise test who will in the course of interviewing me consider any obvious reasons which could make it undesirable or unsafe for me to take the exercise test. Consequently, I understand that it is important that I provide complete and accurate responses on the health history questionnaire and to the interviewer, and recognize that my failure to do so could lead to possible unnecessary injury to myself during the exercise test.

The graded exercise test will be performed to evaluate the functional performance and capacity of the heart, lungs, blood vessels, and skeletal muscles. The graded exercise test is a physical work test, usually performed on a treadmill or bicycle. The test begins at a low level of exertion and then gradually increases until the limits of fatigue, breathlessness, or any symptoms of severity which the examining team considers significant to terminate the test, are reached. I recognize that I may stop the test at my discretion at any time. These test results will be used in developing a personalized physical fitness program. The test procedures may take place on two separate days and will take approximately one and a half hours to complete.

There exists a possibility of adverse changes occurring during the exercise test. I have been informed that these changes could include muscle or joint injury, abnormal blood pressure, fainting, disorders of heart beat, rare instances of heart attack or stroke, as well as death. I understand that reasonable efforts will be made to minimize problems by preliminary examination and by observation during the testing. I also understand that trained personnel will be available to deal with foreseeable situations which may arise.

The results of this test may or may not benefit me. Potential benefits relate mainly to my personal motives for taking the test, e.g., knowing my exercise capacity in relation to the general population, understanding my fitness for certain sport, recreational and occupational activities, planning my physical conditioning program or evaluating the effects of my current lifestyle and/or exercise habits. Although my cardiorespiratory fitness level might also be evaluated by alternative means, such as a step test, outdoor run or walk test, or other submaximal tests, such tests do not provide as accurate a fitness assessment as the above mentioned treadmill or bike test, nor do these options allow equally effective monitoring of my responses.

The information which is obtained during the fitness assessment will be treated as privileged and confidential, and will not be released or revealed to any person other than Program Staff, without my consent. The information obtained, however, may be used for a statistical or scientific purpose.

I have read the above information, and I have full understanding of the risks, benefits, and safeguards of the test procedures. I have been given an opportunity to ask questions as to the procedures. Any questions that I might have had, have been answered to my satisfaction. I acknowledge that I have read this document in its entirety or that it has been read to me if I have been unable to read same. I consent to participate in all services and procedures as explained herein by all program personnel.

Participant _____   Date _____

Testing Staff _____   Date _____

Physician _____   Date _____

****

I hereby authorize the Preventative Exercise Program to release my test information obtained during the laboratory evaluation to my physician.

Participant _____   Date _____

****

I hereby authorize **Dr.** _____ to release my medical records that are relevant to cardiorespiratory fitness and exercise training, to the Preventative Exercise Program. Furthermore, I authorize **Dr.** _____ to discuss these medical records with the Director and/or staff of the Preventative Exercise Program.

Participant _____   Date _____

Form D

PREVENTATIVE/REHABILITATIVE EXERCISE PROGRAM

EXERCISE TEST DATA SHEET

Name _____ Age _____ Sex _____ Date _____ Time of test _____

Rest HR _____/_____ Rest BP _____/_____ Weight _____ lb _____ kg Height _____ in _____ cm
      supine/standing   supine/standing

RISK FACTORS: _____

Hours since last meal? _____ List food and/or beverages: _____

MEDICATIONS:

Name   Dose   Time last taken

ACTIVITY/EXERCISE HISTORY: _____

PAST ET INFO: Date: _____ HRmax _____ BPmax _____ $\dot{V}O_2$max _____ Test time _____

            Protocol _____ ECG _____

Protocol: _____ Chest Auscultation _____ Checked : Yes   No   Findings _____

Time (min)	Speed (mph)	Grade (%)	HR (bpm)	BP (mmHg)	RPE	Comments
0 - 1				/		
1 - 2				/		
2 - 3				/		
3 - 4				/		
4 - 5				/		
5 - 6				/		
6 - 7				/		
7 - 8				/		
8 - 9				/		
9 - 10				/		
10 - 11				/		
11 - 12				/		
12 - 13				/		
13 - 14				/		
14 - 15				/		

Immediate Post-Test Symptoms: Chest Pain   Shortness of Breath   Lightheadness   Other:

RECOVERY						
0 - 1				/		
1 - 2				/		
2 - 3				/		
3 - 4				/		
4 - 5				/		
5 - 6				/		
6 - 7				/		

Time started running _____   Total Test Time _____   Peak Speed/Grade _____/_____

REASON for STOPPING TEST: _____ Supervisor Review _____

FOLLOW-UP PLAN: _____

ECG TECH _____   BP/Spotter TECH _____   PHYSICIAN _____

PREP TECH _____   METABOLIC TECH _____   SUPERVISOR _____

Form E

PREVENTATIVE/REHABILITATIVE EXERCISE PROGRAM

INCIDENT REPORT FORM — GRADED EXERCISE TESTING

Participant: _____ File No.: _____ Date: _____

CHIEF COMPLAINT: _____

SIGNS & SYMPTOMS: (Angina, dizziness, syncope, ECG changes, etc.)

_____
_____
_____

HOW/WHEN INCIDENT OCCURRED: _____

_____
_____

OBSERVATION/TREATMENT FLOW RECORD

TIME	BP	HR	RHYTHM	SIGNS/SYMPTOMS	TREATMENT

DISCHARGED: HOME _____   TO PERSONAL MD _____   TO HOSPITAL _____

MODE OF TRAVEL: OWN CAR _____   STAFF CAR _____   AMBULANCE _____

RELATIVE NOTIFIED: Yes/No   (Phone, in person - explain) _____

STAFF IN ATTENDANCE: _____

_____

COMMENTS: _____

_____
_____

REPORT PREPARED BY: _____

PROGRAM DIRECTOR'S SIGNATURE _____

Form F

PREVENTATIVE / REHABILITATIVE EXERCISE PROGRAM

PENDING FOLLOW-UP

Name _____   File # _____   Test Date _____

Test # _____

Reason patient must follow-up with physician: _____

_____

Information given to participant: _____

_____

Participant response to referral information: _____

_____

Signed by _____
                    Testing Supervisor

Information forwarded to _____ (participant, M.D.) on _____ (date)

Follow-up Comments (Include any contact with patient and/or patient's physician and date of contact):

DATE

_____

_____

_____

_____

_____

Was patient cleared for participation in the exercise program? _____Yes   Date: _____

                                    _____ No   Reason: _____

                                                      _____

                                                      _____

Form G

GLOSSARY

Body composition: the total amount of adipose tissue in the body relative to the total body weight (i.e., the percentage of body fat)

Cardiorespiratory endurance: the ability of the heart, respiratory, and circulatory systems to supply nutrients and oxygen to and remove waste products from the working muscles (and other organs) efficiently

Flexibility: the ability to move a body part fluidly through a complete range of motion about a joint

Muscular endurance: the ability of a muscle to sustain repeated contractions or to maintain a submaximal contraction

Muscular strength: the ability of the muscles to exert a force to move an object or to develop tension to resist the movement of an object

REFERENCES

1. Caspersen, C.J., K.E. Powell, and G.M. Christenson. 1985. Physical activity, exercise and physical fitness: Definitions and distinctions for health-related research. *Public Health Reports* 100:126–130.

2. Miller, A.J., I.M. Grais, E. Winslow, and L.A. Kaminsky. 1991. The definition of physical fitness. *J. Sports Med. Phys. Fit.* 31:639–640.

3. Eckel, R.H., and R.M. Krauss. 1998. American Heart Association call to action: Obesity as a major risk factor for coronary heart disease. *Circulation* 97:2099–2100.

4. Gordon, C.C., W.C. Chumlea, and A.F. Roche. 1988. Stature, recumbent length, and weight. In *Anthropometric standardization reference manual,* ed. T.G. Lohman, A.F. Roche, and R. Martorell, 3–8. Champaign, IL: Human Kinetics.

5. United States Department of Agriculture, Agriculture Research Service, Dietary Advisory Committee. 1995. Report of the Dietary guidelines for Americans 1995 to the Secretary of Health and Human Services and the Secretary of Agriculture. Washington, D.C.: U.S. Government Printing Office.

6. Hamwi, G. 1964. Changing dietary concepts. In *Diabetes mellitus and treatment,* ed. T.S. Dankowski, New York: American Diabetes Association.

7. Despres, J.P. 1997. Visceral obesity, insulin resistance, and dyslipidemia: Contribution of endurance training to the treatment of the plurimetabolic syndrome. In *Exerc. and Sport Sci. Rev.,* ed. J.O. Holloszy, 271–300. Baltimore: Williams & Wilkins.

8. Expert Panel on the Identification, Evaluation and Treatment of Overweight and Obesity in Adults. 1998. *Clinical guidelines on the identification, evalua-tion and treatment of overweight and obesity in adults.* Pub. no. 98-4083. Bethesda, Md.: National Heart Lung and Blood Institute Information Center. (Also available online at: **http://www.nhlbi.nih.gov/ guidelines/obesity/ob_home.htm**)

9. Siri, N.E. 1961. Body composition from fluid spaces and density. In *Techniques for measuring body composition,* ed. J. Brozek and A. Henschel, 223–224. Washington, D.C.: National Academy of Science.

10. Lohman, T.G. 1981. Skinfolds and body density and their relation to body fatness: A review. *Human Biol.* 53:181–225.

11. Dempster, P., and S. Aitkens. 1995. A new air displacement method for the determination of human body composition. *Med. Sci. Sports Exerc.* 27:1692–1697.

12. Franklin, B., E. Howley, and M. Whaley, eds. 2000. *ACSM's guidelines for exercise testing and prescription.* 6th ed. Baltimore: Lippincott, Williams & Wilkins.

13. Lohman, T.G. 1982. Body composition methodology in sports medicine. *Physician and Sports Med.* 10:46–58.

14. American Association of Cardiovascular and Pulmonary Rehabilitation. 1999. *Guidelines for cardiac rehabilitation programs.* 3rd. ed. Champaign, IL: Human Kinetics, 281.

15. American Association of Cardiovascular and Pulmonary Rehabilitation. 1998. *Guidelines for pulmonary rehabilitation programs.* 2nd. ed. Champaign, IL: Human Kinetics, 250.

16. American College of Sports Medicine. 2000. Position stand: Exercise and type 2 diabetes. *Med. Sci. Sports Exerc.* 32:1345–1360.

17. American College of Sports Medicine. 1993. Position stand: Physical activity, physical fitness, and hypertension. *Med. Sci. Sports Exerc.* 25:i–x.

18. Golding, L.A., C.R. Myers, and W.E. Sinning, eds. 1989. *Y's way to physical fitness: The complete guide to fitness testing and instruction.* 3rd ed. Champaign, IL: Human Kinetics.

19. Neiman, D.C. 1999. *Fitness and sports medicine: A health-related approach.* 4th ed. Mountain View, CA: Mayfield, 168.

20. Maud, P.J., and M.Y. Cortez-Cooper. 1995. Static techniques for evaluation of joint range of motion. In *Physiological assessment of human fitness,* ed. P.J. Maud and C. Foster, 221–244. Champaign, IL: Human Kinetics.

21. American College of Cardiology / American Heart Association Task Force on Practice Guidelines, Committee on Exercise Testing. 1997. ACC/AHA guidelines for exercise testing. *Circulation* 96:345–354.

22. Myers, J.N., L. Voodi, and V.F. Froelicher. 2000. A survey of exercise testing: Methods, utilization, interpretation and safety in the VAHCS. *Med. Sci. Sports Exerc.* 32:S143.

23. Stuart, R.J., and M.H. Ellestad. 1980. National survey of exercise stress testing facilities. *Chest* 77:94–97.

24. Buchfuhrer, M.J., J.E. Hansen, T.E. Robinson, D.Y. Sue, K. Wasserman, and B.J. Whipp. 1983. Optimizing the exercise protocol for cardiopulmonary assessment. *J. Appl. Physiol.* 55:1558–1564.

25. Myers, J., N. Buchanan, D. Smith, J. Neutel, E. Bowes, D. Walsh, and V.F. Froelicher. 1992. Individualized ramp treadmill: Observations on a new protocol. *Chest* 101:236S–241S.

26. Myers, J., N. Buchanan, D. Walsh, M. Kraemer, P. McAuley, M. Hamilton-Wessler, and V.F. Froelicher. 1991. Comparison of the ramp versus standard exercise protocols. *J.A.C.C.* 17:1334–1342.

27. Myers, J., and V.F. Froelicher. 1990. Optimizing the exercise test for pharmacological investigations. *Circulation* 82:1839–1846.

28. Kaminsky, L.A., and M.H. Whaley. 1998. Evaluation of a new standardized ramp protocol: The BSU/Bruce ramp protocol. *J. Cardiopul. Rehabil.* 18:438–444.

29. Foster, C., A.S. Jackson, M.L. Pollock, M.M. Taylor, J. Hare, S.M. Sennett, J.L. Rod, M. Sarwar, D.H. Schmidt. 1984. Generalized equations for predicting functional capacity from treadmill performance. *Am. Heart J.* 107:1229–1234.

30. McConnell, T.R., and B.A. Clark. 1987. Prediction of maximal oxygen consumption during handrail supported treadmill exercise. *J. Cardiopul. Rehabil.* 18:438–444.

31. Pollock, M.L., R.L. Bohannon, K.H. Cooper, J. Ayers, A. Ward, S. White, and A. Linnerud. 1976. A comparative analysis of four protocols for maximal treadmill stress testing. *Am. Heart J.* 92:39–46.

32. Pollock, M.L., C. Foster, D. Schmidt, C. Hellman, A.C. Linnerud, and A. Ward. 1982. Comparative analysis of physiologic responses to three different maximal graded exercise test protocols in healthy women. *Am. Heart J.* 103:363–373.

33. Bailey, R.H. J.H. Bauer. 1993. Ambulatory blood pressure measurement. *Arch. Intern. Med.* 153:2741.

34. Whaley, M.H., L.A. Kaminsky, G.B. Dwyer, and L.H. Getchell. 1992. Age and other fitness parameters as predictors of maximal heart rate in adult men and women. *Res. Q. Exerc. Sport* 63:A30.

35. Myers, J.N. 1996. *Essentials of cardiopulmonary exercise testing.* Champaign, IL: Human Kinetics, 177.

36. Brubaker, P.H., A. Kiyonaga, B.A. Matrazzo, W.E. Pollock, M. Shindo, H.S. Miller, and H. Tanaka. 1997. Identification of the anaerobic threshold using double product in patients with coronary artery disease. *Am. J. Cardiol.* 79:360–362.

37. Greiwe, J.S., L.A. Kaminsky, M.H. Whaley, and G.B. Dwyer. 1995. Evaluation of the ACSM submaximal cycling ergometer test for estimating $\dot{V}O_2$max. *Med. Sci. Sports Exerc.* 27:1315–1320.

38. Cahalin, L.P., M.A. Mathier, M.J. Semigran, G.W. Dec, and T.G. DiSalvo. 1996. The six-minute walk test predicts peak oxygen uptake and survival in patients with advanced heart failure. *Chest* 110:325–332.

CHAPTER 7

Exercise Prescription in Coronary Artery Disease Prevention and Rehabilitation Programs

BEHAVIORAL OBJECTIVES

- To be able to describe basic exercise prescription principles for both cardiorespiratory endurance and musculoskeletal resistance training in both the primary and secondary prevention settings

- To be able to develop individualized cardiorespiratory endurance and musculoskeletal resistance-exercise prescriptions for adult participants in primary or secondary prevention programs

Exercise training prescriptions should include an individualized intensity, frequency, duration, mode, and rate of progression. Exercise professionals in the primary or secondary **exercise** setting should possess the knowledge to develop and modify exercise prescriptions for both **cardiorespiratory** (CR) endurance and **musculoskeletal** (MS) resistance training. This process involves much more than the use of the target heart rate formulas presented later in the chapter. This chapter describes general exercise prescription principles for both CR endurance and MS resistance training. Several case studies illustrate the use of physiological data from an exercise test in the development of the initial exercise prescription. The discussion emphasizes the importance of considering the total **energy expenditure** within the exercise prescription. And finally, we address how to develop an exercise prescription in the absence of maximal exercise test data.

The optimal exercise prescription should be determined from an objective evaluation of an individual's responses to exercise and should take into account an individual's health status (chapter 3), chronic disease risk factors (chapter 1), fitness evaluation (chapter 6), behavioral readiness for change (chapter 10), personal goals, and exercise preferences. Other chapters describe methods for obtaining this information from individuals who present for an exercise prescription. The purposes of an individualized exercise prescription are to (1) enhance some facet of **physical fitness** (e.g., CR endurance, muscular strength/endurance), (2) promote health by modification of chronic disease risk factors (e.g., decrease excess body fat, normalize blood lipids or blood pressure), and (3) ensure safety during exercise participation (i.e., decrease incidence of cardiovascular complications and/or MS injuries). Exercise professionals should evaluate each of their individualized exercise prescriptions in light of these criteria before subjecting their clients or patients to the regimen. The American College of Sports Medicine (ACSM) and the American Association of Cardiovascular and Pulmonary Rehabilitation (AACVPR) each publish guidelines (1-3) for exercise prescription that all professionals should review when designing such programs. The following two sections review these national guidelines and provide some insight into the application of these principles for exercise prescription in both the primary and secondary prevention settings.

PRINCIPLES OF EXERCISE PRESCRIPTION— PRIMARY PREVENTION

For the most part, participants in primary prevention programs are at lower risk for exercise-related cardiovascular events than are those with CAD, and as discussed in chapter 6, the level of sophistication of the preparticipation screening is generally lower. In addition, the level of monitoring during the program can be much lower than within secondary prevention programs. However, the individualized exercise prescription in either type of program is still based on objective information obtained during the pre-participation screening. The following sections cover exercise prescription principles for both CR endurance and MS resistance training for participants in primary prevention exercise programs.

Cardiorespiratory Endurance Exercise Prescription

A physically active lifestyle has numerous documented physiological and psychological benefits. Chief among these is the reduction in risk for chronic diseases such as cardiovascular disease, diabetes mellitus, and certain site-specific cancers. Most of the **physical activity** reported by subjects in the epidemiological studies presented in chapter 1 was aerobic; therefore, to lower chronic disease risk, the prescription for exercise training should be primarily based on aerobic or CR endurance training principles. Musculoskeletal resistance training is also important but should always be a supplement to activities that develop the CR systems. When designing a CR endurance training regimen, the exercise program professional should define a training mode(s), intensity, frequency, duration, and progression that are suited to the individual's goals (e.g., increased $\dot{V}O_2$max, body fat loss, improved lipid profile, etc.). The following sections provide a rationale for development of these components of the CR endurance exercise prescription.

Mode

An endurance exercise prescription should include a variety of physical activities that are aerobic (i.e., rely on the aerobic energy system to provide the energy needed). These activities use large-muscle groups, can be maintained rather continuously (i.e., 15-60 min), and are rhythmical in nature. Traditionally, activities such as walking, jogging, cycling, swimming, cross-country skiing, and aerobic dancing have been the main modes for endurance exercise training. More recently, newer designs for indoor exercise machines such as various stair climbers, recumbent leg cycles, and elliptical trainers have provided for a wider variety of activities for CR endurance training. Exercise professionals should have a sense of the pros and cons of the various activities and be able to match an individual's preferences with one or more modes that will allow for an optimal training outcome (i.e., achievement of training goals). The ACSM Guidelines (1) define three categories of endurance training activities as presented in table 7.1. Group 1 activities are those that allow for maintenance of a constant energy expenditure and should be the basis for most initial exercise prescriptions. The primary activities in this category are brisk walking and cycling. As individuals progress through the training program, they can probably safely add activities that fall into groups 2 and 3 to complement the primary activity. When selecting modes from group 2 or 3, exercise program professionals are strongly encouraged to make use of published metabolic equivalency tables that provide estimates of the energy cost of various physical activities of interest to program participants (4). In summary, there are several keys to recommending appropriate modes for CR endurance training. First, you'll need to recommend activities that are enjoyable to the participant and within that person's capabilities, and second, recommend activities that if performed habitually will produce the desired training adaptations.

Intensity

Exercise training intensity refers to how hard one is exercising. For several reasons, training intensity is often considered the most important variable in the prescription. First, many research studies have documented that a threshold training intensity exists—that an individual has to exercise above a given threshold intensity before significant improvements in CR endurance will accrue. However, the minimal threshold for training adaptations will likely vary among individuals, with perhaps less fit or older persons having a lower threshold for adaptation than their younger, more fit counterparts. On the other end of the intensity spectrum, individuals who exercise too intensely may increase their risk of injury or untoward events during training and may be less likely to adhere to the training program. Therefore, an individualized exercise prescription should define an exercise intensity range that is suited to the participant. The ACSM position stand on exercise training (2) defines broad intensity ranges that are summarized in table 7.2. These ranges should be further delimited for the individual, especially during the initial phases of training. These ranges should also be viewed within the context of structured exercise training and therefore not be seen as inconsistent with or contradictory to physical activity recommendations for the general public, which encourage daily activity of a light to moderate intensity (5).

The exercise training intensity ranges recommended by the ACSM are defined using physiological ranges of heart rate (HR) or **oxygen uptake** ($\dot{V}O_2$). The theoretical basis for these measures as indicators of exercise intensity is a simple sequence of physiological adjustments made during exercise stress. These are described in detail in chapter 2 but are reviewed briefly here to establish HR and $\dot{V}O_2$ as indicators of exercise intensity. Readers should review the section in chapter

Table 7.1
ACSM Grouping of CR Endurance Activities

Group	Description
Group 1	Activities that can be readily maintained at a constant intensity and interindividual variation in energy expenditure is relatively low. Desirable for more precise control of exercise intensity, as in the early stages of a rehabilitation program. Examples include walking and cycling, especially treadmill and cycle ergometry.
Group 2	Activities in which the rate of energy expenditure is highly related to skill, but for a given individual can provide a constant intensity. Such activities may also be useful in early stages of conditioning, but individual skill levels must be considered. Examples include swimming and cross-country skiing.
Group 3	Activities where both skill and intensity of exercise are highly variable. Such activities can be very useful to provide group interaction and variety in exercise, but must be cautiously employed for high-risk, low fit, and/or symptomatic individuals. Competitive factors must also be considered and minimized. Examples include racquet sports and basketball.

Reprinted, by permission, 2000, *ACSM's Guidelines for Exercise Testing and Prescription.* 6th ed. (Philadelphia: Lippincott, Williams, and Wilkins), 144.

Table 7.2
Elements of the Aerobic Exercise Prescription

Variable	Recommendation
Mode	Aerobic: rhythmical and continuous in nature
Intensity	55/65 to 90% maximal HR 40/50 to 85% maximal $\dot{V}O_2R$ or HR reserve
Frequency	3 to 5 sessions per week
Duration	20 to 60 min of continuous or intermittent aerobic activity
Progression	Individualized based on tolerance and adaptation Optimally, maintenance programs should include energy expenditure threshold of >1500 kcals per week.

HR = heart rate; $\dot{V}O_2R$ = oxygen uptake reserve.

2 if the concepts here are not clear. First, as workload increases during exercise, the skeletal muscle's need for O_2 increases. During aerobic exercise, this increase in O_2 demand is met by an increase in cardiac output in an attempt to deliver the O_2 to the active muscle (see figures 2.9 and 2.10). The increase in cardiac output is achieved by increases in both HR and stroke volume. Now, as shown in figure 2.10, the increase in HR is fairly linear in relation to the increase in cardiac output, whereas the increase in stroke volume typically plateaus at approximately 50% to 60% of maximal $\dot{V}O_2$. Therefore, the increased HR mirrors the increased cardiac output, and the increased cardiac output mirrors the increased $\dot{V}O_2$ during incremental aerobic exercise. However, remember that the initial physiological stimulus is the increase in the O_2 required by the exercising muscles. This is the reason aerobic exercise intensity is often defined in terms of the amount of oxygen ($\dot{V}O_2$) required to perform the task. Now, because of the linear relationship between increased HR and increased cardiac output, when cardiac output rises sufficiently to match the O_2 requirement of the working muscles (i.e., steady state exercise), the HR response can be used as a surrogate measure of the metabolic rate ($\dot{V}O_2$) of the exercise.

In summary, then, the HR response during aerobic exercise may serve as a marker of the metabolic rate, and by targeting a given HR response during exercise (i.e., target HR) we are actually attempting to target a certain metabolic rate (i.e., target $\dot{V}O_2$). Herein lies the importance of these two physiological variables in defining exercise intensity. Examples of how to calculate the target HR or $\dot{V}O_2$ are provided in the next section. However, the student should re-

member that the HR:$\dot{V}O_2$ relationship described is most accurate during steady state exercise and under standardized environmental conditions (i.e., those encountered in the exercise test laboratory).

Traditionally, the optimal exercise training intensity has been defined in relative terms, meaning a percentage of the individual's measured maximal HR or maximal $\dot{V}O_2$. These variables are measured during a maximal graded exercise test as described in chapter 6. The concept of using a relative exercise intensity for training has its roots in the pioneering work of Karvonen and colleagues (6), who studied a group of young medical students in the late 1950s and concluded that a threshold intensity of approximately 60% of maximal heart rate reserve (MHRR) was required to elicit a physiological training effect. Karvonen and his colleagues used a reduction in the HR response to a standardized submaximal treadmill workload after the training program as the marker of a physiological training effect. As presented in table 7.2, the ACSM recommends an intensity range for CR endurance training between 55/65% and 90% of the maximal heart rate (MHR), or between 40/50% and 85% of maximal $\dot{V}O_2$ reserve ($\dot{V}O_2R$) or MHRR. The term reserve, used with the ranges above, refers to the difference between an individual's maximal value (HR or $\dot{V}O_2$) and that person's resting value as shown in the following equations.

$$\text{maximal } \dot{V}O_2 \text{ reserve} = \text{maximal } \dot{V}O_2 - \text{resting } \dot{V}O_2$$

$$\text{maximal HR reserve} = \text{maximal HR} - \text{resting HR}$$

As a general practice, older or less fit individuals should initiate exercise training at the lower end of these ranges (40-50% $\dot{V}O_2R$) and progress with gradual increases in intensity as they adapt during the training program. We'll look more closely at progression of the exercise plan later in the chapter. In summary, exercise training intensity should be defined using $\dot{V}O_2$ or HR responses from a graded exercise test. The following sections describe the prescription of exercise training intensity using $\dot{V}O_2$ and HR. The chapter provides several case study examples showing how to determine the target intensity for training.

Prescribing intensity using $\dot{V}O_2$

The concept of maximal oxygen uptake reserve ($\dot{V}O_2R$) has recently been introduced into exercise prescription recommendations (1, 2, 7). As already explained, the $\dot{V}O_2R$ is the difference between the maximal and resting $\dot{V}O_2$, and as such defines the available metabolic range—above resting metabolic rate—that one can utilize during exercise. The inclusion of the $\dot{V}O_2R$ in recent prescription guidelines stems from work by Swain and colleagues, who reported that a percentage of the MHRR matched more closely with the percentage of the $\dot{V}O_2R$ during leg cycling than a straight percentage of $\dot{V}O_2$max did (7). Substitution of the $\dot{V}O_2R$ for a straight percentage of the $\dot{V}O_2$max appears to make the agreement between HR and $\dot{V}O_2$ more scientifically accurate (2). However, many exercise program professionals prefer to use a straight percentage of $\dot{V}O_2$max (rather than of $\dot{V}O_2R$), and this is certainly acceptable. As shown in table 7.2, the recommended training intensity for aerobic exercise ranges between 40/50% and 85% of $\dot{V}O_2R$. Therefore, to define training intensity using $\dot{V}O_2$, one needs a measured or predicted $\dot{V}O_2$max and an estimate of resting $\dot{V}O_2$ (e.g., 3.5 ml·kg^{-1}·min^{-1}). Because of the considerable error associated with predicting $\dot{V}O_2$max from submaximal tests, we highly recommend using a directly measured $\dot{V}O_2$max or a predicted value from a maximal exercise test. These issues and procedures are discussed in detail in chapter 6. When a predicted $\dot{V}O_2$max from a submaximal test is all that is available, it becomes important to consider principles for prescribing exercise in the absence of exercise test data as explained later in the chapter. If a measured or reasonably accurate predicted $\dot{V}O_2$max is available, an individualized intensity can be calculated using the following equation:

$$\text{target } \dot{V}O_2 =$$
$$(\dot{V}O_2\text{max} - \dot{V}O_2\text{rest}) \times \% \text{ intensity} + \dot{V}O_2\text{rest}$$

Let's look at an example of how this method works. Table 7.3 contains data on a 67-year-old man who completed a maximal exercise test at the laboratory at Ball State University (BSU). He had a measured $\dot{V}O_2$max of 36.4 ml·kg^{-1}·min^{-1}. What would his exercise prescription intensity (i.e., target $\dot{V}O_2$) be using 50% to 85% of $\dot{V}O_2R$? Use the equation just presented with data from table 7.3 to calculate the answer as follows:

$$\text{target } \dot{V}O_2 \text{ ml·kg}^{-1}\text{·min}^{-1} \text{ at } 50\% \text{ } \dot{V}O_2R =$$
$$(36.4 - 3.5)(0.50) + 3.5$$
$$= (32.9)(0.50) + 3.5$$
$$= 16.5 + 3.5$$
$$= 20 \text{ ml·kg}^{-1}\text{·min}^{-1}$$

$$\text{target } \dot{V}O_2 \text{ ml·kg}^{-1}\text{·min}^{-1} \text{ at } 85\% \text{ } \dot{V}O_2R =$$
$$(36.4 - 3.5)(0.85) + 3.5$$
$$= (32.9)(0.85) + 3.5$$
$$= 28.0 + 3.5$$
$$= 31.5 \text{ ml·kg}^{-1}\text{·min}^{-1}$$

Table 7.3
Physiological Data for 67-Year-Old Man

Resting variables	Value
Body weight (kg)	68.9
BMI (kg · m^{-2})	24.0
Resting HR (bpm)	62
Resting BP (mmHg)	104/58
Exercise variables	
Exercise time* (min:sec)	11:35
Peak workload (mph/%)	4.2/15.6%
$\dot{V}O_2$max (ml·kg^{-1}·min^{-1})	36.4
RER$_{max}$	1.16
HR$_{max}$ (bpm)	167
Peak BP (mmHg)	166/96
Peak RPE (6-20 scale)	20

BMI = body mass index; HR = heart rate; BP = blood pressure; VE = pulmonary ventilation; RER = respiratory exchange ratio; RPE = rating of perceived exertion.
BSU/Bruce ramp protocol: reference (35).

As shown, this man's target $\dot{V}O_2$ range for aerobic exercise training would lie between 20 and 31.5 ml·kg^{-1}·min^{-1} based on the $\dot{V}O_2R$ concept. Many practitioners in the fitness center setting prefer to use the relative $\dot{V}O_2$ unit of METs. In this case, MET units could have been entered into the original equation (36.4 ml·kg^{-1}·min^{-1} = 10.4 METs); one could simply convert the equation solutions from ml·kg^{-1}·min^{-1} to METs by dividing each by 3.5. When using the unit of METs in the equation, you need to remember to enter the value 1.0 for the resting $\dot{V}O_2$ (1 MET = 3.5 ml·kg^{-1}·min^{-1}). The target $\dot{V}O_2$ range would be 5.7 to 9.0 METs. Once the target metabolic range is determined (ml·kg^{-1}·min^{-1} or METs), the metabolic equations in appendix D of the ACSM Guidelines (1) can be used to estimate exercise training workloads from the target $\dot{V}O_2$. We provide an example of this process with the case studies at the end of the chapter.

Rather than using the $\dot{V}O_2$ method to define training intensity, many exercise program professionals prefer to use HR methods. While this is certainly acceptable, exercise prescriptions defined solely by HR do not directly yield estimates of energy expenditure (kcal). With use of the $\dot{V}O_2$ methods described, it is easy to make estimates of the energy expenditure during exercise training. Why is this an important aspect of exercise prescription? Remember from chapter 1 that many of the health benefits associated with habitual physical activity appear to be linked to the total volume of activity or exercise. Estimating the caloric expenditure of a client's prescription allows a comparison with the energy expenditure thresholds shown to be protective in the studies reviewed in chapter 1. Therefore, regardless of whether prescriptions are based on a target HR or $\dot{V}O_2$, exercise program professionals should estimate the weekly energy expenditure of each client's exercise program to ensure that the individual is completing a sufficient dose of exercise to reap health benefits. More on caloric thresholds is presented later in the chapter.

A few precautions are in order when one is prescribing exercise intensity based on $\dot{V}O_2$ units. The oxygen cost of most aerobic activities is independent of environmental stressors such as high ambient heat or high altitude. During exercise in hot or humid conditions and at altitude, an individual's HR response will be higher for a given $\dot{V}O_2$, and therefore workloads need to be adjusted downward to stay within a calculated target HR range. In addition, if patients have an HR threshold they need to stay below during training (e.g., angina patients with a defined angina threshold), the $\dot{V}O_2$ prescription should always be evaluated to ensure that the HR response is below the critical threshold.

Prescribing intensity using heart rate
The most common method of defining exercise intensity is through use of a target HR range. Exercise program professionals have been providing target HR ranges for their fitness clients and cardiac patients for years. In this context, the target HR serves as a surrogate marker of the desired metabolic intensity ($\dot{V}O_2$) during training. As shown in table 7.2, the ACSM recommends a range of 40/50% to 85% of MHRR or 50/60% to 90% of MHR as the appropriate intensity range for CR endurance training. There are several methods for calculating the HRs associated with these ranges, including (1) use of a regression plot of HR and $\dot{V}O_2$ data collected during an exercise test, (2) use of the MHRR formula, and (3) calculation of a straight percentage of the MHR. This section describes and illustrates each of these methods, and in addition stresses the importance of using a measured MHR for these calculations.

Let's look first at the method of calculating a target HR range that uses the HR:$\dot{V}O_2$ plot. The best way to illustrate the linear relationship between HR and $\dot{V}O_2$ during an incremental exercise is by plotting the HR data as a function of the $\dot{V}O_2$ each minute during an incremental graded

exercise test (GXT). This type of plot serves as a direct method for relating a specific $\dot{V}O_2$ range to a specific HR range for the individual. This relationship is illustrated in figure 7.1, *a* and *b*, where the submaximal HR and $\dot{V}O_2$ data from the maximal GXT on our 67-year-old male case study have been plotted in both *absolute (a)* and *relative (b)* units. As shown in table 7.3, this man had a measured MHR of 167 bpm, and as discussed earlier, his $\dot{V}O_2$max was 36.4 ml·kg^{-1}·min^{-1}. In figure 7.1a, our case's measured $\dot{V}O_2$ (ml·kg^{-1}·min^{-1}) has been plotted as a function of the HR response (bpm) each minute throughout the stages of the GXT. Figure 7.1b contains the data after they have been converted to percentages of MHRR and $\dot{V}O_2$max. As you can see, both plots reveal very linear relationships between HR and $\dot{V}O_2$, which illustrates why we can use a target HR as a surrogate measure of the target $\dot{V}O_2$ during training. Now, within the context of determining an appropriate target HR for training, figure 7.1b illustrates that a given percentage of HR reserve on the y-axis matches fairly closely the same percentage of $\dot{V}O_2$max from the x-axis. On the figure we've chosen a lower and upper end for the training intensity range of 50% and 85% of $\dot{V}O_2$max, respectively. As you can see, the range of 50% to 85% of $\dot{V}O_2$max matches very closely with 50% to 85% of MHRR. The ACSM Guidelines (1) actually recommend this sort of plot (using the raw data as shown in figure 7.1a) as the most direct method for calculating a target exercise HR range for training. Let's return to the data for our 67-year-old man in figure 7.1a and see how this works. The first step is to calculate 50% and 85% of our subject's $\dot{V}O_2$max[1]:

$$50\% \text{ of } \dot{V}O_2\text{max: } 36.4 \text{ ml·kg}^{-1}\text{·min}^{-1} \times 0.50 = 18.2 \text{ ml·kg}^{-1}\text{·min}^{-1}$$

$$85\% \text{ of } \dot{V}O_2\text{max: } 36.4 \text{ ml·kg}^{-1}\text{·min}^{-1} \times 0.85 = 30.9 \text{ ml·kg}^{-1}\text{·min}^{-1}$$

Next, return to the plot of the raw data in figure 7.1a and find these two points on the x-axis. Then draw a line from the x-axis up to the line that passes through the data points on the graph. Finally, draw a line from the data points back to the y-axis to determine the HR response associated with 50% and 85% of our subject's $\dot{V}O_2$max. With this method, the appropriate target HR range for our subject is at 115 to 150 bpm. Now, rather than taking the time to plot each data point on graph paper, some practitioners actually prefer to use the equation for the straight line in figure 7.1a to calculate the target HRs. All commercially available statistical soft-

---

1 If one wanted to use the $\dot{V}O_2$R concept, the values for 50% and 85% $\dot{V}O_2$R would be 16.5 and 28.0, respectively.

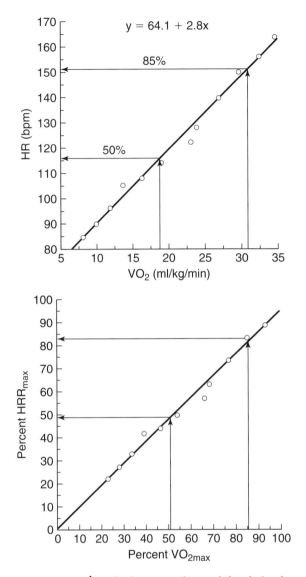

Figure 7.1 HR : $\dot{V}O_2$ plot for *(a)* raw data and *(b)* relative data.

ware packages and most handheld electronic calculators include the means to calculate the equation using the HR and $\dot{V}O_2$ data points. As shown in figure 7.1*a*, the equation for the line of best fit for our subject's HR:$\dot{V}O_2$ data is y = 64.1 +2.8x. Now, by plugging our two target $\dot{V}O_2$s into the equation as the "x" variable, we can calculate the target HRs using the equation as follows:

Target HR at 50% of $\dot{V}O_2$max: 64.1 + 2.8(18.2) = 115 bpm

Target HR at 85% of $\dot{V}O_2$max: 64.1 + 2.8(30.9) = 151 bpm

If you took care in constructing the data plot, visual inspection of the plot should yield an HR range similar to that calculated from the equations,

so it's no surprise that the two ranges are identical.

Although the HR:$\dot{V}O_2$ plot for calculating a target HR range is the most precise when we are matching a percentage of maximal $\dot{V}O_2$ to the same percentage of HR reserve, it is time-consuming to use. Most clinicians rely on another formula that yields HR values similar to those derived from the HR:$\dot{V}O_2$ plot, which brings us to our second method—maximal heart rate reserve. This formula, often referred to as the heart rate reserve (HRR) or Karvonen formula, is based on the study by Karvonen, Kantala, and Mustala (6) described earlier. The HRR formula determines the target HR (THR) by multiplying the difference between the maximal and resting exercise HR by the desired relative exercise intensity (%) and then adding the resting HR to the result. This is the formula:

target HR (bpm) = (maximal HR – resting HR) × (% intensity) + resting HR

As you recall, our case study's MHR was 167 bpm, and his seated resting HR (table 7.3) was 62 bpm. Using the formula just presented, let's calculate 50% and 85% of our subject's MHRR.

THR at 50% MHRR = (167 – 62)(.50) + 62 = 115 bpm

THR at 85% MHRR = (167 – 62)(.85) + 62 = 151 bpm

The THR range derived from the MHRR or Karvonen formula of 115 to 151 bpm matches very closely with the range derived from the HR:$\dot{V}O_2$ plot in figure 7.1*a*. The matching of the THR ranges will not always be as close as this example indicates, but it will usually be close when the HR and $\dot{V}O_2$ data are collected and plotted accurately. Because it is easy to use, most clinicians apply the Karvonen formula rather than plotting the results from the GXT. Again, either method will yield an appropriate THR range for training. Occasionally in our programs we encounter individuals whose THR ranges from these two methods do not match very well at all. In these cases we typically use the THR range determined from the MHRR formula as the individual's training intensity, because this method is less likely to be affected by data collection errors than the HR:$\dot{V}O_2$ method described earlier (e.g., imprecision in measurement of $\dot{V}O_2$). Furthermore, most exercise programs do not measure $\dot{V}O_2$ during an exercise test, which means they would be using *predicted* $\dot{V}O_2$s with *measured* HRs to construct the HR:$\dot{V}O_2$ plot. This could introduce addition error into the calculation of the THR and is therefore not recommended.

A third and final method for determining a THR is to simply calculate a straight percentage of the MHR—the percent HRmax—rather than using the HRR. Obviously, this method eliminates one step in the mathematical process (i.e., we don't subtract resting HR before multiplying by the intensity factor). With use of this method, the recommended target range as shown in table 7.2 is 55/65% to 90% of the measured HR max. Using the MHR of 167 from our 67-year-old in the case study, the THR range would be calculated as follows:

THR at 65% HRmax = 167(0.65) = 109 bpm

THR at 90% HRmax = 167(0.90) = 150 bpm

Why is the percentage range within this method (i.e., 65-90%) higher than the range associated with the HRR method (i.e., 55-85%)? The answer lies within the HR:$\dot{V}O_2$ relationship discussed earlier. Remember, THRs are useful because they represent surrogate markers of the target $\dot{V}O_2$. Once the target $\dot{V}O_2$ is established (i.e., between 50% and 85% of $\dot{V}O_2R$), we identify the HR response (bpm) associated with it. In our case study example, the HR response associated with the target $\dot{V}O_2$ was 115 to 150 bpm. The appropriateness of this HR range doesn't change just because we use a different formula. Therefore, in order to match this HR range using the straight percentage of MHR method, we have to use higher percentages in the equation (i.e., 65-90%). Research suggests that we would need to adjust the percentage up 10% to 15%, especially at the lower intensities, to match the HR responses between the methods (2). As the matching of HR response to a target $\dot{V}O_2$ is best defined using the MHRR formula, the MHRR is the preferred method for calculating the THR for training because it accounts for individual differences in resting HR.

Before moving to the next method of prescribing exercise intensity, the use of ratings of perceived exertion, we should consider what happens when we use a predicted MHR instead of measured MHR. Target HR calculations are most accurate when they are based on a measured MHR rather than a predicted value. As illustrated in figure 2.11, the range of measured MHRs at any given age is considerable. Within the several thousand apparently healthy individuals who completed a maximal treadmill test at Ball State University, one standard error of the estimate for MHR was approximately 11 bpm. What does this mean in the context of exercise prescription? Let's look at an example. As you can see from the graph in figure 2.11, individuals who were 40 years of age had MHRs ranging from 158 up to 205 bpm. That's a range of almost 50 bpm for individuals the same age! But if a predicted MHR had been used for calculating the THR range, all the 40-year-olds on the graph would have been assigned 180 bpm as their MHR. This error in prediction would have resulted in substantial error in the calculated THR range for many of the adults tested. This is why we discourage the use of predicted MHRs as end points during exercise testing as well as for THR calculations. To illustrate this point more directly, let's return to our 67-year-old man (data in table 7.3). This individual had a measured MHR of 167 bpm, which is 14 bpm higher than the 157 bpm predicted for his age (220 − 67 = 153). Now, if we were to calculate his THR as 50% to 85% of his MHRR using 153 as the MHR rather than 167, the HR range would have been 108 to 139 bpm, as the following calculations show. As figure 7.1a illustrates, this HR range (bpm) equates with a lower metabolic rate range ($\dot{V}O_2$) than would be optimal for our case study's training program.

THR at 50% MHRR = (153 − 62)(.50) + 62 = 108 bpm

THR at 85% MHRR = (153 − 62)(.85) + 62 = 139 bpm

Our case study example illustrates the error created when the predicted MHR lies below the true MHR. As the calculations show, the result is a lower metabolic intensity than desirable, which equates with a less-than-optimal training stimulus. In contrast, using a predicted MHR in the THR equation that exceeds the measured value will lead to overexertion during training. As the actual degree of overexertion (i.e., how much over the target $\dot{V}O_2$ the exertion is) will not be known, this kind of error is a more serious one in the context of exercise prescription. Obviously, when using a predicted MHR, the exercise program professional will not know which type of error she is making (under- or overexertion). For this reason, we strongly advocate calculating THRs using measured MHR. At the same time, we concede that the only way to attain a measured MHR—performing a maximal exercise test—may not be technically or financially feasible in all settings where exercise prescriptions are prepared. Therefore, many exercise professionals must rely on other means to define and monitor the intensity of endurance training. When a measured MHR from a GXT is not available, we advocate prescribing moderate activities (e.g., brisk walking) for initial training sessions in sedentary adults. Obviously, selecting a moderate intensity provides a safety buffer during initial exercise training, but also doesn't force the practitioner to guess about the individual's predicted MHR. These initial sessions could be used to assess HR, symptoms, and/or ratings of perceived exertion even without a designated *predicted* HR value as the target for the exercise session. During subsequent exercise sessions, the exercise workloads could be modified (increased or decreased) depending on the physiological responses and any symptoms observed during the initial sessions.

Prescribing intensity using rating of perceived exertion

Although we advocate the use of HR or $\dot{V}O_2$ as objective markers of exercise training intensity, rating of perceived exertion (RPE) may be an additional marker of intensity to use in conjunction with physiological measures during training. The concept of perceived exertion during exercise was pioneered by a Swedish physician named Gunnar Borg in the 1960s (8). Over the years, Dr. Borg published several iterations of his RPE scale, but the version most frequently used for exercise prescription is the 15-point scale shown in table 7.4. Recent exercise prescription guidelines (2) recommend a generalized RPE range of 12 to 16 as the perceptual range associated with a physiological training effect, as this numeric range is thought to correlate with the appropriate physiological range during exercise (i.e., 50-85% of $\dot{V}O_2$max). Regarding the matching between RPE and metabolic rate during exercise, Drs. Bruce Noble and Robert Robertson—noted researchers in the field of perceived exertion—state in their text on the topic (9):

> *Perceptual regulation of exercise intensity is considered physiologically and clinically valid if HR, V.O$_2$, RPP [rate-pressure product], or ECG criteria do not differ when comparisons are made at similar levels of exertion (RPE) between GXT and training session.*

In other words, for RPE to be a useful marker of physiological intensity during exercise training, there should be consistency in the RPE value reported at a given HR or $\dot{V}O_2$ across exercise modes or conditions. As reviewed by Noble and Robertson in their recent text (9), this has been the topic of considerable research in recent years, and results have been mixed. While some studies have concluded that RPE is valid, others have reported problems with the matching of RPE to physiological markers of exercise intensity in healthy adults and cardiac patients. Several years ago, in order to evaluate the validity of using RPE

Table 7.4
Borg 15-Point RPE Scale

Number	Verbal anchor
6	
7	Very, very light
8	
9	Very light
10	
11	Fairly light
12	
13	Somewhat hard
14	
15	Hard
16	
17	Very hard
18	
19	Very, very hard
20	

Borg RPE scale ©Gunnar Borg, 1970, 1985, 1994, 1998
G. Borg, 1998, *Borg's perceived exertion and pain scales* (Champaign, IL: Human Kinetics), 47.

as a marker of physiological intensity, researchers at Ball State assessed RPE and physiological responses of 30 men and women during three different exercise sessions (10). Two of the three exercise trials were maximal GXTs (Bruce and Balke protocols), with the third bout serving as a simulated steady state exercise session (track). As shown in figure 7.2, when RPEs (Borg 15-point scale) were compared across the three exercise trials at 75% of MHRR, there were considerable differences among the trials. The mean RPE ranged from as high as 16 during the Balke GXT to a low of 10 during the simulated exercise session. Again, the subjects in the study rated their effort at the same physiological intensity (i.e., 75% MHRR) during all three trials. A similar study was performed with 25 cardiac patients at Wake Forest University (11). In this investigation, patients' RPEs were compared at matched HRs between a GXT and several exercise sessions. As illustrated in figure 7.3, patients' RPEs were significantly higher during the steady state exercise training sessions (gym) than during their GXT. Again, the RPEs were recorded at the same THR between conditions. The results from these and other studies (12-15) indicate that RPEs will not always match with specific physiological values

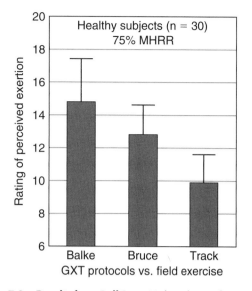

Figure 7.2 Results from Ball State University study on rating of perceived exertion. Data are mean ± standard deviation.
Adapted, by permission, from M.H. Waley and M.S. Wegner, 1991, "Ratings of perceived exertion among standard treadmill protocols and steady state running," *International Journal of Sports Medicine* 12(1):80.

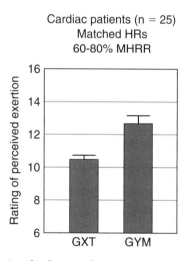

Figure 7.3 Results from Wake Forest University study on rating of perceived exertion. Data are mean ± standard error.

(% MHRR or % $\dot{V}O_2$max) across exercise modes or conditions. Therefore, whether the use of RPEs as markers of exercise intensity passes the validity litmus test cited by Noble and Robertson is not clear.

The important thing to remember about using RPEs for monitoring exercise prescription intensity is that there is considerable inter- and intra-individual variability in the psychophysiological relationship during exercise testing and training (13, 15, 16). In other words, exercise program professionals should not expect a given number on the scale (e.g., RPE of 12) to match with a given physiological intensity (e.g., 50% $\dot{V}O_2$max) in all

individuals, or within the same individual across different modes of exercise or from day to day within the same mode. Therefore, it is best to view RPE as an adjunct to HR and workloads as methods for monitoring intensity during exercise training.

Duration

An endurance exercise prescription should include a duration of exercise per session that, when combined with the intensity and frequency, provides a dose of activity—that is, **kilocalories (kcal)** expended—consistent with achievement of participant goals and meeting or preferably exceeding the minimal dose associated with health benefits. According to the ACSM Guidelines (1), continuous exercise for 20 to 30 min at 60% to 80% of MHRR provides for most health and fitness benefits. Those needing or choosing to exercise at lower intensities should increase the duration of the exercise session to attain a minimal caloric expenditure of 1000 kcal per week. Individuals who are very unfit or people who are attempting to increase the intensity of the exercise sessions will benefit from a discontinuous protocol consisting of multiple short bouts of exercise (e.g., 4-6 min) separated by brief periods of reduced intensity. This type of interval training approach has been shown to be quite successful during the initial stages of training in both apparently healthy and chronic disease patients.

Frequency

An endurance exercise prescription should include a frequency of training (i.e., number of sessions per week) that, when combined with the intensity and duration, provides for a dose of activity consistent with achievement of the participant's goals and the attainment of the dose of activity associated with health benefits. The ACSM Guidelines (1) recommend an optimal exercise training frequency of three to five times per week. However, one needs to consider intensity of training, type of activity, initial fitness level, and orthopedic limitations when selecting the appropriate frequency for an individual's training routine. Numerous research studies have shown that individuals exercising at the middle to upper intensity range (60-80% of MHRR) could maintain or improve aerobic capacity with three sessions per week (2). However, sedentary individuals who are initiating an exercise program will likely be training at a lower intensity and would benefit from more frequent sessions. In addition, many sedentary individuals begin an exercise program with a goal of reducing excess body fat; in these cases, the increased energy expenditure associated with an increased training frequency will help them attain the goal. Exercise prescriptions designed for body fat reduction should be set at a moderate intensity (e.g., 50-65% of MHRR) and should progress as quickly as tolerable to five to six times per week. This may take a month or two, but the increased frequency will enhance the total caloric expenditure of the regimen and help in establishing exercise as part of the individual's lifestyle. Persons who adopt exercise five to six times per week as an integral part of their lifestyle are more effective in maintaining body fat losses, and thus a frequency of five to six times per week should be a goal within the training regimen.

Severely deconditioned patients (MET capacity <5) will likely benefit from multiple, short exercise sessions within the same day (e.g., 5- to 10-min bouts, three to four times daily) when beginning an exercise program. For those participating in vigorous weight-bearing activities, the incidence of lower-extremity injuries rises significantly with frequency above three to four times per week. Therefore exercise professionals should monitor orthopedic symptoms under these conditions and modify training frequency and mode when overuse symptoms arise.

The frequency range of three to five times per week from the ACSM Guidelines should not be viewed as inconsistent with the physical activity recommendations from the U.S. Surgeon General's Report (SGR) on physical activity and health (5) regarding the importance of activity on "most, preferably all days of the week." The general frequency recommendation in the ACSM Guidelines is given within the context of an exercise training regimen in which a major goal of training is to increase aerobic capacity; in contrast, the SGR recommendations are given within the context of health benefits and are based on a dose-response relationship between physical activity and reduction in chronic disease risk. The Surgeon General's recommendation for daily physical activity was also combined with a recommendation for light to moderate intensity (<6 METs). The SGR authors state, "People who maintain a regular regimen of activity that is of longer duration or of more vigorous intensity are likely to derive greater benefit." This means that up to a point, more activity is better than less activity; for the general public whose activity level is rather low, it would make sense to recommend daily activity at a light to moderate intensity as an initial goal to reduce chronic disease risk.

Progression

An initial endurance exercise prescription should include a progression of training (i.e., systematic increase in dose of exercise) that provides for a dose of activity consistent with achievement of the participant's goals and attainment of the dose of activity associated with health benefits. The ultimate goal is to reach a dose of activity that allows for maintenance of the health and fitness benefits associated with regular exercise training. However, one must get there first! This means that exercise professionals need to design routines that allow each individual to progress toward this optimal prescription at a rate that is safe and physiologically sound. Table 7.5 presents a rate of training progression recommended by the ACSM that includes initial, improvement, and maintenance stages (1). These stages differ both in the total volume of exercise completed during

Table 7.5
ACSM Recommended Progression for Apparently Healthy Individuals during Endurance Training

Program stage	Week	Exercise frequency (sessions/wk)	Exercise intensity (%HRR)	Exercise duration (min)
Initial stage	1	3	40–50	15–20
	2	3–4	40–50	20–25
	3	3–4	50–60	20–25
	4	3–4	50–60	25–30
Improvement stage	5–7	3–4	60–70	25–30
	8–10	3–4	60–70	30–35
	11–13	3–4	65–75	30–35
	14–16	3–5	65–75	30–35
	17–20	3–5	70–85	35–40
	21–24	3–5	70–85	35–40
Maintenance stage	24+	3–5	70–85	30–45

HRR = heart rate reserve.
Reprinted, by permission, 2000, *ACSM's Guidelines for Exercise Testing and Prescription.* 6th ed. (Philadelphia: Lippincott, Williams, and Wilkins), 154.

training sessions (i.e., sum of intensity, frequency, and duration) and in the rate at which the training stimulus is increased across weeks and/or months. As illustrated in figure 7.4, the initial phase of training (line A) begins with a low total volume of training and should incorporate gradual increases in the training stimulus. Following this, the improvement stage (line B) allows for more aggressive increases in the training stimulus, with the total volume increasing throughout the stage. The maintenance stage (line C) is characterized by a stable dose of exercise that allows an individual to maintain the improved fitness level. The following sections present more specific information regarding the progression of training frequency, intensity, and duration within each of the stages. Most people presenting for an exercise prescription are able to attain a maintenance dose of exercise within six months from the onset of the training program.

Initial stage
The initial stage of exercise training usually involves a lower intensity, frequency, and duration compared to later stages. As shown in table 7.5, the first week of training might consist of only three sessions at a moderate intensity (i.e., 40-50% of HRR) for no more than 15 to 20 min. Although this is actually less than the minimal dose of physical activity recommended by the U.S. Surgeon General, we've found that patients can tolerate this dose well and that they can complete it with little or no discomfort or muscle soreness. Therefore, individuals are likely to have a good experience during their first few sessions and to gain confidence in their ability to exercise. During the later weeks of the initial stage of training, an extra day may be incorporated into the routine so that the individual is exercising more days per week than not (i.e., four vs. three). The progression also provides for gradual increases in intensity (still moderate at

60%) and duration (now up to the daily recommendation in the SGR—30 min). Perhaps the most important goal of the initial stage is to complete it, and complete it without injury! In other words, you should design a routine with adherence and safety in mind. Use the first few weeks to introduce timid individuals to a lifestyle of physical activity and help them see that accomplishing the goal is possible. Don't be so regimented that you turn people off before they have a chance to develop exercise into a habit. On the other hand, there are many former athletes who've reached middle age and haven't exercised regularly since their late teens or early 20s when they competed on sport teams. These individuals often present a different type of challenge during the early weeks of training. From our experience, many want to pick up right where they left off as athletes and will overdo it during the initial weeks. As an exercise leader, you need to hold tight to the leash and keep such individuals from overdoing it and injuring themselves in the process.

Improvement stage
After the initial stage, the individual is ready orthopedically and physiologically for an increase in the training stimulus that will bring about an increase in aerobic capacity as well as many other physiologic benefits associated with CR endurance training. This stage is often referred to as the improvement stage, because as a consequence of the overall increases in the dose of exercise during this stage, individuals experience a number of physiological improvements. As illustrated in figure 7.4, this stage is characterized by a more rapid progression in the training stimulus, including systematic increases in the frequency (up to five times a week), intensity (up to 85% HRR or $\dot{V}O_2R$), and duration (up to 40 min per session) of training. This is the phase of training in which exercise prescription can become a bit of an art form as the exercise leader is the artist, and the participant is the canvas. The role of the leader in this instance is to create a progression of workouts over the ensuing three to four months that provides for the systematic increases in the exercise stimulus referred to earlier. As illustrated in table 7.5, training intensity, frequency, and duration all increase during this phase. A quick review of the progressions in table 7.5 might suggest that all the exercise leader needs to do is follow the progression "recipe" in the table. Although this is certainly one approach, we've found that mode-specific progression charts are a more effective means of guiding the participant through this phase.

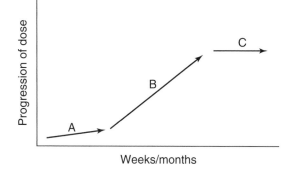

Figure 7.4 Stages of the training program.

Figure 7.5, *a* and *b*, contains two examples of mode-specific progression charts that were designed originally by Leroy "Bud" Getchell, a professor emeritus at Indiana University. Dr. Getchell founded the Ball State University Adult Physical Fitness Program in the 1960s. The walking and run-walk progressions in the charts have been completed by over 1000 adult members of the Ball State University fitness program over the years. The charts contain steps that build the dose of exercise gradually over time. Participants using the charts get to see where they're going from workout to workout, and we've found that this breeds ownership in the process. In addition, as participants record their workout results on the chart each day, they

gain confidence in their ability to exercise (i.e., increased self-efficacy). An additional advantage of the progression charts is that they can be modified to fit other modes of exercise (swimming, cycling, stationary aerobic exercise machines, etc.). Specific instructions for use of the charts are provided at the end of the chapter. Let's take a look at an example of how the progressions in the BSU walking and run-walk charts work.

Table 7.6 contains some physiological data on a 41-year-old man tested prior to joining the adult fitness program at Ball State. This man was considered sedentary, as he reported golf as his only activity (indicating that he rode in a golf cart when playing). He had a measured $\dot{V}O_2$max of

BSU ADULT PHYSICAL FITNESS PROGRAM

WALKING CHART-EXERCISE RECORD

NAME _____   APFP # _____   THR Range _____

STEP	TIME (min)	DISTANCE (Laps)	Date/Pulse	Date/Pulse	Additional Workouts Date/Pulse	Date/Pulse
1	15	5.0 - 6.0	_____/_____	_____/_____	_____/_____	_____/_____
2	**20**	7.0 - 8.0	_____/_____	_____/_____	_____/_____	_____/_____
3	24	8.5 - 9.5	_____/_____	_____/_____	_____/_____	_____/_____
4	28	10.0 - 11.0	_____/_____	_____/_____	_____/_____	_____/_____
5	32	11.5 - 12.5	_____/_____	_____/_____	_____/_____	_____/_____
6	36	13.0 - 14.0	_____/_____	_____/_____	_____/_____	_____/_____
7	**40**	14.5 - 15.5	_____/_____	_____/_____	_____/_____	_____/_____
8	44	16.0 - 17.0	_____/_____	_____/_____	_____/_____	_____/_____
9	48	17.5 - 18.5	_____/_____	_____/_____	_____/_____	_____/_____
10	52	19.0 - 20.0	_____/_____	_____/_____	_____/_____	_____/_____
11	56	20.5 - 21.5	_____/_____	_____/_____	_____/_____	_____/_____
12	**60**	22.0 - 23.0	_____/_____	_____/_____	_____/_____	_____/_____
13	58	23.0	_____/_____	_____/_____	_____/_____	_____/_____
14	56	23.0	_____/_____	_____/_____	_____/_____	_____/_____
15	54	23.0	_____/_____	_____/_____	_____/_____	_____/_____
16	52	23.0	_____/_____	_____/_____	_____/_____	_____/_____

Walking lanes are #3-5; 1 mile ≈ 7.6 Laps in lane #3; 1 mile ≈ 7.5 Laps in lane #4.

Figure 7.5a   Ball State University walking chart.

BSU ADULT PHYSICAL FITNESS PROGRAM

RUN-WALK CHART - EXERCISE RECORD

NAME _____ APFP # _____ THR Range _____

STEP	WALK (min)	RUN-WALKS	WALK (min)	Date/Pulse	Date/Pulse	Date/Pulse
1	20	$1/2 - 1/2 - 1/2 - 1/2$	10	_____/_____	_____/_____	_____/_____
2	17.5	$1/2 - 1/2 - 1/2 - 1/2 - 1/2 - 1/2$	10	_____/_____	_____/_____	_____/_____
3	15	$1/2 - 1/2 - 1/2 - 1/2 - 1/2 - 1/2 - 1/2 - 1/2$	8	_____/_____	_____/_____	_____/_____
4	15	$1/2 - 1/2 - 1/2 - 1/2 - 1/2 - 1/2 - 1$	8	_____/_____	_____/_____	_____/_____
5	10	$1/2 - 1/2 - 1/2 - 1/2 - 1/2 - 1/2 - 1 - 1$	8	_____/_____	_____/_____	_____/_____
6	10	$1/2 - 1/2 - 1/2 - 1/2 - 1 - 1 - 1$	8	_____/_____	_____/_____	_____/_____
7	8	$1/2 - 1/2 - 1/2 - 1/2 - 1 - 1 - 1 - 1$	6	_____/_____	_____/_____	_____/_____
8	8	$1/2 - 1/2 - 1/2 - 1/2 - 1 - 1 - 1 - 1 - 1$	6	_____/_____	_____/_____	_____/_____
9	8	$1/2 - 1/2 - 1 - 1 - 1 - 1 - 1 - 1$	6	_____/_____	_____/_____	_____/_____
10	8	$1/2 - 1/2 - 1 - 1 - 1 - 1 - 1 - 1 - 1$	6	_____/_____	_____/_____	_____/_____
11	6	$1 - 1 - 1 - 1 - 1 - 1 - 1 - 1$	4	_____/_____	_____/_____	_____/_____
12	6	$1 - 1 - 1 - 1 - 1 - 1 1/2 - 1 1/2$	4	_____/_____	_____/_____	_____/_____
13	6	$1 - 1 - 1 - 1 - 1 1/2 - 1 1/2 - 2$	4	_____/_____	_____/_____	_____/_____
14	6	$1 - 1 - 1 1/2 - 1 1/2 - 2 - 2$	4	_____/_____	_____/_____	_____/_____
15	6	$1 - 1 - 2 - 2 - 2 - 2$	4	_____/_____	_____/_____	_____/_____
16	4	$1 - 1 - 1 - 2 - 2 - 2 - 2$	4	_____/_____	_____/_____	_____/_____
17	4	$1 - 1 - 2 - 2 - 2 - 2 - 2$	4	_____/_____	_____/_____	_____/_____
18	4	$2 - 2 - 2 - 2 - 2 - 2$	4	_____/_____	_____/_____	_____/_____
19	4	$2 - 2 - 2 - 2 - 2 - 2 - 2$	4	_____/_____	_____/_____	_____/_____
20	4	$2 - 2 - 2 - 2 - 2 - 2 - 2 - 2$	4	_____/_____	_____/_____	_____/_____
21	4	$2 - 2 - 2 - 2 - 2 - 3 - 3$	2	_____/_____	_____/_____	_____/_____
22	4	$2 - 2 - 2 - 2 - 3 - 3 - 3$	2	_____/_____	_____/_____	_____/_____
23	4	$2 - 2 - 2 - 2 - 3 - 3 - 3 - 2$	2	_____/_____	_____/_____	_____/_____
24	4	$2 - 2 - 2 - 2 - 3 - 3 - 3 - 3$	2	_____/_____	_____/_____	_____/_____
25	2	$2 - 2 - 2 - 2 - 3 - 3 - 3 - 4$	2	_____/_____	_____/_____	_____/_____
26	2	$2 - 3 - 3 - 3 - 3 - 4 - 4$	2	_____/_____	_____/_____	_____/_____
27	2	$3 - 3 - 4 - 4 - 4 - 5$	2	_____/_____	_____/_____	_____/_____
28	2	$4 - 8 - 4$	2	_____/_____	_____/_____	_____/_____
29	2	$2 - 12 - 2$	2	_____/_____	_____/_____	_____/_____
30	2	16	2	_____/_____	_____/_____	_____/_____

1/2 represents 110 yds. or 30-45 sec; 1 represents 220 yds. or 1-1.5 min; 2 represents 440 yds. or 2-3 min; represents 660 yds. or 3-4.5 min; 4 represents 880 yds. or 4-6 min; 8 represents 1760 yds. or 8-12 min.

Jogging lanes are #1-2.

Figure 7.5*b* **Ball State University run-walk chart.**

Table 7.6
Physiological Data for 41-Year-Old Man

Resting variables	Value
Body weight (kg)	73.0
BMI (kg · m⁻²)	24.8
Resting HR (bpm)	70
Resting BP (mmHg)	116/78
Exercise variables	
Exercise time* (min:sec)	12:30
Peak workload (mph/%)	4.4/16.4%
$\dot{V}O_2$max (ml·kg⁻¹·min⁻¹)	39.1
RERmax	1.15
MHR (bpm)	186
Peak BP (mmHg)	166/90
Peak RPE (6-20 scale)	20

BMI = body mass index; MHR = maximal heart rate; BP = blood pressure; VE = pulmonary ventilation; RER = respiratory exchange ratio; RPE = rating of perceived exertion.
BSU/Bruce ramp protocol: reference (35).

39.1 ml·kg⁻¹·min⁻¹ or 11.2 METs, which placed him at about the 60th percentile for his age (1). This means that he was more aerobically fit than 60% of the men his age. Did this man have room for improvement? You bet! Now, as we explain in the instructions for the BSU run-walk progression chart, most healthy adults who have a $\dot{V}O_2$max >8 METs have the physiological ability to start a progressive exercise routine similar to that shown on the BSU run-walk chart (figure 7.5b). This doesn't mean we advocate that everyone with a $\dot{V}O_2$max >8 METs begin this sort of training program; but if people desire to do so and have a normal exercise test, they should be able to handle the progressions well. Again, we are speaking from experience with over 1000 adults who've followed the progressions with great results. Now, our case study man had a normal GXT (i.e., normal blood pressure [BP], ECG, and no symptoms) and expressed a desire to use running as his exercise training mode, so he was started on the BSU run-walk progressions. We started him at step 3 (see figure 7.5b), which includes 15 min of brisk walking followed by eight run-walk intervals (i.e., half-lap jog, half-lap brisk walk) around a 200 m track. The last part of the workout is an 8-min brisk walk. As you can see, even though he's on our run-walk chart, the

majority of his initial workout was brisk walking! Again, it is very important to build up to the jogging sections of the progression charts gradually.

Figure 7.6 illustrates this man's HR response throughout the entire walking, run-walk, walking routine of step 3 on the chart. His HR response was below the calculated THR range during both brisk walking phases. However, his HR quickly increased during each jogging bout and recovered rather quickly during the brisk walking in between each run. This is a very common physiological response to interval-type aerobic training. You should also note that this participant's peak HR during the first four jogging bouts didn't reach his THR range. Does this mean he wasn't running fast enough? No! The reason relates to the length of each jogging bout. As explained in the legend to the chart, the jogging bouts at step 3 are only 100 m, which typically takes 30 to 45 s at the jogging pace we encourage. This short period of time does not allow for achievement of a true steady state HR. Therefore we don't worry about the HR response as much during these early steps on the chart. As our 41-year-old man progressed through the steps—lengthening the jogging distance gradually—his HR response would have been elevated into his THR range for more and more of the workout routine. We have had excellent success with a progression in which individuals complete each step twice (two workouts in a row) and then move on to the next step. Obviously, people adapt at different rates, so exercise leaders need to evaluate the rate of progression on a case-by-case basis. We've found that some adults need to complete each workout three times before moving on to the next step. Keep in mind that the exercise progressions outlined in figure 7.5 can be translated to fit most modes of

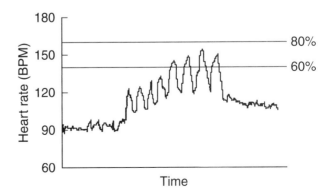

Figure 7.6 Case study heart rate response to the run-walk intervals. Lines represent 60-80% of maximal HRR.

aerobic exercise; specific progression charts for other modes, such as cycling and swimming, are available elsewhere (17).

The improvement stage of the CR endurance program typically lasts between three and six months. Over the years, many of the healthy adults who've participated in the fitness program at Ball State took three to four months to progress through the walking or run-walk charts shown in figure 7.5, *a* and *b*. Chapter 8 describes the various physiological adaptations that occur during this phase of training. Although the magnitude of the adaptation varies considerably, numerous studies have shown that with appropriate intensity, frequency, and duration, individuals typically experience a 15% to 30% improvement in $\dot{V}O_2$max during this stage of training.

Maintenance stage

As adults progress through the initial three to six months of exercise training, they achieve some or perhaps all of their fitness goals. Clearly, some fitness adaptations can be achieved in less time than others. For example, individuals who are obese often attain a significant increase in $\dot{V}O_2$max during aerobic training well before they attain an ideal body weight. However, most adults reach a stable dose of exercise within five to six months after beginning a training program. This stage of the program is often referred to as the maintenance stage (see figure 7.4 and table 7.5). The major goals are to maintain the CR fitness developed during the improvement stage and to continue to work toward the training goals not yet attained (e.g., decreased body fat, normalization of blood lipids, etc.).

Now, what volume or dose of exercise constitutes an appropriate amount within a maintenance program? We can approach this issue in several ways. Many exercise program professionals define an optimal training dose for each participant using the exercise prescription elements from table 7.2. For example, our 41-year-old male (table 7.6) might be given a maintenance exercise prescription of 60% to 80% of MHRR, four to five days per week, 45 min per session. The individual would gradually work up to this volume of exercise during the improvement stage of the program and after reaching this dose would continue at this dose during the maintenance stage. While this is certainly an acceptable and commonly used approach, we encourage exercise leaders to complement this strategy by incorporating the concept of caloric thresholds into their exercise prescriptions.

The concept of the caloric threshold is an attempt to define the optimal volume of training using the amount of energy expended per week as a metric. Why is this important? As discussed in chapter 1, many of the health benefits associated with habitual physical activity have been linked to a volume of activity (e.g., kilocalories per week). For this reason, organizations such as the ACSM and American Heart Association (AHA) have specified energy expenditure recommendations within their guidelines statements (1, 18). The ACSM Guidelines suggest that a minimal dose of physical activity per week should be equivalent to 1000 kcal, with 2000 kcal representing a more optimal dose. Therefore, exercise leaders should estimate the energy expenditure of the prescriptions they provide and consider designing the maintenance dose of activity with a caloric threshold in mind. Using a caloric threshold to define the optimal dose of activity necessitates knowledge of the energy expenditure for a variety of exercise modes. In other words, how much walking, cycling, or swimming would one need to perform to achieve the minimal or optimal caloric threshold? The ACSM publishes metabolic equations that can be used to estimate the energy cost of selected activities (1). In addition, MET values (which can readily be converted to kilocalories of energy expenditure) for over 500 different recreational and occupational activities are available (4).

Let's look at an example of using the concept of a caloric threshold within an individualized exercise prescription. Remember our 67-year-old man from earlier in the chapter? As shown in table 7.3, his fitness level was 36.4 ml·kg^{-1}·min^{-1}, he was not overweight, and he had a normal resting BP. His blood lipid profile and fasting blood glucose were within normal limits (data not shown). As most of his fitness measures and risk factors were within the normal ranges for his age, the primary goal of his training program would be to establish a habitual routine that he could maintain through the years to come. The following is a summary of his initial CR endurance exercise prescription:

Intensity: 50-60% $\dot{V}O_2$R (5.7 to 6.6 METs)

Frequency: 3× week

Duration: 20–25 min

Mode: Walking

Again, we suggest approaching the prescription dose from the perspective of energy expenditure. As our case study man was sedentary when he joined the exercise program, our first energy expenditure goal would be a dose of activity that met the minimal recommended level of 1000 kcal per week. Let's estimate the weekly energy expenditure of his initial workout routine. Remember that energy expenditure during steady state exercise is related to the volume of oxygen consumed. For the purposes of the calculations, we'll use the lower end of the ranges presented earlier. The lower end of the range for his initial exercise prescription intensity was defined as 50% of $\dot{V}O_2R$, which equates with 5.7 METs.[1] The following equation provides an easy method to convert the oxygen cost of exercise (METs) into energy expenditure (1), and can be used to estimate the rate of energy expended (i.e., $kcal \cdot min^{-1}$) during this man's workouts.

$$kcal \cdot min^{-1} = METs \times 3.5 \times body\ weight\ in\ kg/200$$

Based on our man's 5.7-MET target for his initial prescription and his body weight of 73.0 kg, his rate of energy expenditure would be approximately $7.3\ kcal \cdot min^{-1}$. This would translate into approximately 146 kcal each 20-min exercise session and 437 kcal per week using the three times per week training frequency. Now, although these are clearly estimates, they do provide some insight into the dose of exercise. Even though this man is exercising three times per week for 20 min at an appropriate target intensity (50% $\dot{V}O_2R$), he's well below the minimal caloric threshold of 1000 kcal per week. Therefore, as mentioned in the earlier section on the stages of a CR training program, one of the initial goals for this man would be to increase his dose of exercise to 1000 kcal per week. This could be accomplished in several ways; however, a gradual increase in exercise duration and frequency during the first three to four weeks would be the most appropriate means. Given this, five 30-min sessions at the intensity specified would equate with the minimal goal of 1000 kcal per week. Obviously, the exercise leader can manipulate the training intensity, frequency, and duration in a variety of ways; but it is a good idea to keep the concept of the caloric threshold in mind.

Within the context of a maintenance exercise program, national guidelines suggest that a more optimal energy expenditure goal is closer to 2000 kcal per week (1). Now, we submit that there may be differences of opinion among exercise program professionals as to the optimal dose of exercise for our 67-year-old man. It's possible that the optimal dose may be lower than 2000 kcal per

week. Perhaps somewhere between 1500 and 2000 kcal per week would be appropriate for this 67-year-old. However, whether one recommends 1500 or a value closer to 2000, our point is that the maintenance dose of exercise should be defined with a caloric threshold in mind. What combination of intensity, frequency, and duration would allow him to achieve a maintenance dose of 1500 kcal per week?

To speculate on this we fast-forward through the improvement stage of his program; and, for the purposes of these calculations, let's arbitrarily assume a 15% increase in $\dot{V}O_2$max during this stage of his training. Thus, our man arrives at the doorstep of his maintenance stage with an increased $\dot{V}O_2$max of approximately $42\ ml \cdot kg^{-1} \cdot min^{-1}$, or 12 METs. He also been able to increase his relative training intensity during the improvement stage to approximately 75% of $\dot{V}O_2R$. Using the $\dot{V}O_2R$ equation presented earlier, we can estimate that his target $\dot{V}O_2$ during exercise is now approximately 9.3 METs.[2] So, what would the training frequency and duration need to be for this man to expend 1500 kcal per week during his maintenance program? Using the caloric expenditure equation cited earlier (assuming no significant change in body weight for this man), his current caloric expenditure rate would be appropriately 12 kcal/min ($12 = 9.3 \times 3.5 \times 73/200$). Now, this new value warrants a comment. This increase in the energy expenditure rate for his exercise sessions (12 vs. 7 kcal/min) is due to both the increased $\dot{V}O_2$max following the improvement stage and an increase in his tolerable training intensity (50% vs. 75%). Thus, compared to his initial training value, his new value of 12 kcal/min allows for a significantly higher energy expenditure rate during his training routine. Exactly why is this important? If during the course of a maintenance program our man was willing to commit to four exercise sessions per week, he would need to expend approximately 375 kcal per session to achieve the 1500 weekly goal. This would mean a duration of 31 min for each workout ($375/12 = 31.3$ min). In summary, our case study man could achieve the weekly caloric threshold with four 30-min exercise sessions per week at an intensity of 9 METs. His increased CR fitness level allows for greater energy expenditure during training, reducing the number of minutes required each week to achieve the desired caloric threshold.

---

1 The MET value for 50% $\dot{V}O_2R$ for this man was calculated using his $\dot{V}O_2$max of 36.4 (i.e., 10.4 METs) and the equation for $\dot{V}O_2R$ presented earlier in the chapter.

2 (12 METs – 1 MET)(.75) + 1 MET = 9.3 METs

To summarize, the maintenance phase of the training program should include a dose of exercise consistent with the attainment of energy expenditure thresholds that are associated with maintenance of CR fitness and reduction in chronic disease risk (1,19). The optimal dose of energy expenditure will vary from person to person, but, as we've seen, generally lies between 1000 and 2000 kcal per week. Use of the equations and the logic illustrated in this discussion will help exercise program professionals design exercise prescriptions that take caloric thresholds into account.

Phases of the Exercise Training Session

An enjoyable and safe exercise training session should consist of three distinct phases—a warm-up, a stimulus, and a cool-down. Figure 7.7 illustrates these phases within the context of the physiological transition from rest to exercise, through the stimulus phase, and back again to rest during the cool-down phase. We turn now to recommendations for each of the phases.

Warm-up phase

In a general sense, the purpose of the warm-up phase is to allow a gradual physiological transition from the resting state to the higher metabolic rate required during the stimulus phase of the exercise session. Therefore, warm-up activities should be designed to provide for a gradual increase in the metabolic rate of, and blood flow to, the skeletal muscles to be used during the stimulus phase (i.e., upper body and/or lower body). The increased metabolic rate and blood flow will warm the skeletal muscle bed, which will enhance muscular performance and perhaps decrease the risk of MS injury during the subsequent exercise bout, although this latter effect lacks clear scien-

tific support (20). In addition, a proper warm-up may also have a cardiovascular-protective effect in susceptible individuals because of the decreased risk of an ischemic response (21), ventricular arrhythmias, and left ventricular dysfunction (22) during subsequent strenuous exercise.

The warm-up period may be as short as 5 min to as long as 20 min. In general, the more vigorous the intensity during the stimulus phase, the longer the warm-up should be. Traditionally, exercise leaders have incorporated a variety of physical activities into the warm-up period. We advocate a low-intensity aerobic activity as the initial and most important element of the warm-up phase. This might mean brisk walking for those who will proceed to running (or other vigorous activities) during the stimulus phase, but might also be slower walking or stationary cycling against a low resistance for those intending more moderate exercise. The important point is to start the warm-up intensity well below the intensity planned for the stimulus phase and to gradually raise the intensity through 5 to 10 min of activity.

Over the years it has become commonplace for exercise leaders to incorporate 5 to 10 min of range of motion (ROM), calisthenics, and/or flexibility exercises into the warm-up phase. The beginning of the exercise session is a convenient time to fit these important activities in. However, exercise program professionals debate whether it would be more appropriate to include these activities in the cool-down phase because muscles and joints might be more responsive to these activities following the more strenuous phase of the exercise session. Unfortunately, the scientific data on this issue are not clear. If these activities are included in the warm-up phase, though, we strongly suggest sequencing them after the low-level aerobic activity just described. A wide variety of ROM/calisthenics routines are available, as no one routine will fit all clients or patients. Over the years, hundreds of participants in the adult fitness program at Ball State completed Dr. Getchell's "Basic Twelve" exercises before starting on their walking or run-walk routine. Table 7.7 contains the twelve exercises, which include a series of ROM/calisthenics starting with the shoulder girdle and moving downward to finish with the legs. This routine takes approximately 5 to 10 min and was always preceded by 3 to 5 min of brisk walking. The routine is described in detail in Dr. Getchell's book, *Being Fit: A Personal Guide* (17). Again, no single routine will fit everyone, and exercise leaders at Ball State would frequently modify this routine

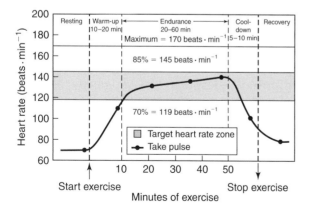

Figure 7.7 Phases of the cardiorespiratory endurance exercise session.

Reprinted, by permission, 2000, *ACSM's Guidelines for Exercise Testing and Prescription.* 6th ed. (Philadelphia, PA: Lippincott, Williams, and Wilkins), 141.

Table 7.7

Getchell *Basic Twelve* Exercises for Warm-Up

Exercise	Description
Arm circles	Starting position: Stand with your feet shoulder-width apart and your arms at your sides.
	Movement: Start with circles across the front of the body, proceed to circles forward (as in a crawl swimming motion), finish with backward circles (as in backward swimming crawl motion).
Trunk bender	Starting position: Stand with your feet 5-6 in. apart and parallel to each other.
	Movement: Bend forward at the waist, allowing your arms, trunk, and head to hang freely. Reach to touch the floor, slowly. Then twist the trunk and reach for the outside of one shoe and slowly return to an upright position by coming up from the side. Again bend forward from the waist and alternate your movement to the other side.
	Alternate directions: Large sweeping circles with the waist as the center of rotation.
Trunk twister	Starting position: Stand with your feet shoulder-width apart, arms extended to the sides at shoulder level.
	Movement: While keeping your heels flat on the floor, twist your trunk to the right slowly as far as you can turn comfortably, then return to the starting position. Then, twist in the opposite direction and return to starting position.
Side stretcher	Starting position: With your feet shoulder-width apart with one arm extended upward (palm facing inward) and the other arm extended downward (palm touching the side of your thigh).
	Movement: Bend your trunk to the side of the lower extended arm. Reach with your lower hand and stretch, sliding the hand down your thigh to the knee or lower. The other arm should be stretched over your head and in the direction of body's lean. Return to the starting position and repeat the exercise on the other side.
Leg-overs	Starting position: Lie on your back with your legs extended, and your arms extended at shoulder level (palms up).
	Movement: Keep the knee extended as you raise your leg to a vertical position (point your toes). The opposite leg should remain on the floor in extended position; keep the back of that leg on the floor. While keeping your shoulders, arms, and back on the floor, reach with the vertically extended leg across your body to the extended opposite hand. Stretch to touch your toe to the floor in the area of the extended hand, then return your leg first to the vertical position and then to the floor. Follow the same procedure with the other leg.
Side leg raises	Starting position: Lie on your right side, in extended position, with your head resting on your right forearm and hand.
	Movement: Raise your left leg upward from the floor (keeping the knee extended and toes pointed away) to a position well above the horizontal, then return to starting position. Keep your pelvis perpendicular to the floor. After completing repetitions for one side, repeat the exercise on the other side.
Low-back stretcher	Starting position: Lie on your back with knees straight.
	Movement: Pull one knee to your chest. Grasp the leg just below the knee and pull the knee toward your chest. Hold for 5 s. Then, curl your shoulders and head toward the knee. Hold for 5 or more s. Return to starting position and repeat exercise with other leg.
Arm and leg lifter	Starting position: Lie face down (prone position) with your arms extended over your head and your legs extended.
	Movement: Raise your right arm and left leg simultaneously and keep them extended for a few s. Then return to starting position. Now raise the left arm and right leg simultaneously.
	*Do this exercise slowly; do not jerk your legs and arms.

(continued)

Table 7.7 *(continued)*

Exercise	Description
Stride stretcher, forward and lateral	Starting position (forward): Move your leg forward so that it is flexed under your chest, knee directly over the ankle, and your other leg stretched out behind. Movement: With your hands on the floor and your forward heel on the floor, roll your body forward while pushing your hips down toward the floor. Hold for five or more s. Repeat the exercise with the other leg forward. Starting position (lateral): Spread your legs in a wide straddle position, toes pointing straight ahead. Movement: Shift your weight sidewards so that most of your weight is on one leg. Hold this position for five s or more, feeling a moderate stretching discomfort on the inner muscles of the thigh. Then shift weight over to the other foot for the same interval of time.
Hamstring stretcher, standing or leaning	Starting position (standing): Stand and cross one leg in front of the other. The toes of the front leg should touch the floor, heel up. Movement: Slowly bend forward from the waist, keeping your rear leg straight (heel on floor). Try to stretch until you feel a slight discomfort in the muscles of your rear leg. Hold the position for five or more seconds and return to the starting position. Stretch the other leg in a similar manner. Starting position (leaning): Raise one leg and rest the heel of the foot on a solid object such as a table or chair, toes pointing up. Movement: Reach and lean toward the raised foot until you feel an easy stretch and hold for a few s. While holding the stretch, you can also slowly roll the heel forward (pointed toes moving away) to an extended position; then slowly roll heel back, drawing toes as close as possible to your body. Be careful not to over-stretch. Repeat a few times and then stretch the other leg.
Achilles and calf stretcher*	Starting position: Stand facing a wall an arm's distance away with your knees straight, toes slightly inward, and your heels flat on the floor. Movement: (a) With hands resting on the wall, lean forward, bending your elbows slowly. Keep legs and body straight and heels on the floor. Hold for five or more s then return to the starting position. (b) Then, do the same exercise but bend the knees slightly and hold for five or more s before returning to starting position. * This exercise can also be performed with one leg forward (knee bent) and the other leg back (knee straight). In this case, alternate weight from leg to leg.
Quad stretcher	Starting position: While standing erect bend the right knee and lift the right foot directly behind the body. Hold the toes of the foot with the left hand. Use your right hand to balance on a wall or chair. Movement: Bend the lifted right knee and draw the leg up and back. Pull up the right leg until you feel a slight discomfort in the upper front thigh (quadriceps). Balance and hold firmly for five or more s (it is important to stand erect while holding the stretch). Repeat with the other leg.

Reprinted, by permission, from B. Getchell, 1982, *Being fit: A personal guide* (New York: John Wiley & Sons). This material is used by permission of John Wiley & Sons, Inc.

to fit specific individual needs. We encourage exercise leaders to be creative in individualizing this component of the warm-up phase.

Another important element of the warm-up phase is the interaction between program staff and clients or patients. These few minutes before the start of the stimulus phase afford the program staff an opportunity to assess each person's readiness for exercise that day. In addition, exercise leaders should spend time talking and listening to participants during the warm-up phase to enhance the socialization aspect of the program.

Stimulus phase

As described in detail earlier in the chapter, the stimulus phase of the exercise session is the phase that stresses the cardiovascular and respiratory systems and leads to an improvement in CR fitness. This phase should include physical activities that are aerobic and should last between 20 and 60 min. Although recent exercise prescription guidelines (1, 2, 5) indicate that the stimulus phase may be completed either as one continuous session (i.e., 20-60 min) or as multiple shorter sessions throughout the day (i.e., several 10-min bouts), we strongly encourage most individuals to complete it in a continuous fashion. However, when time constraints are a barrier to participation in a continuous exercise session several times per week, several shorter bouts of exercise throughout the day will increase one's total energy expenditure and contribute to a negative energy balance over time.

Cool-down phase

Physiologically, the purpose of the cool-down phase is opposite that of the warm-up phase. A proper cool-down should allow the cardiovascular system's response to the stimulus phase (e.g., increases in HR, BP, cardiac output, etc.) to return to near resting values. In addition, the greater venous return associated with an active recovery period lessens the risk of a hypotensive response postexercise. We will look more closely at the potential consequences of this in a moment. Furthermore, an active recovery facilitates the removal of lactate from the exercising muscle and aids in the dissipation of body heat, returning the core temperature to a pre-exercise value. As illustrated in figure 7.7, it's very important to reduce the intensity of activity gradually throughout a 5- to 10-min period. A simple method is to decrease the intensity of the activity performed during the stimulus phase (e.g., slowing to a walk from a jogging pace, or slowing the walking pace for walkers). Individuals who exercise on stationary aerobic equipment (e.g., leg cycles, stair climbers, rowing machines, etc.) should be instructed to continue exercising at a reduced pace following the stimulus phase, rather than hopping off the equipment suddenly.

What are the potential consequences of an improper cool-down? An abrupt cessation of vigorous exercise can lead to a cascade of cardiovascular responses and their subsequent complications, which are illustrated in figure 7.8. The cascade is thought to begin with the drop in venous return associated with pooling of blood in the legs when exercise is stopped too abruptly. The decrease in venous return leads to a drop in cardiac output and ultimately a drop in mean arterial pressure. As discussed in chapter 2, adequate coronary blood flow is, in part, dependent on an adequate perfusion pressure (i.e., BP). The drop in BP postexercise—often referred to as postexercise hypotension—may lead to a decrease in perfusion through the coronary arteries. This results in myocardial ischemia and may contribute to an increase in ventricular arrhythmias. The cascade of events shown in figure 7.8 is further exacerbated by the rise in catecholamines during the postexercise period. A more detailed description of this sequence of events is beyond the scope

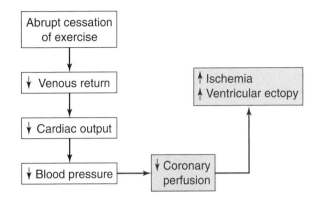

Figure 7.8 Cardiovascular responses to abrupt cessation of vigorous exercise.

of this text and can be found elsewhere (23). We should note here, though, that in a report on cardiovascular complications during cardiac rehabilitation exercise sessions, nearly three-fourths (44/61) of the complications occurred during either the warm-up or the cool-down phase of the exercise session (24) which is discussed further in chapter 10. Thus it's very important to watch patients during these time periods. Individuals taking direct-acting vasodilators (see table 4.5) are especially prone to postexercise hypotension and must be instructed on proper cool-down procedures. Program staff should observe participants following the exercise session to ensure that they recover properly.

In summary, a few minutes of reduced-intensity activity following the stimulus phase is a very important element of the exercise session. In our experience, many exercisers often disregard this advice unless (a) program staff provide specific instructions for a proper cool-down and (b) staff remain vigilant in observing program participants during this phase of the exercise session.

Exercise Prescription for Muscular Strength and Endurance

Exercises for development of muscular strength and endurance are considered an important part of a well-rounded exercise program. Because of the nature of the overload applied during training, this type of exercise is often referred to as resistance training. When we take the time to think about it, we realize that most tasks in daily life require some amount of muscular effort. However, while aerobic exercises contribute to the overall health and function of the CR system, they do little for developing and maintaining muscular strength and muscular endurance. During the 1960s and 1970s when aerobic exercise was finding its way back into the American culture (a trend fostered by books such as Ken Cooper's *Aerobics*, as well as the vision of American Frank Shorter winning the Olympic marathon in Munich, Germany), resistance training was often de-emphasized in fitness programs for adults.

However, as observational studies of our aging population began to show, losses in muscle function and lean body mass during the aging process often left older adults with less muscular strength and muscular endurance than necessary to complete many daily tasks. These losses eventually led to a lower quality of life for many older Americans, who became more dependent on others to take care of their daily needs. To counter this public health problem, which is still increasing, we need to encourage all adults to maintain muscular strength and muscular endurance throughout the life span. This section outlines specifics for a resistance-training routine recommended for healthy adults in the fitness center environment. The reader is referred elsewhere for more elaborate or advanced routines for sport performance enhancement (25).

Dose

Muscular strength and endurance are defined in chapter 6. Components of an exercise prescription for development and maintenance of muscular strength and endurance should include an individualized mode, intensity, frequency, duration, and rate of progression. Table 7.8 contains general resistance-training recommendations from the ACSM (1). The minimal dose of resistance training recommended by ACSM is one set of 8 to 12 repetitions for each of 8 to 10 exercises completed two times per week. Now, this dose is considerably lower than in the traditional weight-training regimens of three sets three times per week that are performed in many athletic training settings. When the current guidelines were first published by ACSM in 1990 (26), considerable debate arose among exercise program professionals about whether the minimal dose of training described was adequate to produce increases in muscular strength and endurance. However, studies have shown that this minimal dose can provide for significant improvements in strength/endurance for adults participating in fitness programs (27). In fact, in a research study within the Adult Physical Fitness Program at Ball State that used a single-set, twice-a-week routine, we found increases in strength (i.e., 1-RM) ranging from 15% to 33% across eight different exercises following 10 weeks of training (28).

Clearly, we can conclude that the minimal dose does produce results. Moreover, we found that promotion of the ACSM minimal dose—which usually takes less than 30 min per session—actually increased the number of adults in our fitness program who began resistance training. The reason? Many of our participants were reluctant to commit the extra time necessary to complete the traditional routine of three sets, three times per week, over and above their aerobic workouts. When we showed them how to incorporate the minimal resistance workout into their overall routine in <30 min, twice a week, many were very receptive. Does this mean that we (or for that matter the ACSM) discourage a more intensive program (i.e., greater number of sets and/or higher training frequency)? Certainly not. But while the addition of more sets and/or more workouts per week may lead to greater gains in strength and endurance, the additional improvements associated with a greater dose of training do not appear to be substantial for most adult participants in fitness programs (27). Therefore, we recommend an initial resistance-training prescription consistent with the dose defined in table 7.8.

As mentioned earlier, resistance-training prescriptions should be individualized based on the goals of the participant. Depending on the empha-

Table 7.8

Elements of the Resistance Training Exercise Prescription for Healthy Adults

Variable	Recommendation
Mode	Dynamic, concentric 8-10 exercises using all the major muscle groups (arms, shoulders, chest, abdomen, back, hips, legs)
Intensity	1 set with load allowing completion of 8-12 repetitions for healthy individuals < 50-60 years of age Load allowing completion of 10-15 repetitions for those > 50-60 years of age or more frail individuals.
Frequency	Minimum of 2 to 3 times per week
Duration	< 60 min per session needed (usually <30 min)
Progression	Individualized based on tolerance and adaptation In general, when one can complete 12 repetitions with a load, an increase of 5-10 lbs would be appropriate to provide further overload

sis (development of muscular strength or endurance) within an individualized prescription, one can modify the resistance and number of repetitions as illustrated in figure 7.9. The underlying principle is a variation of the interrelationship between exercise intensity and duration. Higher intensity leads to shorter duration and vice versa. Individuals who desire to focus more on strength development (as opposed to muscular endurance) would increase the load during resistance training to one that they can lift only a few times each set (≤6 repetitions). Conversely, those whose goal is to develop more muscular endurance would lower the load to allow for completion of >12 repetitions per set. It would be advisable for most healthy, middle-aged adults to select loads that they can complete in 8 to 12 repetitions as described in table 7.8, as this loading scheme contributes to development of both muscular strength and endurance.

Modes

A wide range of resistance-training equipment is available in the marketplace. Individuals or facilities may choose from traditional free weights, various weight machines, or even the elastic bands (Therabands) that have become popular in rehabilitation settings. In addition, a series of calisthenics without any special equipment or machines can often provide for significant improvements in muscular strength and endurance. During the past decade, most fitness centers have invested in some brand of machine weights; typically, the design of these allows the user to be comfortably seated during the exercise. With regard to training outcomes (i.e., increases in muscular strength and/or endurance), choices such as that between free weights and machines are not all that important; what is important is to produce

an overload on the skeletal muscles. Any of the available modes for resistance training can usually accomplish this for most beginners. When safety is an issue, however, machine weight units typically provide a better margin of safety because the weight stacks don't have to be balanced by the lifter.

Most commercially available series have a full complement of machines that allow for exercises of the major muscle groups. About 10 years ago in our fitness center, we installed a series of 10 weight machines that provided exercises for the major muscle groups listed in table 7.8. We arranged the machines in a circuit that would allow individuals to alternate muscle groups from machine to machine and that individuals could complete in 20 to 25 min. The circuit incorporated the following exercises:

Overhead press

Vertical fly

Lat pull-down

Hip flexion/extension, abduction/adduction

Bench press

Lower back extension

Tricep extension

Leg extension

Abdominal curl

Leg curl

Safety

Regardless of the initial resistance-training dose or mode, individuals need to receive instruction on certain precautions about lifting technique in order to ensure safe participation in this form of training. This is especially important with free weights, as this form of resistance training necessitates balancing the load during the exercise routine. Individuals beginning a resistance-training program should be taught the following guidelines:

- Adhere as closely as possible to specific techniques for performing a given exercise. (Note that even though these instructions are often printed on the machines, professionals should still demonstrate the proper technique for beginners before they perform the exercise.)

- Use a load that allows for a full ROM for each exercise.

- Perform both the lifting (concentric) and lowering (eccentric) phases of the exercise in a controlled manner.

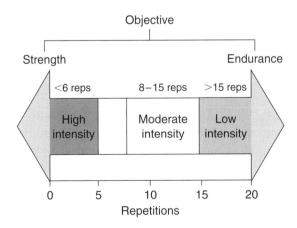

Figure 7.9   Weight-lifting intensity classification.
Reprinted, by permission, 2000, *ACSM's Guidelines for Exercise Testing and Prescription.* 6th ed. (Philadelphia, PA: Lippincott, Williams, and Wilkins), 179.

- Maintain a normal, controlled breathing pattern throughout the exercise with the exhalation occurring during the lifting (concentric) phase. Avoid breath-holding, which can induce unnecessary increases in BP.
- Progress at a rate that is safe and comfortable. If possible, exercise with a partner who can provide spotting when appropriate.

Summary

Resistance training is an integral part of a comprehensive exercise program and should be an element of all exercise prescriptions unless the individual has a contraindication to this form of activity. However, resistance training should be a complement to CR endurance exercise and not the sole form of training. People can achieve significant improvements in muscular strength with as low a dose as one set of 8 to 12 exercises two times per week. This type of routine can usually be completed in less than 30 min per week.

PRINCIPLES OF EXERCISE PRESCRIPTION— SECONDARY PREVENTION

As pointed out in chapter 1, more than 1 million myocardial infarctions occur in the United States each year. When we add to this the number of patients who undergo the coronary **revascularization** procedures described in chapter 4, we realize that there are literally millions of cardiac patients eligible for secondary prevention programs. Furthermore, although cardiac rehabilitation programs in the 1970s catered mostly to post-MI patients, the list of eligible patients continues to expand, now including those recovering from coronary revascularization (coronary artery bypass graft surgery, percutaneous transluminal coronary angioplasty, etc.), cardiac transplantation, heart valve replacement, and implantation of pacemakers and automated defibrillators, as well as persons with clinically stable heart failure. The AACVPR (3), ACSM (1) and AHA (29) have each published exercise prescription guidelines for cardiac patients participating in secondary prevention programs. A review of these documents would reveal that the basic principles related to exercise prescription for primary prevention as described earlier in this chapter generally apply to patients in secondary prevention programs. At the same time, there are some important differences in the application of the guidelines for prescription of CR and MS endurance activities for cardiac patients; this section of the

chapter describes and illustrates these important differences. We begin by looking at the current model for cardiac rehabilitation programs and finish by discussing how the exercise prescription principles described earlier apply in the cardiac rehabilitation setting.

Structure of Contemporary Secondary Prevention Programs

Beginning in the 1970s, cardiac rehabilitation programs were often divided into four sequential phases (I, II, III, and IV) based on the need for medical supervision and patient monitoring during exercise sessions. Phase I related to rehabilitative activities during the inpatient stay (1-2 weeks). Phase II, following hospital discharge, consisted of two to three months of medically supervised, continuous ECG-monitored exercise training that typically took place in the hospital setting. After completing Phase II, patients might have continued exercise training in a Phase III program that was usually medically supervised but that entailed either intermittent or no ECG monitoring. Some rehabilitation programs considered Phase III an ongoing phase that patients stayed in indefinitely, whereas others targeted completion of the Phase III program about a year after hospital discharge. Phase IV cardiac rehabilitation programs typically included little medical supervision and no ECG monitoring. Phase IV programs were often located in a community setting, occasionally in conjunction with structured adult fitness programs. Although most cardiac rehabilitation programs still contain the essential elements of these traditional phases, the time periods for the phases have become much less distinct in recent years; and for the most part the terms *inpatient* and *outpatient rehabilitation* have replaced the Phase I-IV terminology.

The combination of cost containment measures by medical insurance providers, along with the realization that many low-risk cardiac patients don't necessarily need the more costly elements of the rehab program (i.e., direct medical supervision and continuous ECG monitoring) for extended periods of time, has led to a new paradigm for delivery of cardiac rehabilitation services (3). A contemporary approach to the management of cardiac patients focuses more attention and resources on modification of CAD risk factors (described in chapter 1) in an attempt to lower the patient's risk for disease progression and recurrent cardiac events. This new model for secondary prevention begins with an initial risk stratification for each patient that is then used to optimize risk factor management and individualize the degree of medical supervision and ECG monitoring during the training program. Thus, the process of risk stratification relates to the risk for progression of coronary disease as well as the risk of untoward events during participation. Obviously, a major goal of the rehabilitation program is to prevent either of these occurrences, and the elements of the program are designed to promote safety and to slow the progression of the disease. Here we focus on the exercise prescription guidelines for inpatient and outpatient cardiac rehabilitation programs. Other elements of a comprehensive rehabilitation program (patient education and counseling, risk factor intervention strategies, etc.) are discussed in detail in chapter 10.

Cardiorespiratory Endurance Prescription for Secondary Prevention

Although guidelines for exercise prescription in the secondary prevention setting incorporate all the basic principles discussed earlier in relation to primary prevention, there are also more specific guidelines based on the clinical status of the patient and the environment of the program (i.e., inpatient vs. outpatient). Therefore, we begin with a discussion of exercise prescription guidelines for patients who are in the hospital following a cardiac event (e.g., myocardial infarction) or procedure (e.g., revascularization).

Inpatient Cardiac Rehabilitation

The recommended physical activities and length of hospital stay for cardiac patients will vary depending on the nature of the clinical event precipitating hospitalization (e.g., MI, revascularization, etc.). Historically, Phase I typically lasted from 7 to 14 days and involved a gradual but systematic increase in activities of daily living (ADLs) and low-intensity exercise. While ADLs and low-intensity exercise are still an important part of inpatient rehabilitation, the length of hospitalizations has shortened considerably in recent years, and in many cases patients are seen in the hospital for less than a week. Thus the amount of time available for inpatient rehabilitation is considerably shorter, and the goals for the program focus more on educating the patient about the disease process, offsetting the deleterious effects of prolonged bed rest, and assessing the patient's ability to complete ADLs safely prior to discharge.

Readers will find extensive inpatient guidelines for physical activity and education in the AACVPR and ACSM *Guidelines* documents (1, 3), and exercise program professionals should review these carefully. Table 7.9 provides recommendations for the type, intensity, frequency, duration, and progression of physical activities during the inpatient stay (1). In addition, table 7.10 presents an activity classification guide for inpatients that can be used to assess a patient's functional status and progression from day to day in ADLs, as well as exercise tolerance. Although structured, multistep inpatient exercise routines are available and have been used within rehabilitation programs for years (30), many patients are now being discharged well before they could typically complete such routines. Furthermore, such routines may not enhance a patient's functional capacity over that achieved through standard medical care (31).

Table 7.9
Elements of the Exercise Prescription for Inpatient Cardiac Rehabilitation*

Variable	Recommendation
Mode	Self care activities, ROM, postural changes, walking (hallway or treadmill), stationary cycling, stair climbing
Intensity	Post-MI: HR < 120 bpm or HRrest + 20 bpm (arbitrary upper limit) Post surgery: HRrest + 30 bpm (arbitrary upper limit) RPE < 13 (Borg 6-20 scale) To tolerance if asymptomatic
Frequency	Early mobilization: 3 to 4 times per day (days 1-3) Later mobilization: 2 times per day (beginning on day 4)
Duration	Intermittent bouts lasting 3 to 5 min Rest periods at patient's discretion, last 1 to 2 min (shorter than exercise bout duration) Total duration of up to 20 min
Progression	Initially increase duration to 10 to 15 min, then increase intensity

HR = heart rate; ROM = range of motion; RPE = rating of perceived exertion.
*Modified from *ACSM Guidelines for Exercise Testing and Prescription* (1).

Table 7.10
Activity Classification Guide for Inpatient Activities*

Activity class	Activities
I	Sits up in bed with assistance Does own self-care activities, seated or may need assistance Stands at bedside with assistance Sits up in chair 15 to 30 min, 2 to 3 times per day
II	Sits up in bed independently Stands independently Does self-care activities in bathroom, seated Walks in room and to bathroom (may need assistance)
III	Sits and stands independently Does own self-care activities in bathroom, seated or standing Walks short distances (50 to 100 ft) in halls with assistance as tolerated, up to 3 times per day
IV	Does own self-care and bathes Walks in halls short distances (150 to 200 ft) with minimal assistance, 3-4 times per day
V	Walks in halls independently, moderate distances (250-500 ft), 3-4 times per day
VI	Independent ambulation on unit, 3-6 times per day

Reprinted, by permission, 2000, *ACSM's Guidelines for Exercise Testing and Prescription*. 6th ed. (Philadelphia: Lippincott, Williams, and Wilkins), 168.

Therefore, as already noted, the purposes of physical activities during inpatient rehab are to offset the decline in physical function associated with prolonged bed rest and to gradually return the patient to ADLs prior to hospital discharge. Before hospital discharge, patients should receive instructions outlining physical activities that are appropriate while they are at home, as well as any restrictions in physical activity based on their clinical status. They should also leave the hospital with an outline of physical activities including progressions for completion at home. Finally, all patients should be apprised of outpatient rehabilitation opportunities and encouraged to participate if at all possible.

Outpatient Cardiac Rehabilitation

Soon after hospital discharge, eligible cardiac patients should enter a structured outpatient rehabilitation program designed to help them meet the following goals:

- Optimal management of CAD risk factors to maximize secondary prevention
- Implementation of a safe and effective exercise program that is ultimately self-monitored
- Return to pre-event vocational and/or recreational activities with modifications when necessary

An additional goal of the outpatient program is to provide appropriate medical surveillance for detection of a significant deterioration in the patient's clinical status, whereupon the program staff could alert the appropriate medical professional for assessment and treatment of the patient if necessary. Although the outpatient program goals just outlined are rather generic, the combination of interventions necessary for accomplishing these goals will vary from patient to patient. In other words, each patient is unique with regard to risk factor interventions during outpatient rehabilitation. Some cardiac patients may not need medical management for hypertension or a smoking cessation program, but others will. All of this means that elements (i.e., interventions) of the rehabilitation program must be individualized. This having been said, most, if not all, patients will benefit from a structured exercise program—so this intervention is a common thread within most secondary prevention settings.

How do professionals in secondary prevention programs individualize the elements of the rehab program? Although there are many ways to do this, the AACVPR promotes a process of risk stratification as the initial step in designing an individualized secondary prevention program. This process addresses two major issues within the rehab program. First, patients are stratified according to their risk of events based on their clinical status as described in table 7.11. Then they are stratified for the risk of disease progression as described in table 7.12. Let's take a closer look at each process.

Table 7.11
AACVPR Stratification for Risk of Cardiac Events*

Lowest risk	Moderate risk	Highest risk
No significant left ventricular dysfunction (ejection fraction >50%)	Moderately impaired left ventricular function (ejection fraction = 40–49%)	Decreased left ventricular function (ejection fraction <40%)
No resting or exercise-induced complex dysrhythmias	Signs/symptoms including angina at moderate levels of exercise (5-6.9 METs) or in recovery	Survivor of cardiac arrest or sudden death
Uncomplicated MI; CABG; angioplasty, artherectomy, or stent	**Moderate risk is assumed for patients who do not meet the classification of either highest or lowest risk.**	Complex ventricular dysrhythmia at rest or with exercise
Absence of CHF or signs/symptoms indicating post-event ischemia		MI or cardiac surgery complicated by cardiogenic shock, CHF, and/or signs/symptoms of post-procedure ischemia
Normal hemodynamics with exercise or recovery		Abnormal hemodynamics with exercise (especially flat or decreasing systolic blood pressure or chronotrophic incompetence with increasing workload)
Asymptomatic including absence of angina with exertion or recovery		Signs/symptoms including angina pectoris at low levels of exercise (< 5.0 METs) or in recovery
Functional capacity ≥ 7 METs[a]		Functional capacity < 5.0 METs[a]
Absence of clinical depression		Clinically significant depression
Lowest risk classification is assumed when each of the risk factors in the category is present.		**Highest risk classification is assumed with the presence of any one of the risk factors included in this category.**

a: If measured functional capacity is not available, this variable is not considered in the risk-stratification process.

*Reprinted by permission, 1999, Outpatient cardiac rehabilitation and secondary prevention. In *Guidelines for cardiac rehabilitation and secondary prevention program*, edited by ACVPR (Champaign: Human Kinetics), 45, 42.

Table 7.12
AACVPR Stratification for Risk of Disease Progression*

Risk factor	Lowest risk level	Moderate risk level	Highest risk level
Smoking	None Quit ≥ 6 months or never smoked	Smoker Quit < 6 months	Smoker
Lipids/Diet	Diet ≤ 20% fat ≤ 7% saturated fat ≤ 150 mg chol Lipids LDL < 100 mg / dl	Diet 21–29% fat 8–9% saturated fat 151–299 mg chol Lipids LDL < 100-129 mg / dl	Diet ≥ 30% fat ≥ 10% saturated fat ≥ 300 mg chol Lipids LDL ≥ 130 mg / dl
Diabetes mellitus	Hb A_1c ≤ 7% or FBG ≤ 120 mg / dl	Hb A_1c = 8-9% or FBG = 121-180 mg / dl	Hb A_1c > 9% or FBG > 180 mg / dl
Weight (kg · m⁻²)	BMI ≤ 27	BMI = 28–29.9	BMI ≥ 30
HTN (mmHg)	SBP ≤ 130 DBP ≤ 85	SBP = 131–159 DBP = 86-99	SBP ≥ 160 DBP ≥ 100
Depression	No clinical depression	Evidence of moderate clinical depression	Evidence of significant clinical depression
Exercise	> 1500 kcal/wk	500-1499 kcal/wk	< 500 kcal/wk

mg = milligrams; LDL = low-density lipoprotein; FBG = fasting blood glucose; BMI = body mass index; SBP = systolic blood pressure; DBP = diastolic blood pressure; HbA₁c = glycosylated hemoglobin; HTN = hypertension.

*Reprinted by permission, 1999, Outpatient cardiac rehabilitation and secondary prevention. In *Guidelines for cardiac rehabilitation and secondary prevention program*, edited by ACVPR (Champaign: Human Kinetics), 45, 42.

How are patients stratified for risk of cardiac events? Using clinical information as outlined in table 7.11, patients can be categorized into one of three risk levels. The three categories provide a continuum from lowest to highest risk for recurrent cardiac events based on a patient's clinical data. This information can then be used to make appropriate decisions regarding the extent of medical supervision and monitoring during the exercise training component of the program. Keep in mind that all of these patients are candidates for outpatient rehabilitation, meaning that participation per se is not contraindicated for even those patients in the highest risk category. Once patients have been categorized, there are supervisory and ECG monitoring recommendations for each risk stratum as shown in table 7.13.

In addition to being stratified for risk of events, cardiac patients should be stratified for risk of CAD progression. In doing this, we are taking the longer view. In other words, based on his collective risk factors (e.g., high low-density lipoprotein cholesterol, smoking, hypertension, etc.), what is the patient's risk for a worsening of his CAD in the future? In a qualitative sense, the more risk factors (and also the more abnormal each risk factor is), the greater the risk for disease progression. On average, CAD lesions progress (i.e., get

larger) at a rate of 1% to 4% per year, but this is known to be highly variable within cardiac patients (32). Obviously, the major purpose of secondary prevention programs is to prevent the worsening of the disease process. This means more than keeping patients from having another myocardial infarction: it also includes slowing down or even reversing the atherosclerotic process described in chapter 2. How does this process work? The AACVPR Guidelines suggest the risk stratification scheme outlined in table 7.12. The three categories provide a continuum from lowest to highest risk for disease progression based on a patient's number and degree of abnormal risk factors.

Let's take a look at how these risk stratification processes work by applying them to a patient who presented to the cardiac rehabilitation program at Ball State University. You may need to review the discussions of coronary pathophysiology and diagnostic cardiac procedures in chapters 2 and 3 while evaluating this case. Table 7.14 contains some CAD risk factor and clinical data on a 44-year-old male cardiac patient. According to available medical records, this man had suffered an anterior MI two years prior to his arrival at our doorstep, with an uncomplicated hospital course. Three months after the MI, he experienced

Table 7.13

AACVPR Recommendations for ECG Monitoring and Close Supervision During Exercise*

Risk category	Recommendations
Lowest	Patients are at the lowest level of risk for complications during exercise. They may be monitored for 6-18 sessions, beginning with continuous ECG monitoring along with close clinical supervision initially, decreasing the intensity of ECG monitoring to intermittent during sessions 8-12. Hemodynamic response to exercise should be normal[a] and progression of the exercise prescription should be regular[b] during those sessions. Close clinical supervision, which may include direct supervision of exercise sessions, should continue for at least 30 days post-event.
Moderate	Patients are at moderate risk for complications during exercise. They may be monitored for 12-24 sessions, initially with continuous ECG monitoring along with close clinical supervision, decreasing the intensity of ECG monitoring to intermittent during latter sessions. Hemodynamic response to exercise should be normal[a] and progression of the exercise prescription should be regular[b] during those sessions. Close clinical supervision, which may include direct supervision of exercise sessions, may be required for up to 60-90 days post-event.
Highest	Patients are at the highest level of risk for complications during exercise. They may be monitored for 18-24 sessions or more, initially with continuous ECG monitoring along with close clinical supervision, decreasing the intensity of ECG monitoring to intermittent during latter sessions. Hemodynamic response to exercise should be normal[a] and progression of the exercise prescription should be regular[b] during those sessions. Close clinical supervision, including direct supervision of exercise sessions, may be required for 90 days or more post-event.

a = Normal hemodynamic response as defined by appropriately increasing SBP, level or falling DBP, appropriately increasing HR, and no symptoms indicating exercise intolerance.

b = Regular progression of the exercise prescription is defined by periodic (e.g., daily to weekly) progression of the exercise prescription such that functional capacity is increasing and exercise is well tolerated without undue fatigue.

*From reference (3).

Table 7.14
Clinical and Risk Factor Data for 44-Year-Old Male Cardiac Patient

Clinical data	Value or measurement
LVEF (%)	40%
Cardiac arrhythmias	None significant
Resting HR (bpm)	74
Medications	Lipitor, ASA
GXT data	
Protocol (time)	Bruce ramp (9:48)
Peak workload	2.8 mph/ 12.7%
Peak HR (bpm)	192
Peak $\dot{V}O_2$ (ml/kg/min)	29.9
Peak BP (mm Hg)	170/92
RPE (6-20 scale)	18
ECG	normal
Risk factor data	
Smoking	Never smoked
Lipids	TC = 163 mg/dl
	LDL = 88 mg/dl
	HDL = 42 mg/dl
	TG = 167 mg/dl
Diabetes mellitus	FBG = 116 mg/dl
	History of glucose intolerance
Weight (lbs)	197
BMI (kg/m²)	33.5
Body fat (%)	31.8
Waist girth (cm)	108.5
Blood pressure (mmHg)	136/98 & 134/96
Depression	No data available
Exercise history	Jogger, 2-3 times/wk; 60 min

a recurrence of chest pain, and a repeat coronary angiogram revealed an 80% stenosis of his left anterior descending (LAD) coronary artery. This was not surprising considering the history of the anterior MI. However, no significant lesions were observed in his other coronary arteries; thus the LAD lesion was implicated in the recurrence of his chest pain. His cardiologist performed a percutaneous transluminal coronary angioplasty, placing a stent at the site of the LAD lesion. The patient tolerated the procedure well and experienced no complications. During an annual follow-up evaluation with his cardiologist, this man indicated that he no longer had any chest pain, and he also had a normal stress perfusion study (see chapter 3 for a detailed description of this procedure). Following his annual checkup, he had been on his own for about six months before seeking entry into our exercise program. Yes, we agree that he should have been with us much sooner, but that's another discussion!

Now, let's evaluate this man's status for the clinical variables in table 7.11 and stratify him for risk of cardiac events according to the guidelines from the AACVPR (3). First, his ejection fraction was measured at 40%, which falls into the moderate risk category in the AACVPR scheme. However, he has no complex arrhythmias, is symptom free, had a normal ECG response during the exercise test, and had a functional capacity greater than 7 METs (29.9/3.5 = 8.5 METs). We did not have any data pertaining to an evaluation for clinical depression. On the basis of the analysis just presented, our cardiac patient would fall into the moderate risk stratum according to the AACVPR Guidelines. What's the practical significance of this stratification process? Table 7.13 contains recommendations for the amount of supervision and ECG monitoring during exercise training based on the three risk strata. As our cardiac patient is in the moderate risk category, the AACVPR Guidelines suggest some initial exercise sessions with continuous ECG monitoring and close clinical supervision. Monitoring and supervision would gradually be decreased provided he has normal responses during the exercise sessions. Note that this is one example of how the AACVPR Guidelines can be applied. Not all cardiac rehabilitation programs use this process to determine the amount of ECG monitoring and clinical supervision for their patients. However, we feel it's important for students to be acquainted with this process, as it represents a logical, systematic approach to stratification for risk of cardiac events.

Finally, let's evaluate our case study patient's CAD risk factors (table 7.14) and stratify his risk for disease progression using the variables and thresholds in table 7.12. Our cardiac patient never smoked, and his low-density lipoprotein cholesterol is below 100 mg/dl (the antilipidemic, Lipitor, appears to be working well), placing him at the lowest risk level for these risk factors. Although his medical history is positive for glucose intolerance, his fasting blood glucose is below the 120 mg/dl threshold. We did not have any data on his glycosylated hemoglobin level (Hb A_1c). However, this patient is hypertensive and obese and therefore would clearly benefit from interventions to normalize these risk factors. Again, we had no data with which to evaluate clinical depression. Finally, his self-reported exercise habits would most likely result in a weekly energy expenditure above 500 kcal per week. On the basis of this analysis, our cardiac patient would be stratified at a moderate risk for disease progression according to the AACVPR Guidelines (3). Can we use the information we have to individualize his intervention program? You bet! In summary, he would benefit from interventions for hypertension, obesity, and impaired fasting glucose. Hygienic interventions aimed at reducing his excess body fat (diet and exercise) could also help to normalize his BP and glucose tolerance. Therefore, the cardiac rehabilitation team should design a set of interventions that target all of his abnormal risk factors and should work toward achieving the lowest risk level threshold for each risk factor.

Mode

Just as within primary prevention programs, endurance exercise prescriptions for patients in secondary prevention programs should include activities that are aerobic. Therefore, the concepts on training modes covered in relation to primary prevention are applicable to patients in secondary prevention programs. Exercise leaders should review the activity categories described in table 7.1 when evaluating the appropriateness of a given activity; and when incorporating group recreational activities with a variable-intensity component (group 3), they should modify the rules to avoid overexertion during participation. In addition, it is important to emphasize activities that allow ease of monitoring ECG, BP, and symptoms (e.g., treadmill, stationary cycling) during the early stages of the program in which monitoring is more intensive. And finally, as already mentioned, a major goal for patients within secondary prevention programs is to return them to their pre-event employment status. Thus, the physical demands of their occupation should be assessed during the early stages of the outpatient program, and physical activities that will improve their functional abilities related to job performance should be incorporated into the exercise routine whenever possible.

Intensity

Guidelines for defining an appropriate exercise training intensity for patients in secondary prevention programs vary depending on the setting of the training program (i.e., inpatient vs. outpatient) and the clinical status of the patient (low, moderate, or high risk for exercise complications). Inpatient intensity guidelines are presented in table 7.9 and have already been discussed. Once patients are considered clinically stable and have left the hospital, they are ready for an outpatient program in which a primary focus of the exercise regimen is to improve functional capacity. With this in mind, most of the same concepts discussed in the section on exercise intensity are applicable here. However, as the risks associated with exercise are greater for those with CAD, exercise prescriptions must provide for safe participation. In this context, we strongly encourage exercise leaders to incorporate the concept of risk stratification presented earlier and at a minimum to divide their patients into one of two groups: (1) those with normal ECG and **hemodynamic** responses during exercise and (2) those with abnormal signs or symptoms induced by exercise. For patients with normal responses to graded exercise, one can usually define the appropriate intensity by using the concept of relative intensity range described earlier (i.e., percentage of MHRR or $\dot{V}O_2R$). However, for patients who have exercise-induced signs or symptoms, exercise training intensity needs to be set below the intensity at which the abnormal response occurs in order to provide a safety buffer during training. We'll now consider appropriate exercise intensity for each scenario (i.e., normal exercise response vs. abnormal response).

First, let's look at the exercise prescription intensity for cardiac patients who have normal ECG and hemodynamic responses to graded exercise. For these patients, the ACSM Guidelines (1) indicate that the endurance training intensity should be sufficient to produce a physiological "training effect." Table 7.2 contains the recommended intensity range from the ACSM Guidelines, indicating that a minimal-intensity threshold lies between 40% and 50% of a patient's MHRR or $\dot{V}O_2R$, with the upper end of the range set at approximately 85%. Once the relative intensity is defined (% $\dot{V}O_2R$), a target $\dot{V}O_2$ and/or HR range can be calculated using the equations for $\dot{V}O_2R$ and MHRR presented previously. To illustrate this point, let's calculate a target MET and HR range for our 44-year-old male cardiac patient by using the data in table 7.14. Remember, defining his training intensity as a percentage of his $\dot{V}O_2R$ or MHRR is appropriate because he had a normal ECG and hemodynamic response during his GXT. If we were to define his relative exercise intensity range as 50% to 60% of $\dot{V}O_2R$ or MHRR, his individualized ranges would be calculated as follows:

target $\dot{V}O_2$ ml·kg^{-1}·min^{-1} at 50% $\dot{V}O_2R$ =
(29.9 – 3.5)(0.50) + 3.5 = 16.7 ml·kg^{-1}·min^{-1}

target $\dot{V}O_2$ ml·kg^{-1}·min^{-1} at 60% $\dot{V}O_2R$ =
(29.9 – 3.5)(0.60) + 3.5 = 19.3 ml·kg^{-1}·min^{-1}

THR at 50% MHRR =
(192 – 74) (.50) + 74 = 133 bpm

THR at 60% MHRR =
(192 – 74) (.60) + 74 = 145 bpm

Thus our 44-year-old cardiac patient would have a target $\dot{V}O_2$ of 16.7 to 19.3 ml·kg^{-1}·min^{-1}, which translates to a target MET range of 4.8 to 5.5. His THR range would be 133 to 145 bpm.

However, as mentioned in the previous section, knowledge of MHR and/or $\dot{V}O_2$ is implicit to the use of a relative range for defining intensity. If this information is available and the patient has normal responses during the GXT, then it would be appropriate to use the approach to defining exercise intensity just explained. However, this information would be available only if the patient had completed a sign/symptom-limited maximal GXT. Obviously, if the patient has not completed a GXT, these ranges could not be computed and thus the patient's intensity could not be defined in this way. There are several alternative approaches in such cases. First, one could define exercise intensity using the inpatient intensity guidelines for THR listed in table 7.9. Exercise prescription intensities formulated in this way have been shown to be both safe and effective in the outpatient setting (33). Another approach would be to perform a submaximal exercise assessment during one of the first outpatient exercise sessions and use HR and MET levels derived from this evaluation as target intensities for early training sessions. The appropriate workloads for the exercise assessment could be based on the patient's activity level (i.e., METs) during the inpatient program or on the MET estimates from her home exercise program. Application of either alternative approach to defining a target intensity should be conservative, meaning that it should start with loads well within the patient's documented abilities.

Just as described in relation to primary prevention programs, RPEs may be used as an adjunct to the physiological measures of HR and $\dot{V}O_2$ when we are monitoring exercise intensity in cardiac patients (1, 3). The 15-point RPE scale presented in table 7.4 is typically used for this purpose. The ACSM Guidelines (1) provide recommendations regarding the use of RPEs for monitoring exercise intensity during outpatient cardiac rehabilitation exercise sessions. Perceived

exertion values of 11 to 13 are recommended for early outpatient exercise sessions, whereas a range of 12 to 15 is recommended for the higher training intensities during subsequent exercise training sessions. Use of such generalized RPE ranges for monitoring training intensity, such as those reflected above, is likely based on the assumption that a number on the RPE scale equates with a relative physiological intensity (% $\dot{V}O_2$max or MHRR). However, as discussed in the previous section on primary prevention, specific RPE values do not always match with a given relative physiological intensity during exercise. We assessed this issue—matching of an RPE to a specific physiological intensity—in a study of 680 adults (463 healthy adults; 217 cardiac patients) who underwent exercise testing at Ball State and Wake Forest (16). We asked subjects to rate their effort during progressive stages of a GXT and then analyzed the RPE values reported at both 60% and 80% of MHRR within the cohort. The results of the study are illustrated in figure 7.10, a and b. Figure 7.10a shows the range of RPEs reported

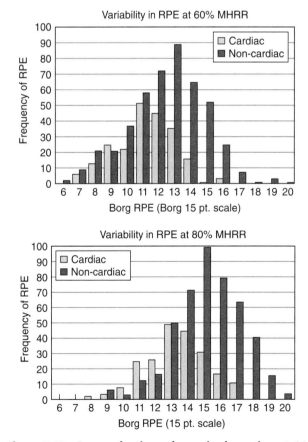

Figure 7.10 **Range of ratings of perceived exertion at** *(a)* **60% and** *(b)* **80% maximal heart rate reserve.**

Reprinted, by permission, from M.H. Whaley et al., 1997, "Validity of rating of perceived exertion during graded exercise testing in apparently healthy adults and cardiac patients," *Journal of Cardiopulmonary Rehabilitation* 17:264.

by the healthy (i.e., noncardiac) and cardiac patients when exercising at 60% of their MHRR, and figure 7.10b shows the range of RPEs reported by each group at 80% of MHRR. Overall, the figures reveal considerable variability in the matching between an RPE number and a relative physiological intensity. The results clearly challenge the validity of the assumption that a given number on the RPE scale equates with a given physiological intensity.

What does this mean in the context of using RPE to monitor exercise training intensity? Because of the significant interindividual variability in RPE at the physiological intensities commonly used for training prescriptions (i.e., 60-80% of MHRR), RPE prescriptions should be individualized when used to monitor training intensity (1). This is easy to accomplish by trial and error during the early stages of a training program. We recommend the following procedures. First, have the patient exercise at the desired intensity for several minutes. Once the patient reaches a steady state level, have the individual rate his perceived exertion using the RPE scale. If over the course of several exercise sessions the patient reports a consistent RPE at the same physiological intensity, that RPE may be used, in conjunction with physiological markers, for monitoring the patient's training intensity. On the other hand, if the patient's RPEs vary considerably from day to day (at the same physiological intensity), perceived exertion may not be an appropriate means for monitoring physiological intensity for this patient.

What about exercise prescription intensities for cardiac patients who have abnormal ECG and/or hemodynamic responses to graded exercise? Some of these patients might be referred for further diagnostic testing, as described in chapter 3, before entering the outpatient program. However, a number of these patients will be permitted to begin exercise training and may be referred to outpatient rehabilitation. Thus, you will need to define an appropriate exercise intensity for their training sessions. In such cases, according to the ACSM Guidelines (1), the endurance training intensity should be set at least 10 bpm below the exercise HR associated with any of the signs or symptoms listed in table 7.15. In addition, careful monitoring of the patient's symptoms, HR, BP, and ECG is recommended to ensure that the intensity of exercise remains at a safe level. Whether the relative exercise intensity (% $\dot{V}O_2$ or MHRR) is above the minimal threshold associated with a training effect is irrelevant at this point. Safety is the primary concern. Over time, a patient's sign/symptom threshold may

Table 7.15

Signs and Symptoms For Which an Upper Limit for Exercise Intensity Should Be Set*

Onset of angina or other symptoms of CV insufficiency

Plateau or decrease in SBP, SBP > 240 mmHg, or DBP of > 110 mmHg

$\geq$ 1 mm ST-segment depression, horizontal or downsloping
Radionuclide evidence of LV dysfunction or onset of moderate-to-severe wall motion abnormalities during exertion

Increased frequency of ventricular arrhythmias

Other significant ECG disturbances (e.g., 2 or 3 degree AV block, atrial fibrillation, supraventricular tachycardia, complex ventricular ectopy, etc.)

Other signs or symptoms of intolerance to exercise

* Reprinted, by permission, 2000, *ACSM's Guidelines for Exercise Testing and Prescription.* 6th ed. (Philadelphia: Lippincott, Williams, and Wilkins), 173.

improve to the point where higher exercise intensities are possible. In the meantime, the patient will still be expending energy during the exercise sessions, and many of the health benefits associated with regular exercise are achievable at moderate intensities.

Duration

The recommended exercise duration for patients in outpatient cardiac rehabilitation programs is similar to that for apparently healthy participants in primary prevention programs. Although 20 to 60 min of continuous aerobic exercise is the standard recommendation, several recent guideline statements suggest that an accumulation of shorter exercise sessions throughout the day (i.e., three 10-min bouts) is comparable to a single, continuous session (1, 2). Either of these scenarios provides for an increase in one's daily energy expenditure and can lead to improvements in functional capacity as well as other physiological training benefits. However, there is a need for more studies that compare the two training models (i.e., continuous vs. intermittent) in a variety of patient populations before it will be possible to reach a clear conclusion about comparable training adaptations. We advocate continuous training sessions whenever possible but concede that intermittent sessions are more feasible for some patients, and we would certainly advocate this over a sedentary lifestyle.

Exercise program professionals should also keep in mind that training duration is inversely related to the training intensity. In other words, the lower the training intensity, the longer each session needs to be to achieve the same adaptation. The converse is also true. The higher the training intensity, the shorter the duration required to achieve the same adaptation. As discussed in relation to primary preventive programs, the major theme operating here relates to the prescribed dose or volume of exercise for each patient. The appropriate training duration for each patient will be the one that allows the individual to attain her weekly goal for energy expenditure. Based on the association between intensity and duration we have described, the appropriate duration will depend on each patient's intensity and number of training sessions per week. We recommend that exercise program professionals first establish the desirable dose or volume of exercise for each patient. The next step, given the intensity prescription, is to determine the number of minutes the patient will need to exercise each session to accumulate the weekly goal. Naturally, the weekly goals are estimates and will get progressively larger during the first few months of the outpatient program. Typically, 45 to 60 min of continuous aerobic activity is the upper limit for training duration in outpatient cardiac rehabilitation programs.

Frequency

The recommendation for exercise training frequency for primary prevention programs—three to five days per week—is also appropriate for outpatient cardiac rehabilitation. Most outpatient programs offer two to three supervised exercise sessions per week but encourage their patients to be physically active—within prescribed limits—on most days of the week. The appropriate frequency for a given patient will depend on the individual's goals for the program. Most cardiac patients can achieve improvements in functional capacity (increased $\dot{V}O_2$max; decreased HR at given workload) with two to three sessions per week, provided that the intensity and duration of these sessions are adequate. However, as discussed in the context of primary prevention, patients in need of risk factor intervention (e.g., to decrease obesity or hypertension, normalize blood lipids, increase glucose tolerance, etc.) will likely benefit from a higher volume of exercise on a weekly basis. Increasing the number of sessions per week (to four or five) will help to modify these risk factors over time. The next chapter provides more details on training adaptations, but we add one last word on frequency here. Since conventional wisdom suggests that the risk of MS injury increases as a function of exercise intensity and frequency, it is wise to monitor MS symptoms in patients participating in vigorous, weight-bearing activities such as jogging. Using several different modes of exercise throughout the week (some of which are non-weight bearing) will decrease the risk of injury.

Progression

The general concepts concerning progression of the training program that we considered in connection with primary prevention apply in the outpatient cardiac rehabilitation setting as well. First, it's important to remember that as a general rule, increases in training duration, and perhaps frequency, should precede increases in intensity. More specifically, most patients should achieve a duration of 20 to 30 min of continuous aerobic exercise before increasing the intensity (1). Second, the goal within primary prevention programs of progressing beyond a minimal dose of exercise equal to 1000 kcal per week is also important in the secondary prevention setting. However, achieving this volume of exercise usually takes longer for cardiac patients (perhaps between three and six months, depending on functional capacity and clinical status) compared to their healthy, sedentary counterparts in primary prevention programs. We now look at these issues in more detail.

First, what about the rate of progression in outpatient cardiac rehabilitation programs? Several characteristics of patients with cardiovascular disease necessitate a modification of the rate of progression early in the outpatient program. Because many cardiac patients begin outpatient programs with significantly lower functional capacities compared to their healthy, sedentary counterparts, the rate of progression during the early weeks needs to be slower. In fact, as a consequence of extremely low functional capacity or limiting symptoms (e.g., claudication), some patients may need exercise to be intermittent during the early stages. Table 7.16 provides recommendations for work/rest intervals for intermittent exercise sessions within the first few weeks of training. The goal is to gradually work toward 15 to 20 min of continuous exercise at the target intensity. Once patients achieve this level of exercise, some will be able to progress at a rate consistent with that presented in table 7.5 for healthy adults. However, patients limited by symptoms will continue to need a more conservative rate of progression indefinitely.

As already mentioned, the ultimate goal for progression of the training volume within secondary prevention programs is a weekly energy

Table 7.16
Example of Exercise Progression for Intermittent Exercise

Functional Capacity (FC) > 4 METs					
Week	%FC	Total min at %FC	Min exercise	Min rest	Reps
1	50–60	15–20	3–5	3–5	3–4
2	50–60	15–20	7–10	2–3	3
3	60–70	20–30	10–15	Optional	2
4	60–70	30–40	15–20	Optional	2
Functional Capacity (FC) ≤ 4 METs					
Wk	%FC	Total Min at %FC	Min Exercise	Min Rest	Reps
1	40–50	10–15	3–5	3–5	3–4
2	40–50	12–20	5–7	3–5	3
3	50–60	15–25	7–10	3–5	3
4	50–60	20–30	10–15	2–3	2
5	60–70	25–40	12–20	2	2
6	Continue with 2 reps of continuous exercise, with one rest period, or progress to a single continuous bout				

Reprinted, by permission, 2000, *ACSM's Guidelines for Exercise Testing and Prescription*. 6th ed. (Philadelphia: Lippincott, Williams, and Wilkins), 173.

expenditure exceeding 1000 kcal (1). Weekly energy expenditures exceeding 1000 kcal are more effective in modifying risk factors associated with obesity (hypertension, impaired glucose tolerance) and, as discussed in chapter 1, may also contribute to a slower progression of coronary disease. Hambrecht and colleagues (34) assessed the relationship between leisure-time physical activity and CAD progression in 62 cardiac patients in Heidelberg, Germany. After a year of intervention, the authors grouped the patients according to changes in the size of their CAD lesions (i.e., progression, no change, or regression). Results showed an inverse dose-response relationship between the amount of physical activity and disease progression, which simply means that the greater the amount of physical activity, the slower the progression of disease. Patients who reported >2200 kcal of activity per week were found to have some regression of their CAD lesions. This amount of activity equated to approximately 5 to 6 h of physical activity per week. Patients who reported ≤1000 kcal per week were found to have progression of their lesions. The middle group of patients—those reporting an average of 1500 kcal per week—showed no progression of CAD. It should be noted that the physical activity estimates in the study were derived from activity-recall instruments that rely on the patient's self-report of activity habits. Thus, there may be potential problems with the precision of the measurement (i.e., precise number of kilocalories expended per

week). More studies on this issue are needed before the definitive dose of physical activity associated with regression of CAD can be identified. Nevertheless, because the results from the Hambrecht et al. study suggest that a threshold of approximately ≥1500 kcal per week can slow disease progression in cardiac patients, exercise program professionals should be encouraging patients who are able to do so to meet this caloric threshold. Obviously, patients need to progress to and ultimately beyond this volume of exercise at their own rate and in a safe manner.

Let's return to our 44-year-old male cardiac patient to emphasize the concept of an energy expenditure threshold for exercise prescription. Remember that his exercise prescription intensity was set at approximately 5 METs (4.8 METs = 50% of $\dot{V}O_2R$). If we started with an energy expenditure goal of 1000 kcal per week, how many minutes of exercise per week would he need—at his target intensity—to achieve this threshold? As described earlier, the first step in determining this is to estimate the patient's net energy expenditure rate per minute during exercise. For this we need the patient's net MET intensity (5 METs – 1 MET for resting = 4 METs) and his body weight in kilograms (89.3). We estimate his net energy expenditure rate by substituting the data into the following equation:

$$kcal/min = METs \times 3.5 \times body\ weight\ in\ kg/200$$

$$6.3 = 4 \times 3.5 \times 89.3/200$$

His exercise intensity and body weight indicate that our patient will expend about 6.3 kcal/min above resting metabolism during his exercise routine. Our next step is to determine the number of minutes it will take him per week—at this net energy expenditure rate—to achieve the goal of 1000. Simply divide the 1000 by 6.3 kcal/min, and the answer is 159 min per week. Now, if the patient decides to exercise four times per week, he will need to exercise about 40 min each session to accumulate the weekly goal of 1000 kcal (159/4≈40). If he wanted to exercise only three days per week, he would have to increase the duration of his sessions to reach the threshold; on the other hand, increasing his frequency to five sessions per week would allow for shorter sessions (32 min). Is the 1000 kcal per week goal within his capacity? It certainly is! In addition, our patient could increase his overall energy expenditure by being more physically active throughout the day, most days of the week. These calories also contribute to the weekly goal for energy expenditure. Now, as we saw earlier, a more optimal goal would be >1500 kcal per week of activity. At his current fitness level (i.e., $\dot{V}O_2max$) he would have to exercise over 200 min per week to achieve the 1500 threshold. Most patients are not prepared to commit to this volume of exercise on a weekly basis. However, as our patient's fitness level improves during the course of the training program, he will be able to exercise safely at a higher absolute energy expenditure rate as a function of increases in both his relative intensity (say 70% vs. 50% $\dot{V}O_2R$) and $\dot{V}O_2max$. This is one of the reasons an increase in functional capacity is a goal for his program; it will allow him to exercise at higher energy expenditure during training. The higher energy expenditure will help him to modify several of his risk factors for disease progression. The next chapter takes a closer look at training adaptations.

There is one final issue relating to progression within outpatient cardiac rehabilitation programs. Not all patients wish or are able to afford to continue participation in a supervised program. When is it prudent to decrease the level of monitoring and supervision for cardiac patients in outpatient programs? While this decision ultimately rests with the physician, members of the rehab team, and the patient, table 7.17 provides recommendations from the ACSM to help the exercise program professional in this regard. However, patients and program staff should bear in mind that CAD is by nature a progressive disease and that therefore patients who graduate to less supervised settings for exercise should remain vigilant about any signs or symptoms that may signal a progression of the disease state. When such symptoms arise, patients should seek medical attention immediately.

Resistance Prescription for Secondary Prevention

Beginning in the 1970s, almost all cardiac rehabilitation programs focused on aerobic exercise. However, for many of the same reasons cited in the primary prevention section, MS resistance-exercise training provides many important benefits for cardiac patients in secondary prevention programs. In a general sense, skeletal muscle is skeletal muscle regardless of whether the individual is a cardiac patient or not. So the basic prescription principles for resistance training described

Table 7.17
Guidelines for Progression to Independent Exercise With Minimal or No Supervision.

- Functional capacity of ≥ 8 METs or twice the level of occupational demand

- Appropriate hemodynamic response to exercise (increase in systolic blood pressure with increasing workload and recovery

- Appropriate ECG response at peak exercise with normal or unchanged conduction, stable or benign arrhythmias, and nondiagnostic ischemic response (i.e., <1 mm ST-segment depression)

- Cardiac symptoms stable or absent

- Stable and/or controlled baseline heart rate and blood pressure

- Adequate management of risk factor intervention strategy and safe exercise participation such that the patient demonstrates independent and effective management of risk factors with favorable changes in those risk factors

- Demonstrated knowledge of the disease process, abnormal signs and symptoms, medication use, and side effects

Reprinted, by permission, 2000, *ACSM's Guidelines for Exercise Testing and Prescription.* 6th ed. (Philadelphia: Lippincott, Williams, and Wilkins), 175.

for primary prevention apply to cardiac patients as well. Because of the higher risk of complications during exercise for those with CAD, though, program staff should address important issues regarding who should participate (i.e., patient eligibility) and when they should participate (i.e., time course following a cardiac event), as well as specific prescriptive guidelines. The following section presents information on these issues.

Most cardiac patients can participate in MS resistance programs safely, as long as they have received instruction on appropriate lifting techniques and use loads appropriate for their capacity. The decision to initiate a resistance-training routine should be made by the program staff in consultation with the medical director and/or surgeon. However, resistance training is generally contraindicated for patients with the following clinical conditions (1):

Unstable angina

Uncontrolled arrhythmias

Left ventricular outflow obstruction

Symptomatic congestive heart failure

Severe valvular disease

Uncontrolled hypertension (i.e., systolic BP >160; diastolic BP ≥105 mmHg)

In addition to not having these clinical conditions, it is also advisable for patients to have moderate to good left ventricular function and a functional capacity >5 METs before starting a resistance-training regimen.

As described in the section on inpatient exercise, cardiac patients often begin ROM exercises during the inpatient stage of rehabilitation. The physical effort associated with active ROM exercises incorporates a muscular endurance component using the weight of the limb as the resistance. During the early outpatient stage (i.e., first few weeks), many cardiac rehabilitation programs incorporate low-intensity resistance exercise using elastic bands, wall pulleys, and so on. Most low-risk patients tolerate these activities without any problems. But when is the appropriate time for eligible patients to begin a traditional resistance-training routine following a myocardial infarction or revas-cularization procedure? A traditional resistance-training routine is defined as one that would have the patient lifting ≥50% of her 1-RM. The ACSM and AACVPR Guidelines recommend the following:

- Post-MI patients should wait four to six weeks following the event before engaging in traditional resistance training.

- Postsurgical patients should wait a minimum of 8 to 12 weeks following surgery to allow for healing of the sternum.

In addition, both the ACSM and AACVPR Guidelines recommend that patients complete a minimal period (i.e., several weeks) of endurance training before starting traditional resistance training.

The resistance-exercise prescription guidelines shown in table 7.8 represent a minimal dose of exercise that is associated with a training effect (i.e., increased muscular strength and/or endurance). These guidelines are generally suitable for most low-risk cardiac patients provided that they adhere to all the safety techniques discussed earlier. In addition, cardiac patients should be instructed to avoid the excessive isometric contraction associated with gripping the weight bars or dumbbells too tightly. A well-rounded program should include one to two sets of 8 to 10 exercises that work all the major muscle groups, with a minimal training frequency of two times per week. Readers can refer back to the section on primary prevention for a listing of specific exercises that may be used in a resistance-training routine. Within the context of resistance training, the exercise intensity is often defined as a percentage of an individual's 1-RM. The procedures for measuring a 1-RM are presented in chapter 6 (box 6.1). However, prescribing training intensity using a percentage of 1-RM requires knowledge of a patient's 1-RM. While some cardiac rehabilitation programs do indeed use a 1-RM test for each exercise to determine specific loads for their patients, we advocate a more conservative approach. Rather than defining the initial load as a percentage of 1-RM, we suggest that patients start with a fairly light load—one that they can perform for 12 to 15 repetitions—and focus on performing each exercise using correct technique. Once patients master the correct form, they can progress to heavier loads gradually. The rate of progression will vary from patient to patient. Although most commercially available resistance-training machines use weight stacks, with 10- to 15-lb (4.5-6.8 kg) plates, these machines can be modified to provide increments as low as 2.5 to 5 lb (1.1-2.3 kg) when smaller progressions are necessary.

SUMMARY

In this chapter we presented a number of basic exercise prescription principles pertaining to CR endurance and MS strength and endurance programs. The chapter initially focused on the basic principles as they apply to generally healthy adults in primary prevention programs, then addressed the modification of these basic principles of exercise prescription for patients in secondary prevention programs. We emphasized using objective data from a GXT to develop the prescription, whenever possible, but also discussed designing programs in the absence of GXT data. We also stressed defining an appropriate volume or dose of exercise using energy expenditure thresholds and then designing a routine (mode, frequency, intensity, and duration) that would eventually—through a proper progression of exercise—help individuals achieve the threshold. After reading this chapter, students should be able to describe the basic elements of exercise prescriptions for CR and MS strength and endurance programs. By following the case study examples to be presented, students should be able to design appropriate exercise prescriptions for participants in either primary or secondary exercise programs.

CASE STUDIES

This section contains the initial exercise prescriptions for the three case studies that appear throughout the book. We provide a rationale for the *individualized* elements of each prescription based on the principles discussed throughout this chapter. Keep in mind that the purposes of an individualized exercise prescription are to

- enhance some facet of physical fitness (e.g., CR endurance, muscular strength/endurance),

- promote health by modification of chronic disease risk factors (e.g., decrease excess body fat, normalize blood lipids and BP), and

- ensure safety during exercise participation (i.e., decrease incidence of CV complications and/or MS injuries).

The exercise prescriptions developed for each case will reflect each of these purposes. Pertinent data for each case, along with a summary of each exercise prescription, are presented in table 7.18. Exercise professionals need to evaluate every individualized exercise prescription in light of the criteria listed before subjecting their clients or patients to the regimen. Finally, we want you to keep in mind that the prescriptions described here are based on how we would develop them for participants in our respective primary and secondary prevention programs. However, exercise program professionals must draw on their clinical judgment when designing programs, and we certainly concede that our prescriptions could be adapted in a number of ways and still meet established, scientifically sound guidelines for exercise prescription. Remember, exercise prescription is as much an art as it is a science. On to the case studies!

Table 7.18
Pertinent Exercise Prescription Data for Case Studies 1, 2, and 3

Resting variables	Case 1	Case 2	Case 3
Age (years)	38	50	61
Resting HR (bpm)	59	60	67
Resting BP (mmHg)	144/100	118/68	120/80
Body weight (kg)	91.6	163.7	100.7
BMI (kg/m²)	28.0	43.9	29.3
Peak exercise test variables			
Test mode/protocol	Treadmill BSU/Bruce ramp	Treadmill Individualized ramp	Treadmill Modified Bruce
HRpeak (bpm)	187	103	136
$\dot{V}O_2$peak (ml·kg⁻¹·min⁻¹)	45.2	16.1	32.6[a]

(continued)

Table 7.18   *(continued)*

Peak exercise test variables	Case 1	Case 2	Case 3
Peak BP (mmHg)	186/86	142/68	na
Peak RPE (6-20 scale)	20	17	na
ECG/signs-symptoms	Negative	Negative	Negative
Termination criteria	Fatigue	Leg fatigue	Fatigue
Initial cardiorespiratory exercise prescription			
Modes	Walking/cycling	Walking/cycling	Walking/cycling
Intensity range (% of MHRR)	50–65	50–60	40–50
Target HR MHRR (bpm)	123–142	82–86	95–102
Target $\dot{V}O_2$ (METs)	6.5–8.4	2.3–2.8	3[b]
Duration (min)	20–25	15–20	15–20
Frequency (days/week)	3–4	3	3
Energy expenditure (kcals/min)[c]	10.4–13.5	6.6–8.0	5.3
Minutes needed for 1000 kcals/week lower intensity	96	152	188
Initial musculoskeletal resistance exercise prescription			
	Initiate routine based on BP control BP monitoring daily until controlled	Defer until stable pattern established with CR exercise Once stable, initiate program with low resistance, high repetitions	Defer until stable pattern established with CR exercise Once stable, initiate program with low resistance, high repetitions
Mode	Machines or free weights	Elastic bands, graduating to free weights (i.e., dumbbells) as tolerated	Elastic bands, graduating to free weights (i.e., dumbbells) as tolerated
Intensity	Resistance equal to 12–15 RM	Resistance equal to 12–15 RM	Resistance equal to 12–15 RM
Duration	1 to 2 sets of 8–10 exercises Major muscle groups	1 to 2 sets of 8–10 exercises Major muscle groups	1 to 2 sets of 8–10 exercises Major muscle groups
Frequency (days/week)	2–3×	2–3×	2–3×

bpm = beats per minute; BP = blood pressure; na = not available; kg = kilograms; HR = heart rate; BSU = Ball State University; WFU = Wake Forest University; RPE = rating of perceived exertion; MHRR = maximal heart rate reserve; METs = metabolic equivalent units; kcals/min = kilocalories per min; RM = repetition maximum; CR = cardiorespiratory.

a = estimated from treadmill time during GXT

b = Not necessarily 40-50% of VO_2peak as 32.6 ml/kg/min was most likely overestimate. See text for explanation.

c = kcals/min = METs × 3.5 × BW in kilograms / 200

Case Study 1
Primary Prevention: Low Risk

You've become acquainted with this gentleman through our presentations in previous chapters. Here's where we put together the exercise plan to aid this man in achieving his fitness goals. As you recall, our 38-year-old male came to the fitness program at Ball State with several risk factors that are clear targets for modification. Among these are sedentary lifestyle, hypertension, and excess body fat. These risk factors can all be modified with appropriate lifestyle interventions (i.e., exercise and dietary habits). Our focus here is on the exercise plan we would design within the context of our programs.

Let's briefly review this man's exercise test results that were presented and discussed in chapter 6. As you can see from the data in table 7.18, this man reached a peak HR of 187 bpm and a $\dot{V}O_2$peak of 45.2 ml/kg/min. His $\dot{V}O_2$peak represents the 75th percentile for men his age (1). Given his relatively sedentary lifestyle, his $\dot{V}O_2$peak seems a bit high; but if you test enough individuals, you will observe this sort of thing occasionally (i.e., sedentary individual with above-average $\dot{V}O_2$peak). How might this occur? Remember that part of one's aerobic power is genetically determined. On the basis of his sedentary lifestyle, we might conclude that this man has the genetic potential for a high CR fitness. We will discuss this in more detail in chapter 8. For now, let's just conclude that his higher-than-expected $\dot{V}O_2$peak will allow him to exercise at a higher metabolic rate (METs) during the initial phases of his program in comparison to most middle-aged men. The data in table 7.18 also indicate that his exercise BP and ECG responses were within normal limits, and he didn't report any abnormal signs or symptoms during the exercise test. Therefore, as discussed in earlier chapters, we consider his exercise test negative, meaning normal, and he's ready to initiate an exercise program. We did discuss his resting hypertension with his personal physician, and collectively we decided to initiate an exercise program to see whether the increased exercise, and perhaps accompanying weight loss, could lower the resting BP into the normal range without the use of antihypertensive medications. We discussed this plan with our case study and indicated that we would be monitoring his BP on a systematic basis within the program and providing his physician with the measurements on a regular basis. Now, with his fitness assessment results in order, let's take a look at his initial exercise prescription.

In a general sense, the exercise training goals for this man would parallel those cited earlier (i.e., increase CR and MS fitness and modify CAD risk factors). Although his CR fitness level is at the 75th percentile, there is still room for improvement; and this man reported no involvement in activities that would enhance his muscular strength or endurance, so this would also be a focus of his exercise

prescription. In addition to his sedentary lifestyle, the other risk factors of hypertension and moderate obesity represent additional goals for his program. Therefore, we need to design an exercise prescription that will improve his overall fitness level and help normalize his hypertension and obesity. The initial plans for both CR and MR resistance training are summarized in table 7.18.

His initial CR prescription includes walking and leg cycling as the primary modes; however, as this man has no overt orthopedic limitations, we prefer that he spend the majority of the time walking during the early phase of his training. This will enhance his energy expenditure during the sessions. His exercise training intensity should be set within the 50% to 85% range described earlier in the chapter, and we would generally use the lower end of the range for the first few weeks (i.e., 50-60%). Using the formulas presented earlier in the chapter, his target MET and HR levels at 50% to 65% of $\dot{V}O_2$peak/MHRR are shown in table 7.18. This target metabolic rate would provide for an energy expenditure range during the initial sessions of 10 to 13 kcal/min. Rounding out his initial CR endurance plan would be a training duration of 20 to 25 min and a frequency of three to four sessions per week. These are consistent with the ranges suggested in table 7.5 from the ACSM (1).

As you recall from our discussions earlier in the chapter, it is important to evaluate the exercise plan in light of currently recommended caloric thresholds from the ACSM (1). Based on the elements of our initial exercise prescription, where would our gentleman be relative to the minimal threshold of 1000 kcal per week? If we multiply an energy expenditure rate of 13.5 kcal/min (i.e., upper end of his energy expenditure range from table 7.18) by 25 min and three sessions per week, he would expend approximately 1000 kcal per week within this initial exercise plan. One could obviously use various combinations of the elements within the individualized prescription (intensity, frequency, duration) depending on how each was modified within the plan. However, because of this man's higher-than-expected baseline $\dot{V}O_2$peak, he can attain the minimal caloric threshold from the outset of the program without having to supplement his formal workouts with additional light/moderate recreational activities. Incidentally, we would still encourage him to take up several recreational activities, as this would enhance the overall energy balance model for this man and aid in his goal of losing excess body fat.

What kind of workload would our case study need to maintain during his walking or leg cycling routines to achieve a metabolic intensity of 6 to 8 METs? While it would seem simple enough to have our case study begin walking on the treadmill and gradually increase the workload until such point as he reaches his THR, we advocate estimating the initial workload using metabolic equations when they are available. Here's where the ACSM metabolic equations can come in handy. We encourage the reader to review the information presented in appendix D of the ACSM Guidelines (1) text if necessary. Let's calculate workloads for both the treadmill and leg cycle based on the middle of our case's initial MET intensity range presented in table 7.18. This would be approximately 7.5 METs. Before working through the calculations, it's worth noting that our case could not achieve a 7.5-MET level by just walking on a level surface. Therefore, we would need to combine a walking speed with some amount of incline on the treadmill in order to achieve the 7.5-MET intensity with our case. In this instance, it would be wise to select a treadmill speed, determine the MET requirement for that speed, and then use the vertical component of the ACSM walking equation to account for the remainder of the 7.5 METs. We would generally determine this walking speed by trial and error with the participant during the first few training sessions. For the sake of this example, let's say our case study was comfortable walking at 3.5 mph (5.6 km/h) and then proceed with the calculations to determine the amount of incline needed for the treadmill to achieve 7.5 METs. Remember to convert the METs into ml/kg/min (7.5 METs × 3.5 = 26.3 ml/kg/min) and the speed from miles per hour to meters per minute (3.5 mph × 26.8 = 93.8 m/min) prior to using these terms in the equation. The ACSM metabolic equation for walking is as follows:

ACSM Walking Equation

$$\dot{V}O_2 \text{ ml/kg/min} = 0.1(\text{speed}) + 1.8(\text{speed})(\text{fractional grade}) + 3.5$$

Computational Steps
1. multiply expressions:
   26.3 = 0.1(93.8) + 1.8(93.8)(grade) + 3.5
2. subtract 3.5:
   26.3 = 9.38 + 168.8(grade) + 3.5

3. subtract 9.38:
   22.8 = 9.38 + 168.8(grade)
4. divide by 168.8:
   13.5 = 168.8(grade)
5. result:
   0.08 = grade

On the basis of these calculations, we see that if we have our subject walking on the treadmill at 3.5 mph (5.6 km/h), we would need to use an 8% grade to achieve the 7.5-MET target. Of course, if you had chosen a different walking speed to start with, there would be a different % grade value in combination. The ACSM Guidelines actually contain a series of tables in appendix D that present MET equivalents for various speed/grade combinations. These tables should come in handy when exercise leaders are calculating workloads for clients or patients during workouts. Now, we don't advocate focusing on the workloads in a vacuum, without information about other physiological variables. You should always be monitoring the individual's HR response during the exercise and making adjustments in the workload when needed to stay within the THR range.

Let's turn our attention to the other mode of aerobic exercise we chose for our case study, which was leg cycling. What workload would this man need on the leg cycle to achieve a 7.5-MET intensity?

ACSM Leg Cycling Equation

$$\dot{V}O_2 \text{ ml/kg/min} = 1.8(\text{kgm/min})\cdot\text{body weight}^{-1} + 7$$

Computational Steps
1. subtract 7:
   $26.8 = 1.8(\text{kgm/min})\cdot 91.6^{-1} + 7$
2. divide by 91.6:
   $19.8 = 1.8(\text{kgm/min})\cdot 91.6^{-1}$
3. divide by 1.8:
   1815.7 = 1.8(kgm/min)
4. result:
   1009.0 = kgm/min

In this case, our subject's target workload to achieve 7.5 METs on a leg cycle ergometer would be approximately 1000 kgm/min. Once again, we advocate the use of HR monitoring throughout to ensure that he maintains his exercise level within his THR range. In summary, we assume that the reader has had some exposure to the ACSM metabolic equations. If this is not the case, it would be wise to review that section of the ACSM Guidelines while working through the calculations in this section.

The other important segment of this case's exercise prescription would be MS resistance training. As you can see in table 7.18, we suggest a general prescription consistent with the ACSM dose recommendations discussed earlier in the chapter. This routine would consist of one set of 8 to 10 exercises, two to three times per week. There are several methods for selecting the initial loads for each exercise. A very common method is to perform the 1-RM test for each lift and then use a percentage of this load for training. This would be akin to using a percentage of one's $\dot{V}O_2$max for aerobic training. However, we advocate an alternative approach to defining the initial loads. If the goal is simply to identify a load that the individual could perform for 12 to 15 repetitions, we suggest starting with a very light load, one the individual can obviously handle, and have the person complete a set of up to 12 reps if possible. The focus is on correct lifting and breathing techniques throughout the set. If the individual reaches a fatigue threshold at the end of 12 reps, this would represent an approximate 12-RM load and would be an appropriate load for training. If the person can't reach 12, or could continue well beyond 12 reps, the exercise leader can adjust the load accordingly for the subsequent workout. Our 12-RM method for identifying the initial load will not provide maximal strength data for a baseline evaluation. However, we feel that people will be able to note improvements in strength and endurance by simply realizing that after a few weeks of training they are lifting a heavier load compared to the initial load.

What about progression of resistance exercise for our case study? We advocate that he increase the load for a given lift when he can comfortably complete 12 to 15 repetitions. The next logical question is how much he should increase the load. That would depend on the amount of muscle mass involved. Load increases for exercises that involve large-muscle groups (e.g., leg press or bench press) can be advanced by 10 to 15 lb (4.5-6.8 kg) in some cases. Load increases for smaller muscle group exercises (tricep extension, bicep curls) would be smaller (e.g., 5-10 lb [2.5-4.5 kg]) for most individuals.

One final note on resistance training: as you recall, our case study has hypertension. In this situation we would typically delay the start of this type of routine for a few weeks, until the individual establishes a regular pattern of aerobic exercise as a baseline for his program. Furthermore, consistent with the ACSM Guidelines (1), resistance training should not be viewed as the primary form of exercise for those with hypertension. We would also be careful to monitor his resting BP prior to his workouts to detect any elevation that might necessitate postponing the workout session that day. Although guidelines for postponing resistance exercise due to hypertension are not readily available, we have used a threshold of 160/100 mmHg as a cutoff point at which we would defer resistance training on that day.

In summary, we've discussed initial exercise prescriptions for both CR endurance and MS resistance training. These prescriptions have been based on the ACSM Guidelines (1, 2), with a spin learned from the experience of hundreds of participants in the collective exercise programs at Ball State and Wake Forest University. Now, the important thing is to get this man moving and keep him moving. Behavioral strategies for keeping him motivated to continue training are discussed in more detail in chapter 10 on program management. We will pick up this man's story in the next chapter when we discuss his adaptations to the training program.

Case Study 2
Primary Prevention: High Risk

Here we pick up the story of our 50-year-old member of the Cardiac Rehabilitation Program at Wake Forest University. As you recall from previous discussions, this gentleman had all of the major CAD risk factors discussed in chapter 1 except cigarette smoking, and he was being treated medically for several of these (i.e., hypertension, hyperlipidemia, diabetes). He is definitely a candidate for risk factor modification, and participation in a regular exercise program would be an important component of his intervention. Our focus in this chapter is the exercise plan we would design within the context of our programs. In addition to the prescription described here, exercise program professionals would need to review the diabetes section of chapter 9, as well as other references such as the ACSM Guidelines (1) for special considerations for exercise training based on his diabetic status.

Let's review his exercise test results briefly. As you can see from the data in table 7.18, this man reached a peak HR of 103 bpm and a $\dot{V}O_2$peak of 16.1 ml/kg/min. His peak HR is low for men his age; but remember, he's taking atenolol (a beta blocker that significantly lowers HR response). His $\dot{V}O_2$ peak is extremely low at <10th percentile for men his age (1). One of the reasons is the fact that this man weighs 361 lb (163.7 kg). When you express the $\dot{V}O_2$ peak value relative to body weight (i.e., milliliters O_2 per kilogram), the large denominator (i.e., kg) reduces the value considerably. The excess body weight/fat will be an important target for his intervention program, as a reduction in body fat mass can have a favorable effect on most of his other CAD risk factors. As reported in earlier chapters and summarized again in table 7.18, his exercise test BP and ECG responses were within normal limits, and he didn't report any abnormal signs/symptoms during the test. Therefore, we consider his exercise test negative, meaning normal, and he's ready to initiate an exercise program. Now let's take a look at his initial exercise prescription.

Based on his fitness assessment, the goals for his exercise training program would parallel those cited earlier (i.e., increase CR and MS fitness and modify CAD risk factors). There is considerable room for improvement in his CR fitness, and he reported no involvement in muscular strength or endurance activities. In addition to considering his sedentary lifestyle and other risk factors, we need to design an exercise prescription that will improve his overall fitness level and help normalize/control his hypertension, hyperlipidemia, obesity, and diabetic status. The initial plans for his CR and MS resistance training are summarized in table 7.18.

Because of his excessive body weight and history of orthopedic problems, the primary exercise mode during his first few months of training was stationary cycling. Walking became a more viable mode for this man as he began to lose weight during the program. On the basis of his obesity, hypertension, and diabetes collectively, we recommend that his exercise training intensity be set between 50% and 60% of $\dot{V}O_2$peak/MHRR at the start of the program. Using the formulas presented earlier in the chapter, his target MET and HR levels at 50% to 60% of $\dot{V}O_2$peak/MHRR are shown in table 7.18. This target metabolic rate would provide for an energy expenditure range during the initial sessions of 6.6 to 8.0 kcal/min. Rounding out his initial CR endurance plan would be a training duration of 15 to 20 min and a frequency of three sessions per week. These are consistent with the ranges suggested in table 7.5 from the ACSM (1). Using the formulas for cycling and walking already presented and a target of approximately 2.5 METs in intensity, his initial cycling workload would be approximately 160 kgm/min and his walking pace would be approximately 2.0 mph (3.2 km/h).

We recognize that these are low absolute workloads. As the exercise specialist, you would be wise to initiate his exercise session at either of these two loads and then adjust the load based on HR feedback and/or subjective feelings of exertion from this man. Remember, the calculations (e.g., METs, THR, etc.) are a guideline, not a strict rule in most cases. It may well be that our case study man tolerates these workloads quite easily and would prefer to walk a little faster or pedal a bit more vigorously. However, remember that total volume of exercise (intensity + frequency + duration) is more important than intensity alone and that you will likely have to maintain a more moderate intensity within his exercise prescription while increasing the duration and frequency.

Based on the elements of our initial exercise prescription, where would our gentleman be relative to the minimal threshold of 1000 kcal per week? If we multiply an energy expenditure rate of 7 kcal/min (i.e., middle of his energy expenditure range from table 7.18) by 20 min and three sessions per week, he would expend approximately 420 kcal per week within this initial exercise plan. While this level is below the minimal recommendation of 1000 kcal per week from ACSM, we need to remember that this man is just starting and that he has a very low fitness level. His initial prescription is a moderate dose of exercise, and he will be increasing his exercise training volume during the initial stage of training. If he were to exercise at the lower end of his intensity range (i.e., 6.6 kcal/min), he would have to accumulate approximately

152 min of activity per week to meet the 1000 kcal recommendation. His structured exercise plan provides for less than half of this total initially. However, the focus on progression within his program would center on increasing minutes per session and adding another day of training when possible. And, as mentioned for Case 1, we would also encourage him to take up some low- to moderate-intensity recreational activities, as this would enhance the overall energy expenditure for this man and aid in his goal of losing excess body fat.

What about MS resistance training for this individual? As you can see in table 7.18, we suggest a general prescription consistent with the ACSM dose recommendations discussed earlier. However, before initiating a traditional routine involving weight machines, we would usually have this man complete several weeks of resistance exercises using lighter equipment such as elastic bands. This would allow the program staff to assess how he tolerates this form of activity. Most likely he could graduate to a more traditional program using weight machines within a month or so. There's no need to get in a hurry here, as the main emphasis for his overall program is increasing his energy expenditure, and the focus would clearly need to be on aerobic activities in this case. Once he's cleared to use weight machines, we would recommend a regimen consisting of one set of 8 to 10 exercises, with a load equivalent to 12- to 15-RM initially, two to three times per week. This dose

should sound familiar, as it's exactly what we recommended in Case Study 1. There are several methods for selecting the initial loads for each exercise. A very common method is to perform the 1-RM test for each lift and then use a percentage of this load for training. Follow the steps described for Case 1 to define the initial 12- to 15-RM load and make progressions within the program.

One final note on resistance training: as you recall, our case study has hypertension and diabetes. The ACSM Guidelines (1) indicate that resistance training should not be the primary form of exercise for hypertensive patients. We would be careful to monitor his resting BP and fasting blood glucose systematically. Specific recommendations for patient monitoring are discussed in chapter 11. In addition, this man's diabetic status would pose unique challenges for the prescription of resistance training. The major concern would relate to the potential for microvascular disease secondary to the elevations in arterial pressure associated with this form of exercise. More on this in the section on diabetes in chapter 9.

In summary, we've discussed initial exercise prescriptions for both CR endurance and MS resistance training. Again, we want to get this man moving and keep him moving, using behavioral strategies to help him maintain motivation as discussed further in chapter 10. We'll return to this man's story in the next chapter.

Case Study 3
Secondary Prevention

Here we continue the story of our 61-year-old patient from the Cardiac Rehabilitation Program at Wake Forest University. As you'll recall, this patient had experienced an anterolateral MI and subsequently underwent an angioplasty procedure to place a stent in his circumflex coronary artery. This patient was inactive at the time he entered the Cardiac Rehabilitation Program at Wake Forest and had several other modifiable risk factors that were targets for intervention (e.g., lipids, body composition). All of his medical assessment information is interpreted in chapter 3, and specific interventional strategies are detailed in chapter 4. His exercise test responses were reviewed in chap-

ter 6. In this chapter we turn attention to the initial exercise plan we would design for this patient.

Let's briefly review some results from his initial exercise test (the exercise echo test discussed in chapters 3 and 6). As you can see from the data in table 7.18, this man reached a peak HR of 136 bpm and an estimated $\dot{V}O_2$peak of 32.6 ml/kg/min. These data warrant some interpretation before we discuss his exercise prescription. First, he's taking atenolol (a beta blocker that decreases HR response), which would explain the fact that his peak HR is significantly lower than expected for men his age. However, from the standpoint of his training intensity prescription, the 136 bpm is still his peak HR for use in the THR formulas discussed earlier in the chapter. Second, his oxygen consumption was not directly measured during the exercise test (stress echo described in detail in chapter 3), as he was tested initially in another facility before coming to the Wake Forest Cardiac Rehabilitation Program. Therefore, the $\dot{V}O_2$peak value reported in table 7.18 is a predicted value determined through use of the peak workload attained on the treadmill with the ACSM metabolic equation for walking. However, as the ACSM metabolic equations are meant for use during steady state exercise (a physiological state not met during peak effort at the end of a GXT), using this equation, with peak workloads, will invariably overestimate the patient's $\dot{V}O_2$peak. As discussed in chapter 6, we suspect this is what happened with our patient. It's very unlikely that this man has a functional $\dot{V}O_2$peak of 9.3 METs (32.6/3.5 = 9.3). Therefore, because of problems inherent in predicting $\dot{V}O_2$peak in this case, we will rely on the validity of the HR:$\dot{V}O_2$ relationship described earlier in the chapter (refer to conceptual basis for figure 7.1, a and b) and use the HRR formula to define his training intensity.

As reported in table 7.18, this man's BP and ECG responses were within normal limits during the exercise test, and he didn't report any abnormal signs or symptoms during or following the test. Therefore, as with the other two cases, we consider his exercise test negative, meaning normal, and he's cleared to initiate an exercise program. Risk stratification guidelines for cardiac patients were discussed earlier in the chapter; and on the basis of the diagnostic information presented on this patient in chapter 3, he would be stratified as low risk for cardiac events, which would have a bearing on the initial environment for his training program. Chapter 11 includes a more detailed discussion on medical clearance and monitoring issues for this patient. Now, let's look at his initial exercise prescription.

His initial CR prescription includes walking and leg cycling as the primary modes. As discussed with the first two cases, we would prefer to have the majority of the exercise time spent walking during the early phase of his training. However, again, if necessary because of orthopedic or other problems, he may have to resort to leg cycling or some other mode of weight-supported activity. We set this patient's initial exercise training intensity between 40% and 50% of MHRR. Using the formulas presented previously, his THR at this relative intensity would be 95 to 102 bpm. His initial training frequency would be three days per week with a 15- to 20-min initial duration. The program staff would assess how he responds to this dose of exercise and quantify the walking pace that elicits his THR range of 95 to 102 bpm.

Based on the elements of our initial exercise prescription, where would this man be relative to the minimal threshold of 1000 kcal per week? As he will be walking during his initial exercise sessions, an estimate of approximately 3 METs would allow for some speculation on his energy expenditure. As you can see from table 7.18, his estimated kcal/min rate during training would be approximately 5.3 kcal/min at a 3-MET intensity. Combining this intensity estimate with a training duration of 15 to 20 min and a frequency of three sessions per week, he would expend approximately 240 to 320 kcal per week during his training sessions.

Just as we discussed with the previous case study, although this level is below the minimal recommendation of 1000 kcal per week from ACSM, this patient is just starting and has a very low fitness level. His initial prescription represents a moderate dose of exercise, and he will be increasing his training volume on a systematic basis—perhaps consistent with the volume progression described in the Ball State University walking chart (see figure 7.5a). According to table 7.18, he would need to walk approximately 188 min per week to achieve the 1000-kcal threshold at his current intensity. As mentioned earlier in the chapter, this would be a goal for his first few months of training. If he were to work up to 45 min of walking per session, and ultimately add a fourth day of training, he would have achieved the minimal threshold of 1000 kcal per week. And as mentioned in connection with Cases 1 and 2, we would also encourage this patient to take up some low- to moderate-intensity recreational activities—provided he remains stable with regard to his disease status. This would enhance this patient's accumulated energy expenditure and contribute to a decrease in his excess body fat.

What about MS resistance training for this individual? As shown in table 7.18, our prescription is quite consistent with that for the second case study. We suggest a general prescription consistent with the ACSM dose recommendations discussed previously. However, before beginning a traditional routine involving weight machines, patients in the Wake Forest University Cardiac Rehabilitation Program complete several months of resistance exercises using lighter equipment such as elastic bands. This represents a gradual introduction to resistance training while allowing the program staff to assess how they tolerate this form of activity.

To sum up, we've provided an initial outpatient exercise prescription for both CR endurance and MS resistance training for this cardiac patient. Once again, these prescriptions were based on the ACSM Guidelines (1, 2), combined with some exercise prescription policies from the exercise programs at Ball State and Wake Forest Universities. We'll continue this patient's story in the next chapter when we discuss his adaptations to the training program.

GLOSSARY

Cardiorespiratory: relating to the heart and lungs; typically defines a form of exercise or physical fitness dealing with areas of aerobic metabolism or aerobic power

Energy expenditure: the amount of energy used during exercise defined as a total amount or rate (e.g., energy per minute)

Exercise: a subclass of physical activity consisting of planned, structured, and repetitive bodily movement done to improve or maintain one or more components of physical fitness

Hemodynamic: relating to the mechanics of blood circulation; commonly used hemodynamic measures during exercise include heart rate and blood pressure

Kilocalorie (kcal): a large calorie, which is the amount of heat energy required to raise the temperature of one liter of water one degree Celsius; this unit typically used to quantify the amount of energy expended during exercise

Musculoskeletal: having to do with the skeleton, skeletal muscle, and/or joint structures; typically describes a form of exercise or physical fitness dealing with areas of strength, endurance and/or flexibility

Oxygen uptake: the volume of oxygen ($\dot{V}O_2$) used or consumed by the body at rest or during physical activity; usually expressed in liters per minute (liters·min^{-1}) or milliliters per kilogram body weight per unit of time (ml·kg^{-1}·min^{-1})

Physical activity: bodily movement that is produced by the contraction of skeletal muscle and that substantially increases energy expenditure

Physical fitness: a set of attributes that individuals have or achieve that relates to the ability to perform physical activity

Revascularization: various medical procedures for restoring blood flow to a tissue bed (e.g., coronary bypass surgery, percutaneous transluminal coronary angioplasty)

REFERENCES

1. American College of Sports Medicine. 2000. *ACSM's Guidelines For Exercise Testing And Prescription.* 6th ed. B.F. Franklin, M.H. Whaley, and E.T. Howley, eds. Baltimore: Lippincott, Williams & Wilkins.

2. American College of Sports Medicine. 1998. The recommended quantity and quality of exercise for developing and maintaining cardiorespiratory and muscular fitness and flexibility in healthy adults. *Med. Sci. Sports Exerc.* 30:975–991.

3. American Association of Cardiovascular and Pulmonary Rehabilitation. 1999. *Guidelines For Cardiac Rehabilitation And Secondary Prevention Programs.* 3rd ed. Champaign, IL: Human Kinetics.

4. Ainsworth, B.E., W.L. Haskell, A.S. Leon, et al. 1993. Compendium of physical activities: Classification of energy costs of human physical activities. *Med. Sci. Sports Exerc.* 25:71–80.

5. U.S. Department of Health and Human Services. 1996. *Physical activity and health: A report of the Surgeon General.* Atlanta: U.S. Department of Health and Human Services, Centers for Disease Control and Prevention, National Center for Chronic Disease Prevention and Health Promotion.

6. Karvonen, M., K. Kentala, and O. Mustala. 1957. The effects of training on heart rate: A longitudinal study. *Annales Medicinae Experimentalis Biologial Fennial.* 35:302–315.

7. Swain, D.P., and B.C. Leutholtz. 1997. Heart rate reserve is equivalent to %$\dot{V}O_2$ reserve, not to %$\dot{V}O_2$max. *Med. Sci. Sports Exerc.* 29:410–414.

8. Borg, G.A.V. 1973. Perceived exertion: A note on "history" and methods. *Med. Sci. Sports* 5:90–93.

9. Noble, B.J., and R.J. Robertson. 1996. *Perceived Exertion.* Champaign, IL: Human Kinetics.

10. Glass, S.C., M.H. Whaley, and M.S. Wegner. 1991. Ratings of perceived exertion among standard

treadmill protocols and steady state running. *Int. J. Sports Med.* 12:77–82.

11. Brubaker, P.H., W.J. Rejeski, H.C. Law, W.E. Pollock, M.E. Wurst, and H.S. Miller. 1994. Cardiac patients' perception of work intensity during graded exercise testing: Do they generalize to field settings? *J. Cardiopul. Rehabil.* 14:127–133.

12. Moreau, K.L., M.H. Whaley, J.H. Ross, and L.A. Kaminsky. 1999. The effects of blood lactate concentration on perception of effort during graded and steady state treadmill exercise. *Int. J. Sports Med.* 20:269–274.

13. Shephard, R.J., T. Kavanagh, D.J. Mertens, and M. Yacoub. 1996. The place of perceived exertion ratings in exercise prescription for cardiac transplant patients before and after training. *Br. J. Sports Med.* 30:116–21.

14. Whaley, M.H., and G. Forsyth. 1990. The value of traditional intensity feedback for self-regulation of initial exercise training. *J. Cardiopul. Rehabil.* 10:98–106.

15. Zeni, A.I., M.D. Hoffman, and P.S. Clifford. 1996. Energy expenditure with indoor exercise machines. *J.A.M.A.* 275:1424–1427.

16. Whaley, M.H., P.H. Brubaker, L.A. Kaminsky, and C.R. Miller. 1997. Validity of rating of perceived exertion during graded exercise testing in apparently healthy adults and cardiac patients. *J. Cardiopul. Rehabil.* 17:261–267.

17. Getchell, B. 1982. *Being Fit: A Personal Guide.* New York: Wiley.

18. American Heart Association. 1992. Statement on exercise. Benefits and recommendations for physical activity programs for all Americans. *Circulation* 86:340–344.

19. Whaley, M.H., and L.A. Kaminsky. 2001. Epidemiology of physical activity, physical fitness and selected chronic diseases. In *ACSM's Resource Manual For Guidelines For Exercise Testing And Prescription,* 4th ed., J. Roitman, ed. 17–33. Baltimore: Lippincott, Williams & Wilkins.

20. Pope, R.P., R.D. Herbert, J.D. Kirwan, and B.J. Graham. 2000. A randomized trial of preexercise stretching for prevention of lower-limb injury. *Med. Sci. Sports Exerc.* 32:271–277.

21. Barnard, R.J., R. MacAlpin, A.A. Kattus, and G.D. Buckberg. 1973. Ischemic response to sudden strenuous exercise in healthy men. *Circulation* 48:936–942.

22. Foster, C., D.S. Dymond, J. Carpenter, and D.H. Schmidt. 1982. Effect of warm-up on left ventricular response to sudden strenuous exercise. *J. Appl. Physiol.* 53:380–383.

23. Dimsdale, J.E., H. Hartley, T. Guiney, J.N. Ruskin, and D. Greenblatt. 1984. Postexercise peril: Plasma catecholamines and exercise. *J.A.M.A.* 251:630–632.

24. Haskell, W.L. 1978. Cardiovascular complications during exercise training of cardiac patients. *Circulation* 57:920–924.

25. Fleck, S.J., and W.J. Kraemer. 1997. *Designing Resistance Training Programs.* 2nd ed. Champaign, IL: Human Kinetics.

26. American College of Sports Medicine. 1990. The recommended quantity and quality of exercise for developing and maintaining cardiorespiratory and muscular fitness in healthy adults. *Med. Sci. Sports Exerc.* 22:265–274.

27. Feigenbaum, M.S., and M.L. Pollock. 1997. Strength training: Rationale for current guidelines for adult fitness programs. *Phys. Sports Med.* 25:44–64.

28. Kaleth, A.S. 1997. Effects of volume of resistance training on muscular strength and endurance. Unpublished master's thesis. School of Physical Education, Ball State University.

29. American Heart Association. 1994. Cardiac rehabilitation programs: A statement for healthcare professionals. *Circulation* 90:1602–1610.

30. Pollock, M.L., M.A. Welch, and J.E. Graves. 1995. Exercise prescription for cardiac rehabilitation. In *Heart Disease And Rehabilitation,* ed. M.L. Pollock and D.H. Schmidt, 243–276. Champaign, IL: Human Kinetics.

31. Sivarajan, E.S., R.A. Bruce, M.J. Almes, et al. 1981. In-hospital exercise after myocardial infarction does not improve treadmill performance. *N. Engl. J. Med.* 305:357–362.

32. Haskell, W.L., E.L. Alderman, J.M. Fair, et al. 1994. Effects of intensive multiple risk factor reduction on coronary atherosclerosis and clinical cardiac events in men and women with coronary artery disease. *Circulation* 89:975–990.

33. McConnell, T.R., T.A. Klinger, J.K. Gardner, C.A. Laubach, C.E. Herman, and C.A. Hauck. 1998. Cardiac rehabilitation without exercise tests for post-myocardial infarction and post-bypass surgery patients. *J. Cardiopul. Rehabil.* 18:458–463.

34. Hambrecht, R., J. Niebauer, C. Marburger, et al. 1993. Various intensities of leisure time physical activity in patients with coronary artery disease: Effects on cardiorespiratory fitness and progression of coronary atherosclerotic lesions. *J. Am. Coll. Cardiol.* 22:468–477.

35. Kaminsky, L.A., and M.H. Whaley. 1998. Evaluation of a new standardized ramp protocol: The BSU/Bruce ramp protocol. *J. Cardiopul. Rehabil.* 18:438–444.

SUGGESTED READINGS

American College of Sports Medicine. 2000. *Guidelines For Exercise Testing And Prescription.* 6th ed. B.F. Franklin, M.H. Whaley, and E.T. Howley, eds. Baltimore: Lippincott, Williams & Wilkins.

American College of Sports Medicine. 2000. *ACSM's Resource Manual For Guidelines For Exercise Testing And Prescription.* 4th ed. J. Roitman, ed. Baltimore: Lippincott, Williams & Wilkins.

American Association of Cardiovascular and Pulmonary Rehabilitation. 1999. *Guidelines For Cardiac Rehabilitation And Secondary Prevention Programs.* 3rd ed. Champaign, IL: Human Kinetics.

Getchell L. 1982. *Being Fit: A Personal Guide.* New York: John Wiley & Sons.

Verrill, D.E. & P.M. Ribisl. 1996. Resistive exercise training in cardiac rehabilitation: An update. *Sports Medicine.* 21:347-383.

CHAPTER 8

Adaptations to Chronic Exercise Training in Coronary Artery Disease Prevention and Rehabilitation Programs

BEHAVIORAL OBJECTIVES

- To be able to describe general principles related to exercise training (e.g., overload, specificity, individuality, detraining)
- To be able to describe typical physiologic and health-related adaptations to exercise training in both primary and secondary prevention settings

One of the central themes in this text has been the significant fitness and health benefits associated with a physically active lifestyle. Chapter 1 presented the current state of evidence for a reduction in CAD risk associated with habitual physical activity; chapter 7 provided exercise prescription recommendations designed to yield improvements in aerobic and muscular fitness as well as reductions in various chronic disease risk factors. Based on these foundations, this chapter discusses the typical health and fitness adaptations that occur following chronic exercise training. We begin the chapter with a discussion of several key training principles that influence an individual's responses to training; we then review the physiological adaptations and health-related risk factor changes to both cardiorespiratory (CR) endurance and musculoskeletal resistance training. Several case study examples illustrate the potential for improvement in fitness and risk factors with real data from clients or patients in our primary or secondary prevention programs. These case studies should increase the exercise program professional's understanding of the impact that regular exercise can have on the health and fitness status of their clients or patients.

At the same time, this text is not intended to be an all-inclusive exercise physiology text, but rather an introductory one, with emphasis on practical application to participants in primary or secondary prevention programs. For more detailed discussions of the various physiological and biochemical adaptations to exercise training, and the underlying mechanisms for these adaptations, we encourage the reader to review the recommended resources listed at the end of the chapter.

GENERAL PRINCIPLES OF EXERCISE TRAINING

Several general principles of exercise training apply to any form of exercise (e.g., aerobic or resistance) and within any population (e.g., low- to high-risk cardiac patients, elderly, etc.). Here we discuss issues related to progressive overload, **training specificity,** individuality of responses, and consequences of inactivity. These principles are important within the context of formulating the initial exercise prescription, in determining the appropriate adjustments to the training intensity and volume throughout the course of training, and in evaluating outcomes from the training program.

Progressive Overload

In a general sense, the principle of overload suggests that in order for adaptation to occur (i.e., improvement in physiological function in response to training), a training regimen must work the body (e.g., skeletal muscles, CR system) harder than it's accustomed to working. For many sedentary individuals, this type of overload is likely to be achieved initially with a low to moderate dose of activity—perhaps 15 to 20 min of brisk walking, three times per week. However, for more active individuals, or those who are more physically fit prior to the onset of training, the overload required in order for adaptation to occur will be of greater intensity and/or volume. The concept of progressive overload implies that once some initial adaptation occurs, the training stimulus must be adjusted (i.e., increased) to provide for a renewed overload on the muscles or CR system. In theory, this cycle of systematic increases in the training stimulus should continue until the desired training adaptation is achieved (e.g., increases in $\dot{V}O_2$max or one repetition-maximum, etc.). However, exercise professionals should remember that there are physiological limits to each individual's ultimate adaptation to chronic exercise training and should help clients set realistic goals for the training program with this in mind. In other words, it would be unrealistic for a sedentary middle-aged man with a $\dot{V}O_2$max of 40 $ml \cdot kg^{-1} \cdot min^{-1}$ to aspire to compete with age-matched elite marathoners whose maximal aerobic power may be in the high 60s ($ml \cdot kg^{-1} \cdot min^{-1}$), as no amount of progressive training will result in an adaptation of this magnitude (i.e., increase in $\dot{V}O_2$max of 70%).

A key element within the progressive overload principle is the rate of progression of the training stimulus. As the rate of adaptation during exercise training is highly variable from person to person, the rate of overload progression must be individualized. Many professionals often suggest a rate of progression in relative terms (i.e., 5% per week, etc.). However, this manner of progression lacks the requisite detail one needs in order to make precise changes in a workout regimen from day to day, or even week to week. Therefore, many experienced exercise leaders rely on subjective observations of the individual's responses to workouts and objective data from periodic fitness evaluations to guide adjustments in the training load. When possible, we advocate the use of some type of standardized progression chart to guide day-to-day modifications in workout routines. We'll look at the concept of progression of the exercise prescription later in the chapter.

Specificity of Training

The principle of specificity of training suggests that adaptations to chronic exercise training occur in the specific muscle groups (e.g., arms vs. legs) or organ systems (e.g., skeletal muscle vs. CR) that are stressed or overloaded during training. This principle has application in several contexts. First, in a general sense, muscular resistance or strength training will not lead to significant adaptations in CR function and vice versa. Hurley et al. (1) studied 13 healthy, middle-aged males who completed a 16-week progressive, high-intensity resistance-training program. Following the training, the subjects had an average 40% to 50% improvement in muscular strength across the various lifts used to evaluate adaptation, but the measure of CR fitness ($\dot{V}O_2$max) did not change. Again, the training adaptations were specific to the organ systems that were overloaded or stressed with training. Other studies of this type confirm the results of Hurley and colleagues (2). Even further, aerobic training adaptations do not appear to transfer from one mode of training to another (e.g., from running to swimming), even though the modes are both aerobic and provide stress to the CR system (3).

Another example of the concept of specificity of training comes from studies assessing the transfer of training adaptations between limbs (i.e., arms vs. legs). For example, individuals who primarily exercise train their arms will not incur training adaptations in the leg muscles. Figure 8.1 illustrates this concept. The data are from a series of studies reported by Clausen (4). Within these studies, subjects were assigned to exercise train only their arms or their legs. The graph illustrates

the reduction in **submaximal exercise** heart rate (HR) (i.e., a marker of training adaptation) following the training program. During acute arm exercise, subjects who exercise trained with the arms had a reduction in HR of 19 bpm, whereas those who trained their legs had a reduction in HR of only 8 bpm. In other words, training adaptations are specific to the muscles undergoing the training stimulus.

Individuality of Responses

The principle of individuality of responses relates to both the rate and magnitude of the training adaptation. Individual responses to chronic exercise training are highly variable and most likely related to genetic factors, gender, age, and the overall training dose. In recent years, researchers in exercise science have begun to ask and answer questions related to a genetic predisposition to training adaptation. Professionals within the field have long known, through observations, that while most individuals within exercise training programs seem to respond in a predictable manner, others may not experience much adaptation at all. These observations led to considerable discussion about the potential influence of genetics on the trainability of individuals. Studies by Bouchard and colleagues (5-8) have increased our understanding of the role that genetic factors may play in individualized training adaptations. In one study, Bouchard et al. (5) measured $\dot{V}O_2$max in a sample of 42 sets of brothers as well as 66 homozygotic and 106 dizygotic sets of twins. The authors concluded that the proportion of $\dot{V}O_2$max that could be attributed to an inheritable component was approximately 40% when $\dot{V}O_2$max was expressed as $ml \cdot kg^{-1} \cdot min^{-1}$, but only about 10% when expressed relative to fat-free body weight (FFW) as $ml \cdot kg\ FFW^{-1} \cdot min^{-1}$. However, in another study, Lesage et al. (6) measured $\dot{V}O_2$max in a sample of 137 individuals—parents and children from a set of 38 families—to assess familial resemblance for $\dot{V}O_2$max. The authors concluded that the genetic variance in $\dot{V}O_2$max was quite low and that the father-child resemblance for $\dot{V}O_2$max was not statistically significant. These data suggest that the familial resemblance for $\dot{V}O_2$max is probably limited to first-degree relatives of the same generation. In an excellent review of the literature related to this issue (9), Bouchard et al. stated that the data on the inheritable component of $\dot{V}O_2$max are not entirely conclusive but that this value probably lies between 10% and 50%. What about the genetic influence of other chronic exercise training adaptations? Poehlman, et al. (7)

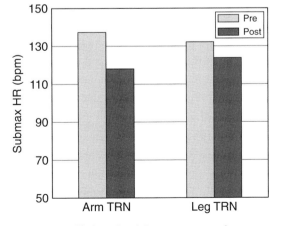

Figure 8.1 Specificity of training: arm versus leg.

reported a genetic influence on numerous hormonal changes from short-term training in six pairs of male monozygotic twins, and Simoneau et al. (8) reported a significant genetic influence on skeletal muscle enzyme changes following high-intensity training in 14 pairs of monozygotic twins. These studies, along with many more, clearly suggest that one's genotype may predispose one to adaptations or the lack thereof following exercise training.

Do other factors such as gender, age, or initial fitness level influence the overall adaptation or the rate of adaptation to endurance or resistance-exercise training? In some cases yes, in others no. While many morphological and physiological differences exist between men and women, most studies of adaptations after either aerobic or resistance training reveal similarities in the relative responses for men and women. We compared the relative (i.e., percentage) improvement in $\dot{V}O_2max$ between men and women following three to four months of aerobic training within the Ball State University Adult Physical Fitness Program. This analysis included 546 middle-aged adults (326 men, 220 women; mean age 43 ± 10 years) who trained at 75% maximal HR reserve for approximately four months. For the majority of subjects the mode of training was a progressive walk-jog routine. Maximal oxygen uptake was measured on a motorized treadmill under standardized laboratory conditions. As illustrated in figure 8.2, the average improvement in $\dot{V}O_2max$ was 18% for both men and women. These results are consistent with those of other studies comparing men and women and suggest that gender does not influence improvement in $\dot{V}O_2max$ subsequent to traditional aerobic exercise training (2).

Does age affect the body's adaptability following exercise training? Years ago the conventional wisdom was that older individuals would gradu-

ally lose their ability to adapt to exercise training. This notion paralleled the scientific data—mostly from cross-sectional studies—that showed declines in muscular strength and CR endurance across the life span. However, recent studies that have assessed the training adaptation in older individuals have shown that despite the inevitable decline in function that comes with aging, older persons can adapt to training and can even improve function, in a relative sense, as much as younger individuals (10-12). However, aging may influence the rate of adaptation (2, 13). We investigated this issue using a large group of adult participants in the Ball State University Adult Physical Fitness Program (297 men; 197 women) ranging in age from 20 to 72 years (14). We compared the improvement in $\dot{V}O_2max$ following the training program across the age range to determine whether the older individuals had a slower rate of improvement. The CR endurance training program consisted of a walk-jog routine for most participants and lasted approximately 16 weeks. The exercise training intensity was 75% to 85% of maximal HR reserve with a mean frequency and duration of four times per week for 30 to 50 min. As illustrated in figure 8.3, the older subjects (those >60 years of age) had an increase in aerobic power comparable to that of the younger subjects when expressed in relative terms (% increase). Now, we did not make serial measurements of $\dot{V}O_2max$ every few weeks during the training period to directly assess the rate of improvement per se, but the data in figure 8.3 suggest that the increase in $\dot{V}O_2max$ observed in older adults can occur within the first few months of training just as it does in

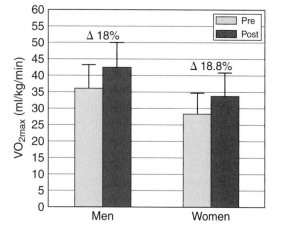

Figure 8.2 Adaptations in $\dot{V}O_2max$ for men and women following cardiorespiratory training.

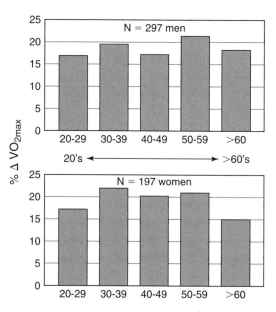

Figure 8.3 Influence of age on changes in $\dot{V}O_2max$ following cardiorespiratory training.

younger individuals. However, when the results illustrated in figure 8.3 were further adjusted for initial or baseline fitness levels among the subjects in the study, age was indeed inversely associated with the percentage increase in $\dot{V}O_2$max for both men and women, suggesting that older subjects may respond to training a bit more slowly. So, age may influence the rate of adaptation, but older adults can still improve their fitness to a degree similar to that for younger adults.

When one is assessing the amount of improvement in various physiological variables after a training program (change in $\dot{V}O_2$max, serum cholesterol, resting blood pressure, etc.), the initial or baseline measurement should be considered. Why is this important? The amount of physiological adaptation observed during an exercise training regimen is influenced by each individual's baseline training status. For example, studies show that the lower an individual's fitness level is at the beginning of a training program, the more it is likely to improve—provided there is a sufficient stimulus or **training overload.** Conversely, if you were to take a well-trained marathon runner and assess her change in $\dot{V}O_2$max following a few months of continued training, you might find very little, if any, change in aerobic power. Therefore, the further an individual is from his or her optimal physiological level, the more room the person has for improvement during training! This kind of association has been shown in study after study, across a wide range of physiological outcomes from exercise training. A simple illustration of this phenomenon is shown in figure 8.4. The data depict the changes in total serum cholesterol in a large group of male participants in

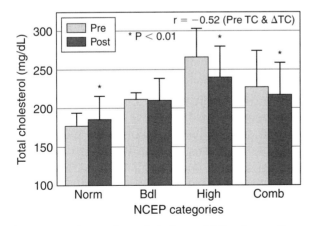

Figure 8.4 Changes in total cholesterol following cardiorespiratory training.
Reprinted, by permission, from M.H. Whaley, L.A. Kaminsky, L.H. Getchell, et al., 1992, "Changes in total cholesterol following endurance training: A function of initial values," *Journal of Cardiopulmonary Rehabilitation* 12:42-50.

the Ball State University Adult Physical Fitness Program (15). The training program consisted of 12 to 16 weeks of aerobic training, and each man had his fasting lipids measured before and after the program. As shown in the figure, those with the highest baseline concentrations for total cholesterol (National Cholesterol Education Program high-risk category) were the men who tended to have the largest declines in serum total cholesterol (10%) following the training program. In summary, when interpreting training adaptations, be sure to consider the baseline value before concluding that the observed change is as expected or not.

Consequences of Inactivity or Detraining

The principle of **detraining** reflects the adage, "Use it or lose it!" Following a period of exercise training, adaptation occurs. However, if training stops, the adaptations are lost over time. The fact that we lose our adaptation to training makes sense to most, but the often asked question is "How long will it take for me to lose the adaptation?" There is considerable interindividual variability in the rate at which we lose improvements in muscular strength or CR endurance. Coyle and colleagues showed that significant losses in CR endurance are apparent after only two weeks of detraining (16). Following an exercise training program, a decline in fitness to pretraining levels may take as little as 10 weeks (17). However, as professionals, we strongly advocate habitual physical activity. Therefore, the important question is not how long it would take to lose a training adaptation if we became totally sedentary. The important question is how much do we need to do during periods of reduced activity in order to maintain our muscular or CR fitness. The rate of loss in function depends, in part, on how much of a couch potato we become.

In a series of studies, Hickson and colleagues (18-20) evaluated the rate of loss of training adaptations during periods of reduced training. They reported that during periods of reduced training volume (decreased duration and frequency), the residual exercise training intensity is critical for maintenance of CR endurance. Their results showed that $\dot{V}O_2$max could be maintained for up to 15 weeks despite a reduction in training volume by as much as two-thirds. The critical issue was the training intensity. When the researchers altered the experiment by reducing training intensity while keeping the frequency and duration constant, the subjects experienced a significant reduction in $\dot{V}O_2$max. What about maintenance of muscular strength and endurance during periods of reduced training? Graves and colleagues (21) studied the effects of reduced frequency of resistance training in young men and women and concluded that muscular strength could be maintained for up to 12 weeks of reduced training with as little as one workout per week. So it would appear that the adage is correct—use it or lose it! However, according to a recent stand from the American College of Sports Medicine, missing a workout now and then, or reducing training for periods of two to three months, will not greatly affect maximal capacity as long as the training intensity remains adequate (2).

Summary

On the basis of the preceding discussion, it should be apparent that exercise training regimens need to be designed with specific outcomes in mind, and that there is considerable interindividual variability in the health and fitness adaptations following chronic participation in CR and muscular resistance-training regimens. You need to appreciate this type of variability when interpreting an individual's results from an exercise training program. The remainder of the chapter presents a discussion of training adaptations with a few case study examples to illustrate what you can realistically expect.

CHRONIC EXERCISE TRAINING ADAPTATIONS

As covered in chapter 7, the goals of an individualized exercise prescription are to enhance physical fitness (e.g., CR endurance, muscular strength/endurance) and promote health by modification of chronic disease risk factors (e.g., decrease excess body fat, normalize blood lipids or blood pressure). In fact, we often talk to potential participants in our programs about these benefits and encourage them to participate based on an expectation that they will experience some, if not all, of these improvements. But, although this sounds great in theory, the obvious question many of our participants ask is, "Can I really achieve these improvements if I follow your advice and initiate a regular exercise program?" In other words, can participants in our primary or secondary prevention programs really expect these adaptations to occur following a period of training?

We need to be careful extolling the virtues of habitual activity and not overstep what the research literature can support. What do the scientific studies tell us? Exercise training studies clearly support that a number of morphological and physiological adaptations occur subsequent to chronic aerobic or resistance-exercise training. These adaptations include both central and peripheral improvements in cardiovascular system function, changes in skeletal muscle structure and function, and improvements in various coronary artery disease risk factors. Of course, these adaptations are in line with the general principle of specificity of training. That is, adaptations in the cardiovascular system will result from a training regimen that stresses the aerobic metabolic pathways, putting an overload on the cardiovascular system. This section overviews typical adaptations to both CR endurance and musculoskeletal resistance-exercise training.

Cardiorespiratory Endurance Training

For reasons discussed in chapter 7, the primary form of exercise used in preventive or rehabilitative programs should be aerobic in nature. This form of exercise stresses the cardiorespiratory systems and has been associated with improvements of many CAD risk factors. This section of the chapter will present a summary of the changes in physiological function and risk factors associated with this form of exercise training.

Basic Physiological Changes

Numerous adaptations occur in the cardiovascular and skeletal muscle systems following chronic CR endurance training that rises to the intensity, frequency, and duration levels described in table 7.2 (2, 22-24). These collective adaptations—often referred to as a "training effect"—not only increase the CR system's ability to meet the demands of acute exercise; they also contribute to many of the long-term health benefits (decrease in CAD risk factors) associated with an active lifestyle. Moreover, these physiological adaptations generally follow a dose-response pattern, with greater exercise training intensity, frequency, and duration producing larger adaptations. Individuals who participate in light-to moderate-intensity physical activity—below the quality and quantity described in chapter 7 (table 7.2)—may certainly benefit by a reduction in risk for several chronic diseases (CAD, stroke, type II diabetes mellitus, etc.), but will probably not accrue most of the physiological adaptations described in table 8.1. Dr. Per-Olaf Astrand, a Swedish physician and noted exercise physiologist, sums it up this way:

Physical activity is not synonymous with physical training. The training stimulus must be of a certain intensity and duration to produce any training effect.

Therefore, when designing an exercise training program in which the desired outcome is both improvement in aerobic power and reduction in CAD risk factors, you will need to incorporate a threshold dose of exercise (i.e., intensity + frequency + duration) that has been shown to result in the physiological adaptations outlined in table 8.1.

A major goal for most adults participating in aerobic exercise programs is an improvement in their CR fitness defined as the maximal amount of oxygen ($\dot{V}O_2$max) one can utilize during exhaustive exercise (26). As presented in table 8.1, the increase in $\dot{V}O_2$max following training ranges between 10% and 30% in previously untrained adults (2). This improvement is inversely related to the initial or baseline value—meaning that af-

ter adjustment for other variables known to influence the training response (e.g., training intensity, duration), the lower an individual's fitness prior to the training program, the larger the potential for an improvement in fitness. As reviewed in the previous section, older individuals have the ability to improve their $\dot{V}O_2$max to a relative degree similar to that for younger individuals, but the rate of improvement may be slower. Thus, older individuals may take a longer training duration (months) to achieve the adaptation.

Adaptations at Maximal Exercise

What contributes to the increase in $\dot{V}O_2$max following training? Several key physiological adaptations are summarized in table 8.1. These adaptations are often referred to as either **central adaptations** (changes in the central circulation leading to an increase in cardiac output) or **peripheral adaptations** (changes in the peripheral delivery and utilization of oxygen). However, whether the adaptations are central or peripheral, they collectively contribute to the increase in $\dot{V}O_2$max and a significant reduction in the CR strain felt during submaximal exercise. As you learned in chapter 2, $\dot{V}O_2$max is the product of cardiac output (HR × stroke volume) and the

Table 8.1

Typical Physiological Adaptations to CR Endurance Training in Previously Untrained Individuals

Variable	Unit of measure	Training change	Range of change
Maximal exercise			
$\dot{V}O_2$max	ml/kg/min	↑	≈10–30%
Cardiac output	liters/min	↑	≈10–20%
HR_{max}	beats/min	↔ or ↓	Very little if any
Stroke volume	mls/beat	↑	Varies
a-$\bar{v}$ O_2 diff	mls O_2/100 mls blood	↑	Varies
Submaximal exercise			
Cardiac output	liters/min	↔ or ↓	Minimal
Heart rate	beats/min	↓	≈10–30 bpm
Stroke volume	mls/beat	↑	Varies
a-$\bar{v}$ O_2 diff	mls O_2/100 mls	↑	8–10%
Systolic/diastolic BP	mmHg	↔ or ↓	Varies
Rate pressure product	HR × SBP	↓	Varies
Resting values			
Cardiac output	liters/min	↔	
Heart Rate	beats/min	↓	Varies (≈10 bpm)
Stroke volume	mls/beat	↑	Varies
Systolic/diastolic BP	mmHg	↔ or ↓	Varies

↑ = increase; ↓ = decrease; ↔ little if any change; a-$\bar{v}$ O_2 diff = arteriovenous oxygen difference.

amount of oxygen extracted from the arterial circulation at peak exercise. The increase in cardiac output is brought about primarily by an increase in left ventricular stroke volume, which is the result of several factors (increased plasma volume, increased preload, decreased peripheral vascular resistance) (22). Maximal HR does not appear to change much with chronic training, but some might encounter a slight decline (3-4 bpm). Oxygen extraction is referred to as the **arteriovenous oxygen difference (a-$\bar{v}$ O_2 diff)** and is typically measured as the number of milliliters of O_2 extracted from 100 ml of arterial blood passing across an active skeletal muscle bed.The increase in maximal a-$\bar{v}$ O_2 diff is brought about primarily by an increase in oxidative capacity and capillary density within the recruited skeletal muscle mass (22). So, increases in both cardiac output and a-$\bar{v}$ O_2 diff at **maximal exercise** contribute to the overall improvement in $\dot{V}O_2$max following an aerobic training program. However, it's important to remember that these two factors may not contribute equally in all individuals or at the same rate within an individual. Physiological changes that contribute to an increase in O_2 extraction by skeletal muscle (increased a-$\bar{v}$ O_2 diff) may occur sooner during the training program than the adaptations that contribute to an increase in blood flow (increased cardiac output) (22).

Adaptations During Submaximal Exercise

Several important cardiovascular adaptations that contribute to a more efficient cardiovascular response to submaximal exercise loads are summarized in table 8.1. So that comparisons before and after training can be made, these adaptations are usually expressed as changes at a standardized or given submaximal workload or oxygen consumption. To fully appreciate the mechanisms responsible for these adaptations, you will need to recall some of the basic cardiovascular physiology covered in chapter 2. That is, cardiac output is a function of HR and stroke volume, and the increase in cardiac output during exercise is in response to the increased metabolic demands of the skeletal muscle (increased $\dot{V}O_2$). Now, how does this change after CR endurance training? One of the most apparent cardiovascular adaptations following training is the reduction in HR at a given submaximal workload or $\dot{V}O_2$. Figure 8.5a illustrates this phenomenon throughout the submaximal stages of a graded exercise test for a 38-year-old man after six months of training in the adult fitness program at Ball State. During most of the exercise test, the man had a 15 to 20

bpm lower HR at the same workload following training. The lower HR is brought about by the combination of increases in left ventricular stroke volume and skeletal muscle a-$\bar{v}$ O_2 diff. So, the reduction in HR during submaximal exercise reflects both central (i.e., increased stroke volume) and peripheral (i.e., increased a-$\bar{v}$ O_2 diff) adaptations following the training program. In fact, the decline in HR at standardized submaximal workloads following training is an excellent way to document an improvement in CR fitness, especially when it's impractical to repeat a maximal exercise test to assess $\dot{V}O_2$max.

Reduction in Submaximal Heart Rate

The reduction in submaximal HR after training has several important ramifications. First, recall from our discussion of target HRs in chapter 7 that the target HR served as a surrogate marker of the target metabolic rate for training (i.e., $\dot{V}O_2$). Again, it's important to remember that the bottom-line variable was the target $\dot{V}O_2$. Now, let's take another look at the submaximal data for our 38-year-old man. Even though the x-axis on the graph represents time on the test protocol, it essentially represents a specific oxygen demand within the "graded" exercise test. Now, in the preceding

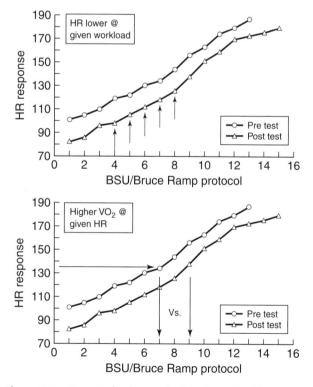

Figure 8.5 Case study changes in *(a)* submaximal heart rate following cardiorespiratory training and *(b)* $\dot{V}O_2$ following cardiorespiratory training.

paragraph, we focused attention on the lower HR for a given $\dot{V}O_2$ following training. However, for the purposes of understanding the impact of the training adaptation on this man's exercise prescription, let's reshuffle the deck, so to speak, and consider the higher $\dot{V}O_2$ at any given submaximal HR. To do this, start at any submaximal HR value on the y-axis of figure 8.5b and move across the graph to the right, noting the pre- versus posttest values for $\dot{V}O_2$. The posttest $\dot{V}O_2$ is shifted to the right, meaning it's higher following the training program. Is this an important adaptation? You bet it is! It means that at the same target HR, this person's metabolic rate, and thus energy expenditure, will be higher during future exercise sessions. For our case study man, his metabolic rate is about 2 METs higher at a HR of 135 bpm following the training program. For this man, the 2 MET increase in metabolic rate translates into 3 more kcals expended each minute of exercise when compared to his pre-training value. This has clear implications for other risk factor changes after the training (e.g., decreased body fat, hypertension, etc.). A later section of the chapter has more on changes in CAD risk factors.

In addition to the reduction in HR, both systolic blood pressure and diastolic blood pressure are generally reduced following a training regimen, and the product of HR and systolic pressure—known as the **rate-pressure product (RPP)** or double product—is therefore lower as well. This adaptation has clinical implications, as the RPP correlates well with myocardial oxygen demand, and reductions in the RPP following CR endurance training reflect a reduction in myocardial stress during submaximal exercise. So, this reduction in RPP reflects a decline in the overall workload of the heart during exercise. Although this adaptation is beneficial for everyone, it is especially important to cardiac patients who have an ischemic threshold that must be considered when the training intensity is being defined. As discussed in chapter 7, cardiac patients with exercise-induced myocardial ischemia must have their exercise training intensity set below their ischemic threshold (by approximately 10 bpm). While this provides for an important safety buffer during training, it unfortunately imposes a ceiling on the energy expenditure rate during training (kcal·min^{-1}) for such patients. However, as a patient's ischemic threshold is usually associated with a given RPP, the reduction in the RPP at a given workload following training allows cardiac patients to exercise at a higher absolute workload before reaching their ischemic threshold.

Adaptations at Rest

Table 8.1 also presents cardiovascular adaptations at rest following chronic CR endurance training. Although the degree of these changes varies considerably from person to person, one can typically expect a reduction in resting HR coupled with an increase in stroke volume. These changes result in a fairly stable resting cardiac output. Adaptations in resting blood pressure depend on the baseline or pretraining value, with little or no change for people with normal pretraining blood pressure. However, there can be clinically significant reductions in both systolic and diastolic pressure for those with mild to moderate hypertension (27). See chapter 9 for more details.

Coronary Artery Disease Risk Factor Changes

In addition to the improvement in $\dot{V}O_2$max and the cardiovascular adaptations just described, CR endurance exercise training can result in favorable changes for a number of the CAD risk factors identified in chapter 1. A listing of CAD risk factors and their potential adaptation to endurance training is presented in table 8.2, along with some key references for review. As discussed in the previous section on training principles, there is considerable variability among individuals regarding the amount of change in most of the risk factors listed in table 8.2. Some people will have rather large changes in their risk factor profile following exercise training, whereas in others the exercise will have little effect. In addition, favorable changes in each of the risk factors listed in table 8.2 are seldom due to the exercise intervention alone. The majority of studies have shown that changes in lipids, blood pressure, obesity, and glucose tolerance following training are affected by baseline values, the overall exercise dose, other lifestyle factors such as nutritional habits, and changes in body composition. Therefore, an individual's response to training is, at best, hard to predict.

Literally hundreds of research studies have reported favorable changes in the blood lipid profile following chronic exercise training (28-30). Increases in high-density lipoprotein cholesterol along with decreases in low-density lipoprotein cholesterol and triglycerides are the changes most commonly reported. The studies are mixed with regard to changes in total cholesterol, with many reporting no change and others reporting slight reductions. However, as mentioned earlier, the alteration in the lipid profile following endurance training is dependent on a number of factors, one being the baseline or pretraining value. For

Table 8.2
**Potential Changes in CAD Risk Factors Associated With Chronic
CR Endurance Training in Previously Untrained Individuals**

Risk factor	General direction of adaptation	Approximate magnitude of adaptation
Lipids[1] Total cholesterol LDL-C HDL-C Triglycerides	→ or ↓ ↓ ↑ ↓	Varies depending on pretraining value, and changes in diet, BW, BF, medications, etc.
Hypertension[2] Systolic BP Diastolic BP	→ or ↓ → or ↓	Varies depending on changes in BW and diet, total exercise dose, etc. SBP & DBP ↓ ~ 10 mmHg in persons with mild to moderate HTN
Body composition[3] Body fat % Regional obesity	↓ ↓	Varies depending on obesity status & combination of total exercise dose (kcals) and dietary changes
Glucose tolerance[4]	↑	Varies depending on glycemic status, obesity status, combination of total exercise dose (kcals) and dietary changes, etc.
Clinical depression[5]	↓	

LDL-C = low-density lipoprotein cholesterol; HDL-C = high-density lipoprotein cholesterol; BF = body fat; BW = body weight; HTN = hypertension
1. Reference (28-30, 33).
2. Reference (27); moderate hypertension as defined in chapter 3.
3. Reference (33, 37).
4. Reference (33).
5. Reference (33, 38).

instance, we found a correlation of –0.51 between the baseline total cholesterol and the change following training in a study of 552 individuals in the adult fitness program at Ball State (15). This means that individuals with "normal" lipid profiles might not experience much of a change following training, but that those with the most abnormal values are more likely to see favorable changes. Therefore, view all clients or patients who have abnormal lipid profiles as potential responders to exercise training.

Research has also shown a favorable effect of CR endurance training on mild to moderate hypertension, with mean reductions in both resting systolic and diastolic pressures of approximately 10 mmHg in well-controlled trials (27). Figure 8.6 illustrates the changes in resting blood pressure following four to five months of CR endurance training within a large group of participants in the adult fitness program at Ball State. The 550 individuals represented in the figure are stratified into hypertensive (n = 60 systolic blood pressure [SBP] >140 mmHg; n = 110 diastolic blood pressure [DBP] >90 mmHg) and nonhypertensive groups. Each subject completed four to six months of CR endurance training; the regimen consisted

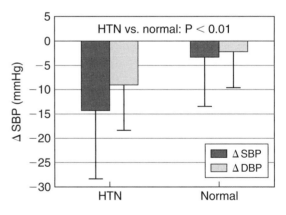

Figure 8.6 Changes in resting blood pressure following cardiorespiratory endurance training. Note the rather large standard deviation around the mean group change.

of walking or walk-jogging four times per week for 30 to 45 min at an intensity of 60% to 80% of maximal HR reserve. As illustrated in the figure, subjects who were hypertensive before the study were much more likely to achieve reductions in both systolic and diastolic pressures than subjects who were not hypertensive. The magnitudes of the mean reductions for the hypertensive individuals (–14 mmHg SBP and –9 mmHg DBP) are consistent with the results reported in the review paper cited earlier. So, the potential for reductions in both systolic and diastolic pressure following CR endurance training clearly exists; however, as illustrated in the figure (i.e., large standard deviation associated with the mean group change), the response varies considerably from individual to individual.

Although the increases in energy expenditure associated with initiating an exercise program are very important for body weight and fat reduction, the amount of energy typically expended during the initial months of training does not contribute to large weight or fat reductions for most people. In a review of 17 CR endurance training studies (32) including 342 subjects, Dr. Michael Pollock reported a mean body weight loss across the studies of 0 to 2 kg (0-4.4 lb) and a mean body fat loss of 0% to 3.8%. The training programs included in the review were typically four to five months in duration, with the mode of exercise usually jogging. Therefore, significant decreases in body weight and fat are clearly achievable, but should be viewed as long-term goals within both primary and secondary prevention programs. Given this, one of the goals during the first few months of training is to increase an individual's functional capacity so that the energy deficit during training sessions increases. Again, as discussed in chapter 7, many less fit clients or patients will need to "get in shape" before they are ready to use exercise as a means for weight loss.

So far we have considered typical physiological and risk factor adaptations to chronic CR endurance training. However, it's important to remember—on the basis of the principle of individuality discussed earlier in the chapter—that not all participants achieve these changes to the same degree or at the same rate during a program. Nevertheless, the changes do represent the potential for adaptation for individuals who participate in our primary or secondary prevention programs. And furthermore, we have collectively evaluated, trained, and counseled several thousand clients or patients following their participation in our adult fitness and cardiac rehabilitation programs during the past 20 years and have come to appreciate the varying responses to the same dose of exercise during training. The student can obtain some insight into the interpretation of exercise training responses by reviewing physiological and risk factor adaptations for our three case studies at the end of this chapter. We hope this will help to amplify the readers' understanding of the typical training adaptations described in this discussion, and also—through the use of real data from our programs—provide ex-

amples of realistic expectations for training outcomes.

Musculoskeletal Resistance Training

As discussed in chapter 7, resistance exercise is an important component of a well-rounded exercise program, provided the individual is cleared for participation in this type activity. This section of the chapter will present a summary of the changes in physiological function and risk factors associated with this form of exercise training.

Basic Physiological Changes

As outlined in chapter 7, a complete well-rounded exercise program should include a musculoskeletal resistance-training component. Within both primary and secondary prevention programs, the major goals for participation in this mode of activity are as follows:

- Muscular strength
- Muscular endurance
- Maintenance of fat-free mass during periods of weight reduction
- Maintenance of functional independence during later years of life

The physiological adaptations to resistance training tend to follow a dose-response pattern, with higher-volume/higher-intensity regimens yielding greater adaptation. In addition, because a wide array of training regimens is available (e.g., isotonic vs. isokinetic; straight sets vs. pyramid protocols, free weights vs. machines, etc.), it's important to remember that musculoskeletal training adaptations are also likely to be specific to the type and intensity of the regimen selected for training. However, no criterion reference norms are available that describe how much muscular strength and/or endurance a participant in a primary or secondary prevention program needs. Therefore, most guideline statements (34, 35) recommend a dose of training that represents the minimal amount associated with meeting the first two of the training goals just listed (i.e., strength and endurance).

Musculoskeletal Adaptations Increasing Strength and Endurance

After as little as 8 to 10 weeks of resistance training using the minimal dose characterized in chapter 7, adults can experience significant increases in both muscular strength and endurance. The magnitude of the improvements can typically range between 15% and 30% for commonly used exercises (see chapter 7). These adaptations are independent of gender and age. In other words, women respond similarly to men, and older individuals can achieve adaptation as much as their younger counterparts when the adaptation is expressed in relative terms (i.e., percentage improvement). However, as previously mentioned, the amount of improvement depends on several factors, such as the training volume and the individual's initial strength and endurance levels. Most adults who have never participated in resistance training and who start a regimen of 8 to 10 exercises, with a dose of one set of 8 to 12 reps performed twice a week, will have noticeable improvements during the first months of training. They may choose to slow the progression at this point and just maintain their new strength/endurance level, or some may want to increase the dose of training, seeking further improvements.

Health-Related Changes

While one can find resistance-training studies that report improvements in selected CAD risk factors following several months of training (e.g., decreased lipids, increased glucose tolerance, etc.), the magnitude of the adaptations is generally less than that reported after CR endurance training. In addition, we do not advocate resistance training as the sole mode of exercise. Resistance training should be viewed as one part of a program that contains an appropriate dose of CR endurance exercise as the base. Therefore, although it is possible for resistance-training regimens to contribute to an improvement in selected CAD risk factors, these adaptations are likely to occur in response to the CR endurance training that serves as the base for the overall exercise program. However, resistance training remains an integral component of the well-rounded exercise program because of its unique role with respect to overall muscular strength and endurance, maintenance of lean body mass during periods of weight reduction, and functional independence in later years.

SUMMARY

In this chapter we discussed several general principles that influence the type and magnitude of exercise training adaptations within primary and secondary prevention programs. We then addressed expected physiological and health-related adaptations that occur after participation in CR or muscular resistance regimens. Finally, we provided three exercise training case studies that illustrate not only the training adaptations, but also the ways in which these adaptations lead to a reduction in risk for CAD in both the primary and secondary prevention settings. After reading this chapter, students should have a better understanding of the range of benefits that participants in primary and secondary prevention programs can achieve through regular participation.

Case Study 1
Primary Prevention: Low Risk

Table 8.3 contains pre- and posttraining data for our 38-year-old man who participated in the Ball State University Adult Physical Fitness Program. This man reported participation in a recreational basketball league one to two nights per week but no other regular physical activity at the time he joined the program. A review of his health history questionnaire revealed no signs or symptoms of cardiac, pulmonary, or metabolic disease. He had never smoked, and he denied any family history of CAD. He was not taking any medications at the time he presented for entry into the program. A review of the risk factor data in table 8.3 reveals hypertension (both SBP and DBP) and hyperlipidemia (LDL-C >130 mmHg) as positive CAD risk factors within the risk stratification guidelines from the ACSM (34). While his body composition would not place him in the obese category (BMI <30), he is overweight for his height (BMI >25) and overfat (24% body fat) by the body fat standards presented in chapter 6. In addition, his waist girth and waist:hip ratio reflect an abdominal obesity pattern. Thus, he's a definite candidate for a regular exercise program and potentially other interventions targeting his hypertension, hyperlipidemia, and obesity. Regular exercise would be a key intervention for this man, as each of these risk factors can be favorably affected by CR endurance exercise training (table 8.2). Thus, modification of each of these risk factors became a focus within his primary prevention program.

Table 8.3
Pre/Post Training Data for Case Study 1

Resting variables	Pretraining	Posttraining	% change
Resting HR (bpm)	65	54	↓ 17
Resting BP (mmHg)	144/100 148/106	124/72	↓ 14 SPB ↓ 28 DBP
Body Composition			
Body weight (kg)	92.1	81.6	↓ 11
BMI (kg · m^{-2})	28.0	24.9	↓ 11
Percent body fat*	23.9	16	
Waist circumference (cm)	95.8	85.5	↓ 11
Waist/hip ratio	0.90	0.83	↓ 8
Blood values			
Total cholesterol (mg / dl)	238	222	↓ 7
HDL-C (mg / dl)	45	55	↑ 22
LDL-C (mg / dl)	169	154	↓ 9
Triglycerides (mg / dl)	120	67	↓ 44
Glucose (mg / dl)	108	101	↓ 6
Peak exercise variables			
Exercise time** (min:sec)	13:20	15:11	↑ 14
Peak workload (mph/%)	4.6/16.8	5.1/18.0	↑
$\dot{V}O_2$max (ml·kg^{-1}·min^{-1})	45.2	57.6	↑ 27
RERmax	1.19	1.15	na
MHR (bpm)	187	183	↓ 2
Peak BP (mmHg)	186/86	196/68	↑ SBP/↓ DBP
Peak RPE (6-20 scale)	20	20	→

HR = heart rate; bpm = beats per minute; BP = blood pressure; kg = kilograms; BMI = body mass index; cm = centimeters; mg% = milligrams percent; HDL-C = high-density lipoprotein cholesterol; LDL-C = low-density lipoprotein cholesterol; RER = respiratory exchange ratio; RPE = rating of perceived exertion; MHR = maximal heart rate.

* Body density determined using the sum of 7 skinfolds (39) and converted to % fat using Siri equation (40).

**BSU-Bruce Ramp treadmill protocol (41).

On the basis of his preliminary data, this man would have been categorized in the moderate risk category according to the ACSM Guidelines (34). Although he could have begun a moderate-intensity exercise regimen without having completed an exercise test, he underwent a maximal exercise test in our laboratory, which provided maximal HR and $\dot{V}O_2$ data for exercise prescription purposes as well as a baseline for evaluating training adaptations. A summary of the peak exer-

cise data is presented at the bottom of table 8.3. His GXT responses were within normal limits (i.e., no anginal symptoms, normal BP and ECG responses), and he was cleared to participate in the fitness program. His pretraining CR fitness level ($\dot{V}O_2$max of 45.2 ml/kg/min) was at the 75th percentile for men his age, which is a good level of CR fitness level but one that could be improved with training. Following a discussion of his risk factors and exercise testing results, he was given an exercise prescription consistent with the concepts presented in chapter 7. He participated in the training program on a very consistent basis for six months, at which time he was re-evaluated in the lab to assess his responses to the training program.

This patient's training adaptations are summarized in table 8.3. He showed a significant improvement in his fitness as well as in each of his CAD risk factors following the six months of training. His $\dot{V}O_2$max increased almost 30% to 57 ml/kg/min, which places him above the 90th percentile for men his age. He lost 23 lb (10.4 kg) during the six months, and both his whole-body (% fat) and regional fat (waist girth and waist:hip ratio) measures were significantly reduced. His posttraining resting blood pressures were within the normal range (<140 SBP, <90 DBP), and his lipid profile was markedly improved with a total cholesterol:HDL ratio of 4.0 compared to the pretraining value of 5.3. His fasting glucose measure, although not considered abnormal at baseline, was improved as well. Therefore, after six months, this man essentially had a normalization of all of his CAD risk factors! Now, can every patient expect these kinds of results during six months? The answer, unfortunately, is no. For this man, however, these were real changes that definitely reduced his risk for CAD.

We can quantify his CAD risk reduction using the Framingham risk score concept presented in chapter 1 (figure 1.14a for men). Once we have this estimate, we can compare it to the average risk for others of the same age. (At this point you may want to review the concepts of absolute and relative risk discussed in chapter 1.) Using this 38-year-old man's CAD risk factor data (table 8.3), what's the likelihood he will develop CAD by the time he's 48? And more importantly, based on the improvement in his risk factors following training, how much was his CAD risk reduced? The CAD probabilities using his pretraining and posttraining risk factors are shown in table 8.4.

This man's 10-year CAD risk based on pretraining levels of his risk factors was 7%. As described in chapter 1, this means that 7 of 100 men with his set of risk factors will develop CAD within the next 10 years. Using step 9 in figure 1.14a, we would estimate the average risk for men our case's age at 5% during the next 10 years.

Table 8.4

Pre/Post Training Framingham Risk Scores for Case Study 1

Risk factor	Pretraining FRS points	Posttraining FRS points
Age	0	0
LDL-C	1	0
HDL-C	0	0
Resting BP	3	0
Diabetes mellitus	0	0
Smoking	0	0
Total points	4	0
10 yr risk[1] (%)	7%	4%

FRS = Framingham Risk Score; LDL-C = low-density lipoprotein cholesterol; HDL-C = high-density lipoprotein cholesterol; BP = blood pressure.
1 = absolute CAD risk.

Therefore, our man's relative risk would be defined as follows:

Pretraining CAD Risk

Individual's absolute risk = 7%

Average absolute risk = 5%

Relative risk (RR) = 7/5 = 1.4

The 1.4 RR statistic reflects that before training, our 38-year-old man had a 40% greater CAD risk than the average man his age. But let's look at what happened to his risk estimate as a consequence of the risk factor changes following the training program. Calculation of the Framingham risk score using his posttraining data yields a total of 0 points, which translates into a 4% absolute CAD risk as we follow the steps in figure 1.14a. When we compare our case's posttraining 4% CAD risk to the average for men his age (i.e., 5%), the RR is now <1.0 (see calculations below). A RR of <1.0 means that our man's 10-year CAD risk is now less than the average risk for men his age.

Posttraining CAD Risk

Individual's absolute risk = 4%

Average absolute risk = 5%

RR = 4/5 = 0.80

So, normalization of CAD risk factors can have a quantifiable benefit, and we will often use these data to illustrate the benefits of risk factor modification to our program participants.

Now, it's worth repeating that not all partici-pants will achieve these kinds of results following six months of risk factor intervention. However, taking up a more active lifestyle, and modifying other lifestyle factors (smoking, nutrition, etc.) known to increase one's risk for CAD, can clearly have an impact on disease risk. We certainly wish that all of the participants in our programs could lower their CAD risk to the degree illustrated by our 38-year-old case study, but realistically, that's not likely to happen. Because the potential is there, though, we will continue to promote regular exer-cise as well as the other important interventions discussed in chapter 4.

Case Study 2
Primary Prevention: High Risk

Table 8.5 contains pre- and posttraining data for the 50-year-old man with a history of multiple CAD risk factors who participated in the Wake Forest University Cardiac Rehabilitation Program. In ad-dition to his other risk factors, he also presented to the program with a medical history of type 1 dia-betes, hypertension, peptic ulcer, sleep apnea, and a prior knee injury. He was a nonsmoker and led a rather sedentary lifestyle. A cardiac catheterization performed immediately prior to program entry re-vealed a normal left ventricular ejection fraction of 60%, with mild CAD lesions in the left anterior descending artery and left circumflex artery (LCX), but these were not of the magnitude to warrant any interventional procedure. This man was asymp-tomatic at rest and had a normal resting ECG, and his chart revealed the medications in the follow-ing list at the time of program entry. (Refer to the medication tables in chapter 4 for specific infor-mation about each medication.)

Medication	Dose Change Following Training
Atenolol	→
Accupril	↓
Lasix	→
K-Dur	↓
Lipitor	→
ASA (aspirin)	→
NTG (nitroglycerine) (prn)	↓
Insulin	↓

Because of his subclinical disease status (mild CAD lesions without symptoms), some programs would choose to risk-stratify this individual according to the procedures from the AACVPR Guidelines that were described in chapter 7. On the basis of the data provided, he would be stratified as low risk for cardiac events (table 7.11), but as high risk for disease progression (table 7.12) because of his obesity, hyperlipidemia, diabetes, and sedentary lifestyle. Thus, this man is a definite candidate for a regular exercise program with primary goals fo-cused on reducing body weight/fat, normalizing the lipid profile, reducing the reliance on medica-tions to control his blood pressure, and perhaps lowering the dosage of insulin required to control his blood glucose. Just as with our previous case study, regular exercise will be a key intervention for this man, as each of his risk factors can be fa-vorably affected by CR endurance exercise train-ing (table 8.2).

This gentleman completed a maximal treadmill exercise test with an individualized ramp protocol (36). A summary of his peak exercise data is pre-sented at the bottom of table 8.5. His GXT responses were within normal limits (i.e., no angina symptoms, normal BP and ECG responses), and thus he was cleared to participate in the cardiac rehabilitation program. You'll note that his peak HR response dur-ing the test was significantly lower than the age-pre-dicted value. This is mostly due to the medication, atenolol, which is a beta adrenergic blocker. Beta blockers lower HR and blood pressure at rest and during exercise. The test termination criterion was leg fatigue, and the patient reported an RPE of 17 (Borg 6-20 scale) at the end of the test. The test was considered a fatigue-limited test with no abnormal responses. Following a discussion of his risk factors and exercise test results, he was given the exercise prescription described in chapter 7. He participated in the Cardiac Rehabilitation Program at Wake For-est University on a very consistent basis for three months, at which time he was re-evaluated in the lab to assess his responses to the training program.

Table 8.5
Pre/Post Training Data for Case Study 2

Resting Variables	Pretraining	Posttraining	% change
Resting HR (bpm)	60	47	↓ 22
Resting BP (mmHg)	118/68	120/70	→
Body Composition			
Body weight (kg)	163.7	145.6	↓ 11
BMI (kg · m⁻²)	43.9	39.1	↓
Percent body fat	na	31.1	
Blood values			
Total cholesterol (mg / dl)	243	123	↓ 50
HDL-C (mg / dl)	35	31	↓ 11
LDL-C (mg / dl)	178	77	↓ 57
TC/HDL-C	6.9	3.9	↓ 43
Triglycerides (mg / dl)	152	75	↓ 51
Hb A₁c (%)	11.3	7.5	↓ 34
Peak exercise variables			
Peak workload (mph/%)	2.5/7.0	2.5/8.5	↑
V̇O₂peak (ml·kg⁻¹·min⁻¹)	16.1	17.5	↑ 9
MHR (bpm)	103	102	→
Peak BP (mmHg)	142/68	136/70	→
Peak RPE (6-20 scale)	17	17	→
ECG	Negative	Negative	→
Angina (0-5)	0	0	→
Termination criteria	Leg fatigue	Knee pain	

HR = heart rate; bpm = beats per minute; BP = blood pressure; kg = kilograms; mg% = milligrams percent; HDL-C = high-density lipoprotein cholesterol; LDL-C = low-density lipoprotein cholesterol; HbA₁c = gylcosylated hemoglobin concentration; RPE = rating of perceived exertion; MHR = maximal heart rate.

What happened to this man after three months of participation in the cardiac rehabilitation program? Did he reach any of his goals? His posttraining data are also summarized in table 8.5. Let's focus on his CAD risk factors first. This cardiac patient had a significant reduction in body weight (losing 40 lb [18 kg]) and fat during the three months of training. In addition, both his waist girth and waist:hip ratio decreased (data not shown), reflecting a reduction in the abdominal fat mass. A reduction in excess abdominal fat is often associated with an improvement in the metabolic profile (decreased lipids and increased glucose tolerance). In addition to the changes in his body composition, he had rather impressive improvements in his lipid profile. There is little doubt that his antihyperlipidemic medication, Lipitor, was responsible for part of the improvement in his lipid profile; but we certainly can't discount the collective impact of the increase in physical activity and the decrease in abdominal fat mass. While he did incur a slight reduction in HDL-C, his LDL-C is now <100 mg/dl, which is the treatment goal for cardiac patients; and his total cholesterol:HDL ratio decreased by about 40%. Therefore, his lipid profile was much improved. His resting blood pressure was controlled well with medication at baseline, so a significant decrease was unlikely following training. However, one of his antihypertensive medications (Accupril) was reduced, perhaps reflecting less reliance on the medications to control his pressure. And finally, his diabetic status was favorably affected after three months of intervention as evidenced by a decline in his glycosylated hemoglobin level (7.5% posttraining) and a reduction in the amount of insulin needed to regulate his blood glucose.

What happened to this patient's CR fitness level after three months of exercise training? He had a 9% increase in $\dot{V}O_2$peak; but this may not reflect the true adaptation, as his posttraining treadmill test was stopped due to leg pain rather than overall fatigue. However, a 9% increase is a significant improvement, and most likely during the next three months he will continue to improve his fitness. But another way to assess improvement is to look at HR and BP responses to standardized workloads during the test. As you recall from earlier in the chapter, a lower HR and/or SBP following training reflect a lower overall workload on the heart at any level of submaximal exercise. Figure 8.7 shows this patient's pre- and posttraining RPP data, and the figure illustrates the training adaptation quite

nicely. At comparable submaximal MET levels, his RPP was lower after the training program.

Therefore, after three months of participation in the secondary prevention program, this patient had improved his CAD risk factor profile considerably (decreased obesity, lipids, diabetes). However, we would all agree that he is not done yet. He can't afford to rest on his laurels! He could benefit from a further reduction in body weight and fat, as well as from further increases in his functional capacity. These goals will be pursued as he continues with the program.

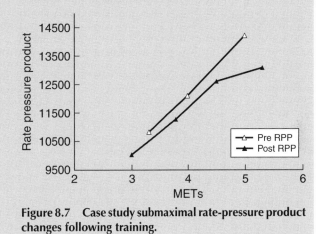

Figure 8.7 **Case study submaximal rate-pressure product changes following training.**

Case Study 3
Secondary Prevention: Post-MI and PTCA/Stent

Table 8.6 contains pre- and posttraining data for our 61-year-old cardiac patient. This patient attended the cardiac rehabilitation program exercise sessions on a consistent basis during the three-month period between his lab evaluations. As you recall from previous discussions, this patient had a history of MI, and PTCA with stent. He was being treated with a number of the medications reviewed in chapter 4. On the basis of his assorted risk factors, he would have been stratified as moderate risk for disease progression at baseline (table 7.12). Risk factor targets for the rehabilitation program were his sedentary lifestyle, excess body fat, and hyperlipidemia. As with our previous cases, regular exercise would be a key intervention for this man, since each risk factor can be favorably affected by CR endurance exercise training (table 8.2).

What happened to this man after three months of participation in the Cardiac Rehabilitation Program at Wake Forest? Did he improve his CR endurance or modify any of his risk factors for disease progression? We'll look first at his CAD risk factors. This patient had a modest reduction in body weight (losing 6 lb [2.7 kg]); but his body composition, assessed using the skinfold technique, did not show a change after three months of training. While this might be disappointing to some, it's not an atypical result after only three months of participation in the program. Remember, during the first month or so, his overall energy expenditure during the exercise sessions was rather low (<1000 kcal per week), and in this situation weight loss targets are more difficult to achieve by exercise alone in the initial months of training. Once he progresses to a higher volume of exercise, the

Table 8.6
Pre/Post Training Data for Case Study 3

Resting variables	Pretraining	Posttraining	% change
Resting HR (bpm)	67	60	↓ 22
Resting BP (mmHg)	130/72	138/80	↑
Body composition			
Body weight (kg)	100.7	98.0	↓ 2.7
BMI (kg · m⁻²)	29.3	28.6	↓ 2.3
Percent body fat	25.3	25.3	→
Blood values			
Total cholesterol (mg / dl)	186	112	↓ 40
HDL-C (mg / dl)	36	37	→
LDL-C (mg / dl)	131	58	↓ 56
TC/HDL-C	5.1	3.1	↓ 39
Triglycerides (mg / dl)	98	86	↓ 12
Peak exercise variables			
Peak workload (mph/%)	na	3.0/15	—
V̇O₂peak (ml·kg⁻¹·min⁻¹)	32.6	33.3 (22.4)	—
MHR (bpm)	136	128	↓ 6
Peak BP (mmHg)	na	144/80	—
Peak RPE (6-20 scale)	na	17	—
ECG	Negative	Borderline	
Angina (0-5)	0	0	→
Termination criteria	Fatigue	SOB	

HR = heart rate; bpm = beats per minute; BP = blood pressure; kg = kilograms; mg% = milligrams percent; HDL-C = high-density lipoprotein cholesterol; LDL-C = low-density lipoprotein cholesterol; RPE = rating of perceived exertion; SOB = shortness of breath.

weight loss target will be a more realistic goal. In these cases, we would focus more on the six-month and one-year outcomes.

This patient's other major risk factor was his baseline lipid profile. He was started on an antihyperlipidemic medication after his PTCA. As presented in table 8.6, he had rather impressive improvements in his lipid profile at the three-month evaluation. Almost certainly his antihyperlipidemic medication, Lipitor, was responsible for much of the improvement in his lipid profile, but we can't discount the collective impact of the increased physical activity. The most remarkable changes were the reductions in LDL-C (now <100 mg/dl, which is the treatment goal for cardiac patients)

and total cholesterol:HDL ratio. Therefore, his lipid profile was much improved. You will also note from table 8.6 that this man had a slight increase in resting blood pressure at the three-month assessment. However, as his posttraining values were still within the normal range, they do not represent a clinically important outcome at this time. His blood pressure should be monitored on a routine basis within the program and should the values begin to exceed the upper limit of normal, a consultation with his physician would be prudent.

What about this patient's CR fitness level following three months of exercise training? As you recall from our discussion in chapter 7, his baseline treadmill test did not include measurement of

$\dot{V}O_2$peak because of the nature of the test (i.e., stress echo), and therefore his baseline fitness level was estimated as 32.6 ml/kg/min using the ACSM equation. As already discussed, this was very likely an overestimate and makes the comparison with the posttest data problematic for several reasons. First, the baseline and follow-up treadmill tests involved different treadmill protocols, and this can lead to differences in the estimated value from the test. Second, you will note that there are two values in table 8.6 for $\dot{V}O_2$peak for the posttest. The first one (33.3) is the estimated value from the peak workload attained during the ramp treadmill test, whereas the second value (22.4) is the measured $\dot{V}O_2$peak from the same exercise test. Just as we thought, the estimated value is, in fact, a significant overestimate of this patient's CR fitness level. We suspected that this was the case with the pretest value and therefore didn't use the 9.3-MET value for his exercise prescription.

However, our issue here relates to the interpretation of his training response. As we pointed out in chapter 6, an apples-to-apples comparison with a measured $\dot{V}O_2$peak isn't possible because we don't have a measured value from the pretest. In addition, an apples-to-apples comparison between the estimated $\dot{V}O_2$peak isn't all that desirable because the values were derived from different protocols using different prediction equations. So where does this leave us? Most exercise program professionals would look back over the patient's exercise logs and evaluate the increase in the total volume and intensity of exercise completed by the patient. This would provide some insight into the increase in functional capacity that the patient experienced during the three months. A true apples-to-apples comparison with a measured $\dot{V}O_2$peak would be made after the next evaluation, three months down the road.

Finally, we want to look at the hemodynamic and diagnostic responses during the posttest GXT. As you can see in table 8.6, the patient's peak HR response was slightly reduced (i.e., –8 bpm) compared to that in the pre-test. While this is not an unusual finding following CR endurance training (see table 8.1), it may well be the result of the test end point, which was shortness of breath. The sensation of respiratory distress is often a termination criterion for cardiac patients, and this man's lower HR response during the second GXT may be associated with the onset of the symptom rather than a chronic adaptation. The other interesting finding is the ECG result at peak exercise (see figure 5.53). This patient's ECG response during the pre-training GXT was interpreted as normal; however, there was 1-2 mm of ST-segment depression on the peak tracing during the posttest. The attending physician interpreted the ECG as "borderline," but in light of the fact that the patient denied having any chest pain, and had had a normal stress echo exam three months earlier, the test was ruled "clinically negative." The ECG response was noted, and the patient would be followed during the subsequent training period for any changes in symptoms that might shed light on the ECG change noted on the GXT. As discussed in chapter 7, his exercise training intensity prescription would be set safely below the level that elicited the ST changes observed during the GXT. The target HR range presented in table 7.18 reflects this intensity.

Therefore, after three months of participation in the secondary prevention program, this patient had improved his CAD risk factor profile considerably by increasing his physical activity level and normalizing his lipid profile. However, we would all agree that he is not done yet, as he still has goals for decreasing his body fat and improving his CR fitness level. These goals will be pursued as he continues with the program.

GLOSSARY

Arteriovenous oxygen difference (a-$\bar{v}O_2$ diff): the difference between the oxygen content of arterial and venous blood, which represents the oxygen extracted or used by the body tissue; usually measured or estimated as whole-body difference using mixed venous blood returning to the heart, but can also be measured across smaller tissue areas (skeletal muscle group, heart, etc.)

Central adaptation: an adaptation following chronic exercise training that relates to the heart or central circulation

Detraining: a period of reduced exercise training or total cessation of exercise

Maximal exercise: activity at the highest intensity possible during exhaustive exercise

Peripheral adaptation: an adaptation following chronic exercise training relating to an increase in skeletal muscle function (i.e., strength or endurance) or extraction of oxygen (a-$\bar{v}O_2$ diff)

Rate-pressure product (RPP): the product of the heart rate and systolic blood pressure, related to the oxygen requirement of the heart muscle at rest and during exercise; also referred to as the double product

Submaximal exercise: exercise at an intensity of effort that is less than maximal; standardized submaximal intensities are often used to describe workloads (e.g., 50% of $\dot{V}O_2$max) or to evaluate a training response

Training overload: principle reflecting the concept that one must work against a greater load than what one is accustomed to before achieving training adaptations

Training specificity: principle reflecting the concept that training adaptations will occur in the specific organ systems or muscle groups involved in the training program

REFERENCES

1. Hurley, B.F., D.R. Seals, A.A. Ehsani, et al. 1984. Effects of high-intensity strength training on cardiovascular function. *Med. Sci. Sports Exerc.* 16:483–488.

2. American College of Sports Medicine. 1998. The recommended quantity and quality of exercise for developing and maintaining cardiorespiratory and muscular fitness, and flexibility in healthy adults. *Med. Sci. Sports Exerc.* 30:975–991.

3. McArdle, W.D., J.R. Margel, D.J. Delio, M. Toner, and J.M. Chase. 1978. Specificity of run training on $\dot{V}O_2$max and heart rate changes during running and swimming. *Med. Sci. Sports* 10:16–20.

4. Clausen, J.P. 1976. Circulatory adjustments to dynamic exercise and effect of physical training in normal subjects and in patients with coronary disease. *Progressive Cardiovasc. Dis.* 18:459–495.

5. Bouchard, C., R. Lasage, G. Lortie, et al. 1986. Aerobic performance in brothers, dizygotic and monozygotic twins. *Med. Sci. Sports Exerc.* 18:639–646.

6. Lesage, R., J.A. Simoneau, J. Jobin, J. Leblanc, and C. Bouchard. 1985. Familial resemblance in maximal heart rate, blood lactate and aerobic power. *Human Heredity* 35:182–189.

7. Poehlman, E.T., A. Tremblay, A. Nadeau, J. Dussault, G. Theriault, and C. Bouchard. 1986. Heredity and changes in hormones and metabolic rates with short-term training. *Am. J. Physiol.* 250:E711–7.

8. Simoneau, J.A., G. Lortie, M.R. Boulay, M. Marcotte, M.C. Thibault, and C. Bouchard. 1986. Inheritance of human skeletal muscle and anaerobic capacity adaptation to high-intensity intermittent training. *Int. J. Sports Med.* 7:167–171.

9. Bouchard, C., F.T. Dionne, J. Simoneau, and M.R. Boulay. 1992. Genetics of aerobic and anaerobic performances. In *Exercise and Sports Science Reviews*, ed. J.O. Holloszy, 27–58. Baltimore: Williams & Wilkins.

10. Meredith, C.N., W.R. Frontera, E.C. Fisher, et al. 1989. Peripheral effects of endurance training in young and old subjects. *J. Appl. Physiol.* 66:2844–2849.

11. Kohrt, W.M., M.T. Malley, A.R. Coggan, et al. 1991. Effects of gender, age and fitness level on response of $\dot{V}O_2$max to training in 60-71 yr olds. *J. Appl. Physiol.* 71:2004–2011.

12. Fiatarone, M.A., E.C. Marks, N.D. Ryan, C.N. Meredith, L.A. Lipsitz, and W.J. Evans. 1990. High-intensity strength training in nonagenarians: Effects on skeletal muscle. *J.A.M.A.* 263:3029–3034.

13. Seals, D.R., J.M. Hagberg, B.F. Hurley, A.A. Ehsani, and J.O. Holloszy. 1984. Endurance training in older men and women. I. Cardiovascular responses to exercise. *J. Appl. Physiol.* 57:1024–1029.

14. Nustad, J.K., M.H. Whaley, L.A. Kaminsky, and L.H. Getchell. 1991. Changes in aerobic power following an endurance training program as a function of age. *Med. Sci. Sports Exerc.* 23:S141.

15. Whaley, M.H., L.A. Kaminksy, L.H. Getchell, M.D. Kelly, and J.H. Treloar. 1992. Changes in total cholesterol following endurance training: A function of initial values. *J. Cardiopul. Rehabil.* 12:42–50.

16. Coyle, E.F., W.H. Martin, D.R. Sinacore, M.J. Joyner, J.M. Hagberg, and J.O. Holloszy. 1984. Time course of loss of adaptation after stopping prolonged intense endurance training. *J. Appl. Physiol.* 57:1857–1864.

17. Fringer, M.N., and A.G. Stull. 1974. Changes in cardiorespiratory parameters during periods of training and detraining in young female adults. *Med. Sci. Sports* 6:20–25.

18. Hickson, R.C., and M.A. Rosenkoetter. 1981. Reduced training frequencies and maintenance of increased aerobic power. *Med. Sci. Sports Exerc.* 13:13–16.

19. Hickson, R.C., C. Kanakis, J.R. Davis, A.M. Moore, and S. Rich. 1982. Reduced training duration effects on aerobic power, endurance, and cardiac growth. *J. Appl. Physiol.* 53:225–229.

20. Hickson, R.C., C. Foster, M.L. Pollock, T.M. Galassi, and S. Rich. 1985. Reduced training intensities and loss of aerobic power, endurance, and cardiac growth. *J. Appl. Physiol.* 58:492–499.

21. Graves, J.E., M.L. Pollock, S.H. Leggett, R.W. Braith, and D.M. Carpenter. 1988. Effect of reduced training frequency on muscular strength. *Int. J. Sports Med.* 9:316–319.

22. Rowell, L.B. 1986. *Human Circulation Regulation During Physical Stress.* New York: Oxford University Press.

23. Wilmore, J.H., and D.L. Costill. 1994. *Physiology of Sport and Exercise.* Champaign, IL: Human Kinetics.

24. Franklin, B.A., and J.L. Roitman. 1998. Cardiorespiratory adaptations to exercise. In *ACSM's Resource Manual for Guidelines for Exercise Testing and Prescription.* 3rd ed. J. Roitman, ed. Baltimore: Lippincott, Williams & Wilkins.

25. Astrand, P.O., and K. Rodahl. 1976. *Textbook of Work Physiology: Physiological Bases of Exercise.* 2nd ed. New York: McGraw-Hill.

26. Pollock, M.L., and J.H. Wilmore. 1990. *Exercise In Health And Disease: Evaluation And Prescription For Prevention And Rehabilitation.* 2nd ed. Philadelphia: Saunders.

27. Gordon, N.F. Hypertension. 1997. In *ACSM's Exercise Management For Persons With Chronic Diseases And Disabilities,* ed. J.L. Durstine, 269. Champaign, IL: Human Kinetics.

28. Durstine, J.L., and G.E. Moore. 1997. Hyperlipidemia. In *ACSM's Exercise Management For Persons With Chronic Diseases And Disabilities,* ed. J.L. Durstine, 101–105. Champaign, IL: Human Kinetics.

29. Lokey, E.A., and A.V. Tran. 1989. Effects of exercise training on serum lipid and lipoprotein concentrations in women. *Int. J. Sports Med.* 10:424–429.

30. Tran, Z.V., A. Weltman, G.V. Glass, and D.P. Mood. 1983. The effects of exercise on blood lipid and lipoproteins: A meta-analysis of studies. *Med. Sci. Sports Exerc.* 15:393–402.

31. Whaley, M.H., L.A. Kaminsky, M.D. Kelly, and J.H. Treloar. 1990. Changes in total cholesterol following endurance training: A function of initial values. *Med. Sci. Sports Exerc.* 22:S48.

32. Pollock, M.L. 1973. The quantification of endurance training programs. In *Exercise and Sports Science Reviews,* ed. J.L. Wilmore, 155–188. New York: Academic Press.

33. U.S. Department of Health and Human Services. 1996. *Physical activity and health: A report of the Surgeon General.* Atlanta: U.S. Department of Health and Human Services, Centers for Disease Control and Prevention, National Center for Chronic Disease Prevention and Health Promotion.

34. American College of Sports Medicine. 2000. *ACSM's Guidelines For Exercise Testing And Prescription.* 6th ed. B.F. Franklin, M.H. Whaley, and E.T. Howley, eds. Baltimore: Lippincott, Williams & Wilkins.

35. American Association of Cardiovascular and Pulmonary Rehabilitation. 1999. *Guidelines For Cardiac Rehabilitation And Secondary Prevention Programs.* 3rd ed. Champaign, IL: Human Kinetics.

36. Myers, J., N. Buchanan, D. Smith, et al. 1992. Individualized ramp treadmill: observations on a new protocol. *Chest* 101:236S–241S.

37. Wallace, J.P. 1997. Obesity. In *ACSM's Exercise Management For Persons With Chronic Diseases And Disabilities,* ed. J.L. Durstine, 106–111. Champaign, IL: Human Kinetics.

38. Skrinar, G.S. 1997. Mental illness. In *ACSM's Exercise Management For Persons With Chronic Diseases And Disabilities,* ed. J.L. Durstine, 230–232. Champaign, IL: Human Kinetics.

39. Jackson, A.S., and M.L. Pollock. 1978. Generalized equations for predicting body density of men. *Br. J. Sports Med.* 40:497–504.

40. Siri, N.E. 1961. Body composition from fluid spaces and density. In *Techniques for measuring body composition,* ed. J. Brozek and A. Henschel, 223–224. Washington, D.C.: National Academy of Science.

41. Kaminsky, L.A., and M.H. Whaley. 1998. Evaluation of a new standardized ramp protocol: The BSU/Bruce ramp protocol. *J. Cardiopul. Rehabil.* 18:438–444.

SUGGESTED READINGS

American College of Sports Medicine. 2001. *ACSM's Resource Manual For Guidelines For Exercise Testing And Prescription.* 4th ed. J. Roitman, ed. Baltimore: Lippincott, Williams & Wilkins.

Astrand, P.O., and K. Rodahl. 1976. *Textbook Of Work Physiology: Physiological Bases Of Exercise.* 2nd ed. New York: McGraw-Hill.

U.S. Department of Health and Human Services. 1996. *Physical activity and health: A report of the Surgeon General.* Atlanta: U.S. Department of Health and Human Services, Centers for Disease Control and Prevention, National Center for Chronic Disease Prevention and Health Promotion.

Verrill, D.E. & P.M. Ribisl. 1996. Resistive exercise training in cardiac rehabilitation: An update. *Sports Medicine.* 21:347-383.

Wilmore, J.H. & Costill D.L. 1988. *Training For Sport And Activity: The Physiological Basis Of The Conditioning Process.* 3rd ed. Champaign, IL: Human Kinetics.

CHAPTER 9

Related Medical Conditions Within Coronary Artery Disease Prevention and Rehabilitation Programs

BEHAVIORAL OBJECTIVES

- To be able to describe the prevalence of chronic obstructive pulmonary disease, diabetes, heart failure, hypertension, obesity, and peripheral arterial disease

- To be able to describe the basic pathophysiology of chronic obstructive pulmonary disease, diabetes, heart failure, hypertension, obesity, and peripheral arterial disease

- To be able to describe the exercise testing and training modifications required for patients with chronic obstructive pulmonary disease, diabetes, heart failure, hypertension, obesity, and peripheral arterial disease

- To be able to describe the common medications taken by patients with chronic obstructive pulmonary disease, diabetes, heart failure, hypertension, obesity, and peripheral arterial disease and their influence during exercise

Although CAD can occur in younger individuals, it is more common after age 45. There are also other diseases that are similarly associated with increasing age. Since it is common to have patients with comorbidities in exercise programs, it is important for exercise program professionals to have a general understanding of the unique needs of each individual. This chapter presents a brief overview of the following common diseases: chronic obstructive pulmonary disease, diabetes, heart failure, peripheral arterial disease, hypertension, and obesity. In many patients, these comorbidities may present more limitations than CAD. We focus specific attention on additional requirements for evaluating, monitoring, and modifying the exercise prescription for patients with different diseases. For each of the diseases we will provide data on prevalence. To put these data in context it will be helpful to know that as of June 2001, the United States population was estimated by the Census Bureau to be approximately 284 million people. Of this number approximately 209 million were adults (> 18 years old) and approximately 100 million were older than 44 years of age.

CHRONIC OBSTRUCTIVE PULMONARY DISEASE

According to estimates from the 1995 National Health Interview Survey, 16.4 million people had COPD. This total consisted of 14.5 million with chronic bronchitis and 1.9 million with emphysema. Prevalence of chronic bronchitis is approximately 50% higher in women than in men, whereas prevalence of emphysema is approximately 30% greater in men. The prevalence of both of these diseases increases with age. Emphysema is common only in older adults (93% of the cases occur after age 45), whereas chronic bronchitis is seen throughout the age spectrum. An additional 14.9 million people (approximately 36% of whom are children under age 18) suffer from asthma. Chronic obstructive pulmonary disease is the fourth leading cause of death in the United States. The most alarming concern is that both the mortality (41%) and morbidity rates (64% for chronic bronchitis) associated with COPD have increased over the last two decades.

Pathophysiology of COPD

The pathophysiology of chronic obstructive pulmonary disease (COPD) varies according to the type. The basic distinctions are as follows: chronic bronchitis is a condition that entails excess mucous production, emphysema is a condition in which some of the alveolar walls are destroyed, and asthma is a condition in which airway size is reduced as the result of constriction of the smooth muscle covering the airways. Regardless of the type, the consequence of COPD is a limitation to airflow.

Normally, there is a good matching of fresh air delivered to the alveoli (ventilation) and blood flow (perfusion) through the adjoining pulmonary capillaries in the lungs. Whenever an airflow limitation occurs, the ventilation-to-perfusion ratio is compromised, and this in turn can lead to **hypoxemia.** Patients with COPD have obvious limitations in delivering fresh air to the alveoli because of the enlarged air sacs in emphysema and because of the reduction in size of the bronchiole lumen in chronic bronchitis. However, blood flow through the lungs can also be abnormal. In emphysema, portions of capillary beds are destroyed, and the smooth muscle of the small pulmonary arteriole walls can become hypertrophied (thus restricting blood flow). Perfusion is also reduced as a result of pulmonary arteriole vasoconstriction, which is caused by a local response to low oxygen levels in the alveoli. The degree of hypoxemia depends on the type and severity of the disease. Reviewing the relationship between oxygen and hemoglobin and transit time of blood flow in the pulmonary capillaries, as described in a physiology text, would be helpful to further your understanding of how hypoxemia develops.

Some patients with COPD also have problems in removing carbon dioxide from their lungs (CO_2 retention), leading to an increased arterial partial pressure of carbon dioxide (PCO_2). This excess CO_2 results in increased ventilatory rates (via chemoreceptor stimulation) and increased acid (hydrogen ion) concentration. The kidneys function to counteract the increased acid concentration by retaining bicarbonate. However, if CO_2 retention occurs more suddenly, or gradually accumulates beyond the kidneys' ability to compensate, respiratory failure can occur.

Unique Concerns Related to Exercise Testing and Training

A comprehensive overview of exercise testing and prescription for COPD patients is found in *Guidelines for Pulmonary Rehabilitation Programs* (1). Here we overview some of the basic issues related to exercising patients with COPD.

Pulmonary Function Testing

It is important to have a basic understanding of pulmonary function testing, which is routinely performed in pulmonary patients to aid in the diagnosis and to assess the progression of the disease. Computer-interfaced **spirometry** systems provide the assessment of many different expressions of pulmonary volumes and airway flow rates. However, in most cases the exercise program professional needs to consider only a few of these measurements. Of primary importance are the measures of **forced vital capacity** (FVC), **forced expiratory volume** in the first second ($FEV_{1.0}$), and the ratio between $FEV_{1.0}$ and FVC. We interpret pulmonary function testing results by comparing the actual measured volumes to norms for an individual that are influenced mostly by gender, age, and body size (height). Generally, test results are considered abnormal if they are less than 80% of the expected (norm) value. The hallmark pulmonary function testing feature of the patient with COPD is a reduced $FEV_{1.0}/FVC$ ratio that results from a reduced $FEV_{1.0}$ (figure 9.1). Forced vital capacity may also be reduced—and commonly is as the disease becomes more severe.

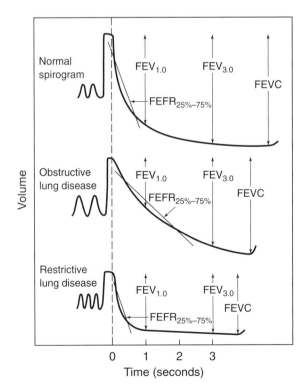

Figure 9.1 Typical volume versus time curves from pulmonary function testing showing normal, obstructive, and restrictive patterns.

Exercise Prescription Modifications

It is important to understand that chronic pulmonary disease is irreversible. An important goal of medical management is to improve airflow (evidenced by increased $FEV_{1.0}$) enough to reduce symptoms. As discussed in chapter 7, the primary goal of exercise training is to maintain or improve physical fitness. This is no different for the COPD patient, with the exception that improvement potential is limited and the maintenance of functional ability is a primary goal. Ventilation is the limiting factor in exercise capacity for individuals with COPD. This ventilatory limitation can be observed by the lack of breathing reserve at maximal exercise in these patients (box 9.1).

> ### Box 9.1 Breathing Reserve
>
> Breathing reserve (BR) = maximal voluntary ventilation (MVV) – maximal exercise ventilation (VE_{max})
>
> MVV can be measured via spirometry, although it is a difficult procedure for many patients to perform. Thus it is usually predicted by:
>
> $$MVV = FEV_{1.0} \times 40$$
>
> VE_{max} is measured as highest ventilation value during an exercise test. Normally, at peak exercise individuals have a BR that is 20-50% of their MVV; however, COPD patients have a BR < 20% and often as low as 0%.

Since pulmonary patients are limited by ventilation, as opposed to the more typical limitation of the cardiovascular system, modifications to the exercise prescription are necessary. The severity of the disease and the patient's level of deconditioning are also important considerations in developing the exercise prescription.

Exercise intensity

The aspect that is most different about the exercise prescription for pulmonary patients is setting the exercise intensity. Both the American Association of Cardiovascular and Pulmonary Rehabilitation (AACVPR) and American College of Sports Medicine (ACSM) Guidelines acknowledge that there is no one universally accepted method. The following is an important statement from AACVPR:

In general, the standard heart rate ranges or targets used in normal populations have little application to ventilatory limited individuals with disabling chronic lung disease. These patients usually stop exercise at low peak heart rates. Using any arbitrary submaximum percentage heart rate target often results in selecting target intensities that are too low for such individuals. (1)

The following are some suggested methods for setting the exercise intensity:

- Exercising at 50% of peak oxygen uptake
- Exercising at or above the anaerobic threshold
- Exercising at the highest level tolerated by symptoms

Which method to use is partially determined by the severity of the disease. For patients with mild to moderate pulmonary impairment (FVC and $FEV_{1.0}$ between 50% and 80% of predicted), setting the intensity at the anaerobic threshold or using a percentage of exercise capacity is generally appropriate. However, for patients with severe pulmonary impairment (FVC and $FEV_{1.0}$ <50% of predicted), the usual approach is to exercise to the point of symptom limitation. The most common symptom is dyspnea, which definitely is the limiting factor for most pulmonary patients. It is important to teach these patients a breathing technique, called pursed-lips breathing, to help them decrease their frequency of breathing and thus maintain a sense of control of their breathing. This technique has patients breathe in through the nose and out through the mouth while keeping the lips pressed together except in the center of the mouth. Patients should be guided to exhale with a firm, steady effort and at a controlled rate (twice as long as the inspiration).

Since COPD patients are limited to using lower exercise intensities, it is important to make complementary increases in the exercise duration, frequency, or both in order to obtain the desired total training volumes. Generally, because of the deconditioned state of many pulmonary patients, the initial approach is to use high exercise frequencies (five to seven days per week) and gradually build exercise session duration. Some patients may not be capable of performing exercise at the desired intensity for a prolonged period of time, and thus it may be necessary to use an interval training approach (alternating work and rest intervals) during the exercise session as discussed in chapter 7.

Upper-body exercise

Another important aspect of the training program for pulmonary patients is upper-body exercise. This component is important because many activities of daily living (bathing, cleaning, cooking, etc.) require lifting, carrying, and moving objects with the arms. Upper-body exercise can and ideally should include both endurance and strength training. Many ergometers are available that incorporate the use of the arms to assist or complement the work being done by the legs during exercise. These are appropriate for all patients capable of using them. In addition, strengthening exercises should be a part of every program. Patients can do strengthening exercises using traditional methods (free weights, dumbbells, and machines) or alternate methods—elastic bands (of variable tension) or handheld weights (e.g., food cans). Circuit-type programs (described in chapter 7) work well for groups of pulmonary patients and, when administered by staff group leaders, also serve to add a reinforcing behavioral aspect to the program.

Special Considerations

Pulmonary patients can safely participate in exercise programs; however, exercise program professionals should be aware of a few special considerations. In addition to the standard emergency equipment, programs that serve patients with moderate to severe pulmonary disease should ensure that patients have their bronchodilator medication and that supplemental oxygen is available. It is also important for program staff to understand the importance of helping patients avoid exposure to upper respiratory illness (URI) germs. These illnesses cause a variety of respiratory problems, including restriction of airflow. Since COPD patients already have limitations in their ventilatory abilities, the additional restriction of airflow resulting from a URI may create situations in which patients are totally disabled or may potentially develop acute respiratory failure. Thus, staff members who have URI must practice good personal hygiene habits to prevent the possible spread of URI germs.

Because exercise performance is limited by the symptom of dyspnea in many COPD patients, this is something that should be monitored. A variety of tools can be used to monitor dyspnea, including a Borg scale (2), the visual analog scale (3), and, as shown in figure 9.2, a modified angina scale. Typically in patients limited by dyspnea, an exercise bout is terminated at a predetermined level (for example +3 on the scale shown in figure 9.2).

Supplemental Oxygen Use

Patients with severe pulmonary disease may also require supplemental oxygen (figure 9.3). In some cases the use of supplemental oxygen must be continuous, whereas in other patients it is necessary only during exercise. In working with these patients, it is important to be able to monitor their blood level of oxygen saturation; typically this is done with an oximeter. The AACVPR recommends that exercise be terminated if the cutaneous oximetry reading of oxygen saturation drops below 90%. This value is set somewhat conservatively because of the measurement error of most oximeters, which ranges from ±3% to ±5%. It is permissible to resume exercise when the oxygen saturation increases above 90%.

Medications

Common medications for patients with pulmonary disease include bronchodilators, steroids, antibiotics, and psychotropic agents (table 9.1). The effects of these medications on heart rate, blood pressure (BP), and electrocardiographic responses during exercise depend on the specific medication used. Although many of these types of medications have no effect on exercise responses, some can cause an increase in heart rate, increase in BP, or increase in number of prema-

ture ventricular contractions. The most notable effect is the potential to increase exercise performance with the use of bronchodilators (when $FEV_{1.0}$ is improved).

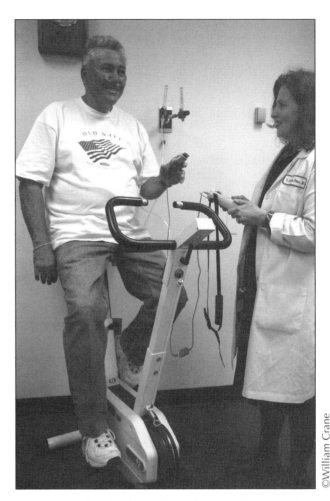

©William Crane

Figure 9.3 Chronic obstructive pulmonary disease patient on supplemental oxygen who is having oxygen saturation monitored.

0	None
+1	Light, barely noticeable
+2	Moderate, bothersome
+3	Moderately severe, very uncomfortable
+4	Most severe or intense dyspnea ever experienced

Figure 9.2 Perception of dyspnea rating scale.

Table 9.1
Common Medications Used in the Treatment of COPD (by class)

Generic name	Brand name	Mechanism and benefit
Bronchodilator agents		Relaxes the smooth muscle surrounding the bronchial tubes.
Anticholinergic		
Ipratropium Bromide	Atrovent	
Beta agonists		
Albuterol	Ventolin, Proventil	
Metaproteronol	Alupent, Metaprel	
Terbutaline	Brethine	
Methylxanthines		
Theophylline	Theo-24, Theo-Dur	

(continued)

Table 9.1 *(continued)*

Generic name	Brand name	Mechanism and benefit
Anti-inflammatory agents		Reduce the inflammation in the airways to lessen the swelling and mucus production.
Cromolyn Sodium		
Corticosteroids		
Antidepressants		Function to reduce symptoms of depression.
Amitriptyline	Elavil	
Amoxapine	Axendin	
Bupropion	Wellbutrin	
Clomipramine	Anafranil	
Desipramine	Norpramin	
Fluoxetine	Prozac	
Imipramine	Tofranil	
Nortriptyline	Pamelor	
Paroxetine	Paxil	
Serrealine	Zoloft	
Trazodone	Desyrel	
Anxiolytic agents		Functions to reduce symptoms of anxiety.
Alprazolam	Xanax	
Buspirone	BuSpar	
Chlordiazepoxide	Librium	
Diazepam	Valium	
Hydroxyzine	Atarax	
Lorazepam	Ativan	
Oxazepam	Serax	

Review Case 9.1
Chronic Obstructive Pulmonary Disease

Janice is a 55-year-old patient who has been exercising in your program for the past year. Janice has severe COPD and requires supplemental oxygen (flow rate of 2 l O_2/min at rest, increasing to 4 l O_2/min during exercise), which maintains her oxygen saturation (O_{2sat}) levels above 93% via oximetry. During her pre-exercise session assessment today, Janice's O_{2sat} was 94%. Janice's regular routine has been to exercise on a treadmill set at 1.9 mph (3 km/h) for 30 min (dyspnea rating +2). After 5 min of exercise today Janice reports that her dyspnea rating is a +3, and you perform a check of her O_{2sat} and obtain a reading of 86%.

Given this information, respond to the following:

1. What should your immediate response be?

2. What could have caused this to occur?

3. Should Janice continue to exercise today?

DIABETES

According to estimates from the American Diabetes Association (ADA), 15.7 million Americans (5.9%) have diabetes. However, about a third of these people (5.4 million) have not yet been diagnosed and thus are not being treated. Type II diabetes (90-95%) is far more common than type I diabetes (5-10%). Prevalence of diabetes is ≈10-12% in African American, Hispanic American, and Native American populations and is much higher in elderly (>65 years old) populations (18.4%) versus younger ones. Diabetes is the seventh leading cause of death in the United States. Concerns exist that with the rising incidence of obesity, diabetes rates will also increase and that the disease will begin at earlier ages.

Pathophysiology of Diabetes

There are three principal forms of diabetes: type I, type II, and gestational. Type I diabetes usually results from immune system dysfunction that causes destruction of the beta cells of the pancreas. The body's ability to produce insulin is lost, and survival is dependent on daily injections of insulin. Type I diabetes most commonly develops during childhood (peak incidence is around the age of puberty), but it can begin during adulthood. Type II diabetes occurs as a consequence of resistance of the body's cells to the action of insulin. As this type of the disease progresses, the ability of the pancreas to produce insulin may be diminished, leading to a relative degree of insulin deficiency. Gestational diabetes, which occurs in up to 5% of all pregnancies, is a temporary disorder that results from either excessive hormone production or a failure of the pancreas to produce enough insulin. Although the condition resolves after pregnancy, women who have had gestational diabetes are at increased risk for developing type II diabetes later in life.

Diabetes leads to a number of pathological complications that result from chronically elevated blood glucose (and in many cases insulin) concentrations. Specifically, individuals with diabetes may develop **retinopathy,** which can lead to blindness (29 times more likely in those with diabetes than in those without); **nephropathy,** which can lead to end-stage renal disease; **neuropathy,** which may cause loss of various sensory signals; and hypertension and dyslipidemias, which lead to accelerated atherosclerosis. Recently, a clustering of abnormalities that appear to result from insulin resistance has been receiving increased attention. This disorder is called syndrome X, the deadly quartet, or (most commonly) the metabolic syndrome. As described in chapter 1, the characteristics of the metabolic syndrome are upper-body obesity, hypertension, hypertriglyceridemia (and low high-density lipoprotein), and hyperinsulinemia (with associated glucose intolerance). Recently, an association between low cardiorespiratory fitness and the metabolic syndrome has been identified (4). Individuals with the metabolic syndrome are much more likely to develop cardiovascular disease than are people with none or only one of the characteristics of the metabolic syndrome.

Unique Concerns Related to Exercise Testing and Training

A comprehensive overview of exercise testing and prescription for individuals with diabetes appears in the technical reviews and position stands of the ADA and ACSM (5-8). The following sections of this chapter overview some basic issues related to exercising patients with diabetes.

Comprehensive Medical Evaluation

Because of the many potential pathological complications associated with diabetes, the ADA and ACSM state that individuals with diabetes "should undergo a detailed medical examination with appropriate diagnostic studies"(8). The National Kidney Foundation now recommends that physicians take an aggressive approach to controlling hypertension in patients with diabetes, since diabetes is the primary cause of renal failure requiring dialysis (9). The new goal for treatment of resting BP is <130/80 mmHg. Exercise testing is an important part of this examination. Individuals with diabetes are at increased risk for CAD, and those with autonomic neuropathy may have the silent type of ischemia. In general, individuals with diabetes can undergo exercise testing using the same modes and protocols as low-risk patients. However, individual health status may necessitate modifications. For example, those with peripheral neuropathy should usually be tested on a non-weight-bearing mode to prevent ulceration or other potential injuries to the feet. Other factors to consider in modifying the exercise testing procedures are retinopathy (need to be concerned about excessive BP response), autonomic neuropathy (greater potential for abnormal heart rate and BP responses; also, optimally controlled testing environment required for thermoregulatory deficiencies), and obesity.

Monitoring Blood Glucose

One additional monitoring consideration for both exercise testing and training situations is that of measuring blood glucose prior to exercise. This is essential for all individuals with type I diabetes and for most individuals with type II diabetes when they are beginning an exercise program or increasing the intensity of the program. From a diagnostic standpoint, blood glucose is measured in the fasting state, and results are classified according to the recommendations of the ADA as presented in figure 9.4. For individuals with diabetes, additional monitoring criteria exist that differ between the types of diabetes.

It is recommended that all individuals with diabetes self-monitor their blood glucose using small, portable monitors requiring only a small drop of blood (figure 9.5). Although most patients can be trained to monitor their own glucose status and report it to the exercise staff, it is important for exercise facilities to have a blood glucose monitor available. For individuals with type I diabetes, the most common concern is prevention of hypoglycemia. Thus, the recommendation is that if a pre-exercise glucose test shows a value of <100 mg/dl, the exercise be delayed until adequate carbohydrate (20-30 g) can be consumed. On the other hand, individuals with type II diabetes are more commonly prone to develop extreme hyperglycemia. When a pre-exercise measurement reveals a glucose value between 250 and 299 mg/dl, urinary **ketones** should be measured. Exercise testing or training should be postponed for those with blood glucose values >300 mg/dl or those who have values >250 mg/dl with ketones present.

Exercise Prescription Modifications

Exercise prescription recommendations vary for persons with type I versus type II diabetes. Certainly many unique modifications to the exercise plan are necessary for individuals who have diabetes and in addition some of the pathological considerations mentioned earlier. Although we will address some common issues faced by exercise program professionals working with indi-

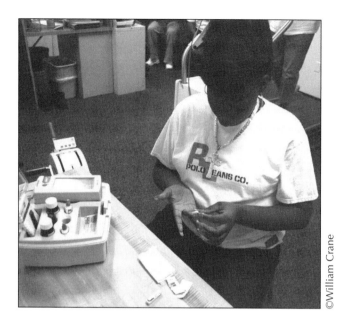
©William Crane

Figure 9.5 Diabetes patient self-monitoring blood glucose.

viduals who have diabetes, a complete discussion of these special considerations is beyond the scope of this chapter. More discussion of these issues appears in the reviews referred to earlier in this section.

In general, the exercise prescription for individuals with type I diabetes is no different than for low-risk adults, as discussed in chapter 7. The exercise plan is essentially based on the patient's goals and interests, but there are a number of unique concerns related to exercise. A primary goal for individuals with type I diabetes is balancing their carbohydrate use (energy expenditure) and supply (energy intake) with appropriate amounts of insulin. The ideal approach to maintain this balance, and thus maintain desirable control of blood glucose concentrations, is to develop a consistent daily routine. One way to do this is to have a higher frequency of exercise than one would have otherwise (i.e., 4-6 days per week) and to perform a similar type and amount of exercise each day. It is also desirable if the time of day (preferably earlier in the day) and exercise environment are similar each day. This type of approach, sometimes referred to as pattern management, allows the individual with type I diabetes to develop a consistent adjustment in the timing and amount of insulin injected. The patient develops the approach over time through regular monitoring of blood glucose before, during, and after exercise. Any variation in the routine or involvement in any significant amount of additional physical activity requires the individual with type I diabetes to adjust the insulin dosage or carbohydrate intake. Exercise facilities should have either glucose tablets or cans of fruit

<110 mg/dl	Normoglycemia
110-125	Impaired fasting glucose
≥126	Diagnostic for diabetes

Any abnormal value should be confirmed by a repeat test on a separate day.

Figure 9.4 Criteria for classification of fasting plasma glucose.

juice available for individuals who develop symptoms of hypoglycemia. Persons with type I diabetes generally must be highly motivated to participate in regular exercise, since managing the disease requires a significant amount of effort (i.e., adjusting doses of insulin to match variations in energy expenditure and intake). Therefore, it is imperative for exercise program professionals to be as supportive and helpful as possible.

The exercise prescription for individuals with type II diabetes includes some modifications distinct from those for the low-risk individual because of the common finding of multiple comorbidities (i.e., characteristics of the metabolic syndrome). Specific recommendations of the ADA are presented in figure 9.6 (6). The intensity is capped at a lower level because of the different comorbidities, the most common of which is obesity (85% of individuals with type II diabetes are obese). The major focus of the exercise prescription for obesity, as presented later in this chapter, is to maximize caloric expenditure by emphasizing increased duration and frequency of exercise. Higher intensity levels, with the associated higher systolic BP levels, may also have adverse consequences (e.g., potential for retinal damage) in those with retinopathy. Thus, the ADA recommends that systolic BP not rise above 180 mmHg during exercise. Certainly, other modifications to the exercise prescription may be necessary depending on the comorbidities present. If the screening of an individual with type II diabetes

reveals no significant concerns, it may be appropriate for the person to exercise at higher intensities, i.e. the intensity can be set anywhere within the range of intensity recommended in the ACSM Guidelines (50-85% $\dot{V}O_2$max) (10). Although regular monitoring of blood glucose is important for people with type II diabetes, monitoring does not have to take place daily if the patient's blood glucose is reasonably well controlled (<180 mg/dl) throughout the day.

Special Considerations

Some research studies have demonstrated that insulin sensitivity of the skeletal muscles can be improved with resistance training; thus this type of training is recommended for most individuals with type II diabetes. It is important to emphasize good technique, particularly in relation to breathing patterns, to avoid exaggerated BP responses associated with the **Valsalva maneuver.** Generally, the exercise prescription guidelines in chapter 7 should be modified to use lower resistance (not to maximum) and a higher number of repetitions (e.g., 10-15). Resistance training may be contraindicated in some patients with retinopathy and should not be performed without physician approval.

A number of special concerns or considerations related to individuals with either type of diabetes are dictated by their comorbidities. Some of these are avoidance of weight-bearing exercise (peripheral neuropathy), the need to regularly inspect the feet (peripheral neuropathy), possible use of perceived exertion as an alternative indicator of intensity (autonomic neuropathy), and avoidance of exercise in hot or cold environments (autonomic neuropathy).

Medications

Common medications for individuals with diabetes include insulin and oral hypoglycemic agents, which are used to control blood glucose levels (table 9.2). These medications have no

Intensity	50–70% $\dot{V}O_2$max (limit so SBP does not exceed 180 mmHg)
Duration	20–45 min session
Frequency	At least 3 days/week, ≥5 days/week if weight reduction is a goal

Figure 9.6 ADA recommendations for exercise prescription for Type II diabetes.

Table 9.2
Common Medications Used in the Treatment of Diabetes (by class)

Generic name	Brand name	Mechanism and benefit
Insulin		Binds with cell receptors; stimulates the uptake of glucose by the cells.
Rapid Acting	Humulin R	
Intermediate Acting	Humulin L, Lente	
Long Acting	Humulin U, Ultralente	
Oral hypoglycemic		Stimulates the release of insulin from the pancreas.
Glyburide	Diabeta, Micronase	
Chlorpropamide	Diabetinese	
Glipizide	Glucotrol	
Tolbutamide	Orinase	
Tolazamide	Tolinase	

specific effects on heart rate, BP, or ECG responses during exercise. Obviously these individuals may be on additional medications for the treatment of associated comorbidities. Thus, one must pay attention to any potential influence that such medications may have in association with exercise.

Review Case 9.2
Type II Diabetes and Obesity

Cathy is a 53-year-old woman who was diagnosed with type II diabetes one year ago. Cathy first attempted an at-home exercise program using the "Fat-No-More" abdominal exerciser that she purchased after watching an infomercial on television. After using the Fat-No-More for four months, Cathy became discouraged when she did not lose any weight or feel more fit. At her regular physical her physician referred her to the preventative/rehabilitative exercise program that you direct. The results from her physical fitness evaluation revealed the following:

Resting blood pressure: 134/86 mmHg

BMI: 36.7 kg/m^2

Waist circumference: 41 in. (104.5 cm)

Fasting blood testing results (mg/dl): Total cholesterol 223; HDL cholesterol 37; triglycerides 221; glucose 189

Medications: Diabeta, Vasotec

Maximal exercise capacity: 6.7 METs

Given this information, respond to the following:

1. What mode(s) of exercise would you recommend for Cathy?

2. What would you recommend as a caloric expenditure goal for Cathy in the exercise program? How many minutes of exercise per week would it take Cathy to achieve this goal?

3. If a pre-exercise check of Cathy's blood sugar revealed a value of 228 mg/dl, would you allow Cathy to exercise that day? If so, would you make any specific recommendations?

HEART FAILURE

According to estimates from the National Health and Nutrition Examination Survey III (NHANES III), there are 4.7 million Americans (1.6%) with heart failure. However, the incidence rate is increasing, and it is estimated that approximately 450,000 cases of heart failure are diagnosed each year, due in part to the aging of the population and to increased survival rates of patients following cardiac-related events. Heart failure is a disabling condition that generally has a poor prognosis. Data from NHANES III indicated that six-year mortality rates reached 80% in men and 65% in women with heart failure.

Pathophysiology of Heart Failure

Heart failure is defined as an inability to produce sufficient cardiac output to meet the requirements of the body. There are two types of heart failure, systolic dysfunction and diastolic dysfunction. Systolic dysfunction results from impaired ventricular contractility or elevated afterload, lead-

ing to a higher-than-normal end-diastolic volume. Ejection fraction is reduced in patients with systolic dysfunction. The major causes of systolic dysfunction are uncontrolled systemic hypertension, myocardial infarction, and idiopathic dilated **cardiomyopathy.**

Diastolic heart failure is estimated to account for 30% to 50% of all heart failure cases and is the most common type in patients who are elderly, particularly women. Diastolic dysfunction is the result of reduced ventricular filling, which can be caused by inappropriate relaxation of the ventricle, reduced compliance of the ventricle (increased "stiffness" of the myocardium), or both. Ejection fraction is normal or elevated in patients with diastolic dysfunction. The major causes of diastolic dysfunction are left ventricular hypertrophy, myocardial ischemia, and hypertrophic cardiomyopathy.

As might be expected, the inadequate cardiac performance is sensed by the body's regulatory mechanisms and results in a number of compensatory responses. These responses include activation of the adrenergic nervous system, stimulation of the renin-angiotensin system, and increased production of antidiuretic hormone.

Unique Concerns Related to Exercise Testing and Training

There are no national guidelines or position stands that are specific to exercise testing or training for patients with heart failure. However, there are a number of common practices that have been developed by exercise program professionals, which are reviewed below.

Exercise Testing

Exercise testing is an essential component of the evaluation of patients with heart failure. Because of the relatively low functional capacity levels of these patients and the need to detect small changes in their status, it is highly desirable to obtain gas-exchange measurements during exercise testing. Indeed, measured $\dot{V}O_2$max data are important in determining the prognosis of heart failure patients. One commonly employed criterion for consideration of placement on a heart transplantation list is a $\dot{V}O_2$max of <14 ml·kg^{-1}·min^{-1}. Low-level or modified exercise testing protocols (either incremental or ramp) are required to allow adequate test times. Treadmills and cycle ergometers are both often used; however, some clinicians prefer cycle ergometers for patients who are elderly as these devices are thought to enhance the sense of security, which would translate into better effort. Exercise testing staff need to pay close attention to the multiple medications that heart failure patients are treated with, as will be discussed later in this section, since many of these can have effects on the ECG and BP responses during the test.

Since it is important to regularly assess functional status in heart failure patients, alternatives to the use of maximal exercise testing are desirable. One alternative is submaximal exercise testing, ideally with measurement of the ventilatory threshold. These tests have demonstrated utility in clinical research trials but are less common in clinical practice. Another alternative, which is more practical, is the 6-min walk test. This often-used test is easy to perform and administer, but it is important to standardize the procedures. Studies have shown that patients' performance can be affected by different levels of encouragement during this test. Other results have shown that test performance can improve due to a learning effect. Thus, the recommendation is to perform multiple 6-min walk tests (at least two, preferably three) to establish a baseline result.

Exercise Prescription Modifications

Exercise training has been shown to be an effective therapy for heart failure patients. However, close observation of these patients is essential, as their status can change rapidly. Exercise staff should observe for daily changes in body weight and BP response. They should also be aware of increased dyspnea and fatigue. Any of these signs or symptoms could be suggestive of deterioration into uncompensated heart failure, which is an absolute contraindication for exercise testing or training. Additionally, some heart failure patients are prone to experience ventricular dysrhythmias, which may require regular ECG monitoring. Regular BP monitoring is also desirable.

As a consequence of the low functional capacity of heart failure patients and their typical level of deconditioning, it is usually necessary to begin exercise programs with short durations (10-20 min, possibly divided into smaller work periods separated by rest intervals). A goal for these patients is to be able to exercise continuously for 20 to 40 min. The recommended exercise intensity range is between 40% and 75% of $\dot{V}O_2$max. Use of heart rate as an indicator of intensity may be problematic in some heart failure patients who demonstrate an impaired chronotropic response to exercise. Ideally, one can determine intensity directly by a plot of $\dot{V}O_2$max and work rates from an exercise test as shown in chapter 7. A common factor that may limit exercise is dyspnea, so the use of a perceived dyspnea scale (figure 9.2) is a valuable adjunct to monitoring exercise intensity. Given the limitations with exercise duration and intensity, it is helpful to utilize increased exercise frequency (5-7 days per week) for heart failure patients in order to obtain adequate total training volume (i.e., the caloric thresholds discussed in chapter 7). Walking is the preferred mode of activity because it translates into activities of daily living, but cycling is an acceptable alternative for many patients. These patients can use other modes of aerobic activity as well, particularly ergometers that offer the combination of arm and leg exercise. Resistance training using low resistance and 12 to 15 repetitions per exercise is also recommended to help improve functional status.

Medications

As mentioned earlier, most heart failure patients are on combination pharmacological therapy regimes. Typical medications for patients with either systolic or diastolic dysfunction include diuretics, beta blockers, beta and alpha blockers, calcium channel blockers, angiotensin receptor blockers, and angiotensin-converting enzyme inhibitors (see table 4.5). One drug unique to patients with systolic dysfunction is digoxin (Lanoxin), which functions to increase the strength of myocardial contractions (i.e., increases inotropy). We should point out that the most efficacious medication therapy for patients with diastolic dysfunction is not yet known. Additionally, heart failure patients prone to ventricular dysrhythmias are usually prescribed an antiarrhythmic medication.

Review Case 9.3
Heart Failure

Rhoda is a 74-year-old woman who went to her physician complaining of dyspnea. After a series of medical evaluations, Rhoda was diagnosed with heart failure and was referred to your preventative/rehabilitative exercise program. One of the medical findings you observed in Rhoda's history was an ejection fraction of 72%. You assign your exercise science intern to select an exercise test protocol for Rhoda's baseline evaluation. The intern recommends using the Ball State University/Bruce ramp treadmill protocol.

Given this information, respond to the following:

1. Do you think the diagnosis of heart failure can be incorrect?

2. Do you agree with the mode for the exercise test?

3. Do you agree with the selection of protocol for the exercise test?

HYPERTENSION

According to the sixth report of the Joint National Committee on Prevention, Detection, Evaluation, and Treatment of High Blood Pressure, an estimated 50 million Americans have high blood pressure defined as greater than 140/90 mmHg (11). Higher rates are seen in African Americans and Mexican Americans than in Caucasians, and in middle-aged and younger men compared to women. Lower educational and income levels are also associated with greater incidence of hypertension, and rates are known to increase with age. Hypertension is present in only 4% of those under age 30, whereas it is seen in 54% of people in their 60s.

Pathophysiology of Hypertension

Elevated BP can result from either an increase in cardiac output or an increase in peripheral vascular resistance (see section on control of BP in chapter 2). However, persistent hypertension is usually due to the latter. Regardless of the etiological origin, the physiological consequences are the same.

Peripheral vascular resistance can be modified by the nervous system, by metabolic factors, by hormones, and by local vascular factors. Alteration of baroreceptor sensitivity and increased sympathetic nervous system activity can both lead to increased arterial BP. Likewise, increased circulating catecholamines and angiotensin, as well as abnormalities in vascular smooth muscle function due to defects in sodium and calcium balance or endothelial-derived factors, can cause hypertension.

The vascular derangements of hypertension include CAD, cerebral artery disease, and peripheral artery disease. As noted in chapter 2, hypertension has been associated with causing endothelial damage that results in atherosclerosis. Individuals with hypertension also have an increased likelihood of producing emboli, which can lead to a myocardial infarction or a stroke. Aortic aneurysms and hemorrhagic strokes are also more common consequences among those with hypertension, because of weakening of blood vessels.

Since the myocardial workload is increased as a response to hypertension, it follows that a typical adaptation is left ventricular hypertrophy. Complications from left ventricular hypertrophy include myocardial ischemia, ventricular ectopy, and, in the long term, congestive heart failure.

Unique Concerns Related to Exercise Testing and Training

A comprehensive overview of exercise testing and prescription for patients with hypertension appears in the ACSM's position stand on this topic (13). The normal BP response to exercise is an increase in systolic pressure with little or no change in diastolic pressure. Obviously, if one starts with an elevated resting BP, the absolute BP during exercise will be higher than in people who are normotensive at rest. Although there is some debate about the seriousness of higher absolute BP values during exercise, common sense suggests that avoidance of an exaggerated BP response would be beneficial.

Exercise Testing

Although there are no specific exercise testing protocols or procedures unique to individuals with hypertension, there are a few special concerns. Exercise test technicians should know two BP threshold values recommended by ACSM in relation to individuals with hypertension. First, a pre-exercise BP reading of >200 (systolic) and/ or >110 (diastolic) mmHg is considered a relative contraindication to exercise testing. Second, an excessive rise in BP of ≥260 (systolic) and/or ≥115 (diastolic) mmHg is considered termination criteria for exercise testing. Additionally, during the test the patient must avoid any isometric contractions due to gripping the handrails or handlebars. Finally, it is essential that all technicians be familiar with the potential changes in the heart rate, BP, and electrocardiographic responses during the test that are associated with various medications for hypertension. Unless clinical diagnostic testing issues dictate otherwise, patients should take their medications as scheduled prior to testing. Ideally, it is desirable to test patients at a time of day similar to that of their usual exercise session so that the effects of medications will be consistent in the two situations.

Exercise Prescription Modifications

As reviewed in chapter 4, exercise training is a recommended therapy for patients diagnosed with hypertension, shown to be effective both as a first-line therapy in those with stage I hypertension and in patients taking medications for hypertension. The ACSM has published recommendations for exercise training of hypertensive individuals in a position stand (13) as well as within its guidelines (10). In general, the recommendations are similar to those for low-risk individuals without hypertension. A unique aspect is that BP-lowering benefits may be achieved at lower exercise intensities (40-70% $\dot{V}O_2$max). Thus, hypertensive patients who prefer moderate-intensity exercise may actually obtain the same BP-lowering benefit as those who participate in more vigorous exercise programs. This does not imply that individuals with hypertension should avoid exercise intensities >70% $\dot{V}O_2$max. Rates of caloric expenditure are higher at vigorous versus moderate exercise intensities, making achievement of the energy expenditure goals (chapter 7) more efficient.

Resistance training is an important part of a total physical fitness program. Concerns exist for patients with hypertension who wish to participate in a resistance-training component. First, it is important that these patients have adequate control of their hypertension before beginning resistance training. Recommended modifications to the resistance-training program include avoiding exercises that require isometric hand gripping, or at least making attempts to minimize the degree of the isometric component. Another recommendation is to use lower intensities of training with a complementary increase in the number of repetitions of each exercise in order to obtain the desired training volume. It is not always necessary for all individuals with hypertension to avoid higher-intensity resistance training; however, these patients may require more evaluation, and the overall patient profile forms the basis of decisions.

Special Considerations

One major concern related to exercise testing or training of patients with hypertension is the risk for postexercise hypotension in those taking certain medications (primarily vasodilators). Although an active cool-down is important for everyone, it is especially important for people with hypertension.

Another major concern with individuals who have hypertension is that the condition is not adequately controlled in the majority of patients. Indeed, almost one-third of persons with hypertension do not know they have it, and another 15% are not on any therapy for the condition.

Thus, the exercise program professional can play an important role in educating and counseling patients about hypertension. As reviewed in chapter 4, the Joint National Committee on Prevention, Detection, Evaluation, and Treatment of High Blood Pressure recommends pharmacological therapy for all individuals with stage 2 (BP ≥160/≥100 mmHg) or stage 3 (BP≥180/≥110 mmHg) hypertension. The recommendation is to initiate pharmacological therapy at even lower BP values if the patient has cardiovascular disease, diabetes, renal insufficiency, or heart failure.

Medications

Many different types of medications are used to treat hypertension. Ideally, adequate BP control can be achieved with one medication; however, some patients require a combination of two or more classes of medications. As reviewed in chapter 2, BP control is affected by cardiac output. Thus, to achieve control of BP, some of the medication classes also influence heart rate and as a consquence can affect the ECG. The precise effects on these responses vary between the medication classes and are summarized in appendix A-2 of the ACSM Guidelines (10). Among the classes of medications (see table 4.5) commonly used to treat hypertension are beta blockers, alpha blockers, calcium channel blockers, diuretics, and angiotensin-converting enzyme inhibitors.

Review Case 9.4
Hypertension

Robert is a 58-year-old participant in your preventative/rehabilitative exercise program. Robert has been prescribed Apresoline to treat his hypertension. He has exercised regularly for the past three years and has had good control of his blood pressure (resting pressures range from 116/78 to 124/84 mmHg, and exercise systolic pressures range from 154 to 172 mmHg with diastolic pressures consistently <87 mmHg). Robert enjoys trying new pieces of exercise equipment and asks you (the clinical exercise physiologist) if he can try the new arm/leg elliptical training device that just arrived in your fitness center. You agree to let Robert give it a try but suggest that you check a blood pressure reading on him after 5 min of use. This measurement reveals a blood pressure of 168/98 mmHg.

Given this information, respond to the following:

1. What would your immediate response be?

2. Why do you think Robert's blood pressure was elevated on this piece of exercise equipment? Should Robert not use this equipment, or can the exercise be modified in some way to allow him to use the new trainer?

3. What effect, if any, does the medication have in relation to Robert's exercise training response? Does anything in particular need to be modified in his program?

OBESITY

According to estimates from the NHANES III, 97 million adult Americans (55%) are overweight (BMI: 25-29.9kg/m^2) or obese (BMI ≥30kg/m^2). Rates of obesity are increasing in all age groups, including children. Obesity rates are particularly high (approaching 50%) in African American and Mexican American women. Lower educational and lower income levels are associated with increased incidence of obesity.

Pathophysiology of Obesity

Obesity results from an imbalance between total body energy expenditure and energy intake. Daily energy expenditure has three components: resting metabolism, dietary-induced thermogenesis (i.e., the energy associated with digesting food and processing nutrients), and physical activity. Basically, if energy intake is greater than energy expenditure (i.e., positive energy balance), this excess energy will be stored by the body as excess fat. Even though the energy balance equation seems quite simple (and it is!), the many mechanisms that control energy metabolism are quite complex (figure 9.7).

There are two primary forms of obesity—upper-body (android, or abdominal) and lower-body (gynoid) obesity. Although disease risk increases directly with body mass index (BMI), the risks are much greater in those with the upper-body form of obesity. Another way of characterizing obesity is based on the size and number of adipocytes (fat cells). The number of adipocytes an individual has is important, since once developed they cannot be destroyed. It is generally accepted that there is a genetic influence on the number of adipocytes an individual is born with. It is also believed that adipocyte number can be increased by overfeeding during the first year of life and around the time of puberty. One theory is that adipocytes "desire" a set amount of triglycerides per cell. If the triglyceride level of the adipocyte drops much below this set amount, the body tends to respond so as to increase triglyceride storage. The responses may include lowering metabolism to conserve energy and stimulating appetite. Conversely, adipocytes have a limited capacity to hypertrophy. Initially, when subjected to a positive energy balance, the response of the body is to store more triglycerides in adipocytes (i.e., hypertrophic obesity: existing adipocytes are enlarged). However, if the positive energy balance is maintained and adipocytes have reached their storage limit, then hyperplasia of adipocytes will occur (i.e., hyperplastic obesity: new adipocytes are created).

The pathological complications of obesity are numerous. Among the diseases and conditions that develop from or worsen because of obesity are hypertension, diabetes (type II), hyperlipidemia, cardiovascular diseases, cancer, gallbladder disease, osteoarthritis, and respiratory disease. Particularly noteworthy is the central role that abdominal obesity appears to play in the metabolic syndrome described earlier in this chapter.

Unique Concerns Related to Exercise Testing and Training

Few, if any, modifications to exercise testing procedures are necessary for obesity if it is present by itself. However, it is quite common for individuals who are obese also to have one or more of the associated diseases (e.g., type II diabetes) or conditions (e.g., hypertension) mentioned previously. In these cases, testing modifications are made based on the related disease or condition.

Exercise Testing

Probably the most common testing modification relates to mode. Some exercise program professionals prefer cycle versus treadmill testing for persons who are obese because it is a weight-supported activity. This is particularly the case if the patient has osteoarthritis of a lower-body joint. However, some prefer treadmill testing, as this mode of exercise (i.e., walking) is desirable for training to maximize energy expenditure. A recommendation is to select walking protocols to avoid stress-related injuries that could occur from running. Another factor to consider in selecting a protocol is that the functional capacity of individuals who are obese is generally lower than in those who are not obese. Thus, it is important to use protocols with lower initial workloads and smaller workload increments to assure reasonable test times.

Exercise Prescription Modifications

When one is designing an activity program for an individual who is obese, the major emphasis should be on maximizing energy expenditure (total volume). The total volume of the activity program is primarily a function of its duration, frequency, and intensity, and to a lesser extent of the mode. The optimal activity program is developed on the basis of the individual's characteristics. This is especially true in the case of patients who are obese. It is necessary to achieve a balance between promoting factors that optimize energy expenditure and factors that maximize patient safety

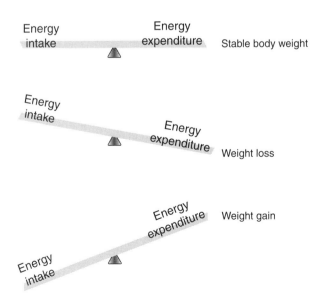

Figure 9.7   The principle of energy balance.

(figure 9.8). Since many patients who are obese also have other diseases or conditions, such as hypertension and type II diabetes, a number of specific safety-related modifications are necessary. Two major concerns are the risks of orthopedic injuries and of hyperthermia. To limit the risk of orthopedic injuries, low-impact (walking) versus high-impact (running) as well as weight-supported (cycling) activities are advisable. Swimming would be considered an excellent choice from an injury prevention viewpoint; but there are questions whether swimming entails adequate amounts of energy expenditure, since the buoyancy advantage that obese individuals have in the water makes them more efficient (less energy required). To limit the risk of hyperthermia it is advisable to avoid exercise in high-temperature or high-humidity environments. It is also important to emphasize wearing clothing that allows heat loss and sweat evaporation. If exercising in a warmer environment, the patient should reduce the exercise intensity and consume plenty of water.

Caloric Expenditure

The ACSM recommends an energy expenditure goal of 300 to 500 kcal per day (1000-2000 kcal per week) to promote body fat loss in individuals who

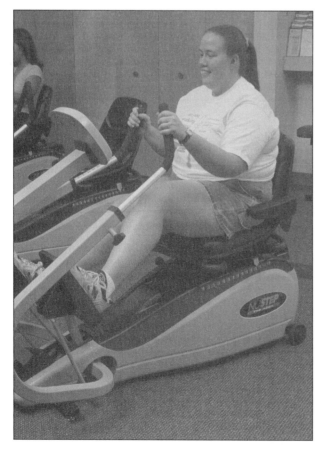

Figure 9.8   Obese patient exercising on a Nu-Step.
Photo courtesy of FCS, Inc.

are obese (10). To achieve this total volume goal, the recommendation is a frequency minimum of five days per week. Ideally, one encourages daily activity. In general, lower intensities (40-70% $\dot{V}O_2$max) are advisable, with durations in the range of 40 to 60 min. Some people may prefer breaking the activity into two shorter daily sessions. Persons who are obese should also be encouraged to increase physical activity throughout the day. The aim is to promote additional energy expenditure and to ward off a tendency to have a compensatory decrease in leisure-time caloric expenditure (i.e., some individuals "reward" themselves for their exercise session with a prolonged period of little to no activity). Resistance training is also recommended for patients who are obese. This type of training can help prevent the potential loss of fat-free mass that accompanies low calorie diets (i.e., 1500 kcal per day for men and 1200 kcal per day for women) used to induce weight loss. Maintenance of fat-free mass is important since this component of the body is known to be the greatest contributor to resting energy expenditure.

Maintenance of Weight Loss

Long-term success rates in maintaining body fat loss are not good. Most studies have shown that initial fat loss is optimized if an activity program is complemented by a reduction in energy intake. Total energy intake should not be reduced below 1000 kcal per day (note that caloric restriction of this magnitude needs to be medically supervised), but does not need to be that extreme. Furthermore, many believe that the potential for long-term success diminishes if the rate of weight loss exceeds 1 kg per week. Finally, it is important to recognize that the factor most associated with long-term maintenance of weight loss is adherence to a regular activity program.

Medications

Persons who are obese have sought over-the-counter remedies for many years. More recently, prescription pharmacological therapy for obesity has become increasingly common. This type of treatment is recommended only for those with BMI >30, or BMI >27 along with two or more CAD risk factors who have not been successful with non-drug therapies. Although new pharmacological treatments are emerging for obesity (see discussion of this topic in chapter 4), caution is warranted prior to widespread acceptance because of the lack of information about side effects and long-term efficacy. A variety of medications are used in the treatment of obesity, most of which do not affect the cardiovascular system. However, some, like sibutramine (an appetite suppressant), can cause increases in BP and heart rate.

PERIPHERAL ARTERIAL DISEASE

According to estimates from the Vascular Disease Foundation , approximately 8 million Americans have PAD. Because PAD is caused by an atherosclerotic process, meaning that it is a progressive disease, rates of PAD are higher as age increases. Likewise, since the risk factors for atherosclerosis are the same (e.g., smoking, hypertension, hypercholesterolemia, diabetes), it is not uncommon for PAD patients to also have CAD.

Pathophysiology of Peripheral Arterial Disease

A number of conditions can result in peripheral vascular reductions in blood flow. Peripheral arterial disease (PAD), the most common of these, results from an atherosclerotic process in the arteries of the lower extremities. The pathophysiology of atherosclerosis is reviewed in chapter 2 in relation to coronary arteries. The process is similar for peripheral arteries, as is the resulting inability to increase blood flow to tissues (i.e., leg muscles in this case). Thus, when leg muscles become active (e.g., in walking), they have an increased demand for blood flow. In patients with PAD, this demand cannot be met with increased blood flow; the leg muscles become ischemic, and patients usually experience symptoms such as leg pain or cramping (intermittent claudication). If PAD becomes severe, ischemia may be present at rest, and the lack of blood flow may cause ulcerations and gangrene. Approximately 100,000 amputations per year result from irreversible damage caused by severe PAD.

Unique Concerns Related to Exercise Testing and Training

Since most individuals with PAD are limited by **claudication** pain prior to reaching a cardiac limitation, a number of modifications to exercise testing procedures are necessary. Also, one should recognize that this peripheral symptom limitation may preclude the diagnosis of a cardiac symptom (i.e., angina) since the test would be stopped prior to this point (i.e., where myocardial demand exceeds myocardial supply). In this situation other forms of testing, such as arm ergometry or pharmacologic stress testing (see chapter 3) are necessary to provide cardiac diagnostic information.

Exercise Testing

The primary rationale of exercise testing in individuals with PAD is to determine their symptom-limited functional capacity. Typically, two indicators of functional capacity are used:

- Time or distance to onset of claudication pain (called initial claudication distance)
- Time or distance to maximal claudication pain, which requires termination of the test (called absolute claudication distance)

These measures of functional capacity are important both for determining the exercise prescription and for assessing the efficacy of treatments and the progression of the disease.

Two different types of treadmill exercise test protocols have been used with PAD patient populations (14). One type is a constant-load test that uses the same speed and grade for all patients (most commonly 2 mph [3.2 km/h] and 12% grade). This type of testing has been in use for a long time and is obviously easy to administer. However, because of the wide range of walking abilities of PAD patients as well as other factors, constant-load tests have been shown to lack reliability and thus have limited utility as a measure of functional capacity. The other type of test uses a graded protocol, typically with a fixed speed (2 mph) and incremental increases in grade (2% every 2 min or 3.5% every 3 min). Graded protocols are more reliable than constant-load tests and are thus better suited to the PAD population. The slow speeds of these protocols is necessary to accommodate the markedly lower average functional capacity ($\dot{V}O_2$max of 10-16 ml·kg^{-1}·min^{-1}) of these patients (12). Because of the importance of documenting the onset and severity of claudication pain, it is essential to use a standardized grading scale. One such scale, presented in the ACSM Guidelines and similar to the angina and dyspnea scales, is shown in table 9.3 (10).

Table 9.3
Claudication Grading Scale

Grade	Description
Grade 1	Definite discomfort or pain, but only of initial or modest levels (established, but minimal)
Grade 2	Moderate discomfort or pain from which the patient's attention can be diverted, for example by conversation
Grade 3	Intense pain (short of grade 4) from which the patient's attention cannot be diverted
Grade 4	Excruciating and unbearable pain

Exercise Prescription Modifications

A primary exercise training goal for patients with PAD is to improve their walking ability (i.e., both increased initial claudication distance and increased absolute claudication distance). Because of the low functional capacity and symptom limitation, exercise prescriptions for individuals with PAD require significant modifications from those for the disease-free populations reviewed in chapter 7. Similar to the situation with patients who have COPD, traditional methods for setting the exercise intensity as a percentage of maximal functional capacity may not apply because of the limiting symptom of claudication. Thus, the principal method of setting exercise intensity for individuals with PAD is to have them exercise at a load that can be maintained with no more than a grade of 2 on the claudication scale. For PAD patients without significant symptom limitations, the recommendation is to set the intensity of exercise between 40% and 70% of $\dot{V}O_2$max. Exercise duration may be relatively short (<10 min), at least initially, due to claudication pain (session should be stopped if grade 3 is reached) and/or the relatively low functional capacity of PAD patients. If a patient cannot perform exercise continuously for the desired 20 to 40 min, then an interval approach is recommended, with the patient resting until the claudication pain subsides. As discussed previously in relation to other populations, the frequency of the exercise program should be increased for individuals with PAD to allow them to reach the training caloric expenditure threshold discussed in chapter 7. Generally, walking, stepping, or a combination of the two is the recommended mode of exercise as these activities have the most transfer to activities of daily living. However, cycling or arm ergometry can be included (in addition to the weight-supported modes) to help increase exercise session caloric expenditure.

Remember that PAD patients are at increased risk for CAD. If present, the CAD may not have resulted in symptoms because of the functional limitations related to claudication. Thus, as PAD patients improve their functional capacity it is important for the exercise program professional to be aware of the possibility that cardiac-related signs and symptoms may emerge.

Medications

Presently, only a few medications are prescribed specifically for PAD. Among the primary pharmacological treatments used are blood-modifying agents (hemorrheologic, anticoagulants, antiplatelet) to decrease blood viscosity (to improve blood flow) and to prevent clotting (table 4.6). These medications have no effect on exercise responses. However, it is not uncommon for individuals with PAD to have other conditions (e.g., diabetes [see table 9.2], hypertension [see table 4.5], or hyperlipidemia [see table 4.3]) that require pharmacological treatments, which may influence exercise responses. Thus, the exercise program professional needs to be aware of all the medications that a PAD patient is on.

Review Case 9.5
Peripheral Arterial Disease

Julia is a 64-year-old patient in your preventative/rehabilitative exercise program. When Julia first joined the program two years ago, she could walk on a treadmill at 1.8 mph (2.9 km/h, no elevation) for only 6 min prior to the onset of claudication pain. She has been a regular exerciser in your program for two years. Julia has increased her absolute exercise intensity to a treadmill pace of 2.7 mph (4.3 km/h) at a 2.5% elevation and can walk continuously for 30 min without claudication pain. Today Julia increased her intensity to 3.0 mph (4.8 km/h) with a 2.5% grade. You observe that Julia seems to be in some distress, and when you question her she reports that she feels some tightness in her chest and left shoulder.

Given this information, respond to the following:

1. What should your immediate response be?

2. What significance (if any) do you think Julia's reported symptom has?

3. Why might this have happened today (as opposed to anytime in the last year)?

SUMMARY

As noted in the introduction, since the majority of cardiac patients are over age 45, many have other health-related concerns commonly associated with middle-aged and older individuals. In this chapter we have reviewed six conditions that are often observed in cardiac rehabilitation programs. Certainly, cardiac patients may have many more conditions than are covered in this chapter. A useful reference text that provides a general overview of many different conditions is *ACSM's Exercise Management for Persons with Chronic Diseases and Disabilities* (15).

We hope that this chapter helps you recognize the importance of having a thorough understanding of each patient's health history. Each patient presents a unique set of characteristics that requires the exercise program professional to make individualized modifications to the evaluation of the patient as well as to the exercise plan.

GLOSSARY

Cardiomyopathy: a disorder or disease of the myocardium

Claudication: limping due to leg pain

Dyspnea: difficulty with breathing

Forced expiratory volume (one second): the amount of air that can be expired in the first second during a forced vital capacity test

Forced vital capacity: the amount of air that can be expired, as rapidly as possible, after a maximal inspiration

Hypoxemia: a condition in which the oxygen supply of the arterial blood is below normal

Ketones: chemical product formed from excess fatty acid oxidation

Nephropathy: a disorder or disease of the kidneys

Neuropathy: a disorder or disease of the nerves

Retinopathy: a disorder or disease of the retina

Spirometry: measurement of lung volumes and capacities

Valsalva maneuver: making an expiratory effort against a closed glottis; results in increased intrathoracic pressure, leading to decreased venous return and cardiac output

REFERENCES

1. American Association of Cardiovascular and Pulmonary Rehabilitation. 1998. *Guidelines for pulmonary rehabilitation programs.* 2nd ed. Champaign, IL: Human Kinetics, 250.

2. Borg, G.A. 1998. *Borg's perceived exertion and pain scales.* Champaign, IL: Human Kinetics.

3. Aitken, R.C.B. 1969. Measurement of feelings using visual analog scales. *Proc. Royal Soc. Med.* 62:989–993.

4. Whaley, M.H., J.B. Kampert, H.W. Kohl, and S.N. Blair. 1999. Physical fitness and clustering of risk factors associated with the metabolic syndrome. *Med. Sci. Sports Exerc.* 31:287–293.

5. American College of Sports Medicine. 2000. Position stand: Exercise and type 2 diabetes. *Med. Sci. Sports Exerc.* 32:1345–1360.

6. Schneider, S.H., and N.B. Ruderman. 1990. Exercise and NIDDM. Technical Review by the American Diabetes Association. *Diabetes Care* 13:785–789.

7. Wasserman, D.H., and B. Zinman. 1994. Exercise in individuals with IDDM. Technical Review by the American Diabetes Association. *Diabetes Care* 17:924–937.

8. Zinman, B., N. Ruderman, B.N. Campaigne, J.T. Devlin, and S.H. Schneider. 1998. Diabetes mellitus and exercise. Joint position statement of the American Diabetes Association and the American College of Sports Medicine. *Diabetes Care* 21:S40–S44.

9. Bakris, G.L. 2000. Lower blood pressure goals for patients with diabetes: The National Kidney Foundation consensus report. *J. Clin. Hypertension* 2:369–371.

10. Franklin, B.F., M.H. Whaley, and E.T. Howley, eds. 2000. *ACSM's guidelines for exercise testing and prescription.* 6th ed. Baltimore: Lippincott, Williams & Wilkins.

11. The sixth report of the Joint National Committee on Prevention, Detection and Treatment of High Blood Pressure. 1997. Bethesda, MD: National Institutes of Health.

12. Regensteiner, J.G., and W.G. Hiatt. 1998. Exercise in the management of peripheral arterial disease. In *ACSM's resource manual for guidelines for exercise testing and prescription,* 3rd ed. J. Roitman, 281–287. Baltimore: Williams & Wilkins.

13. American College of Sports Medicine. 1993. Position stand: Physical activity, physical fitness, and hypertension. *Med. Sci. Sports Exerc.* 25:i–x.

14. Hiatt, W.R., A.T. Hirsch, J.G. Regensteiner, and E.P. Brass. 1995. Clinical trials for claudication. *Circulation* 92:614–621.

15. Durstine, J.L., ed. 1997. *ACSM's exercise management for persons with chronic diseases and disabilities.* Champaign, IL: Human Kinetics, 269.

PART III

Organization and Administration of Coronary Artery Disease Prevention and Rehabilitation Programs

CHAPTER 10

Core Components and Models of Coronary Artery Disease Prevention and Rehabilitation Programs

BEHAVIORAL OBJECTIVES

- To be able to describe the core components of prevention and rehabilitation programs and describe appropriate evaluations, interventions, and expected outcomes for each

- To recognize adherence and compliance problems in prevention or rehabilitation programs and understand the basic theories of behavioral change

- To understand how new and alternative models of prevention or rehabilitation incorporate specific theories of behavioral change to create more effective approaches

It is now recognized that contemporary CAD prevention and rehabilitation programs must utilize a multidisciplinary approach and incorporate specific core components. Participation in such well-designed primary and secondary prevention programs has been shown to result in a number of positive health benefits, including a reduction in sudden cardiac death (figure 10.1). Furthermore, in the current era of health care, documentation of the benefits (later described as "outcomes") is essential and is of use in evaluating the effectiveness of the **intervention** program. Potentially, only programs that can demonstrate successful outcomes for their patients will receive reimbursement for the services they provide. However, dropout and lack of **compliance** are common in preventive and rehabilitative programs and limit their effectiveness. Consequently, many have become interested in understanding how patients make and sustain important lifestyle changes and how current models of primary and secondary prevention can be modified to deliver more effective interventions.

CONTEMPORARY PREVENTIVE AND REHABILITATIVE PROGRAMS: NOT JUST EXERCISE

Exercise training, secondary to the numerous benefits described in earlier chapters, is widely rec-

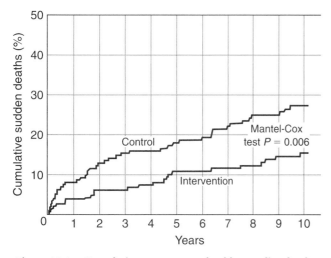

Figure 10.1   Cumulative percentage of sudden cardiac deaths during 10 years of follow-up of multifactorial cardiac rehabilitation intervention and control groups. Participants in multifactorial cardiac rehabilitation had a 46% reduction in risk for sudden cardiac death compared to patients who did not participate in a cardiac rehabilitation program.
Reprinted from *European Heart Journal,* Vol. 15, H. Hamalainen et al., "Long-term reduction in sudden deaths after a multifactorial intervention programme in patients with myocardial infarction: 10-year results of a controlled investigation," p. 55, ©1989, by permission of the publisher W.B. Saunders.

ognized as an important intervention for the prevention and treatment of CAD. Indeed, exercise therapy is the cornerstone of most primary prevention and cardiac rehabilitation programs. However, since the development and progression of cardiovascular disease is multifactorial, an effective primary or secondary intervention program must also address the variety of other factors known to impact disease progression or regression. Exercise training, in combination with other lifestyle changes, has been shown to be more effective than exercise alone in modifying many of the known risk factors for CAD.

In 2000, the American Heart Association and the American Association of Cardiovascular and Pulmonary Rehabilitation released a scientific statement entitled "Core Components of Cardiac Rehabilitation/Secondary Prevention Programs" (1). The AHA and AACVPR recognize that all cardiac rehabilitation/secondary prevention programs should contain specific "core components" that aim to optimize cardiovascular risk reduction, foster healthy behaviors and compliance to these behaviors, reduce disability, and promote an active lifestyle for patients with cardiovascular disease. While this statement was developed specifically for cardiac rehabilitation/secondary prevention programs, we believe that it can be effectively applied to primary prevention programs as well. Although primary and secondary prevention are arbitrarily distinguished on the basis of the clinical presence or absence of CAD, preventive treatment strategies are essentially similar. For example, the need to lower abnormally high blood lipid levels (potentially with lifestyle modification, pharmacologic therapy, or both) in an individual who has experienced a myocardial infarction (MI) is similar (even if target levels are slightly different) to that for an individual who has not shown clinical manifestation of CAD. The purpose of the AHA/AACVPR statement (1) is to provide information regarding specific evaluations, interventions, and expected outcomes for each of the core areas of cardiac rehabilitation and secondary prevention listed in box 10.1.

The recommendations in the AHA/AACVPR statement (1) are intended to assist program staff in the design and development of the program and to help health care providers, insurers and policy makers, and consumers recognize the comprehensive nature of such programs. It was not the intent of this statement to promote a "rote" approach or homogeneity among programs, but rather to foster a foundation of services upon which each program can establish its own spe-

---

cific strength and identity and effectively attain outcome goals for a target population. This chapter presents a brief rationale for each core component; readers can find the detailed recommendations in the published scientific statement (1).

Patient Assessment

Patient assessment is an important part of any prevention or rehabilitation program for three primary reasons: safety, goal setting, and outcome assessment. To ensure safety in the exercise program, each patient should undergo a medical history evaluation, a physical exam, and appropriate testing prior to entering a prevention or rehabilitation program. Details on the medical assessments (history, physical exam, etc.) and rationale for exercise testing are discussed in chapters 3 and 6, respectively. Results of these evaluations, such as initial MET levels and risk factor status, are subsequently used to determine patient-specific goals and identify specific interventions required to attain these goals. For example, the specific interventions for an individual entering the program with abnormal blood lipids should focus on weight loss, dietary changes, and possible pharmacologic therapy. Furthermore, assessment of the patient before and again after participation in the intervention program can yield important outcome measures. That is, did the patient achieve the established goals? In other words, in this example, did the patient's blood lipids improve and/or have they reached defined target levels as the result of the intervention (i.e., lifestyle changes, medication therapy) (described in chapter 4)?

Nutritional Counseling and Weight Management

There is no question that overweight/obesity has become a problem of near epidemic proportions in the United States and other industrialized countries. Over the last two decades, the prevalence of overweight in adults in the United States has risen at a rate of 0.9% per year, and recent estimates (2) suggest classification of more than 35% of Americans as either overweight or obese (see chapter 6 for methods of determination and categorization). Furthermore, obesity is documented in approximately 40% of the 12 million people with CAD (3). While the cause of overweight or obesity is multifactorial and is complicated by a variety of cultural and environmental issues, as well as **socioeconomic status,** there is no question that improper dietary habits play a critical role in this "growing" problem. Since the use of dietary changes alone to produce weight loss is largely ineffective, the American Dietetic Association (ADA) now advocates "weight management" versus "weight loss." Weight management, according to the ADA, is the adoption of healthful and sustainable eating and exercise behaviors necessary to reduce disease risk and improve feelings of energy and well being. According to the ADA (4), the goals of any weight management program should include at least 30 min of daily physical activity and a healthful yet nonrestrictive approach to eating. The focus of weight management is achieving and maintaining good health by stopping weight gain, achieving and maintaining a stable weight, and/or reducing health risks. As described in chapter 1, overweight or obesity and its impact on other risk factors (lipids, blood pressure, diabetes) are strongly related to the development of CAD. Furthermore, the intake of excessive saturated and trans fat, sodium, and refined sugar can potentially alter blood lipids, blood pressure, and blood glucose, respectively, in certain individuals.

A registered dietician typically provides the nutritional evaluations and interventions in a prevention or rehabilitation program; but in certain areas such as physical activity counseling for weight loss, other trained health care providers, specifically exercise physiologists, may play a more significant role. Box 10.2 lists some of the tools that can be used to assess dietary habits. Although feedback of results from these instruments can be effectively disseminated in small patient groups or classes, given the sensitivity of many with respect to weight it may be more desirable to address this information on a one-to-one basis.

It may be helpful to have the patient's spouse, significant other, or family members attend nutritional counseling sessions, particularly if they are heavily involved in meal planning or preparation or if they influence dietary practices (e.g., choosing restaurants, doing grocery shopping, etc.).

Box 10.2 Instruments Commonly Used to Assess Dietary Habits

- Diet Habit Survey
- Harvard-Willett Food Frequency Questionnaire
- Block Food Frequency Questionnaire
- 7-Day Food Diary

Lipid, Hypertension, and Diabetes Management

As described in chapter 1, various blood lipid disorders (i.e., elevated total cholesterol, low-density lipoprotein, or triglycerides; low high-density lipoprotein), hypertension, and diabetes are classified as modifiable risk factors for CAD. Chapter 4 discusses lifestyle and pharmacologic treatments for lipid disorders and hypertension based on goals developed by the National Cholesterol Education Program and Joint National Committee on Prevention, Detection, Evaluation, and Treatment of High Blood Pressure, respectively. Preventive or rehabilitative programs provide an excellent opportunity to assess and intervene on these risk factors. The lipid, hypertension, and diabetes management core components from AHA/AACVPR (1) are consistent with the information presented in earlier chapters, yet the scientific statement from AHA/AACVPR provides clear objectives that programs can focus their efforts on. Blood lipids, glucose, and blood pressure may be measured directly within the program, or information from these measurements may be obtained from outside of the program (physician's office, hospital). In either case, the prevention or rehabilitation program's objective should be to identify lipid disorders, hypertension, and diabetes and intervene with appropriate lifestyle changes. Generally it is acceptable for prevention or rehabilitation professionals to intervene on lipid, glucose, and blood pressure disorders with exercise, dietary, and weight loss recommendations. These recommendations are covered in chapter 4 and are summarized in the core components of the AHA/AACVPR document (1). However, recommendations for medical management (i.e., adding or changing medications for lipid, hypertension, or diabetes) should be left to the discretion of the patient's primary health care provider (physician, physician's assistant, or nurse practitioner). Ideally, the prevention or rehabilitation professional works in concert with the patient's health care provider to obtain an optimal outcome (i.e., achieve target goals) for each risk factor. Generally, health care providers welcome input and recommendations from the preventive or rehabilitative program staff to more effectively manage the risk factors in their patients.

Smoking Management

The relationship between cigarette smoking or secondary exposure to smoke and the risk for cardiovascular disease is well established and is described in chapter 1. Furthermore, patients with heart disease who continue to smoke are twice as likely to experience recurrent cardiac events as patients who do not resume smoking. Thus **smoking cessation** must be a major objective of any primary prevention or cardiac rehabilitation program. Some of the highest cessation rates are noted in patients who were smoking immediately prior to a cardiovascular event. Unfortunately, even in these patients, relapse rates are between 30% and 40% soon after hospital discharge.

An important point in the AHA/AACVPR Statement (1) is that the health care provider (physician, preventive or rehabilitative staff) needs to evaluate the patient's **readiness** to change. This is an important concept in relation to changing any health behavior (exercise, smoking, weight loss) and is discussed in more detail later in this chapter (see "Changing Behaviors for a Healthier Life"—the stages of change or transtheoretical model). Essentially, if the patient is unwilling or has no desire to quit smoking, it is highly unlikely that any of the interventions described here will be effective. For those individuals interested in quitting, the following approaches are commonly used:

- Counseling
- Nicotine-replacement therapies
- Pharmacologic agents

Counseling

For the patient motivated to quit, a number of counseling approaches are relatively successful (5). As with other health behaviors, a strong, unequivocal message about the hazards of smoking by a health care provider, particularly a physician, can have a powerful impact. Statements such as "Quitting smoking now is the most important health advice I can give you" or "You must stop now—let's figure out how you can quit" provide a strong, yet supportive message. Table 10.1 lists several steps that the health care provider can use to facilitate smoking cessation (5).

As with any addictive behavior, "slips," or relapses are common in the early stages of quitting. Marlatt and Gordon (6), in work with addictive behaviors, suggest that health care providers can help people take the following four steps in order to deal with potential relapse to an old behavior:

- Learn how to identify high-risk situations that may result in the old behavior
- Develop skills for managing these high-risk situations
- Develop strategies (such as exercise, relaxation, chewing on vegetables) that provide gratification and that substitute for the addiction
- Learn to implement behavior skills if a relapse occurs

Furthermore, the health care provider should indicate to the patient that

- slips may occur,
- slips do not represent failure and are not necessarily associated with full-blown relapse to smoking, and
- patients should focus on the situation that caused them to smoke (e.g., stress, conflicts, social pressure) and review coping strategies they can use for these high-risk situations.

Nicotine-Replacement Therapies

For several years, researchers have studied the hypothesis that ameliorating nicotine withdrawal symptoms with another form of nicotine might help smokers achieve abstinence from cigarettes. The FDA has approved two forms of nicotine replacement: nicotine gum and the transdermal (skin) patch. Multiple studies have confirmed the efficacy of nicotine-replacement therapy in hospital-based or formal smoking cessation clinics where participants receive counseling in conjunction with the nicotine-replacement therapy. In contrast, nicotine-replacement therapies, particularly gum, without concomitant behavioral counseling have not been found to be very effective (7).

Nicotine-replacement therapies should begin only after the patient stops smoking. Otherwise the nicotine from the cigarettes in addition to the replacement therapy could potentially increase heart rate and blood pressure, subsequently eliciting myocardial ischemia in a patient with coronary disease.

Pharmacologic Agents

The most widely used pharmacologic agent to facilitate smoking cessation, by easing withdrawal symptoms and the urge to smoke, is an antidepressant called Zyban (generic name: bupropion). Zyban appears to work by altering neurochemical pathways including those for norepinephrine and/or dopamine. Its clinical effectiveness has been shown in both depressed and nondepressed smokers, but it has not been adequately studied in patients with CAD. Whether it is more effective than the nicotine patch is not currently known (5).

On the basis of the strength of the evidence in the literature, the Agency for Health Care Policy and Reform (8) has published guidelines that

Table 10.1
Smoking Cessation Methods

Step	Description
1	Help patient select a quit day, normally within 7 days of discussion Write the date down and sign a contract to support the patient
2	Select a quitting method Stop abruptly (i.e., "cold turkey") or cut down in 3 ways: • Gradually reduce number of cigarettes smoked per day • Reduce the amount of nicotine by switching brands every 3 days to one with less nicotine • Reduce the amount of each cigarette smoked (half vs. one-quarter vs. 1-2 puffs)
3	Ask patient to get rid of all cigarette butts, matches, lighters the day before quitting
4	Determine need for nicotine replacement or pharmacological therapy

Adapted from (5).

make four critically important points regarding approaches to smoking cessation:

- Smoking cessation interventions delivered by a variety of providers (medical and non-medical) triple the cessation rate compared to that achieved with an intervention in which there is no provider (e.g., patients who quit on their own or purchase nicotine-replacement devices).

- Smoking cessation interventions using counseling sessions of more than 10 min, compared to briefer sessions, more than double the cessation rate.

- In general, the more prolonged the counseling or treatment, the more effective it is; smoking cessation rates for treatments lasting less than eight weeks and more than eight weeks were 10.4% versus 23.8%, respectively.

- Individualized treatment over four to seven sessions appears to be more efficacious than treatments of fewer than four sessions.

In summary, the Smoking Cessation Clinical Practice Guideline Panel and Staff (8) concludes that multiple health care providers making multiple contacts over time using multiple intervention modalities appear to be the most effective clinical strategy to facilitate smoking cessation. Thus, the prevention or rehabilitation staff should utilize all possible resources to help patients overcome this difficult addiction.

Psychosocial Management

As described in chapter 1, various forms of psychosocial distress, particularly depression, anger, and hostility, have proven to be potent risk factors for the development of CAD. Furthermore, after a cardiac event (e.g., heart attack, surgery), many patients and their families struggle with emotional issues related to the illness and need for lifestyle change. Thus, it is essential for preventive or rehabilitative programs to carefully screen patients for signs of psychosocial distress (box 10.3). This screening can be accomplished with standardized questionnaires or structured interviews performed by a clinical psychologist or other mental health professional. After the initial assessment by the mental health professional, an appropriate intervention is recommended to the patient. Simple interventions, which can often be provided by the rehabilitation staff, may address the following (9):

- Effects of cardiopulmonary illness and medications on mood and sexual response

- Strategies for modifying problem behaviors, such as smoking or overeating

- The dangers of unchecked hostility in relation to health

- The importance of social support in promoting wellness and rehabilitation

- General stress management

- Training in relaxation techniques

Box 10.3 Instruments Commonly Used to Assess Psychosocial Status

- Medical Outcomes Study SF-36 (Short Form 36)
- Health Status Questionnaire
- Beck Depression Inventory
- Nottingham Health Profile
- Symptoms Check List (SCL-90)
- Neo Personality Inventory
- Profile of Mood States
- Ferrins and Powers Health Related Quality of Life
- Spielberger State-Trait Anxiety Inventory

Patients with more significant psychosocial disorders may require referral for psychotherapy, medical therapy, or both. At the Wake Forest Cardiac Rehabilitation Program, approximately one-third of the patients referred to our outpatient cardiac rehabilitation program fall into this category and require referral for extended counseling, medication therapy, or a combination of the two. While the prevention or rehabilitation program may not be capable of providing these types of interventions, it is essential for the program staff to follow up on recommendations and referrals and to document that the patient has received treatment. To assess and educate patients upon entry into a formal prevention or rehabilitation program without follow-up makes no more sense within the psychosocial realm than within any other area of rehabilitation (this would be similar to measuring lipids at entry to a program without measuring again after the intervention). Unfortunately, because of the complexity of many psychosocial disorders, as well as limited knowledge or experience of most prevention or rehabilitation staff in this area, patients' psychosocial needs often remain ignored or undertreated in both inpatient and outpatient programs (9).

Physical Activity Counseling

As we saw in chapter 1, there are distinct differences between "physical activity" and "exercise," yet both provide benefits and should be part of any strategy designed to reduce the risk for CAD. Thus, individuals participating in a preventive or rehabilitative program should receive counseling on how to incorporate physical activity into their daily lives. Furthermore, after a cardiac event, some patients—often at the insistence of their family—avoid returning to domestic, occupational, or recreational activities because of a lack of confidence in their physical ability or fear of further heart damage. One of the many benefits of a cardiac rehabilitation or secondary prevention program is to help patients and their families understand that patients do not have to be "cardiac cripples." Thus it is important to assess the types of domestic, **vocational,** and recreational activities the patient needs or wants to be able to perform. In some cases, simulated work testing can occur along with a consultation with a vocational rehabilitation counselor. Improvement in physical function and resumption of normal activities are best accomplished through physical activity and/or exercise training.

As we noted in chapter 7, exercise training in most structured, center-based preventive or rehabilitation programs takes place three times per week. This practice is based on nearly 30 years of research and clinical application. Readers will recall from chapter 1 that the recommendation according to current views, including the position of the Centers for Disease Control and Prevention and the American College of Sports Medicine, is that individuals should accumulate 30 minutes or more of physical activity on most days of the week (10). This practice represents a departure from the traditional exercise prescription but has been shown to result in positive health benefits in most adult populations. The approach has not been evaluated in a cardiac rehabilitation population, although this topic is currently under investigation. A later section of this chapter deals with current efforts at Wake Forest University to examine this novel approach in a cardiac rehabilitation setting (CHAMP study).

Exercise Training

Obviously, exercise training is the cornerstone intervention in most preventive or rehabilitative programs because of the many potential benefits.

Since exercise testing, prescription, and training are covered extensively in chapters 6, 7, and 8, we provide no further discussion of those topics here. The information in these earlier chapters is consistent with the AHA/AACVPR recommendations for this core component.

Additionally, the core components outlined in the AHA/AACVPR statement provide the framework for certification of cardiac rehabilitation and secondary prevention through the AACVPR. The process of cardiac rehabilitation program certification was actually initiated in the early 1980s in North Carolina (a few other states subsequently established similar models), but it wasn't until the late 1990s that a national certification model was developed. The national certification model ensures that all cardiac rehabilitation and secondary prevention programs adhere to the same standards and guidelines. While national certification of cardiac rehabilitation and secondary prevention programs is still a voluntary process, ultimately certification may be a requirement for receiving referrals and reimbursement for cardiac rehabilitation services. Chapter 11 provides further discussion of the team of health care providers that typically deliver preventive or rehabilitative programs, as well as the process of program certification. At present, there is no equivalent certification process for primary prevention programs.

DOCUMENTATION OF OUTCOMES: WHY AND HOW?

An outcome can be simply defined as what happened to the individual or patient. Thus, the measurement of outcomes provides the basis for assessing the benefit conferred by any type of intervention. During the 1990s, all areas of health care, including cardiac rehabilitation programs, began to emphasize the measurement and documentation of outcomes. Why did this suddenly happen in health care? Essentially, the escalating costs of health care forced the health insurance agencies to question how and why money was being spent. In order to justify the expense of specific medical procedures or services, it is necessary to evaluate the effectiveness (extent of the benefit to the patient) and efficacy (cost in relation to benefit) of a given service. This is accomplished by measuring an "outcome" related to each service. If the outcome from a particular procedure or intervention is cost effective (as measured by an index of treatment benefit per dollar, it is probable that the insurance company will continue to reimburse the health care provider for the service. If a service is not cost effective, the likelihood for reimbursement is questionable.

Moreover, accrediting organizations such as the Joint Commission on Accreditation of Healthcare Organizations (JCAHO) and Medicare use outcomes as a basis for program evaluation. The Joint Commission has recently changed the focus of its on-site inspections to outcomes, emphasizing actual performance and results rather than the capacity to perform and achieve results. Furthermore, the JCAHO expects that hospitals (and their programs, such as cardiac rehabilitation) will develop quality **benchmarks** (allowing for comparison to other institutions), evaluate outcome findings, and make changes using continuous improvement models. The process of examining, redesigning, or refining (often referred to as quality improvement or total quality management) is essential to the management of preventive or rehabilitative programs.

While there are numerous health care-related outcomes, the AACVPR *Guidelines for Cardiac Rehabilitation Programs* (9) addresses three primary outcome "domains" for individuals participating in a preventive or rehabilitative program: Health, Clinical, and Behavioral. Table 10.2 identifies the three primary outcome domains and the specific measures within each that determine the effectiveness

of the prevention or rehabilitation program (9). This document also describes many of the specific tools that are currently available to document outcomes. It is not necessary or feasible to measure each outcome; thus the AHA/AACVPR core components document is helpful in that it identifies and focuses on the more valuable and practical outcomes for prevention or rehabilitation programs to document. The process of certifying cardiac rehabilitation programs through AACVPR (described in more detail in chapter 11) requires documentation of at least one outcome from each of the three domains, but does not stipulate which one.

According to AACVPR (9), selected outcomes should be collected and documented for each patient in the preventive or rehabilitative program at three points: upon admission to the program, at discharge from the program, and at one year after the patient has exited the program. The last data point may be most difficult to obtain, but this outcome is important to measure since maintenance of adaptive or long-term change is a critical measure of program success. Based on the AHA/AACVPR core components document (1), outcomes for CAD preventive or rehabilitative programs can be tracked by means of forms similar to the one used in the Wake Forest Cardiac Rehabilitation Program (figure 10.2).

Table 10.2
Outcome Domains

Health	Clinical	Behavioral

I. Mortality
II. Morbidity
III. Quality of life
	I. Physical
	A. Weight
	B. Blood pressure
	C. Lipids
	D. Oxygenation
	E. Functional capacity
	F. Blood nicotine levels
	G. Blood medication levels
	  1. Theophylline
	  2. Digoxin
	H. Symptom management
	  1. Cough
	  2. Dyspnea
	  3. Angina
	
	II. Psychosocial
	A. Interpersonal function and dysfunction
	B. Psychological status
	C. Return to vocational and avocational independent living
	
	III. Medical utilization
	A. Medication usage
	B. Hospitalizations
	C. Physician/emergency room visits
		I. Medical regime
		II. Diet
		III. Exercise
		IV. Smoking cessation
		V. Breathing retraining
		VI. Relaxation skills
		VII. Social skills
		VIII. Recognition of impending complications

Reprinted, by permission, from AACVPR, *Guidelines for cardiac rehabilitation*, 2nd ed. (Champaign, IL: Human Kinetics), 74.

Wake Forest University Cardiac Rehabilitation Outcomes Tool

Name _____   ID# _____

Date of Entry _____   MDs _____   DOB: _____

Diagnosis _____   Exit Date: _____

	Goals	CRP Entry Date:	Re-Eval ( ) Date:	Change Abs.	Change %	Achieve Goal (Yes or No)
Clinical Outcomes						
LDL (mg/dl)	<100					
Cholesterol (mg/dl)	<200					
HDL (mg/dl)	>40					
TC/HDL Ratio	<4.5					
Triglyceride (mg/dl)	<150					
Blood Glucose (mg/dl)	<110					
Rest Blood Pressure (mmHg)	<140/90					
METs (Estimated)	Add 1 to baseline value					
Health Outcomes						
Quality of Life (overall)	Normal ≥ 23					
Behavior Change						
Smoking (# per day)	0					
Weight (lbs)	Set by Nutritionist					
Waist (inches)	Men <40 Women <35					
Dietary Habits	DPR>65					
Relaxation Training	>2 per week					
Ex. Attendance	>75%					
Activity Outside CRP	>2 days					
Medical Utilization						
Hospitalizations	0					
Emergency Rm. Visits	0					
Unplanned MD Visits	0					

- Quality of life= Ferrans and Powers
- DPR = Diet Pattern Review (a food frequency questionnaire developed and used at Wake Forest University)

Comments:

Figure 10.2   Form used at Wake Forest University to track outcomes in cardiac rehabilitaion.

GOALS AND OUTCOMES OF PREVENTION AND REHABILITATION PROGRAMS

The benefits of participation in a primary prevention program are substantial (discussed in chapter 8). In summary, the goals of a primary prevention program are (1) to improve cardiovascular and respiratory function; (2) to reduce CAD risk factors; (3) to decrease morbidity and mortality; (4) to decrease anxiety and depression; (5) to enhance feelings of well-being; and (6) to enhance performance of work, recreational, and sport activities.

The goals of secondary prevention and cardiac rehabilitation include all those just listed in addition to the following:

- To limit the physiologic and psychological effects of cardiac illness
- To reduce the risk for sudden death or reinfarction
- To control cardiac symptoms
- To stabilize or reverse the atherosclerotic process
- To enhance the psychosocial and vocational status of selected patients

In 1995, the Agency for Health Care Policy and Reform produced The Clinical Practice Guideline for Cardiac Rehabilitation (11). Subsequently, a panel of experts convened to review the existing literature on cardiac rehabilitation and, on the basis of the strength of the supportive evidence, describe the effects of multidisciplinary cardiac rehabilitation.

Readers interested in the extensive body of literature reviewed and cited to support these benefits should refer to the Clinical Practice Guidelines (11), which can be obtained without charge by writing the U.S. Government Printing Office (Superintendent of Documents, Mail Stop: SSOP, Washington, DC 20402-9328). Table 10.3 presents a brief summary of the specific benefits cited in the Clinical Practice Guidelines. On the basis of a comprehensive review of the scientific literature, the panel concluded that cardiac rehabilitation services are an essential component of the contemporary management of patients with CAD and heart failure. However, the guidelines strongly convey that comprehensive cardiac rehabilitation is "not just an exercise program" and that to obtain the benefits described in table 10.3, the rehabilitation program must be a "multifactorial process" that also includes education, counseling, and use of behavioral interventions.

Relationship of Compliance and Outcomes

The benefits of a comprehensive preventive or rehabilitative program, as described earlier, can be expected only when patients comply fully with the various interventions that the program provides. In other words, the patients most compliant to the program components (exercise, weight loss, dietary changes) generally obtain the greatest benefit (12). Furthermore, poor compliance and subsequent lack of benefit constitute one of the many reasons patients decide to drop out of preventive or rehabilitative programs. Oldridge and colleagues (13) have shown that in post-MI trials of rehabilitation that last at least 12 months, the typical dropout curve in cardiac exercise rehabilitation is a negatively accelerating one, with the largest proportion of dropout occurring within the first 6 months. The mean 3-month dropout from 12-month trials is 25% to 30%, increasing to 40% to 50% by 6 months. Box 10.4 presents the numerous variables that are predictive of dropout from exercise programs, and figure 10.3 shows negative and positive variables that affect compliance to exercise programs (14). Obviously, when negative variables outweigh positive ones, the consequence will be poor **adherence,** dropout, or both.

The discouraging dropout rates reported by Oldridge and colleagues (13) are observed in clinical trials (i.e., research studies) involving patients who have volunteered for the study. By definition, these individuals are highly motivated to participate. Furthermore, in these studies there are no fees, so financial issues are not a consideration or cause for dropout. Consider how different this is from "real-world" cardiac rehabilitation programs: patients are often less motivated to participate in these and have to be "pushed into" doing so by a family member or health care provider. Moreover, health insurance and financial issues often impact the duration of participation in cardiac rehabilitation. In fact, at the Wake Forest University Cardiac Rehabilitation Program, we have observed over time that approximately 40% of the patients who enter our program exit after 3 months of participation. By 12 months, nearly 80% of the patients who entered have exited or dropped out. While a number of the factors listed in box 10.4 could relate to why patients drop out of exercise programs, cost (due to lack of extended insurance coverage) appears to be a prominent issue as most people are

Table 10.3
Benefits of Participation in Multifactorial Cardiac Rehabilitation

Benefit	Description
Improvement in exercise tolerance	Cardiac rehabilitation exercise training improves objective measures of exercise tolerance in both men and women, including elderly patients, with CAD and with heart failure. This functional improvement occurs without significant cardiovascular complications or other adverse outcomes. Appropriately prescribed exercise training should be an integral component of cardiac rehabilitation services and particularly benefits patients with decreased exercise tolerance. Maintenance of exercise training is required to sustain improvement in exercise tolerance.
Improvement in symptoms	Cardiac rehabilitation exercise training decreases symptoms of angina pectoris in patients with CAD and decreases symptoms of heart failure in patients with left ventricular systolic dysfunction. Improvement in clinical measures of myocardial ischemia following exercise rehabilitation, as identified by electrocardiographic (ECG) and nuclear cardiology techniques, provides objective support for the reported symptomatic improvement. Exercise training of patients with left ventricular systolic dysfunction provides added symptomatic improvement to that achieved by appropriate medication management.
Improvement in blood lipid levels	Multifactorial cardiac rehabilitation in patients with CAD, including exercise training and education, results in improved lipid and lipoprotein levels. Exercise training as a sole intervention has not effected consistent improvement in lipid profiles. Optimal lipid management requires specifically directed dietary and, when medically indicated, pharmacologic management as a component of multifactorial cardiac rehabilitation.
Reduction in cigarette smoking	Multifactorial cardiac rehabilitation, with well-designed educational and behavioral components, reduces cigarette smoking. Sixteen to 26% of patients can be expected to stop smoking. These smoking cessation rates enhance the spontaneously high smoking cessation rates in most populations following a coronary event. Scientific evidence, consensus reports, and scientific reviews in the non-rehabilitation setting, including the Surgeons General's warning since 1965, lend strong support that education, counseling, and behavioral interventions, particularly when combined, are beneficial for smoking cessation.
Improvement in psychosocial well-being and stress reduction	Exercise training enhances measures of psychological and social functioning, particularly as a component of multifactorial cardiac rehabilitation. Improvement in psychological status and functioning, including measures of emotional stress and reduction of Type-A behavior pattern, is consistent with the improvement in psychosocial outcomes that occurs in non-rehabilitation settings.
Reductions in mortality	A survival benefit for patients who participate in cardiac rehabilitation exercise training is suggested from the scientific data, but this cannot be attributed solely to exercise training because many studies involved multifactorial interventions. Meta-analysis of randomized controlled trials of exercise rehabilitation in patients following myocardial infarction establishes a reduction in mortality approximating 25% at 3-year follow-up. This reduction in mortality approaches that resulting from pharmacologic management of patients following myocardial infarction with beta-blocking drugs or patients with left ventricular systolic dysfunction with angiotensin-converting enzyme (ACE) inhibitor therapy. The reduction in cardiovascular mortality was 26% in multifactorial randomized trials of cardiac rehabilitation and 15% in trials that involved only exercise intervention. The panel concludes that multifactorial cardiac rehabilitation services can reduce mortality in patients following myocardial infarction.
Safety	The safety of cardiac rehabilitation exercise training is inferred from aggregate analysis of clinical experience. None of the more than three dozen randomized controlled trials of cardiac rehabilitation exercise training in patients with CAD, involving more than 4500 patients, described an increase in morbidity or mortality in rehabilitation compared with the control patient groups. A survey of 142 cardiac rehabilitation programs in the United States involving patients participating in exercise rehabilitation from 1980-1984 reported, based on aggregate data, a low rate of nonfatal myocardial infarction of 1 per 294,000 patient-hours; the cardiac mortality rate was 1 per 784,000 patient-hours. A total of 21 episodes of cardiac arrest occurred, with successful resuscitation of 17 patients. Thus safety of exercise rehabilitation is established by the very low rates of occurrence of myocardial infarction and cardiovascular complications during exercise training.

Adapted from (11).

Box 10.4   Variables Predicting Exercise Program Dropout

Personal Factors
- Smoker
- Inactive leisure time
- Inactive occupation
- Blue collar worker
- Type A personality
- Increased physical strength
- Extroverted
- Poor credit rating
- Overweight and/or low ponderal index
- Poor self-motivation
- Depressed
- Hypochondriacal
- Anxious
- Introverted
- Low ego strength

Program Factors
- Inconvenient time and/or location
- Excessive cost
- High-intensity exercise
- Lack of exercise variety, e.g., running only
- Exercising alone
- Lack of positive feedback or reinforcement
- Inflexible exercise goals
- Low enjoyment ratings for running programs
- Poor exercise leadership

Other Factors
- Lack of spouse support
- Inclement weather
- Excessive job travel
- Injury
- Job change and/or move

Reprinted, by permission, from B.A. Franklin, 1999, Program factors that influence exercise adherence: practical adherence skills for clinical staff. In *Exercise adherence: Its impact on public health*, edited by R. Dishman (Champaign, IL: Human Kinetics), 239.

unwilling to pay for this relatively inexpensive, yet beneficial, intervention.

Interestingly, program staff and patients themselves often assume that after dropout from a structured preventive or rehabilitative program, patients will continue to maintain the health behaviors they practiced while in the program (i.e., exercising regularly, eating healthfully). Unfortunately, research at Wake Forest University (15) showed that patients exiting after successful completion of the initial three-month cardiac rehabilitation program were not able to maintain their functional capacity, blood lipids, and body weight/composition (figure 10.4). This study clearly indicated that even after successful participation in a standard (i.e., 3 month) cardiac rehabilitation program, patients were typically unable to avoid losing these benefits after exiting. In contrast, patients who remained in a long-term, center-based maintenance cardiac rehabilitation program continued to benefit or to maintain positive changes in risk factors and functional capacity. Thus, for patients who exit programs after three months, as most do in the current era of reimbursement, we must explore new program models in order to realize the long-term benefits of this type of intervention.

CHANGING BEHAVIORS FOR A HEALTHIER LIFE

To attempt to understand why clients or patients are not more compliant with prescribed medical treatments, including lifestyle changes promoted in CAD preventive or rehabilitative programs, it is necessary to understand how people change health behaviors and maintain new behaviors. Although primary and secondary prevention programs have traditionally provided education and counseling, they typically have not provided the level of behavioral counseling that appears to be necessary for long-term adherence to lifestyle changes. Contemporary approaches to making changes in health behaviors often utilize a combination of education, counseling, and behavioral intervention.

Education can be defined as systematic instruction and is essential, but by itself is insufficient to produce significant behavior change and subsequent risk factor reduction. Indeed, there are many barriers to learning, and efforts to limit these barriers will enhance the patient's learning experience (16). Table 10.4 identifies important barriers to learning that can impact adults in a prevention or rehabilitation program. For effective patient education, program staff must reduce or eliminate these barriers.

In contrast to education, counseling is the act of providing advice, support, and consultation (17). Commonly, a health care provider functions as a consultant to the patient by rendering advice, often in response to specific questions or concerns. Assisting the patient in planning and problem solving is the most commonly utilized counseling technique.

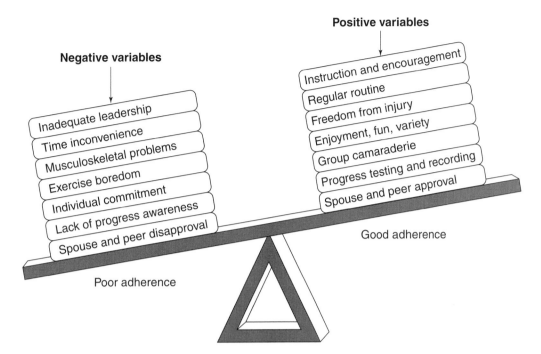

Figure 10.3 **Variables that affect compliance to exercise training programs. Negative variables often outweigh positive ones, resulting in poor adherence (14).**

Reprinted, by permission, from B.A. Franklin, K. Bonzheim, T. Berg, and B. Bonzheim, 1995, Hospital and home-based cardiac rehabilitation outpatient programs. In *Heart disease and rehabilitation*, edited by Pollock and Schmidt (Champaign: Human Kinetics), 222.

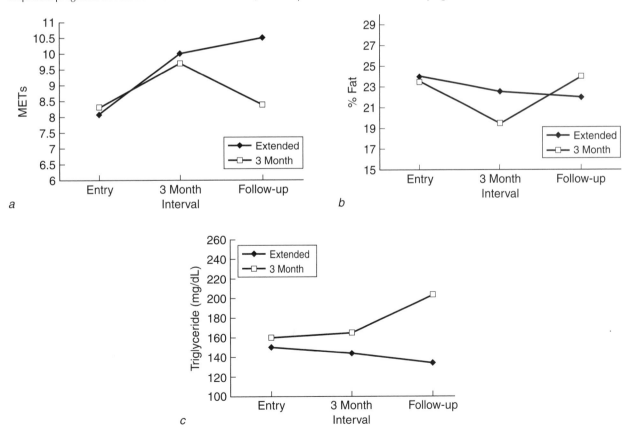

Figure 10.4 **Change in METs, percent body fat, and triglyceride levels in patients who dropped out after participating in a three-month cardiac rehabilitation program compared to patients who remained in the program during the same follow-up period.** *(a)* **MET level (from treadmill test) at entry, after three months in traditional cardiac rehabilitation program, and at follow-up (>1 year, mean = 2.5 years).** *(b)* **Percent body fat level (skinfold measurement) at entry, after three months in traditional cardiac rehabilitation program, and at follow-up (>1 year, mean = 2.5 years).** *(c)* **Triglyceride level (from fasting plasma) at entry, after three months in traditional cardiac rehabilitation program, and at follow-up (>1 year, mean = 2.5 years).**

Table 10.4
Barriers to Adult Learning in Prevention and Rehabilitation Programs

Barrier	Description
Low literacy	Forty to 44 million adults in the United States cannot understand written materials. The average reading level of an American adult is at the eighth-grade level. Twenty percent of adults read at the fifth-grade level or below.
Psychological distress	Anxiety and stress inhibit the ability to learn. Patients in acute distress need emotional support, not cognitive information. Psychological distress that often accompanies a cardiac event must be resolved before effective learning can occur.
Physical instability	Patients must be pain free and in a physical condition that will allow concentration on behavior change. For instance, the day after CABG surgery may be too soon to provide educational materials to a patient.
Sensory impairments	Most common impairments are in sight and hearing. This is especially an issue for elderly individuals, who represent a large percentage of the prevention/rehabilitation population. Thus, it is imperative that appropriate adjustments in the delivery of material be made. For visually impaired, large print, Braille, or audio materials need to be provided. For hearing impaired, a professional interpreter should be involved.
Language differences	Educational materials must be provided for the non-English reading patient, as well as a professional interpreter for oral communication.

Adapted from (16).

A behavioral intervention refers to systematic instruction in techniques to modify health-related behaviors. Most believe that in order for behavior change to take place and be sustained, a behavioral intervention is necessary. A number of widely recognized behavioral intervention theories are applicable to CAD prevention and rehabilitation settings. Several of these theories of behavioral change are listed in box 10.5 and are briefly described in the next section (16).

Box 10.5 Major Theories of Behavior Change

- Health Belief Model
- Theory of Reasoned Action
- Belief in Personal Control: Locus of Control, Self-Efficacy
- Stages of Change Model (Transtheoretical Model)

According to the *health belief model,* the likelihood that an individual will take preventive action (i.e., practice a healthy behavior) depends directly on two patient variables: (1) the value placed on the goal (e.g., the benefits of cholesterol lowering) and (2) the estimate of the likelihood that a given action will achieve a goal (e.g., that changing dietary habits will lower cholesterol). According to another theory, the *theory of*

reasoned action, people decide their intention in advance of most voluntary behaviors, and intentions are the best predictors of what people will do. For instance, to best predict if a person will change his diet or start an exercise program, simply ask the person what he or she intends to do! The health belief model and the theory of reasoned action provide valid explanations for parts of the process that determines people's practice of health-related behaviors. However, both theories assume that people weigh perceived benefits and costs, then behave according to the outcome of their analysis. This view of human behavior is overly simplistic and assumes that people think about the risks of their behaviors in detailed fashion. In theory, individuals know what diseases are associated with different behaviors and can estimate the likelihood of becoming seriously ill. In reality, people may modify their lifestyle—for example, stop smoking cigarettes—for reasons that are quite vague, such as "My doctor said smoking is bad for you."

It is well known in health psychology that an individual's perceived personal control has direct impact on that person's health-related behaviors. The two prevailing theories based on this concept are *health locus of control* and *self-efficacy.* According to the health locus of control theory, patients have an "internal" or "external" locus of control. Individuals with an internal locus of control believe they have a good deal of control over situations and events related to health behaviors. Thus, patients with internal locus of control tend to practice behaviors that prevent illness and maintain good health, such as getting physical exams and dieting and exercising for health benefits. Moreover, these patients are more likely to be successful with a smoking cessation program and are more likely to seek health-related information (read newsletters, watch health programs, etc.). In contrast, individuals with an external locus of control believe that others, such as health care providers (doctors, nurses, etc.), have control and that the individual is not responsible for her overall health status. Do you know someone who tends to blame health problems on someone else (e.g., "My doctor didn't treat me properly!"), unwilling to recognize that her own behaviors caused the problem? An example of someone with an external locus of control might be the lifelong cigarette smoker who blames her doctor for not being able to treat her "end-stage" lung disease.

Self-efficacy theory (often referred to as *social cognitive theory*), defined as a person's belief that he can succeed at something he wants to do, may be an important determinant of whether an individual chooses to practice specific behaviors. Individuals acquire a sense of self-efficacy through their own successes and failures, through observations of others' experiences, and through assessments of their abilities that they hear from others. When deciding to practice a beneficial health behavior, people appraise their efficacy on the basis of the effort required, the complexity of the task, and the amount of help they are to receive from others. Research has shown that self-efficacy clearly influences people's health behaviors. For instance, a cigarette smoker who believes that he is capable of quitting is more likely to succeed than smokers who don't think they can quit. Methods of assessing self-efficacy include having patients rate (on scale from 0% to 100%) their confidence that they can make a behavior change. The lower the rating, the less likely it is that an individual will be able to make and sustain a behavior change. Generally, ratings less than 70% are associated with a lower chance of a successful change. When someone's self-efficacy rating is low, education needs to be directed at discovering the beliefs about and/or barriers to change (18).

The *stages of change theory*, also known as the *transtheoretical model*, has been proposed by Prochaska and colleagues (19) and is beginning to see widespread use in CAD prevention and rehabilitation programs (figure 10.5). This theory addresses individuals' ability to make permanent change based upon their emotional and intellec-

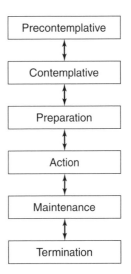

Figure 10.5   Stages of change in the transtheoretical model.

tual "readiness." The model describes six stages of intentional behavior change:

- Precontemplation. People in this stage are not seriously considering changing, at least during the next six months. These people may have never thought about changing or may have decided against it.

- Contemplation. During this stage, people are aware that a problem exists and are seriously considering changing to a healthier behavior in the next six months. But they are not ready to make a commitment to take action.

- Preparation. At this stage individuals plan to pursue a behavioral goal, such as to stop smoking, in the next month and may have tried to reach that goal in the past year without being fully successful. For instance, they may have cut their smoking in half but have not been able to quit completely.

- Action. This stage spans a period of time, usually six months, and represents the individual's active efforts to change a behavior

- Maintenance. People in this stage work to maintain the successful behavioral changes they have achieved. Although this stage can last indefinitely, it is generally assessed in six-month intervals.

- Termination. Few people progress to this stage of behavioral change. People at this point have 100% confidence they will not revert to old habits. Most people will have to continue with maintenance efforts and be prepared to practice **relapse prevention.**

As mentioned earlier, patients referred to or entering a CAD preventive or rehabilitative program should be evaluated on their readiness for change. Individuals in the precontemplation stage are unlikely to participate in the program since they underestimate the benefits of changing behaviors and overestimate the cost of change. Without appropriate intervention, these "precontemplators" are likely to remain at this stage rather than progressing to the next level. Advancement to the contemplation stage occurs only if the individual perceives the benefits of change to be increasing in number. For example, when asked to list all the advantages of an exercise program, the average patient in precontemplation will list four or five. To help move patients to the next stage, prevention or rehabilitation professionals can inform them that there are many more benefits of exercise and can challenge them to double their list of benefits over the next few weeks. The program can provide precontemplators with educational materials to help increase their sense of the value of the program. In the contemplation stage, individuals are aware of the benefits of changing behaviors, but they are also acutely aware of the costs. Thus, for individuals to move to the preparation stage, reasons not to change must decrease.

Individuals who have moved into the preparation stage are ready to take immediate action. They are convinced that the benefits outweigh the costs. Their biggest concern is that they may fail, which unfortunately is a reality for most individuals. People have to know that successful change may require several attempts. Individuals have to be prepared for how long the action stage usually lasts—if action efforts are reduced too soon, relapse is likely. People should be encouraged to commit to six months of concerted effort. After about six months, patients progress into the maintenance stage. Their confidence increases, and temptations to return to unhealthy habits diminish. They don't have to work as hard to prevent relapse, but they have to work to keep progressing. Relapse is possible unless positive coping strategies are in place to deal with periods of emotional distress (anger, boredom, depression). Preventive and rehabilitative programs can help individuals develop healthy ways of coping with distress. Few people progress to the final stage of behavioral change, the termination stage. People at this point have 100% confidence they will not revert to old habits. Realistically, most people will have to continue with maintenance efforts and be prepared to practice relapse prevention.

After one has determined the individual's stage, the goal is to move the person into a stage that will allow for adoption and, ultimately, maintenance of healthy lifestyle behaviors that are promoted in the program. Prochaska and colleagues (19) have identified a number of interventional strategies that can be used in the prevention or rehabilitation setting to facilitate progress of the patient from one stage to the next. Each strategy is briefly described in table 10.5.

Application of the Transtheoretical Model to Prevention and Rehabilitation Programs

As we have seen, the transtheoretical model provides a framework for assessing each patient's readiness for change; the most appropriate intervention can then be utilized to assist the patient through the change process. This section outlines how to apply the model in a preventive or rehabilitative setting—at the patient's entry into the program as well as during and after the program.

After referral to the program, each potential patient meets with a prevention or rehabilitation professional (e.g., exercise physiologist, nurse, etc.) for an intake interview. Data collected at this time include demographics, family history, patient's perspective on her health and illness, lifestyle habits, beliefs and values, and social support. In addition, patients are assessed for depression, denial, or other psychosocial problems. Behaviorally, the interviewer questions the patient to determine readiness for change. Table 10.6 lists examples of questions commonly used for this assessment (in this case the questions refer to smoking behavior, but they could refer to other behaviors such as diet or exercise).

It may seem surprising that not all patients referred for cardiac rehabilitation actually choose to participate. Dr. Ades and colleagues in Vermont (20) analyzed factors that predicted cardiac rehabilitation program enrollment in 226 older patients with documented coronary disease. The strength of the primary care physician's recommendation was by far the single most important factor influencing enrollment. Enrollment was 1.8% when cardiac rehabilitation participation was not mentioned or was only minimally supported by the primary physician. In contrast, enrollment rose to 66% when the recommendation by the primary physician was strong and highly encouraged! Disappointingly, this study showed that only 21% of the referred patients actually participated in the program. A similarly low participation rate has been observed in other studies. Listed in box 10.6 are characteristics (in

Table 10.5
Intervention Strategies to Promote Change in "Stage"

Strategy	Description
Consciousness raising	Through information, education, and feedback, emphasis is placed on increasing awareness about the many benefits that can be derived through a particular behavior change.
Dramatic relief	This approach involves evoking an emotional arousal as a means of motivating patients to progress. Inspiring, scaring, and exciting patients are some ways to help patients break their complacency.
Reevaluation	In this approach, patients are encouraged to imagine how their behavior changes will affect others as well as themselves. Creating positive images that draw patients into the future prepares them for action. For example, walking on the beach is an image that can draw many into preparing for a more active lifestyle.
Self-liberation	This intervention is based on the belief in one's ability to change and the commitment to act on that belief. One strategy used to create self-liberation is to offer choices about how to make the desired change. For initiating exercise, for example, you could offer the patient a variety of types of exercise (bike, treadmill, swimming, etc.) and different combinations of duration and frequency (once a day for 30 minutes vs. 15 minutes twice a day, etc.).
Reinforcement management	In this approach, getting patients to rely on self-reinforcements rather than social reinforcements is the goal. Too often, patients expect to be reinforced (i.e., rewarded) by others much more than others will actually reinforce their changes. This intervention involves rewards contingent on progress, such as resisting temptations to relapse.
Helping relationships	Here the goal is to involve people who care, listen, and are available to support the patient. This is particularly important for the elderly, who are often socially isolated.
Counterconditioning	This intervention focuses on learning how to substitute healthier alternatives for unhealthy behaviors. Nicotine replacement for cigarettes and tasty low fat foods are examples of such substitutes.
Stimulus control	Involves reengineering the environment to add cues for healthy action and remove stimuli that evoke temptations. Placing exercise equipment or exercise shoes by the television can be effective cues for action.

Adapted from (19).

Table 10.6
Sample Questions and Answers Identifying Stage of Readiness in a Smoker

Stage	Assessment question	Answer
Precontemplation	Do you intend to quit smoking in next 6 months?	No
Contemplation	Do you intend to quit smoking in next 6 months?	Yes
Preparation	Do you intend to quit smoking in next month?	Yes
	Have you quit for at least 24 hrs. in past year?	Yes
Action	Did you quit smoking in the last 6 months?	Yes
Maintenance	Did you quit smoking more than 6 months ago?	Yes
Termination	Did you quit smoking more than 5 years ago?	Yes

Adapted from (19).

addition to physician support) of patients less likely than others to participate in cardiac rehabilitation (20).

Box 10.6   Characteristics of Individuals Less Likely to Join a Cardiac Rehabilitation Program

- Female gender
- 62 years of age or over
- Single marital status
- Personal income less than $20,000
- Blue collar work
- Presence of co-morbid disease
- Longer commuting distance to the rehabilitation center
- History of depression
- Denial about disease severity
- Lack of motivation

At the Wake Forest University Cardiac Rehabilitation Program, slightly less than 50% of the patients who are referred to the rehabilitation program actually enroll in the outpatient cardiac rehabilitation program. A recent study from this program (21) examined a variety of demographic, socioeconomic, and medical factors in an attempt to predict participators and nonparticipators. The study did not identify any specific demographic (age, gender, race), socioeconomic (education, income, insurance), or medical (diagnosis, procedures, comorbidities) factor that differed between the patients who joined the program and those who didn't. We were able to determine that the majority of patients electing not to join were simply "precontemplative"—in other words, they lacked readiness to make lifestyle changes at the time. Although the interventions presented by Prochaska and colleagues (19) were not utilized, theoretically they could have enabled these patients to move from the precontemplation stage to the contemplation or action stage and thus become more likely to join the program. To optimize the likelihood for behavior change, it is clear that the treatment and timing (in this case of a cardiac rehabilitation program) must match the person's stage of change or readiness for change. Although patients enter the program in a specific stage, it is not unusual for a patient to move through one stage during the interview itself.

However, prevention or rehabilitation professionals must be cautious not to hurry patients through the stages but to allow them to evolve at their own pace.

Once the patient is in the program, a staff member can be assigned to help the patient progress through the stages of change using the techniques described in table 10.5. The staff member can help the patient identify a specific stage of change for each specific behavior and track changes each week during progression through the program.

After completion of the program, relapse prevention is the priority in terms of interventional strategies. Sincere discussions are in order to advise patients that while a relapse is likely to some extent, it does not have to be catastrophic. Patients should be informed that recycling through the stages is normal and that they should not blame themselves or their caregivers when they are not able to sustain their new behaviors perfectly. When relapse occurs, patients can be encouraged to fall back on the strategies that were helpful in former stages.

ALTERNATIVE MODELS OF CAD PREVENTION AND REHABILITATION

Recognizing the very low referral and high dropout rates associated with traditional preventive and rehabilitative programs, a number of investigators have examined the benefits of alternative models for delivering the critical core components of these programs (22).

Since the mid-1980s, much of the effort at developing alternative models for delivering preventive or rehabilitative services has been initiated by investigators at Stanford University. The innovative approaches for primary and secondary prevention pioneered at Stanford include home-based cardiac rehabilitation (23) and the **lifestyle activity** approach for coronary risk factor modification (24).

Home-Based Cardiac Rehabilitation

Home-based cardiac rehabilitation programs were first developed to eliminate some of the barriers associated with center-based programs, including time and schedule conflicts, travel distance and other transportation problems, cost and lack of third-party reimbursement, lack of referral and support, and dislike for group programs. Debusk and colleagues from Stanford (23) were the first to show the feasibility of home-based exercise training in enhancing the functional capacity of uncomplicated post-MI patients. They used transtelephonic ECG monitoring to enhance the safety of the home-based training. The improvement in functional capacity at six months postevent among patients exercising in a home environment was similar to that of patients exercising in a medically supervised program. This investigation demonstrated that home-based exercise training increased functional capacity by 1.5 to 2.0 METs during the first three to six months following MI or coronary artery bypass graft surgery. No training-induced arrhythmias, MIs, or other untoward events were noted in the home-based group. Furthermore, the cost of this equally effective intervention was essentially one-half that of a traditional cardiac rehabilitation program ($328 vs. $720 per patient per year in 1985). This study emphasized that the components of a well-designed home-based program should be very similar to those of a medically supervised program (i.e., evaluation, intervention, expected outcomes), except for the location of the exercise training. A handful of well-designed studies have since demonstrated that home-based programs can be safe and effective for patients after coronary events.

In the mid-1990s, this same group of investigators developed and studied a physician-directed, nurse-managed home-based case management system for coronary risk factor intervention (24). Patients received either the intervention (n = 293) or usual care (n = 232) during the first year after MI. Specially trained nurses initiated interventions for smoking cessation, exercise training, and diet/medication treatment for hyperlipidemia. Intervention after hospital discharge was primarily by phone and mail. This case management approach resulted in a significantly higher MET level for the intervention (i.e., case managed) group versus the control (usual care) group at 12 months (9.3 ± 2.4 vs. 8.4 ± 2.5). Low-density lipoprotein was significantly lower in the case-managed group (107 ± 30 mg/dl vs. 132 ± 30 mg/dl), and smoking rates were significantly lower in this group (30% vs. 47%). The positive results from this study led the Stanford investigators to create a clinical program, called MULTIFIT, that was available for use by other organizations. The elements of the MULTIFIT model (25), which was based on social learning theory of behavior change, are listed in box 10.7.

Box 10.7 Elements of behavior change incorporated in MULTIFIT

Written agreement: Between patient and healthcare professional

Self-observation forms: Food frequency, smoking history, and self-efficacy questionnaires are used to identify areas of needed change

Goal setting: Short- and long-term goals for health-related behaviors are established by patient and healthcare professional

Contracting: Contracts are used to commit patients to specific behavior changes and to define consequences of not achieving goals

Relapse prevention training: High-risk situations that may trigger relapse are identified and strategies of prevention are discussed

Modeling: Patients receive videotapes of appropriate behaviors (with patient testimonials) to modify each risk factor

Prompting: Calendars and telephone calls by nurses are prompts for behaviors including exercise and medications

Feedback: Positive feedback of exercise logs, tests, etc. are provided by nurse through telephone

Problem solving: Barriers to compliance, getting back on track, and difficulties in initiating behavior change are discussed and solved during phone calls

---

Because of the fairly minimal time spent managing each patient (only about 9 h for a 12-month intervention), the average yearly cost was $541 as compared to $2200 per patient at a traditional cardiac rehabilitation program. Furthermore, the MULTIFIT approach has been shown to result in higher compliance rates for cholesterol and blood pressure medication use, exercise, and smoking cessation than are typically observed in center-based cardiac rehabilitation programs.

Transtelephonic Exercise Monitoring

Although the telephone was invented in 1876, it wasn't until the 1950s that telephone technology and medicine merged into what is known today as "telemedicine." Telemedicine is the use of electronic communication networks for the transmission of information and data related to the diagnosis and treatment of medical conditions (26).

This technology continues to improve and grow in acceptance. Digital imaging, fiber optics, and a variety of new developments now enable clinicians to assess and treat patients from almost anywhere in the world. Although on a somewhat limited basis, this technology has also been used to monitor exercise training sessions of cardiac rehabilitation patients.

Shaw (26) and colleagues identified 32 programs that employed this technology and found the following regarding the use and safety of transtelephonic exercise monitoring:

- More than 500 patients (performing over 14,000 exercise sessions) have been served through transtelephonic exercise monitoring.

- The average distance from the patient to the monitoring location was 72 miles (the longest was 600 miles!).

- There were 141 phone disconnects, but no reported medical emergencies.

Ades and colleagues (27) conducted a multicenter trial to compare the effectiveness of home-based, transtelephonically monitored cardiac rehabilitation with that of standard, on-site, supervised cardiac rehabilitation. The effects of a three-month, home-based, transtelephonically monitored rehabilitation program (n = 83) with simultaneous voice and electrocardiographic transmission to a centrally located nurse coordinator were compared with the effects of a standard on-site rehabilitation program (n = 50). Primary outcome variables were peak aerobic capacity ($\dot{V}O_2$peak) and quality of life. The study indicated that peak aerobic capacity increased to a similar degree in patients in the home-based monitoring program and patients who exercised on site (18% vs. 23% increase in peak $\dot{V}O_2$, respectively). Quality-of-life domains also improved similarly in the two groups. There were no major exercise-related medical events in more than 3000 h of exercise training in either the home-monitored group or the on-site exercise group.

A Home-Based Maintenance Program

In contrast to home-based cardiac rehabilitation programs that begin upon discharge from the hospital, a home-based maintenance program has been successfully employed by investigators from Wake Forest University (28). As described earlier in the section on compliance and outcomes, patients exiting a formal cardiac rehabilitation program were unable to maintain long-term control of important CAD risk factors (15). The disappointing results of that investigation (see figure 10.4a-c) prompted Wake Forest University researchers to experiment with a home-based program for patients electing to exit after successfully completing a traditional three-month center-based (i.e., phase II) cardiac rehabilitation program (28). In short, patients electing to exit (generally because of financial or insurance issues, schedule conflicts, or both) were randomly assigned to either the home-based (HB) program or standard care (SC). The HB patients received

Table 10.7

Components of the Wake Forest University Home-Based Maintenance Exercise Program

Component	Description
Home visit	A single home visit was conducted by a nurse and exercise physiologist to ensure "transfer" of the program to the home setting. Spouse or significant other was encouraged to attend this meeting. Topics/issues covered included: • Safety (how and what to monitor, emergency response) • Exercise prescription (mode, intensity, frequency, duration) • How to complete and return exercise logs • Common barriers to exercise and relapse prevention
Exercise logs	Patients were given exercise logs (with prescribed heart rate ranges) for recording daily exercise/physical activity habits including mode, duration, heart rate, weight, and signs/symptoms. The logs were to be completed weekly and mailed to our center in a supplied stamped envelope.
Phone contact	The exercise physiologist or nurse contacted the patient every other week for the duration of the study (9 months). A checklist of items was used to identify changes in medical status, review compliance to exercise program (based on returned logs), and provide general support and encouragement. The average phone call lasted 15 min. Although infrequent, if medical questions arose (e.g., symptoms, medications issues), the medical director was contacted.

the interventions described in table 10.7. Prior to discharge, the SC group received basic instruction and recommendations from the cardiac rehabilitation program (CRP) staff regarding continuation of the exercise program and other lifestyle habits. Standard-care patients had no further contact with staff until follow-up testing was arranged. The SC patients did, however, learn at time of randomization that they would return to the laboratory for follow-up assessment. This issue was later found to have had a significant impact on the findings of the study. A group of patients who continued to participate in our center-based (CB) program were also studied. Subjects from all three groups were evaluated at the onset of cardiac rehabilitation (0M); after three months in the standard center-based CRP (3M); and after nine months in HB, SC, or CB (12M). The results indicated that the only variables to significantly increase over the 12 months of the study were METs and high-density lipoprotein (figure 10.6a and b). Other lipids and body weight and composition did not significantly change over time. Moreover, there were no differences between the groups: HB patients did as well as CB patients, and SC patients did as well as HB patients. The latter outcome was not expected and was attributed to the lasting effects of the three-month CRP and the knowledge that there would be follow-up testing in the SC group. The conclusions from the investigations were as follows:

- For patients exiting a traditional center-based CRP, a home-based maintenance program was as effective at improving and/or maintaining functional capacity, selected blood lipids, and body weight/composition as the CB maintenance program. Thus, for patients unable or unwilling to attend a center-based CRP, the HB model can be an effective, low-cost, and convenient alternative.

- The fact that the SC patients did as well as HB patients over the nine months of follow-up suggests that follow-up testing alone (i.e., without phone and log component) may be an effective intervention and may help patients maintain health behaviors after exiting a formal program.

A home-based maintenance program similar to the one just described is a part of the Wake Forest Cardiac Rehabilitation Program and is available to patients electing to exit at any time.

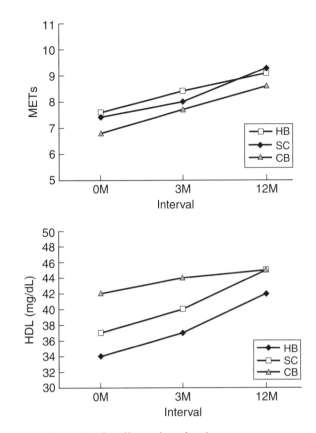

Figure 10.6   Results of home-based maintenance program at Wake Forest University. *(a)* MET level at entry (0M) to cardiac rehabilitation program (CRP), after three months (3M) of participation in CRP, and after nine months of participation (at 12 month follow-up =12M) in either the home-based (HB), standard care (SC), or center-based (CB) condition. *(b)* High-density lipoprotein level (mg/dl) at entry (0M) to CRP; after three months (3M) of participation in CRP; and after nine months of participation (12M) in the homebased (HB), standard care (SC), or center-based (CB) condition.

The Lifestyle Activity Approach

The inability of patients to maintain a desirable amount of exercise after exiting traditional center-based cardiac rehabilitation programs has led health psychologists and exercise physiologists to evaluate models that utilize principles of behavioral changes. One such model, developed by researchers at Wake Forest, is the Lifestyle Activity Program. This approach has been previously shown to be effective in healthy older adults (29) and is currently being evaluated in a study of patients with documented CAD or at high risk for the disease (called the Cardiovascular Activity Maintenance [CHAMP] study).

The primary objective of the Lifestyle Activity Program approach is to provide patients with the behavioral tools that appear necessary for long-term adherence to healthy behaviors. The focus of the intervention in CHAMP is to modify exercise and physical activity behaviors, since we had previously observed that patients had trouble maintaining these behaviors after exiting a formal program. It would be appropriate to use a similar approach to modify other health-related behaviors (e.g., dietary habits or stress management). In addition to participating in traditional center-based exercise sessions, CHAMP patients engaged in group discussions and received assignments designed to gradually build an exercise or physical activity program that became part of their lifestyle. In essence they were learning how to build a physical activity pyramid. The activity pyramid is modeled after the Food Guide Pyramid, with the more common regular activities that should be done everyday (such as walking the dog or taking stairs instead of the elevator) providing the base of the pyramid. Aerobic activities and recreational sports that should be done three to five times a week are one level higher. Leisure activities and stretch/strength exercises (2-3 times per week) are still another level up, and the top of the pyramid consists of sedentary activities (including watching TV and playing computer games), which should be done only sparingly. The idea is that the base of the pyramid should be the base of your activity program, and you should do fewer of the sitting activities at the top of the pyramid. Table 10.8 summarizes specific topics and "homework" assignments included in the 12-week CHAMP program.

The primary outcomes under investigation in the CHAMP study are levels of physical activity and degree of risk factor control, not only after completion of the three-month intervention, but also after nine months of participation when both groups were without contact with the program. The final results from the CHAMP study are not yet available, but we expect that this approach will prove to be a more effective strategy than the "traditional" cardiac rehabilitation model for maintaining long-term exercise and physical activity habits.

The primary limitation of CHAMP and other behavioral change models is the lack of third-party reimbursement for this type of intervention. Most health insurance companies will reimburse for up to 36 sessions of traditional cardiac rehabilitation (i.e., monitored exercise) but not for these behaviorally oriented interventions. As effective as the alternative models we have described appear to be, including those from Stanford and Wake Forest, if there is no mechanism for reimbursement it will be difficult to incorporate these models into mainstream preventive or rehabilitative programs. More information

Table 10.8

Topics Used in CHAMP to Modify Exercise/Physical Activity Behaviors

Topic	Description
Self-awareness and self-monitoring	Patients learned how to become more aware of how much activity they were or weren't doing by monitoring and recording their activity on a specially designed calendar.
Principles of FITT	Patients learned the important components of a physical activity program (FITT = frequency, intensity, type, time).
Goal setting (and resetting)	Patients learned how to set appropriate goals for physical activity habits and, once obtained, how to reset the goals.
Stress-management and relaxation therapy	Patients learned how and when to use basic stress management and relaxation techniques.
Barriers and lapses	Patients discussed various barriers to exercise (weather, lack of time) and how to avoid them, as well as how to prevent lapses in their physical activity habits.
Creating social support	Patients learned the importance of an "exercise support group" and how to create exercise support through family and friends.

Topic	Description
Exercise vs. physical activity	Patients learned the differences between traditional "exercise" and "physical activity" and the importance of both in a healthy lifestyle.
Transition to home exercise	The purpose of this session was to "wean" patients off the center-based program and ensure they were able to exercise safely and effectively on their own.
Exercise affect	Patients learned to evaluate how they felt about exercise and what they could do to make it more positive. They also learned about positive-self talk, such as "I can do this" or "I know I can walk a mile without stopping."
Cues to exercise	Patients were taught to create cues in their daily activity that may prompt them to exercise. Cues could be • putting exercise shoes on the TV, • hanging an exercise calendar on the refrigerator, or • having an encouraging message on the computer screen-saver.
Relapse prevention	Patients were taught that lapses in their physical activity may occur, but that if they revert to the behavioral skills learned, they can reestablish an active lifestyle.

on the status of reimbursement for these programs is presented in chapter 11.

SUMMARY

Comprehensive CAD preventive and rehabilitative programs require a multifaceted approach to effectively modify the risk factors associated with cardiovascular disease development or progression. While short-term participation in traditional preventive or rehabilitative programs usually results in numerous positive health changes (risk factors, functional capacity, quality of life), compliance to long-term behavior change—particularly after people exit formal programs—is disappointingly low. Consequently, a number of models, most utilizing theories of behavior change, have been developed to enhance long-term adherence to healthy lifestyle behaviors. Implementing these approaches is the challenge of current and future programs, particularly when third-party reimbursement for these services is not widely available.

Case Study 1
Primary Prevention: Low Risk

The focus of the lifestyle intervention for this low-risk primary prevention case was primarily exercise training. However, the participant was educated regarding his risk factors for CAD, including hypertension and hypercholesterolemia. Although no formal dietary assessment was conducted, the participant was also educated regarding the benefits of a prudent diet and weight loss (in addition to exercise training) to manage his risk factors. Had more formal dietary interventions been necessary, a fee-for-service session with a dietician would have been arranged. Similar arrangements can be made when psychosocial issues arise. The primary prevention staff worked in concert with the primary care physician to manage risk factors as needed, including possible recommendations to initiate medications had the lifestyle changes been insufficient to bring hypertension and hypercholesterolemia to goal levels. The outcomes for this primary prevention participant are described in chapter 8.

Case Study 2
Primary Prevention: High Risk

Upon entry into a multidisciplinary outpatient cardiac rehabilitation program, this patient underwent the following assessments at the rehabilitation facility:

Patient (Medical) Assessment

- Normal cardiovascular examination (BP, heart sounds, pulses, etc.).
- No contraindications to exercise testing or training.
- Due to obesity, care must be taken to avoid orthopedic problems (use non-weight-bearing activities).
- Monitor blood glucose before and after exercise for several weeks. Be aware of potential for hyperglycemia before exercise and hypoglycemia after exercise.

Exercise Testing Results

- Achieved 5.3/4.6 METs, estimated/measured, respectively (low for age)
- No ischemic changes or significant arrhythmias
- Normal hemodynamic responses, considering medications (beta blockers)
- Limited by leg fatigue

Risk Factor Assessment (Abnormal Findings)

Smoking

- 40 pack/year history (quit in 1988)

Lipids

- LDL = 178 mg/dl
- HDL = 35 mg/dl
- Total cholesterol = 243 mg/dl

Other Relevant Lab Values

- Hemoglobin A_1c = 11.3%

Nutritional Assessment and Weight Management

Assessments

Seven-day food record indicated that patient was eating an AHA Step I Diet (refer to table 4.1):

- Total caloric intake of 1330 kcal
- Carbohydrate intake of 181 g (54% of calories)
- Protein intake of 73 g (22% of calories)

- Fat intake of 36 g (24% of calories)
- 7% saturated, 10% mono-, 3% poly-, and 4% trans fat of total calories
- Cholesterol intake of 120 mg per day
- 0% of calories from alcohol

Recommendations

- Maintain AHA Step I Diet
- Increase intake of polyunsaturated fat
- Maintain caloric intake of 1500 to 1700 kcal per day
- Decrease weight from 361 to 250 lb (163 to 113 kg) through caloric reduction and exercise

Psychosocial Assessment and Interventions

Assessments

NEO Personality inventory indicated:

- Neuroticism—average
- Extroversion—high
- Openness—average
- Agreeableness—average
- Conscientiousness—high
- Very motivated and positive about lifestyle changes
- Health-related quality of life—low
- Stress on job (mechanical engineer at hospital); supervisor not supportive of time off for participation in CAD prevention program
- Vocational assessment: may need intervention to get released time to attend prevention program

Recommendations: No formal psychosocial intervention needed at present time. Lifestyle changes will improve physical and emotional condition.

Multidisciplinary Team Meeting

After completion of all assessments, the multidisciplinary team of health care providers met to review findings for this patient. Those participating in the meeting included:

- Medical director
- Clinical exercise physiologist
- Dietician/nutritionist
- Clinical psychologist

- Vocational rehabilitation coordinator
- Nurse/patient educator

Individualized Goals

Based on the results of the assessments and with input from the multidisciplinary team, the following goals for this patient were defined:

- Improve blood lipids to NCEP goals, particularly LDL and HDL (< 100 and >40 mg/dl, respectively)
- Improve blood glucose to goal (< 110 mg/dl)
- Decrease body weight by nearly 100 lb (45 kg)
- Increase activity levels (3 days per week of exercise in CRP and 2 additional days at home)
- Understand signs and symptoms of hyperglycemia and hypoglycemia and report these to health care providers

Outcomes

The results of the initial and follow-up assessments (patient was re-evaluated after 3 months of participation) are presented in figure 10.8. As you can see, this patient was able to make significant improvements in LDL, total cholesterol, and triglycerides. This was accomplished through lifestyle changes and use of Lipitor (see table 4.3), as well as blood glucose control (hemoglobin A₁c); all these values are now at or below targeted levels. The patient was able to increase his MET capacity (slightly) and improve his dietary habits. He had very successful weight loss (40 lb [18 kg]), but needs to continue to work toward a goal of 250 lb. In a relatively short period of time, patient has made dramatic improvements in most outcomes. Continuation with these lifestyle changes should allow the patient to achieve goals and successfully prevent progression (potentially regression) of CAD.

Wake Forest University Rehabilitation Outcomes Tool

Name: Case Study 2   ID# ********

Date of Entry: 4/19/00   MDs:********   DOB:*******

Diagnosis: Minimal CAD, Risk Factors   Exit Date:****

	Goals	CRP Entry Date: 4/00	Re-Eval (3M) Date: 7/00	Change Abs.	Change %	Achieve Goal (Yes or No)
Clinical Outcomes						
LDL (mg/dl)	**<100**	178	77	-101	-56%	Yes
Cholesterol (mg/dl)	**<200**	243	123	-120	-49%	Yes
HDL (mg/dl)	**>40**	35	31	-4	-11%	No*
TC/HDL Ratio	**<4.5**	6.9	3.9	-3	-43%	Yes
Triglyceride (mg/dl)	**<150**	152	75	-77	-50%	Yes
Blood Glucose (mg/dl)	**<110**	Hb A$_1$c = 11.3	7.5	-3.8	-33%	Not yet (Goal = 4.5-6.4)**
Rest Blood Pressure (mmHg)	**<140/90**	118/63	120/70	Normal	Normal	Yes
METs (Measured/Estimated)	**Add 1/.5 to baseline value**	5.3/4.6	5.8/5.0	0.5/0.4	10%/9%	Not yet***
Health Outcomes						
Quality of Life (overall)	**Normal ≥23**	19.37	29.83	10.46	54%	Yes
Behavior Change						
Smoking (# per day)	**0**	0	0	*****	*****	Yes
Weight (lbs)	**250**	361	321	40	11%	Not yet****
Dietary Habits	**DPR>65**	67	68	1	1.5%	Yes
Relaxation Training	**>2 per week**	********	2x/week	*****	*****	Yes
Ex. Attendance	**>75%**	********	90%	*****	*****	Yes
Activity Outside CRP	**>2 days**	********	2 days	*****	*****	Yes
Medical Utilization						
Hospitalizations	**0**	********	0	*****	*****	Yes
Emergency Rm. Visits	**0**	********	0	*****	*****	Yes
Unplanned MD Visits	**0**	********	0	*****	*****	Yes

- Quality of life= Ferrans and Powers
- DPR = Diet Pattern Review (a food frequency questionnaire developed and used at Wake Forest University)
- Not available

Continues to participate in Cardiac Maintenance Program. Due to improvement in blood glucose control able to reduce insulin.
*HDL dropped from 35 to 31, likely result of dramatic changes in total cholesterol. Expect to rise with weight loss and regular exercise.
**Hb A$_1$c not yet to goal but improved significantly.
***MET level did not increase to goal—limited by leg fatigue/discomfort.
****Weight not to goal after 3 months, making excellent progress.

Figure 10.7   Outcomes for patient in Case Study 2.

Case Study 3
Secondary Prevention: Post-MI and PTCA/Stent

Upon entry into a multidisciplinary outpatient cardiac rehabilitation program, this patient underwent the following assessments at the rehabilitation facility:

Patient (Medical) Assessment

- Two weeks post-MI, stent in LAD.
- Has untreated "moderate" (i.e., 60-80%) lesions in right coronary artery and left anterior descending artery.
- Normal left ventricular function.
- Normal cardiovascular examination (BP, heart sounds, pulses, etc.).
- No contraindications to exercise testing or training.
- Gradually resume normal activities including light lifting.
- Monitor carefully for signs of restenosis (angina, ECG changes).

Exercise Test Results

Functional capacity was determined from stress echo done at hospital prior to discharge.

- Estimated (from treadmill workload) capacity of 9.3 METs (good for age)
- No ischemic changes (on ECG or echo) or significant arrhythmias
- Normal hemodynamic responses, considering medications (beta blockers)
- Limited by general fatigue

Risk Factor Assessment (Abnormal Findings)

Smoking
- 30 pack/year history (quit in 1985)

Lipids
- LDL = 186 mg/dl
- HDL = 36 mg/dl

Other Relevant Lab Results
- Blood glucose = 136 mg/dl

Nutritional Assessment and Weight Management

Assessment

Seven-day food record indicated that patient was eating an AHA Step II Diet (refer to table 4.1):

- Total caloric intake of 1900 kcal
- Carbohydrate intake of 217 g (45% of calories)
- Protein intake of 105 g (22% of calories)
- Fat intake of 41 g (19% of calories)
- 4% saturated, 7% mono-, 6% poly-, and 2% trans fat of calories
- Cholesterol intake of 191 mg
- 13% of calories from alcohol

Recommendations
- Maintain AHA Step II Diet
- Decrease % calories from protein and increase % calories from carbohydrate
- Decrease total caloric intake to 1500 per day
- Decrease alcohol consumption from two to four drinks per day to one to two per day
- Decrease weight from 222 to 195 lb (100 to 88 kg) through caloric reduction and exercise

Psychosocial Assessment and Interventions

Assessments

NEO Personality Inventory indicated:
- Neuroticism—low
- Extroversion—high
- Openness—average
- Agreeableness—average
- Conscientiousness—high
- No evidence of anxiety or depression
- Health-related quality of life—above average
- Family support: excellent from wife and grown children
- Vocational assessment: recently sold business, financially secure
- Recommendations: no psychosocial intervention needed at present time

Multidisciplinary Team Meeting

After completion of all assessments, the multidisciplinary team of health care providers met to review findings for this patient. Those participating in the meeting included:

- Medical director
- Clinical exercise physiologist

- Dietician/nutritionist
- Clinical psychologist
- Vocational rehabilitation coordinator
- Nurse/patient educator

Individualized Goals

Based on the results of the assessments and with input from the multidisciplinary team, the following goals for this patient were defined:

- Improve blood lipids to NCEP goals, particularly LDL and HDL (<100 mg/dl and >40 mg/dl, respectively)
- Improve blood glucose to goal (< 110 mg/dl)
- Reduce caloric intake to 1500 kcal per day
- Decrease alcohol intake to one to two drinks per day
- Decrease body weight by 20+ lb (9+ kg)
- Increase activity levels (3 days per week of exercise in CRP and 2 additional days at home)

- Understand signs and symptoms of restenosis and report these to health care providers

Outcomes

The results of the initial and follow-up assessments (patient was re-evaluated after 3 months of participation) are presented in figure 10.10. This patient was able to make significant improvements in LDL and HDL cholesterol as well as blood glucose, all of which are now at or below targeted levels. The patient was able to increase his MET capacity (slightly) and improve his dietary habits. While he did have some success with weight loss (6 lb [2.7 kg]), he needs to continue to work toward a goal of 195 lb (88 kg). After completion of the initial three-month cardiac rehabilitation program, this patient elected to enter our cardiac maintenance program. He remains clinically stable with no recurrence of CAD symptoms. He will be re-evaluated in a similar fashion in 12 months to ensure that he continues to maintain levels of each of the described outcomes.

Wake Forest University

Name: Case Study 3

Date of Entry: 5/01/00   MDs:********

Diagnosis: S/P/ MI, PTCA w/stent

ID# ********

DOB:*******

Exit Date:****

	Goals	CRP Entry Date: 5/00	Re-Eval (3M) Date: 8/00	Change Abs.	Change %	Achieve Goal (Yes or No)
Clinical Outcomes						
LDL (mg/dl)	<100	131	58	73	55%	Yes
Cholesterol (mg/dl)	<200	186	112	74	39%	Yes
HDL (mg/dl)	>35	36	37	1	2%	Yes
TC/HDL Ratio	<4.5	5.1	3.0	-2.1	41%	Yes
Triglyceride (mg/dl)	<150	98	86	12	12%	Yes
Blood Glucose (mg/dl)	<110	136	97	39	28%	Yes
Rest Blood Pressure (mmHg)	<140/90	140/70	138/80	At goal	At goal	Yes
METs (Estimated)	Add 1 to baseline value	9.3	9.5	0.2	2%	No*
Health Outcomes						
Quality of Life (overall)	Normal ≥ 23	25	27	2	8%	Yes
Behavior Change						
Smoking (# per day)	0	0	0	0	0%	Yes
Weight (lbs)	195	222	216	-6	-3%	Not yet**
Waist (inches)	Men <40	38	37	-1	-2%	Yes
Dietary Habits	DPR>65	56	59	3	5%	Nearly**
Relaxation Training	>2 per week	********	2x/week	*****	*****	Yes
Ex. Attendance	>75%	********	94%	*****	*****	Yes
Activity Outside CRP	>2 days	********	3x/week	*****	*****	Yes
Medical Utilization						
Hospitalizations	0	********	0	*****	*****	Yes
Emergency Rm. Visits	0	********	0	*****	*****	Yes
Unplanned MD Visits	0	********	0	*****	*****	Yes

Comments:
- Quality of life= Ferrans and Powers
- DPR = Diet Pattern Review (a food frequency questionnaire developed and used at Wake Forest University)

Continues to participate in Cardiac Maintenance Program.

*MET level did not increase to goal; however, had high MET capacity and was tested on different protocols (refer to Case Study 3 in chap. 8).

**Needs to continue to work to reduce weight through improved dietary habits and increased exercise.

Figure 10.8   Outcome for patient in Case Study 3.

GLOSSARY

Adherence: degree of cooperation with an intervention; although defined slightly differently, often used synonymously with compliance

Benchmark: a standard or norm for evaluating quality and performance

Compliance: cooperative performance in relation to an intervention (i.e., prescribed therapy or medications)

Intervention: taking actions so as to modify an effect; in our context, cardiac procedures, medications, and lifestyle changes

Readiness: an individual's desire or willingness to make a change

Relapse prevention: systematic efforts made to prevent a recurrence of disease or condition and/or avoid return to inappropriate behaviors

Smoking cessation: quitting smoking

Socioeconomic status: the combination or interaction of sociologic (cultural, environmental) and economic (employment, income) factors that can be used to evaluate the prevalence and incidence of disease

Vocational: referring to work or employment

REFERENCES

1. Balady G.J., P.A. Ades, T. Bazzarre, P. Comoss, M. Limacher, I.L. Pina, D. Southard, and M.A. Willimas. 2000. Core components of cardiac rehabilitation/secondary prevention programs. Statement for healthcare professionals from the American Heart Association and the American Association of Cardiovascular and Pulmonary Rehabilitation. *J. Cardiopul. Rehabil.* 20:310–316.

2. Burt V.L., P. Whelton, E.J. Roccella, C. Brown, J.A. Cutler, M. Higgins. 1995. Prevalence of hypertension in US adult population: Results from the third national health and nutrition examination survey, 1988-1991. 25:305-313.

3. Datillo, A.M. 1999. Weight management and exercise in the treatment of obesity. In *Cardiac rehabilitation. A guide to practice in the 21st century,* ed. N.K. Wenger, L.K. Smith, E.S. Froelicher, and P.M. Comoss. New York: Dekker.

4. Cummings, S.M., G.K. Goodrich, and B.E. Foreyt. 1997. Position statement of the American Dietetic Association: Weight management. *J. Am. Diet. Assoc.* 97:71–74.

5. Houston-Miller, N. 1999. Smoking cessation and relapse prevention: Case management approach. In *Cardiac rehabilitation. A guide to practice in the 21st century,* ed. N.K. Wenger, L.K. Smith, E.S. Froelicher, and P.M. Comoss. New York: Dekker.

6. Marlatt , G.A., and J.R. Gordon. 1980. Determination of relapse: Implications for the maintenance of behavior change. In *Behavioral medicine: Changing healthy lifestyles,* ed. P.O. Davidson and S.M. Davidson, 410–452. Elmsford, NJ: Pergamon Press.

7. Solbert, L.I., P.L. Maxwell, and T.E. Nottke. 1990. A systematic primary care office-based smoking cessation program. *J. Fam. Pract.* 30:647–54.

8. The Smoking Cessation Clinical Practice Guideline Panel and Staff. 1996. The Agency for Health Care Policy and Research Smoking Cessation Clinical Practice Guidelines. *J.A.M.A.* 275:1270–1280.

9. American Association of Cardiovascular and Pulmonary Rehabilitation. 1999. *Guidelines for cardiac rehabilitation programs.* 3rd ed. Champaign, IL: Human Kinetics.

10. Pate, R.R., M. Pratt, S.N. Blair, et al. 1995. Physical activity and public health: A recommendation from the Centers of Disease Control and Prevention and the American College of Sports Medicine. *J.A.M.A.* 273:402–407.

11. Wenger, N.K., E.S. Froelicher, L.K. Smith, et al. 1995. *Cardiac rehabilitation. Clinical practice guidelines no. 17.* AHCPR pub. no. 96-0672, Oct. Rockville, MD: U.S. Department of Health and Human Services, Public Health Services, Agency for Health Care Policy and Research and the National Heart, Lung, and Blood Institute.

12. Oldridge, N.B. 1995. Patient compliance. In *Heart disease and rehabilitation,* ed. M.L. Pollock and D.H. Schmidt. Champaign, IL: Human Kinetics.

13. Oldridge, N.B. 1988. Cardiac rehabilitation exercise program: Compliance and compliance enhancing strategies. *Sports Med.* 6:42–55.

14. Franklin B.A., K. Bonzheim, T. Berg, and S. Bonzheim. 1995. Hospital and home-based cardiac rehabilitation outpatient programs. In *Heart disease and rehabilitation,* ed. M.L. Pollock and D.H. Schmidt. Champaign, IL: Human Kinetics.

15. Brubaker, P.H., J.G. Warner, W.J. Rejeski, D.G. Edward, B.A. Matrazzo, P.M. Ribisl, H.S. Miller, and D.M. Herrington. 1996. Comparison of standard and extended length participation in cardiac rehabilitation on body composition, functional capacity, and blood lipids. *Am J. Cardiol.* 78:769–773.

16. Swails, H.S., and B.H. Southard. 1999. Motivating and empowering patients for self-learning. In *Cardiac rehabilitation. A guide to practice in the 21st century,* ed. N.K. Wenger, L.K. Smith, E.S. Froelicher, and P.M. Comoss. New York: Dekker.

17. Froelicher, E.S. 1999. Multifactorial cardiac rehabilitation: Education, counseling, and behavioral interventions. In *Cardiac rehabilitation. A guide to practice in the 21st century,* ed. N.K. Wenger, L.K.

Smith, E.S. Froelicher, and P.M. Comoss. New York: Dekker.

18. American College of Sports Medcine. 2000. *ACSM's guidelines for exercise testing and prescription.* 6th ed. Franklin, B.F., M.H. Whaley, and E.T. Howley, eds. Baltimore: Lippincott, Williams & Wilkins.

19. Prochaska, J., and K. Congden. 1999. Behavioral change—getting started and being successful. In *Cardiac rehabilitation. A guide to practice in the 21st century,* ed. N.K. Wenger, L.K. Smith, E.S. Froelicher, and P.M. Conness. New York: Dekker.

20. Ades, P.A., M.L. Waldmann, and W.J. McCann. 1992. Predictors of cardiac rehabilitation participation in older coronary patients. *Arch. Int. Med.* 152:1033.

21. Sevensky, K.E. , P.H. Brubaker , H.S. Miller, A.Shutt, W.J. Rejeski. 1994. Characteristics of patients referred to cardiac rehabilitation and factors related to entry. *J. Cardiopulmonary Rehabil.* 14(5) 340.

22. Burke, L.E. 1999. Adherence to a heart-healthy lifestyle—what makes the difference? In *Cardiac rehabilitation. A guide to practice in the 21st century,* ed. N.K. Wenger, L.K. Smith, E.S. Froelicher, and P.M. Comoss. New York: Dekker.

23. Debusk, R.F., W.L. Haskell, N.H. Miller, K. Berra, and C.B. Taylor. 1984. Medically directed at-home rehabilitation soon after clinically uncomplicated myocardial infarction: A new model for patient care. *Am. J. Cardiol.* 55:251–257.

24. Debusk, R.F., N.H. Miller, H.R. Supenko, C.A. Dennis, R.J. Thomas, H.T. Lew, W.E. Berger, R.S. Keller, J. Rompf, D. Gee, H.C. Kraemer, A. Bandura, G. Grandour, R. Shah, M. Clark, L. Fisher, and C.B. Taylor. 1999. A case-management system for coronary risk factor modification after acute myocardial infarction. *Ann. Int. Med.* 120:721–729.

25. Miller, N.H., and C.B. Taylor. 1995. Behavior modification for cardiovascular risk factor reduction. In *Heart disease and rehabilitation,* ed. M.L. Pollock and D.H. Schmidt. Champaign, IL: Human Kinetics.

26. Shaw, D.K., K.E. Sparks, and H.S. Jennings. 1998. Telephonic exercise monitoring. A review. *J. Cardiopul. Rehabil.* 18:263–270.

27. Ades, P.A., F.J. Pashkow, G. Fletcher, I. Pina, L.R. Zohman, and J.R. Nestor. 2000. A controlled trial of cardiac rehabilitation in the home setting using ECG and voice transtelephonic monitoring. *Am. Heart J.* 139 (3): 543–548.

28. Brubaker, P.H., W.J. Rejeski, M.U. Smith, K.H. Sevensky, K.A. Lamb, W.M. Sotile, and H.S. Miller. 2000. A home-based maintenance exercise program of the center-based cardiac rehabilitation: Effects on blood lipids, body composition, and functional capacity. *J. Cardiopul. Rehabil.* 20:50–56.

29. Rejeski W.J., L.R. Brawley. 1997. Shaping active lifestyles in older adults: a group-facilitated behavior change intervention. *Ann. Behav. Med.* 19 (suppl): s106.

CHAPTER 11

Administrative Issues for Coronary Artery Disease Prevention and Rehabilitation Programs

BEHAVIORAL OBJECTIVES

- To be able to describe the qualifications and credentials of personnel in CAD prevention and rehabilitation programs

- To be able to describe appropriate emergency protocols and use of risk stratification models

- To be able to describe budgetary considerations for CAD prevention and rehabilitation programs and understand billing and insurance issues

- To understand basic legal issues in CAD prevention and rehabilitation programs

- To be able to describe the process for program certification through the American Association of Cardiovascular and Pulmonary Rehabilitation

There are two essential objectives of any CAD prevention or rehabilitation program: safety and efficacy. To accomplish both objectives, the preventive or rehabilitative program must have a qualified and well-trained staff, as well as carefully thought-out program policies and procedures. Moreover, all programs must take appropriate steps, including adhering to national standards of care, in order to limit their legal liability. Recently, a national organization (American Association of Cardiovascular and Pulmonary Rehabilitation, AACVPR) has created a certification process to standardize and improve the quality of secondary prevention programs. This certification may eventually be required for reimbursement for preventive and rehabilitative services. Lack of **third-party reimbursement** continues to be a major obstacle for primary and secondary prevention programs.

PERSONNEL

As described in chapter 10, contemporary CAD prevention and rehabilitation programs are multidisciplinary and therefore need to be staffed by a "team" of multidisciplinary health care providers. Preventive and rehabilitative exercise programs range from organizations that are small and narrow in scope to those that are large and multifaceted. Consequently the personnel requirements vary widely and also differ somewhat for primary versus secondary prevention or cardiac rehabilitation programs. This section provides an overview of key personnel that are involved in preventive and rehabilitative exercise programs, presenting a basic job description and outlining necessary qualifications for each role.

Program Director

Ideally, all preventive and rehabilitative exercise programs would be under the direction of an American College of Sports Medicine (ACSM) Health/Fitness Director or Program Director, respectively (box 11.1). The program director of either a primary or secondary prevention program establishes and regularly updates all policies and procedures relative to its operation. This individual also supervises the staff who carry out the program procedures, manages the budget, and oversees the facility and equipment. Minimal requirements for the job of a program director include an academic degree, preferably a **postbaccalaureate degree,** in exercise physiology or a related discipline; experience in fitness assessment, exercise prescription, and exercise lead-

ership; training in administration and personnel management; and experience with facility management. It is highly desirable that this individual obtain either the ACSM Program Director or ACSM Health/Fitness Director certification (1). The AACVPR has also established qualifications for directors of secondary prevention programs (2). In addition to the qualifications just mentioned, the secondary prevention program director should have advanced knowledge in exercise physiology, exercise testing, exercise prescription, and cardiovascular and pulmonary disease management.

Even though the ACSM has established the Program Director certification and the AACVPR has established qualifications for directors, many programs are directed by other licensed clinical professionals (nurses and physical therapists). It is important to understand that clinical exercise physiology is still an evolving profession. In many cases the importance of the clinical exercise physiologist as an allied health professional needs to be "sold" to the hospital or institution administration.

The AACVPR (3) has established **core competencies** for personnel of secondary prevention programs. Students interested in careers in either cardiac or pulmonary rehabilitation should review these position statements of AACVPR to gain a more comprehensive understanding of what is expected of professionals working in secondary prevention programs.

Medical Director

According to AACVPR (2), the medical director is the staff member responsible for assisting with establishing and approving all clinical practice guidelines. This individual works closely with the program director. Minimal qualifications, as established by AACVPR, are that the medical director be a physician with training in cardiology or pulmonology; have experience in exercise testing and prescription; and have experience in emergency procedures, including certification in advanced cardiac life support (ACLS). While the involvement of a medical director is clearly indicated for a secondary prevention or cardiac rehabilitation program, involvement of a physician in a primary prevention program is highly desirable and strongly recommended.

Exercise Physiologist

According to the AACVPR (2), the minimum qualifications for the position of exercise physiologist in a cardiac rehabilitation program are a bachelor's degree in exercise science or a related

Box 11.1 Professional Personnel Certifications of the American College of Sports Medicine

There are many organizations that offer certifications for health and fitness professionals. The leader in the industry, offering what is considered the "gold standard" certifications for professionals working in either preventative or rehabilitative programs, is the American College of Sports Medicine (ACSM). Recently (2000), ACSM celebrated its 25th anniversary of offering certifications to health and fitness professionals. The ACSM certification program is divided into two tracks, Clinical and Health/Fitness.

The Clinical track is designed for professionals who primarily work with moderate and high-risk populations (i.e., secondary prevention programs). This track offers the following two levels of certification:

ACSM Exercise Specialist®—has the knowledge, skills, and abilities to perform exercise testing, exercise prescription, exercise leadership, and patient counseling and education

ACSM Program Director_SM—has the knowledge, skills, and abilities of the Exercise Specialist as well as for administration of secondary prevention programs

The Health and Fitness track is designed for professionals who primarily work with low to moderate-risk populations (i.e., primary prevention programs). This track offers the following three levels of certification:

ACSM Group Exercise Leader_SM—has the knowledge, skills, and abilities to teach safe, effective, and sound methods of exercise in a group setting

ACSM Health/Fitness Instructor_SM—has the knowledge, skills, and abilities of the Exercise Leader and to assess physical fitness and design and implement exercise training programs for individuals or groups

ACSM Health/Fitness Director®—has the knowledge, skills, and abilities of the Health/Fitness Instructor as well as for administration of primary prevention programs

A comprehensive listing of the specific knowledge, skills, and abilities for each level of certification is provided in Appendix F of the ACSM Guidelines or online at **www.lww.com/acsmcrc**.

field, training equivalent to that of an ACSM Exercise Specialist, and experience in cardiovascular rehabilitation programs. Preferred qualifications are a master's degree in exercise science or a related field and ACSM Exercise Specialist certification. These qualifications are also desirable, but not necessarily required, for those working in the primary prevention setting.

Recently, the ACSM established a registry for clinical exercise physiologists (box 11.2). In order to become a Registered Clinical Exercise Physiologist (RCEP), individuals must have a master's degree in exercise physiology with a clinical emphasis, have 1200 hours of experience spread across the six practice areas, and pass the registry exam. This credential is being actively promoted and marketed throughout the country. It is the vision of the Clinical Exercise Physiology Practice Board that the RCEP will become the minimal standard for exercise program professionals in most, if not all, clinical exercise programs (4). It is also possible that the RCEP could lead to licensure of the profession of exercise physiology in many states.

There are a variety of pathways by which exercise program professionals can obtain a credential to verify their professional qualifications, including certifications, registrations, and licenses. A certification can be either an entry-level or an advanced credential that may or may not be essential for employment. Some certifications are offered by national professional organizations that have established standards or guidelines stating that candidates must demonstrate competency (pass an exam) in order to obtain the certification. However, some certifications are offered by independent, and in many cases for-profit, agencies that have less stringent standards. Registry is usually controlled by an autonomous "practice board" of peers who regulate the credential by setting requirements, including qualifications, ethical standards, and discipline. Typically, individuals attain eligibility by meeting specific educational and clinical experience standards and passing a competency-based examination. Generally, registries promote trust in the quality of

Box 11.2 What is a RCEP?

In 1996 the ACSM Board of Trustees approved the following scope of practice for the Registered Clinical Exercise Physiologist:

The Clinical Exercise Physiologist works in the application of exercise and physical activity for those clinical and pathological situations where it (exercise) has been shown to provide therapeutic or functional benefit. Patients for whom (exercise) services are appropriate may include, but are not limited to, those with cardiovascular, pulmonary, metabolic, immunological, inflammatory, orthopedic, and neuromuscular diseases and conditions. This list will be modified as indications and procedures of application are further developed and mature. Furthermore, the Clinical Exercise Physiologist applies exercise principles to groups such as geriatric, pediatric, and obstetric populations, and to society as a whole in prevention activities. The Clinical Exercise Physiologist performs exercise evaluation, exercise prescription, exercise supervision, exercise education, and exercise outcome evaluation. The practice of Clinical Exercise Physiologists should be restricted to cli-

ents who are referred by and are under the continued care of a licensed physician.

A Practice Board governs the practice of Clinical Exercise Physiologists. Among the activities of the Practice Board are: to set and regulate the prerequisite requirements for both academic preparation and clinical experience; to develop and administer the registry examination; to provide professional and public information; and to oversee ethical issues related to the registry. The Practice Board has developed specific knowledge, skills, and abilities for the Clinical Exercise Physiologist. In general the requirements for the RCEP cover the following six defined practice areas: cardiovascular, pulmonary, metabolic, neuromuscular, orthopedic, and immunologic.

Within each practice area the following twelve content domains are present: pathophysiology; clinical exercise physiology; pharmacology; physical examination; medical and surgical treatments; diagnostic techniques; exercise/fitness testing; exercise prescription and programming; education and counseling; emergency procedures; quality assurance, outcome assessment, and discharge planning; and administration.

service through the eligibility standards. Licensure is the legal authority to provide services to the public within a defined scope of practice and jurisdiction. Licensure is established by each state through legislative process and regulated by the state government. A fundamental purpose for establishing a license is to protect the public from potential harm resulting from provision of services by nonqualified individuals. The credentialing process in clinical exercise physiology is presently evolving, and there is no clearly defined or required path. However, many job postings indicate that an ACSM credential (RCEP, Exercise Specialist, or Health/Fitness Instructor) is highly desired.

Nurse

Nurses, given their training in ECG interpretation, medications, and emergency management, often play a substantial role in cardiac rehabilitation programs. Commonly, a nurse draws blood for risk factor assessment; has training in

ACLS and thus provides leadership in emergency situations; provides staff training in emergency management; and educates patients on risk factors, disease status, and medications. The role of a nurse in primary prevention can vary from little to no involvement to the roles just specified. According to the AACVPR, the minimum qualifications for the position of nurse are to be licensed to practice and to have ACLS certification. Preferred qualifications are experience or training equivalent to an ACSM Exercise Specialist certification. It is important to note that few academic nursing curriculums provide any training in exercise physiology, exercise testing, or exercise prescription. Thus, if the exercise program relies on a nurse for exercise physiology-related competencies (i.e., if the program does not have an exercise physiologist on staff), the nurse needs to obtain additional education. Some nurses who choose to work in exercise programs as a career return to school to obtain a master's degree in exercise physiology.

Involvement of Other Allied Health Professionals

As discussed in chapter 10, the ideal preventive or rehabilitative program is much more than just an exercise program. Many other allied health professionals can make a major contribution to the care of program participants. Registered dietitians, mental health professionals, health educators, vocational rehabilitation counselors, physical therapists, occupational therapists, and pharmacists are commonly involved in secondary prevention programs. The recommended qualifications for each of these professionals are described in the AACVPR Guidelines (2).

Primary Prevention Program Staff

Whereas a cardiac rehabilitation program is essentially required to have the involvement of the health care providers just mentioned, their involvement is less clearly defined for primary prevention programs. The diversity of the health status of the clients in the prevention program, as well as the range of services offered by the program, dictates the necessary qualifications of the staff. Some large, comprehensive programs employ the services of a clinical exercise physiologist or exercise specialist. They may also offer consultations with other allied health professionals (e.g., dietitians) as part of the program services. Additionally, primary prevention programs are staffed by a number of "front-line" personnel who have most of the day-to-day contact with the clients. The preferred qualifications for these individuals are a bachelor's degree in exercise science and ACSM certification as either a health/fitness instructor or exercise leader. Typically, health/fitness instructors perform physical fitness assessments and develop the exercise prescription for the clients. They may also be involved in providing personal training services for clients who desire this level of attention. Exercise leaders administer group-based exercise sessions and monitor the clients' performance and progress in these exercise classes.

MANAGEMENT OF MEDICAL EMERGENCIES IN PREVENTIVE AND REHABILITATIVE PROGRAMS

Safety is perhaps the most important consideration of a preventive or rehabilitative exercise program. Clearly there is an increased risk of **untoward events** (heart attack, cardiac arrest, sudden death, etc.) during a vigorous bout of exercise as compared to normal daily activities. However, this transient risk of **cardiac arrest** and other untoward events is significantly lower in individuals who are habitually active compared to those who are sedentary. Overall the risk of cardiac arrest among habitually physically active men is only 40% of that for sedentary men (5). Those at greatest risk for an untoward event during exercise are individuals who get little to no consistent physical activity yet occasionally participate in competitive, high-level sporting activities (basketball, raquetball, running). These individuals, often called "weekend warriors," should be encouraged to reduce their risk of untoward events by improving their overall physical capacity and reducing their risk factors for CAD through regular physical activity. Overall, it is quite clear that the benefits of regular physical activity and/or exercise clearly outweigh the transient risks observed during a bout of exercise (1).

Despite the transient increase in the risk of sudden death during vigorous exercise, the safety of exercise testing and training has been well established. The findings of numerous studies regarding the safety of peak or symptom-limited graded exercise testing, described in chapter 6, can be summarized with the following general statements (1):

- The risk of death during or immediately after an exercise test is ≤0.01%.

- The risk of acute myocardial infarction (MI) during or immediately after an exercise test is ≤0.04%.

- The risk of a complication requiring hospitalization (including acute MI or serious arrhythmias) during or immediately after an exercise test is ≤0.2%.

In more than 10,000 symptom-limited exercise tests conducted on patients with known heart disease at the Wake Forest University Cardiac Rehabilitation Program, there have been no deaths, only one MI, and one cardiac arrest. In more than 5500 symptom-limited exercise tests of apparently healthy individuals at the Ball State University Adult Physical Fitness Program, there have been no deaths, MIs, or cardiac arrests. As would be expected, the risk of untoward events during "submaximal" physical fitness testing often performed in primary prevention settings (methodologies described in chapter 6) are significantly lower than what has been observed during "maximal" testing commonly done in higher-risk populations. In fact, there are no reported cases of a significant cardiac event (MI, cardiac arrest, or death) during a submaximal exercise test, despite the fact that these tests have been given to millions of individuals in a variety of settings including health clubs, work site programs, and schools (1).

The risk of cardiovascular complications during exercise or physical activity in apparently healthy individuals is extremely low. One survey of YMCA sport centers (6) revealed 1 death per 2,897,057 person-hours of activity and 1 cardiac arrest per 2,253,267 person-hours of activity. It should be pointed out that these hours of activity included higher-risk activities (basketball, racquetball) often enjoyed by the "weekend warriors." A five-year retrospective study (7) of cardiac events that occurred during or immediately after exercise in community recreation centers showed fatal and nonfatal cardiovascular complication rates of 1 per 887,526 and 1 per 1,124,200 person-hours of exercise, respectively. At the Ball State University Adult Physical Fitness Program, which has included more than 355,000 participant-hours of exercise training, there have been no exercise-induced complications that required emergency or immediate medical intervention. We should note that most of these participants were classified as low risk and that they underwent preparticipation examinations and exercise testing. These factors, along with staff trained to monitor for warning signs and symptoms, undoubtedly contributed to this outstanding safety record.

As one would expect, the risk of cardiac complications during exercise is considerably higher in individuals with known cardiovascular disease than in those who are apparently healthy. An early survey (8) of 167 cardiac rehabilitation programs (more than 51,000 patients who exercised 2.3 million total hours) reported 29 major cardiovascular events (21 cardiac arrests and 8 MIs) and three fatalities. Accordingly, the reported complication rates from this survey were

- 1 cardiac arrest per 111,996 patient-hours of exercise,
- 1 MI per 293,990 patient-hours of exercise, and
- 1 fatality per 783,972 patient-hours of exercise.

More recent studies indicate that approximately 1 major cardiovascular complication occurs for every 60,000 participant-hours of outpatient cardiac exercise therapy (9, 10). In 25 years (more than 500,000 patient-hours of exercise) at the Wake Forest University Cardiac Rehabilita-

tion Program, there have been just seven cardiac arrests during the exercise program (1 per 71,428 patient-hours of exercise). Interestingly, five of the seven patients who experienced cardiac arrests at Wake Forest were in the cardiac maintenance program (i.e., had been in the program more than 1 year), and only three of the cardiac arrests occurred during the actual exercise training phase. Two occurred during the cool-down phase and two occurred during the warm-up phase. The lesson one should learn from the Wake Forest program is that untoward events (particularly cardiac arrest), although rare, can happen to anyone, at any time, and at any stage (beginning vs. maintenance) of an exercise program.

There has been much interest over the years in identifying those most likely to have exercise-related cardiovascular complications. However, it is very difficult to predict who is going to have an untoward event during exercise. Nevertheless, certain characteristics (presented in table 11.1) associated with exercise-related cardiovascular complications can potentially help the clinician determine the appropriate level of supervision and monitoring.

Steps to Reduce Cardiovascular Complications in Exercise Programs

One reason for infrequent cardiovascular complications during preventive and rehabilitative exercise programs is the availability and application of organizational guidelines to help programs prepare for medical emergencies. Organizations including the ACSM (1) and the AACVPR (2) have described a number of procedures and made recommendations for reducing the risk of untoward events in programs. These pertain to clearances and screening, on-site supervision, emergency planning, participant education, monitoring, and exercise intensities.

Ensure Medical Clearance and Determine Appropriate Level of Monitoring

Prior to participation in an exercise program it is recommended that apparently healthy individuals undergo a preparticipation health screening. The purpose of this screening is to

- identify medical **contraindications** to exercise (i.e., factors or conditions that make exercise unsafe; these are discussed in chapter 6),
- identify individuals who should undergo a medical examination and/or an exercise test

Table 11.1 Characteristics associated with exercise-related cardiovascular complications.

Clinical Status	• Multiple myocardial infarctions
	• Reduced left ventricular function (ejection fraction $\leq$ 30%)
	• Unstable or resting angina pectoris
	• Compromising ventricular or supraventricular arrhythmia
	• Significant ($\geq$ 70% occlusion) multi-vessel coronary disease and/or high-grade stenosis in left main coronary artery system
	• Abnormal serum electrolytes (particularly low potassium)
Exercise Training	• Poor compliance to exercise prescription
	• Lack of adequate warm-up or cool-down
	• Participant in "maintenance" exercise program*
Exercise Test Data	• Low or high functional capacity ($\leq$ 4 or $\geq$ 10 METs)
	• Abnormal hemodynamic responses including inadequate heart rate response (i.e., chronotropic incompetence) and failure of blood pressure to rise with increased workloads
	• Evidence of myocardial ischemia (angina pectoris and/or ST segment changes)
	• Malignant cardiac arrhythmia
Other	• Male gender
	• Cigarette smoker

*Observed at Wake Forest University Program.
Reprinted, by permission, 2000, *ACSM's Guidelines for Exercise Testing and Prescription*. 6th ed. (Philadelphia: Lippincott, Williams, and Wilkins), 27.

prior to participating in an exercise program, and

• identify individuals with medical conditions that require participation in a medically supervised exercise program.

Preparticipation health screening for apparently healthy individuals can be often be accomplished by simple, cost-effective, self-administered questionnaires such as the one developed by the American Heart Association (AHA) and ACSM (figure 11.1). People interested in participating in organized exercise programs should be evaluated for cardiovascular disease risk factors (see chapter 1) and for signs and symptoms of cardiovascular disease (see chapter 3).

After screening for CAD symptoms and risk factors, individuals wishing to participate in an exercise program should be stratified based on their likelihood of untoward events during exercise. As discussed in chapter 6, on the basis of age, health status, symptoms, and risk factors, individuals can be risk stratified into low- to moderate- and high-risk (see table 6.5). Once an individual is stratified, table 11.2 can be used to determine the following for that person:

• Need for a comprehensive medical examination and exercise testing prior to participation

• Need for physician supervision of the exercise test

For individuals with cardiovascular disease, several models for **risk stratification** have been proposed by organizations including the AHA (11) and the AACVPR (1). These models were developed to classify patients based on risk for untoward events during exercise, but are often incorrectly used to determine extent of monitoring and duration of the program, as well as for extent of third-party reimbursement (12). It is important to recognize that these risk stratification systems do not adequately consider **comorbidities** or the impact of risk factors related to the progression of CAD, described in chapters 9 and 10, respectively.

Patient monitoring is an important issue in cardiac rehabilitation settings. While there is little doubt that patients with known cardiovascular disease require some level of monitoring during exercise training, there has been much debate regarding the type and extent of monitoring needed. Most cardiac rehabilitation professionals (and professional standards) agree that all patients should have their vital signs (heart rate and rhythm, blood pressure, cardiac symptoms) assessed before, during, and after an exercise session. What cardiac rehabilitation professionals differ about is how to monitor cardiac rhythm.

AHA/ACSM Health/Fitness Facility Preparticipation Screening Questionnaire

Assess your health needs by marking all *true* statements.

History

You have had:

_____ heart attack

_____ heart surgery

_____ cardiac catheterization

_____ coronary angioplasty

_____ pacemaker/implantable defibrillator/rhythm disturbance

_____ heart valve disease

_____ heart failure

_____ heart transplant

_____ congenital heart disease

If you marked any of the statements in this section, consult your health care provider before engaging in exercise. You may need to use a facility with a **medically qualified staff**.

Symptoms

_____ You experience chest discomfort with exertion.

_____ You experience unreasonable breathlessness.

_____ You experience dizziness, fainting, blackouts.

_____ You take heart medications.

Other health issues:

_____ You have musculoskeletal problems.

_____ You have concerns about the safety of exercise.

_____ You take prescription medication.

_____ You are pregnant.

Cardiovascular Risk Factors

_____ You are a man older than 45 years.

_____ You are a woman older than 55 years or you have had a hysterectomy or you are postmenopausal.

_____ You smoke.

_____ Your blood pressure is greater than 140/90.

_____ You don't know your blood pressure.

_____ You take blood pressure medication.

_____ Your blood cholesterol is > 240 mg/dL.

_____ You don't know your cholesterol level.

_____ You have a close blood relative who had a heart attack before age 55 (father or brother) or age 65 (mother or sister).

_____ You are diabetic or take medication to control your blood sugar.

_____ You are physically inactive (i.e. you get less than 30 minutes of physical activity on at least 3 days/ week).

_____ You are more than 20 pounds overweight.

If you marked two or more of the statements in this section, you should consult your healthcare provider before engaging in exercise. You might benefit by using a facility with **a professionally qualified exercise staff** to guide your exercise program.

You should be able to exercise safely without consulting your healthcare provider in almost any facility that meets your exercise program needs.

_____ None of the above is true.

Figure 11.1 American Heart Association/American College of Sports Medicine Health Fitness Facility Preparticipation Screening Questionnaire.
Adapted with permission Lippincott Williams & Wilkins.

Presently, two approaches are commonly used: (1) continuous ECG monitoring via a hard-wire or telemetry system and (2) intermittent ECG monitoring via defibrillator paddles, periodic rhythm strips, or periodic **telemetry monitoring.** While there is no solid evidence to indicate that continuous monitoring provides any additional safety (8) or efficacy benefit over intermittent monitoring, many programs continue to monitor continuously. Some program administrators are reluctant to reduce or eliminate continuous ECG monitoring since this approach allows for higher billing rates than intermittent monitoring. In response to this controversial issue, AACVPR (2) has developed recommendations for ECG monitoring and patient supervision during exer-

Table 11.2
ACSM Recommendations for (A) Current Medical Examination* and Exercise Testing Prior to Participation and (B) Physician Supervision of Exercise Tests

	Low risk	Moderate risk	High risk
A.			
Moderate exercise†	Not necessary‡	Not necessary	Recommended
Vigorous exercise§	Not necessary	Recommended	Recommended
B.			
Submaximal test	Not necessary	Not necessary	Recommended
Maximal test	Not necessary	Recommended‖	Recommended‖

*Within the past year.

†Absolute moderate exercise is defined as activities that are approximately 3–6 METs or the equivalent of brisk walking at 3 to 4 mph for most healthy adults. Nevertheless, a pace of 3 to 4 mph might be considered to be "hard" to "very hard" by some sedentary, older persons. Moderate exercise may alternatively be defined as an intensity well within the individual's capacity, one which can be comfortably sustained for a prolonged period of time (~45 min), which has a gradual initiation and progression, and is generally noncompetitive. If an individual's exercise capacity is known, relative moderate exercise may be defined by the range 40–60% maximal oxygen uptake.

‡The designation of "Not necessary" reflects the notion that a medical examination, exercise test, and physician supervision of exercise testing would not be essential in the preparticipation screeening; however, they should not be viewed as inappropriate.

§Vigorous exercise is defined as activities of >6 METs. Vigorous exercise may alternatively be defined as exercise intense enough to represent a substantial cardiorespiratory challenge. If an individual's exercise capacity is known, vigorous exercise may be defined as an intensity of >60% maximal oxygen uptake.

‖When physician supervision of exercise testing is "Recommended," the physician should be in close proximity and readily available should there be an emergent need.

cise in a cardiac rehabilitation setting (see table 7.12).

Provide Appropriate or Required On-Site Medical Supervision, Emergency Equipment, and Medications

The degree of medical supervision is generally inversely related to the medical stability of the client. Thus, for apparently healthy individuals stratified into the low-risk category (AHA class A), physician supervision is not required (see table 11.2). However, it is strongly recommended that, from the emergency management perspective (other credentials have been previously described), all personnel directly involved with a primary prevention exercise program have at minimum completed the National Cognitive and Skills examination in accordance with the AHA curriculum for Basic Life Support. Although life-support equipment and drugs may not be required on site in these low-risk settings, the ability to activate and receive rapid response through the emergency medical system (EMS) is still critical. Automatic defibrillators can be potentially very useful (i.e., lifesaving) even in low-risk environments (airplanes, malls, restaurants) and may eventually be required in all exercise facilities.

In cardiac rehabilitation programs, in contrast to the low-risk, primary prevention setting,

it is recommended (2) that all staff directly involved with patient care have completed the National Cognitive and Skills examination in accordance with the AHA curriculum for ACLS. A further recommendation is that at least one supervising staff person with ACLS and appropriate licensure be available to provide appropriate emergency interventions (defibrillation, intubation, administration of medications) during all exercise training sessions. These interventions are typically performed by a physician or nurse, but more programs are beginning to use physician's assistants, nurse practitioners, or paramedics for coverage of emergency situations.

For programs working with high-risk individuals (e.g., cardiac rehabilitation) in which medical personnel must be present during exercise sessions, the emergency medical equipment listed in box 11.3 must also be on site. Obviously it would not make a great deal of sense to require the presence of highly trained individuals without providing them appropriate equipment and medications (box 11.4). In many hospital-based cardiac rehabilitation programs, emergency equipment (as well as personnel to use it) is provided by a **code blue** team. Under these conditions, the staff of the cardiac rehabilitation program are expected to activate the code blue response and perform basic cardiac life support until this assistance arrives. Similarly, health club or other primary prevention

Box 11.3   Emergency equipment for preventive/rehabilitative exercise programs

- Medications (see box 11.4)
- Portable defibrillator with electrocardiographic monitor and printout
- Portable oxygen with nasal cannula, mouth-to-mouth, or bag-to-mouth with tubing
- Portable suction device
- Intravenous fluid access equipment (needles, tubing)
- Method for activating code team, staff, or EMS (code phone, intercom)

- Intubation equipment (including airway devices)
- Blood pressure measurement equipment
- Cart or box for storage of equipment and medications that can be locked or secured out of reach of general public
- Form to document equipment checks and date of medication (see figure 11.2)
- Appropriate personal protective items (gloves, masks, gowns, cleanup kits, sharps containers) to prevent exposure to blood borne pathogens

Reprinted, by permission, from AACVPR, 1999, *Guidelines for cardiac rehabilitation and secondary prevention programs,* 3rd ed. (Champaign, IL: Human Kinetics), 49.

Box 11.4   Primary emergency medications and mechanisms of benefit for myocardial ischemia/infarction and cardiac arrhythmia

- **Aspirin:** To prevent thrombus formation associated with coronary artery plaque rupture. Several aspirin (acetylsalicylic acid, not acetaminophen (Tylenol), ibuprofen (Motrin) or other analgesics) should be chewed if myocardial infarction is suspected.

- **Atropine:** To correct hemodynamically significant bradycardia by suppressing parasympathetic nervous system effect on SA and AV nodes. Administered through IV or endotracheal tube (if IV access not attainable).

- **Beta blockers** (numerous brands; see table 4.5): To reduce myocardial oxygen demand (during myocardial ischemia and/or MI) by reducing heart rate, blood pressure, and contractility. Also used for refractory ventricular and/or supraventricular arrhythmia. Administered through IV.

- **Epinephrine:** To increase blood pressure and cardiac output. Primary benefit is peripheral vasoconstriction (via alpha-receptor stimulation), resulting in improved myocardial and cerebral blood supply. Also, increases myocardial contractility and rate (beta-receptor effect). May enhance automaticity and make fine ventricular fibrillation and/or asystole more amenable to defibrillation. Administered through IV or endotracheal tube (if IV access not attainable).

- **Lidocaine:** To suppress ventricular arrhythmia by decreasing automaticity of cells. Administered through IV or endotracheal tube (if IV access not attainable).

- **Morphine:** To decrease pain during acute myocardial infarction. Also, decreases afterload and preload, which reduces myocardial demand. Administered through IV.

- **Nitroglycerine:** To relax venous and arterial vascular smooth muscle, which results in a decreased myocardial oxygen demand. Thus, used in treatment of myocardial ischemia and/or infarction. Questionable ability to dilate obstructed coronary arteries and improve myocardial blood supply. Administered orally (see table 3.3) and through IV.

- **Oxygen:** To correct hypoxemia (lack of oxygen supply to tissue). Administered by cannula, mask, bag, etc. with goal to maintain oxygen saturation > 90% (PaO_2 = 60-100 mmHg).

- **Vasodilators:** To dilate peripheral arteries and veins (decrease afterload and preload), which is beneficial during hypertensive episodes and with decompensated heart failure. Administered orally (several types; see table 4.5) through IV.

The above are agents initially used for emergency management. Alternative and secondary agents are described in ACLS Guidelines (13).

programs are, at minimum, expected to activate the EMS and provide basic cardiac life support (i.e., cardiopulmonary resuscitation) until EMS arrives.

Establish and Rehearse Emergency Plans

In addition to appropriately trained staff and proper equipment, plans must be in place to respond to minor injuries (cuts, bruises, musculoskeletal problems) as well as life-threatening cardiac conditions. Contemporary programs have a written "plan of action" to define specific staff roles (e.g., perform cardiopulmonary resuscitation, call EMS, operate defibrillator) and appropriate treatments. Treatment **algorithms** for managing various cardiovascular emergencies have been developed by the AHA and are the basis for ACLS (13). Personnel should practice the emergency plan regularly (e.g., at least once per month) and/or whenever there is a change in program staff. During the emergency drill it is important to make and document the following assessments using a form such as that presented in figure 11.2:

- Measure response time (staff or code team)—time to defibrillate is critical!

- Ensure availability of appropriate equipment and drugs.

- Ensure that all equipment is functional and that the drugs are not outdated.

- Ensure that all emergency roles are covered.

- Review appropriate treatment algorithms including drugs (e.g., proper dose and route of administration) and other interventions (e.g., defibrillator settings).

Promote Participant Education

Participants in either primary or secondary prevention programs should receive clear instructions from the staff on how to monitor their exercise intensity (e.g., methods described in chapter 7 such as heart rate range, perceived exertion) and on the potential consequences of exercising outside of their prescribed range. All participants should be educated about major warning signs and symptoms (chest pain, lightheadedness, shortness of breath, unusual fatigue, palpitations) and instructed to inform staff of such changes. Furthermore, participants must be instructed to inform staff of any change in medi-

cal status, including hospital or doctor's office visits, as well as any change in medications. A well-educated and informed program participant will generally be a safer and more successful participant.

Promote Moderate Intensity and Minimize Competition Among Participants

Evidence supports the notion that the lower the exercise intensity, the less likely an exercise-related complication is to occur. This appears to be true in both primary and secondary prevention programs. In fact, several surveys that examined the risk of untoward events during exercise in cardiac rehabilitation programs identified poor compliance to the prescribed intensity level (i.e., patients exercising above determined levels) as a common factor in patients who experienced cardiac arrest (2). Primary and secondary prevention program participants should understand that increasing intensity, frequency, or duration above the recommended levels (discussed in chapter 7) offers little added benefit, but disproportionately increases the risk of orthopedic injuries and reduces long-term adherence. Furthermore, competitive games in preventive or rehabilitative programs should be minimized or closely monitored since intensity is difficult to regulate and varies among participants. Moreover, competitiveness brought out during games may create additional physiologic stimulation and increased risk of untoward events.

Emphasize the Importance of Warm-Up and Cool-Down

As stated earlier, a significant percentage of the cardiac arrests (four of a total of seven) observed in the Wake Forest University Cardiac Rehabilitation program occurred during the warm-up and cool-down phases of exercise. A progressive warm-up period that includes musculoskeletal and cardiorespiratory activities may prevent musculoskeletal injuries and cardiovascular complications. Gradually decreasing the intensity level after vigorous exercise reduces the risk associated with increased sympathetic system activation, that is, **hypotension** and arrhythmias. Medical supervision, in those programs (such as cardiac rehabilitation) where already indicated, should continue until all patients have completed their postexercise cool-down, showered, changed clothes, and exited the facility.

Wake Forest University Cardiac Rehabilitation Emergency Procedure Check List

Program _____   Date _____   Program leader _____

Equipment:	Working	Not working	Date fixed
EMS activation			
Defibrillator			
Oxygen tank/tubing			
Ambu bag			
Airways (nasal & oral)			
Suction pump/tubing			
Emergency drug kit:	**YES**	**NO**	**Expiration date**
Nitroglycerine			
Lidocaine (100 mg/5 ml/inject.) **x2**			
I.V. Lidocaine solution			
Atropine (1 mg/10 ml/inject.) **x2**			
Adenosine (6 mg/2 ml) **x2**			
Epinephrine (1 mg/10 ml/inject.) **x2**			
Dextrose 50% (25 g/50 ml/inject.)			
ASA			
NaCl I.V. solution (0.9%/500 ml)			
I.V. starter kit **x2**			
I.V. tubing			
I.V. needles (angiocath) **x4**			
3 cc injectors **x4**			
disposable syringes (5cc) **x4**			
20-22 gauge needles **x4**			
surgical tape			
conduction gel			
alcohol swabs			
stethoscope			
blood pressure cuff			
gloves			
surgical dressing			
surgical gown			

Emergency procedure:

Satisfactory _____   Unsatisfactory _____

Comments: _____

_____

CPR: _____

ECG: _____

LAB staff: _____

_____ Medical Director

_____ Nurse

_____ Exercise coordinator

Figure 11.2   Emergency procedure/drill check list used at Wake Forest University Cardiac Rehabilitation Program.
Reprinted, by permission, from ACSM and AHA, 1998, "Recommendations for cardiovascular screening, staffing, and emergency procedures at health/fitness facilities," ACSM and AHA Joint Position Statement *Medicine and Science in Sport and Exercise* 30:1012.

Consider the Impact of the Environment (Heat and Cold)

While most preventive and rehabilitative exercise programs are conducted in a controlled indoor environment, people who exercise or conduct normal daily activities outside should be aware of the impact of the environment on the cardiovascular system. Exposure to cold air may result in vasoconstriction of blood vessels of the skin and the coronary arteries. The subsequent increase in peripheral vascular resistance coupled with the reduction in coronary blood flow can precipitate symptoms of myocardial ischemia (angina) and/or arrhythmia in patients with known or subclinical (i.e., not yet manifested) CAD.

Exercise in hot or humid weather also presents a hazard for patients with established or subclinical CAD. Heart rate and myocardial oxygen demand increase disproportionately to keep up with an increasing aerobic requirement. A given exercise level in hot and humid conditions generally results in significantly higher heart rates than it would otherwise. Therefore, in these types of environments patients should be encouraged to reduce exercise levels, dress appropriately, exercise at cooler times of the day, and consume fluids before, during, and after exercise to prevent dehydration.

What to Do in a Medical Emergency

In the unlikely event that a major cardiovascular emergency occurs in the preventive or rehabilitative program, it is essential that all staff members adhere to their assigned roles. Often during emergency codes, several responders will attend to the same task (such as operating the defibrillator) and neglect other vital roles, including basic cardiac life support (BCLS) and blood pressure measurement. Many programs assign each staff member a specific role and distribute a tag or card reminding each person of his responsibility. Since exercise physiologists are not licensed health care providers in most states, they are not typically the primary ACLS provider during an emergency situation. Even so, it is desirable for unlicensed personnel to obtain the ACLS credential so they will better understand the objectives of the ACLS provider and thus be able to offer valuable assistance. Furthermore, since exercise physiologists may have the most direct patient contact, they may be able to provide unique and beneficial information in emergency situations. For example,

during an emergency code that is being managed by a licensed health care provider, the exercise physiologist may assist by

- performing basic cardiac life support;
- describing the nature and time of the event (i.e., precipitating factors);
- providing history on the patient (medications, disease status);
- obtaining measurements of certain vital signs (blood pressure, pulses);
- operating equipment (defibrillator, suction device), particularly if it is unfamiliar to ACLS providers;
- anticipating emergency drugs that may be requested and their location in the "drug box"; and
- recording significant events such as times of defibrillation, drugs and doses, when code team or EMS arrived (a standardized form such as that presented in figure 11.3 should be used to assure that all essential information is gathered and documented; see also form F in chapter 6).

What to Do After a Medical Emergency

After a medical emergency has occurred and the patient has been transferred from the preventive or rehabilitative program to the hospital, the program staff still have a number of important jobs to do, including the following:

- Notifying family of the event and the location and status of the patient
- Notifying the patient's primary medical doctor
- Continuing to follow the patient's status by calling or going to the hospital
- Documenting the event for medicolegal reasons (using a form such as that in figure 11.6)
- Reviewing the incident with staff to discuss appropriate and inappropriate responses
- Restocking emergency supplies and equipment
- Learning from the event and making appropriate changes to more effectively manage future emergencies (after a medical emergency is an excellent time to conduct a staff in-service in an area judged to be substandard)

Wake Forest University Cardiac Rehabilitation Record of Cardiovascular Emergency Event

Event time _____ Participant name _____

Date _____ Program _____ Location _____

Staff arrival time _____ Nurse arrival time _____ MD arrival time _____

Respiratory:	**Y/N : Time**		**Drugs:**	**Dose**	**Time**
Mouth-to-mask	_____		Lidocaine bolus	_____	_____
Intubation	_____		Atropine	_____	_____
Bag-to-mask	_____		Adenosine	_____	_____
Oxygen	_____		Dextrose (50%)	_____	_____

Circulation: Digoxin   _____   _____

Chest compression_____   Epinephrine   _____   _____

ECG: Other:

Initial rhythm: _____   _____   _____   _____

_____   _____   _____   _____

Defibrillation:

Joules _____ Time _____ Rhythm _____

Joules _____ Time _____ Rhythm _____   **Vital signs:**   **Time**

Joules _____ Time _____ Rhythm _____   BP   _____   _____

Joules _____ Time _____ Rhythm _____   _____   _____

Joules _____ Time _____ Rhythm _____   _____   _____

I.V. therapy:

Lidocaine _____   Time _____   Pulse _____   _____

NaCl sol. _____   Time _____   _____   _____

Other _____   Time _____   Resp. _____   _____

Comments/procedure:

_____

_____

_____

_____

_____

Disposition: _____

MD signature _____ Personal MD _____

Nurse signature _____ Time MD notified_____

Staff signature _____ Time family notified_____

(Additional comments on other side)

Figure 11.3   Form to record cardiovascular emergency event used at Wake Forest University Cardiac Rehabilitation Program.

In summary, although the preventive or rehabilitative staff can take a number of steps to decrease the risk of life-threatening medical emergencies, there is always the possibility of an untoward event. Furthermore, it is very difficult to predict when and where these events are going to happen, so it is essential that emergency management plans be in place to deal with any possible scenario. Regular practice (i.e., drills) of emergency plans will help ensure that the staff are prepared and that the emergency equipment is available and operational. Properly credentialed and trained staff, following their defined roles and standard algorithms (such as those developed by AHA for ACLS), should be able to successfully manage the infrequent medical emergencies that occur in preventive or rehabilitative exercise programs.

ECONOMIC ISSUES IN PREVENTIVE AND REHABILITATIVE PROGRAMS

As described throughout this book, the exercise and other lifestyle modifications promoted in primary and secondary prevention programs have numerous proven benefits. Moreover, these lifestyle changes can be made safely and often at relatively little cost. It would seem logical for health insurance companies to pay or reimburse for these effective, low-cost preventive and rehabilitative programs. Unfortunately, they do not always do so, and the lack of third-party support for both primary prevention and cardiac rehabilitation has a negative impact on participation rates. The reality is that many individuals are unable or unwilling to pay for preventive heath service, and thus economics become a barrier to participation.

Cost Effectiveness of Preventive and Rehabilitative Services

As with any medically based procedure or therapy, the preventive or rehabilitative program is under increasing pressure to demonstrate the effectiveness of the service provided. The concept of cost effectiveness is typically used for this purpose. Cost is defined simply as the value of resources used to produce a good or service and is generally expressed in monetary terms (14). *Effectiveness* is the impact of an intervention on medical outcomes (described in chapter 10) in generally accepted practice. Effectiveness should be distinguished from efficacy. *Efficacy* refers to whether an intervention is capable of favorably

affecting outcomes and is most commonly analyzed under ideal circumstances, such as in a controlled research study. In contrast, effectiveness refers to whether an intervention actually favorably affects outcomes in the less ideal circumstances of general practice. While efficacy is the "gold standard" by which new interventions should be judged, effectiveness is generally used to determine the true value of the intervention in clinical practice. Many think of "effectiveness" and "benefit" as interchangeable, but this is not correct. Effectiveness is an attribute of a test or treatment and the delivery system that brings it to the patient; it is most easily expressed when objective outcome measures are available. Benefit is an attribute associated with the patient, relating to an improvement in symptoms or extension of life resulting from a particular diagnostic or therapeutic strategy (14).

Cost-effectiveness analysis is a method in which costs for a medical service are related to a specific medical outcome to establish value. For example, cost effectiveness for smoking cessation could be expressed as cost per smoking quitter; for exercise training it could be expressed as cost per MET increase in capacity. Cost-benefit analysis is a method that defines the relationship between the value of the resources used to produce a medical intervention and the value of the medical outcome produced. Cost-benefit is more complex than cost effectiveness in that it requires that a health benefit, including human life, be given a dollar value. These values are often adjusted for less-than-perfect outcomes using utilities such as quality-adjusted life years (QALYs). The differences between cost effectiveness and cost-benefit are subtle and complex and are beyond the scope of this book. However, to simplify the evaluation of cost-benefit, some recommend comparing the cost-benefit, expressed in dollars per QALY, to an accepted medical intervention, such as treating hypertension. In this approach, very attractive interventions are defined as those that cost less than $20,000 per QALY. Attractive interventions cost $20,000 to $30,000 per QALY, while those that cost more than $60,000 per QALY are considered expensive (14).

Although there is very little literature on the cost effectiveness of comprehensive cardiac rehabilitation programs, it is possible to assess the cost effectiveness of the individual components and interventions of programs. While a detailed review of each component is beyond the scope of this book, table 11.3 summarizes the cost-effectiveness literature on secondary prevention interventions. For the purpose of this summary, each intervention is rated on cost, effectiveness, and benefit. Additionally, the strength of evidence (i.e., the body of literature) is summarized for each intervention.

As table 11.4 shows, most of the interventions provided in secondary prevention or cardiac rehabilitation programs are low cost, with the exception of cholesterol-lowering medications, which have moderate cost. Low-cost interventions even with limited effectiveness are generally attractive, whereas high-cost interventions with limited effectiveness would not be attractive. In the case of cholesterol management, dietary therapy is rated low on effectiveness since dietary changes alone typically lower lipid levels by 10% to 15% and may not result in achievement of established goals, such as those set by the National Cholesterol Education Program (described in earlier chapters). However, dietary therapy is still an attractive intervention in the secondary prevention setting since it is low cost and has other measurable (weight loss, glucose control) and

immeasurable benefits, such as the potential to reduce the dose of cholesterol medication. Drug therapy has been shown to be highly effective in lowering low-density lipoprotein cholesterol levels and concomitantly decreasing morbidity, mortality, and use of medical resources such as angioplasty and coronary artery bypass graft surgery.

Smoking cessation programs, particularly those combining behavioral counseling, nicotine replacement, and pharmacotherapy, are very attractive since they are relatively inexpensive and can have significant benefits. As mentioned in earlier chapters, smoking cessation after MI lowers mortality by 50% in the one to two years following the initial event. Cost-effectiveness studies have shown that smoking cessation interventions in the general population are in the very attractive category, with costs ranging from $1500 to $11,000 per QALY. Remember, interventions under $20,000 per QALY are very attractive (14).

Unquestionably, exercise training has many physiologic and psychosocial benefits for patients

Table 11.3

Cost, Effectiveness, Benefit, and Strength of Evidence of Interventions Offered in Secondary Prevention/Cardiac Rehabilitation

Intervention	Cost	Effectiveness	Benefit	Evidence
Exercise training	Low	Medium	Attractive	Limited
Smoking cessation	Low	High	Very attractive	Strong
Dietary therapy (for hypercholesterolemia)	Low	Low	Attractive	Strong
Drug therapy (for hypercholesterolemia)	Medium	High	Attractive	Strong

Adapted from (14)

Table 11.4

Potential Income Sources For Preventive and Rehabilitative Programs

Items	Fees
Exercise sessions	Can range from $5.00 to $100.00 (or more) depending on the degree of monitoring and supervision
Exercise test	Range is from $200.00 to $1,000.00 depending on location and specific procedures used (measured oxygen consumption, echocardiography or nuclear component)
Laboratory services	Lipids (can range from $25.00 to several hundred dollars depending on analyses that are performed)
	Body composition (varies with type of assessment)
	Pulmonary function ($25.00 to $100.00 depending on extent of tests)
Consultations	Provided by physician, nurse, dietician, psychologist during assessments at entry and various intervals throughout the program. Charges vary based on extent and duration of assessment and consultation

with and without CAD, and these have been presented in earlier chapters. However, establishing the economic benefit of exercise training has not been adequately evaluated. Clearly, larger, long-term studies of the cost effectiveness of exercise training are needed to provide justification for this type of intervention (14). Without such information, preventive and rehabilitative exercise programs have little leverage when approaching third-party payers for coverage of these services.

Budgetary and Reimbursement Issues

Like any business, the preventive or rehabilitative program must have a budget that, at minimum, considers the income and expenses of operation. Income from a preventive or rehabilitative program is generated from the fees charged for services provided directly by the program and its staff members. It's important to recognize that the fee charged for a particular service and the actual income received are not always equal. We will consider this issue later in the section on reimbursement; but for simplification here, we'll assume that fees and income are equal. Each service provided has a corresponding CPT (current procedural terminology) code. The **CPT code** must be used when the insurance claim is filed. If a service or procedure does not have a CPT code, there is no mechanism for reimbursement. The CPT code for exercise training is 93797 or 93798 (noncontinuous and continuous ECG monitoring, respectively) whereas the CPT code for an exercise test (cardiovascular stress test) is 93015.

Reimbursement from third-party payers for various services represent much of the potential revenue or income to a secondary preventive or cardiac rehabilitative program. Other potential sources of income in these programs are listed and briefly described in table 11.4. Additional income to the program can take the form of donations from individuals and corporations or of grant money. These additional sources of income are valuable and often are used to support or underwrite the costs associated with a special event (e.g., lecture program), but rarely are they expected to provide meaningful support for the day-to-day operations of the program.

Who pays the fees for the services provided is another important consideration and one that has direct impact on the income of the program. Ideally, a third-party (e.g., insurance company) would pay all costs associated with the program. This would satisfy the consumer (patient or client), as well as the provider (the program). Un-

fortunately it doesn't always work this way, especially in this era of cost containment in medicine (i.e., managed care). Generally, insurance companies will reimburse for cardiac rehabilitation services (such as those described earlier) only for individuals with a diagnosis indicating the presence of CAD. Diagnoses that usually receive reimbursement by traditional "fee-for-service" providers (particularly Medicare) for cardiac rehabilitation services are as follows:

- Myocardial infarction
- Coronary bypass surgery
- Angina pectoris and/or evidence of myocardial ischemia

Other diagnoses that may potentially qualify for reimbursement of cardiac rehabilitation services include postcoronary interventions (angioplasty, stent), valvular heart disease, arrhythmia, heart failure, and heart transplantation. Each of these medical conditions has an **ICD code** (International Classification of Diseases) that identifies the diagnosis and is necessary for filing an insurance claim. If the appropriate ICD code is not provided, the claim will be rejected and no reimbursement will be received for the services.

When cardiac rehabilitation began in the 1970s, many insurance companies reimbursed (usually at 80% payment rate, i.e., 20% paid by patient) for all cardiac rehabilitation services (exercise therapy, laboratory fees, dietary and psychosocial consultations and assessments) for up to one year of participation. The duration of reimbursable cardiac rehabilitation has gradually decreased and is now generally for 36 sessions (three times per week = 12 weeks), although some regions of the United States may actually receive reimbursement for fewer sessions. Moreover, reimbursement for other services typically provided in secondary prevention or cardiac rehabilitation programs, such as exercise testing, blood lipid assessment, and dietary/psychosocial interventions, has also declined in recent years.

As mentioned in the previous chapter, at this time there appears to be little third-party support, particularly in the traditional fee-for-service type of health insurance, for newer behaviorally-oriented programs such as MULTIFIT and CHAMP (discussed in the previous chapter). However, some managed-care companies have shown more interest in these types of programs, recognizing their potential for long-term behavior change and subsequent reduction in health care costs.

Generally there is no reimbursement for cardiac rehabilitation services (e.g., exercise testing, exercise training sessions, consultations) for low-risk individuals or even for those at moderate risk for CAD (i.e., those who have multiple risk factors). Participation in preventive exercise programs for these individuals is thus dependent on willingness to self-pay or pay out of pocket. Obviously this financial barrier prevents many people from participating in such programs. A recent trend has been for some insurance companies, particularly the managed-care plans, to reimburse individuals, at least in part, for participation in preventive lifestyle modification programs (exercise, diet, stress management), based on the belief that lifestyle changes will reduce long-term health care costs. Unfortunately, at the present time the data are inadequate (studies are too few and too small) to impress the heath insurance companies to the point that they will universally reimburse for these potentially preventive services.

There are a number of expenses associated with operating a prevention or secondary program, many of which are listed in box 11.5. In most programs, salaries represent the largest single budget item and can exceed 80% of the total budget. Obviously, salaries as well as the costs of most supplies and other expenses will continue to rise over time.

Given the increasing costs of operating prevention or rehabilitative programs and the trend for decreased reimbursement rates, a number of programs have had to close or modify their offerings in recent years. Many "traditional" cardiac rehabilitation programs have begun to expand the scope of their practice and to offer their services to a variety of other clinical populations known to benefit from exercise and other lifestyle interventions. Potential target populations include individuals with pulmonary disease, obesity, diabetes, peripheral vascular disease, and musculoskeletal disorders. While the aim of such expansion may be to improve the financial standing of a particular program, expansion is also beneficial for patients who in the past would not have had access to these programs. There is optimism that the near future will witness reimbursement of preventive or rehabilitative services offered to these other populations. Given the medical diversity of patients likely to be seen in preventive or rehabilitative exercise programs in the future, it will become more critical for professionals to have a broad-based education and credentials beyond those now required for working only with pa-

---

Box 11.5 Common expenses associated with CAD prevention/ rehabilitation programs.

- Salary and fringe benefits (full time, part time, consultants)
- Supplies (office, laboratory, educational materials)
- Equipment (purchase, lease, maintenance agreements)
- Facilities (purchase, rent, renovation)
- Service contracts (cleaning, maintenance)
- Program dues and certification fees
- Travel expenses for staff to professional conferences
- Professional memberships and education (organizations, journals, newsletters)
- Marketing (brochures, advertising)
- Liability insurance (Facility and Professional)
- Utilities (phone, electric)

---

tients with known or suspected CAD. It would appear that the ACSM Registered Clinical Exercise Physiologist (box 11.2) is positioned to be such a credential.

LEGAL ISSUES

Law is defined as "all the rules of conduct established and enforced by the authority, legislation, or custom of a community or other group"(15). Thus, laws set the standards by which people and business should conduct themselves. When businesses or individuals do not abide by a standard of conduct, they expose themselves to legal liability for any harm caused by the violation. The harm may be financial loss or physical injury (or death). Preventive or rehabilitative program professionals need to be aware of their potential exposure to legal liability and take steps to manage this liability risk, which may include purchasing liability insurance, available through professional organizations such as ACSM. The aim of this brief section is only to provide an overview of some of the major liability concerns. Legal issues can be quite complex and need to be studied by program administrators in much more depth than permitted in this text. A more comprehensive review of legal issues in exercise programs can be found elsewhere (16).

One legal area of which exercise program professionals need to be aware is contracts made with those served. Sometimes these contracts are formalized in a document with a group or an individual. Often, however, contracts are implied. In a broad sense, any program or service offered by the exercise program professional could be viewed by the patient or client who is paying for that program or service as a contract. Thus, one must take care to clearly and accurately inform patients of the exact nature of the programs or services offered. Another extremely important area is the informed consent process. We emphasize the word "process" to point out that the informed consent is much more than just another form for the patient to sign (see form D in chapter 6). The exercise program professional needs to devote much care to the preparation and wording of the informed consent document, and an attorney should review it. Additionally, the process involves allowing the patient time to thoroughly read the document, orally reviewing key points of the document with the patient, asking the patient if she has any questions, noting any responses given to questions, and then having the client sign the document (which the exercise professional also signs).

Another area of legal concern for the exercise program professional relates to the provision of programs and services to the accepted (and expected) **standard of care.** "A standard of care describes how services should be delivered to clients so as to give reasonable assurance that the desired outcomes will be achieved in a safe manner" (16). Failure to perform to the standard of care that results in harm or injury to the patient can be viewed as an act of negligence. Standards of care for exercise programs and services are in large part influenced by publications (guidelines, position papers, recommendations) of national professional organizations (e.g., AHA, American College of Cardiology, ACSM, AACVPR) and panels of experts such as the Joint National Committee on Prevention, Detection, Evaluation, and Treatment of High Blood Pressure (JNC), or the National Cholesterol Education Program (NCEP). These organizations regularly update their positions as new scientific and clinical findings become available, and it is essential for exercise program professionals to keep current with this type of information. As discussed earlier in this chapter, part of the expected standard of care relates to the qualifications of the exercise program professional. Providers need to be sure that their exercise programs and services are being performed by personnel with the appropriate qualifications.

Hopefully, this brief section has given you an understanding of some of the important legal issues that exercise program professionals face. Certainly the legal issues can be quite complex, and those who will assume administrative roles in exercise programs should study them in greater depth.

PROGRAM CERTIFICATION

As mentioned in chapter 10, the AACVPR has developed a national certification program for cardiac (and separately, pulmonary) rehabilitation programs. At present, the process is completely voluntary, and there is a $300 fee to complete the application. The AACVPR believes that program certification can enhance the overall quality of cardiovascular rehabilitation programs by allowing programs to compare themselves to well-defined, measurable procedures and outcomes. To date, more than 800 programs have completed the process and have been "certified" by AACVPR. By being proactive, cardiac rehabilitation programs can demonstrate that they are dedicated to high-quality, effective interventions. The standards used to create this evaluation tool are as follows:

- AACVPR Guidelines for Cardiac Rehabilitation (2)
- AHCPR Clinical Practice Guidelines for Cardiac Rehabilitation (17)
- AACVPR Core Competencies for Cardiac Rehabilitation Professionals (3)

The process for obtaining certification from AACVPR, as outlined in figure 11.4, begins with a request by the individual program for an evaluation packet from the national office of AACVPR. The packet contains a variety of forms that are used to document the following:

- Size and scope of program (i.e., number of patients, which phases)
- Staff listing with documentation of credentials/licensure
- Appropriate facilities, equipment, supplies
- Documentation of specific policies and procedures
- Medical records and reports of medical emergencies

- Outcomes assessment (select one from each of the three domains: clinical, behavioral, and health)
- Patient care assessment and plan of care
- Intervention and treatment components
- Evaluation, discharge, follow-up

The completed package is forwarded to the AACVPR National Office and then on to the State/Regional Certification Committee for review. If approved by the State/Regional Certification Committee, it is forwarded to a national oversight committee for review. If approved there, the program receives a certificate. This certification is valid for three years, at the end of which time the program must reapply. The process for recertification is still being established but is likely to be more streamlined than the initial process. If the application is not approved by either the state/regional committee or the national oversight committee, then deficiencies are noted and the application is returned to the program.

While certification is currently voluntary, it is conceivable that in the future programs will be judged by whether they are certified or not and that only certified programs will receive third-party reimbursement for the services they provide. Regardless of the financial implications, successful completion of the certification process ensures an acceptable level of competency.

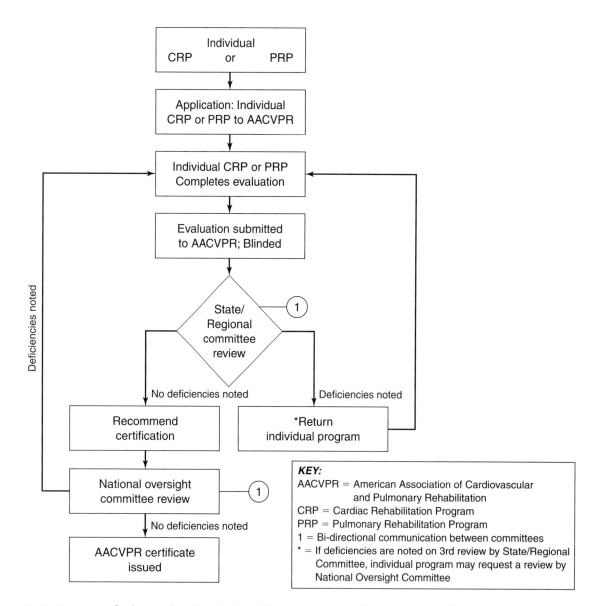

Figure 11.4   Process to obtain American Association of Cardiovascular and Pulmonary Rehabilitation Program certification for either cardiac (CRP) or pulmonary (PRP) rehabilitation programs.

SUMMARY

Since their inception more than 25 years ago, much has been learned regarding the administration and operation of preventive and rehabilitative programs. Although offered in a variety of settings, including hospitals, universities, and health clubs, these programs have essentially the same objective, helping individuals to make risk-reducing lifestyle changes. A number of standards of practice are currently available to assist new and established programs in achieving this objective. Of course, these standards will continue to change and will be updated as new information emerges. In order to offer the safest and most effective program, as well as to limit legal liability, individual programs must adhere closely to these standards even if doing so requires program reorganization or restructuring. Failure of programs to evolve clearly threatens the quality of programs and the profession. An important step in the establishment of standards for cardiovascular rehabilitation programs is the AACVPR certification process, highly encouraged for all secondary prevention or cardiac rehabilitation programs.

Case Study 1
Primary Prevention: Low Risk

Informed Consent and Other Forms

Upon entry into the primary prevention program at Ball State University, the participant signed consent forms for exercise testing, laboratory procedures (blood test), and the exercise training program. The testing form also contained a statement regarding release of medical information (see form D at the end of chapter 6). The purpose of this statement is to document that the client gave his consent to send test results from the primary prevention program to his health care providers and that the program had his permission to obtain his medical records from other health care providers. These instruments were described to the client, and the client was given the opportunity to read them and ask questions before signing. The consent form was also signed by a program staff member.

Risk Stratification and Monitoring

Based on ACSM risk categories (see table 6.5), this individual is classified as moderate risk (young but has 2+ risk factors). Thus, it is recommended that he have a physical examination and maximal exercise test before he participates in a "vigorous" exercise program. Furthermore, it is recommended that a physician be present during the maximal exercise test. For exercise training, the ACSM Guidelines (1) indicate that this individual (due to age, high functional capacity of > 8.0 METs, and relatively low risk) can participate in a medically unsupervised (i.e., with no physician present) exercise program. The primary prevention program at Ball State provides a structured exercise program and has well-trained staff (basic cardiac life support and appropriate credentials) during each session. Furthermore, the staff is well prepared (emergency protocols in place and rehearsed) for dealing with medical emergencies, including activating EMS and providing basic life support. Given this individual's history of hypertension, frequent blood pressure measurements would be obtained, and body weight would be measured regularly in the exercise program. Staff would ensure compliance with the exercise prescription by reviewing exercise logs on a weekly basis.

Reimbursement and Costs

As mentioned previously in this chapter, health insurance companies (particularly Medicare and other fee-for-service programs) rarely pay for primary prevention programs. However, some employers will pay for (or compensate with prizes or time off) for participation in preventive programs. In fact, the employer of this individual paid the annual fee of $240, which included the annual exercise test, exercise prescription, and access to the staffed exercise facility and regular monitoring. Many companies feel that if participation in a prevention program results in healthier, more productive, and satisfied employees, then the money is well spent. It's too bad more health insurance companies don't see it this way!

Case Study 2
Primary Prevention: High Risk

Informed Consent and Other Forms

Upon entry into the Wake Forest University Cardiac Rehabilitation Program, the patient signed informed consents for exercise testing, laboratory procedures (blood test), and the exercise training program. These instruments were described to the patient, and the patient was given the opportunity to read them and ask questions before signing. The consent form was also signed by an exercise physiologist.

A medical release form was also signed by the patient indicating that the cardiac rehabilitation program had his consent to send test results to his health care providers and to obtain his medical records from other health care providers.

Risk Stratification and Monitoring

Based on ACSM risk categories (see table 6.5), this individual is classified as high-risk (older and has 2+ risk factors). Thus, it is recommended that he have a physical examination and maximal exercise test before he participates in a vigorous exercise program, and also that a physician be present during the maximal exercise test. For exercise training, the ACSM Guidelines (1) indicate that this individual (due to presence of risk factors and low functional capacity [~5 METs]) should participate in a medically supervised exercise program. The secondary prevention/cardiac rehabilitation program at Wake Forest is conducted in a free-standing facility that is not connected to a hospital or physician's office. Thus, a physician and an advanced cardiac life support nurse are always present during exercise sessions. All appropriate emergency medical equipment and drugs are on site, and the exercise program staff is well prepared (emergency protocols in place and rehearsed) to deal with minor as well as life-threatening medical emergencies. Prior to each exercise session, this participant would have vital signs (heart rate, blood pressure) measured and recorded. During exercise, the participant would be expected to determine pulse rate twice to ensure compliance to the exercise prescription. This participant would also have his heart rate and rhythm recorded once during each exercise session using the "quick-check" paddles on a defibrillator. This approach of intermittent ECG monitoring has been used by Wake Forest and other programs for many years with excellent safety records.

Reimbursement and Costs

As already mentioned, health insurance companies rarely pay for primary prevention programs. Although this individual exhibits the presence of some CAD (40% blockage in the left anterior descending artery) and numerous risk factors, since he has not had an event he does not have a diagnosis that is normally acceptable for reimbursement of the services offered. However, given the existence of some CAD and several strong risk factors (including diabetes and obesity) in this individual, his health insurance company (actually a health maintenance organization offered through his employment) agreed to reimburse for all preventive testing (blood lipids, exercise testing) and intervention services (exercise therapy sessions, dietary and psychosocial interventions) for an initial three-month period. This provider would also consider longer support if medically necessary and/ or justifiable (i.e., beneficial). Fees for participating in a cardiac rehabilitation program were discussed earlier in this chapter. Because of the limited duration of third-party reimbursement by most providers, most prevention or rehabilitation programs offer a lower-cost maintenance program for continued participation. This individual elected to remain in the Wake Forest maintenance program at a rate of $525 per year (not including annual fees for exercise testing, lipid profile, and dietary and body composition assessments). He will be reassessed (as described in chapter 6) on an annual basis.

Case Study 3
Secondary Prevention: Post-MI and PTCA/Stent

Informed Consent and Other Forms

Upon entry into the cardiac rehabilitation program, the patient signed informed consents for exercise testing, laboratory procedures (blood test), and the exercise training program. These instruments were described to the patient; the patient was given the opportunity to read them and ask questions before signing; and the consent form was also signed by an exercise physiologist.

A medical release form was also signed by the patient indicating that the cardiac rehabilitation program had his consent to send test results to his health care providers and to obtain his medical records from other health care providers.

Risk Stratification and Monitoring

Based on ACSM risk categories (see table 6.5), this individual is classified as high risk (has known CAD). Thus, it is recommended that he have a physical examination and maximal exercise test before he participates in a vigorous exercise program. Furthermore, it is recommended that a physician be present during the maximal exercise test. For exercise training, the ACSM Guidelines (1) indicate that this patient (due to known CAD) should participate in a medically supervised exercise pro-

gram. Staffing, monitoring, and emergency preparation and response at the Wake Forest secondary prevention/cardiac rehabilitation program were outlined above in Case Study 2.

Reimbursement and Costs

As already mentioned, health insurance companies, including Medicare and other fee-for-service programs, will reimburse for cardiac rehabilitation services only for individuals with documented CAD (often only MI, CABG, or angina). Because this individual had an MI and angioplasty/stent, his insurance company would pay 80% (patient paid the other 20%) of the fees associated with his participation in the program, including exercise testing and other lab assessments (blood lipids, body composition), psychosocial and dietary assessments, and exercise therapy sessions. The duration of coverage was three months or 36 exercise sessions, whichever came first. After completion of the initial phase covered by insurance, the patient elected to continue in the maintenance program at the same fee as in Case Study 2. He would also have yearly evaluations (GXT, body composition, lipids) unless he became symptomatic.

GLOSSARY

Algorithms: well-defined procedures and sequences (medications, other interventions) used to treat specific cardiac events

Cardiac arrest: a life-threatening condition that occurs when the heart, due to electrical abnormalities, is unable to provide adequate output to meet the needs of the body

Code blue: a term for the process of alerting a "team" of health care providers (physicians, nurses, paramedics) with their emergency equipment to the scene of a significant cardiac event (myocardial infarction, arrest)

Comorbidities: "other" health-related conditions (in addition to CAD) that have a negative impact on mortality and have potential to alter exercise programming

Contraindications: specific health problems or conditions that increase the risk of an untoward event during exercise

Core competencies: specific education and/or knowledge expected of the competent cardiac rehabilitation professional

CPT code: current procedural terminology, necessary to identify specific medical procedures and for filing insurance claims

EMS: emergency medical services, activated by calling 911

Hypotension: low blood pressure that causes symptoms (lightheadedness)

ICD code: international classification of disease, used to describe various medical conditions and diseases; CPT codes used to identify conditions (myocardial infarction, coronary artery bypass graft, angina) eligible for cardiac rehabilitation services

Postbaccalaureate degree: education beyond a bachelor's degree, generally a master's or doctoral degree

Risk stratification: modeling that attempts to classify individuals (based on health conditions) into low-, moderate-, or high-risk for untoward events during exercise

Standard of care: Any document that describes appropriate and contemporary practice procedures for a given profession

Telemetry monitoring: ECG monitoring that is transmitted by electrical signals to a receiver

Third-party reimbursement: full or partial payment by an individual or company for medical services received by the patient; typically an insurance company or individual's employer

Untoward events: problems that may arise during exercise and that are significant enough to require medical intervention (medications, hospitalization) to manage; commonly include death, myocardial infarction, significant arrhythmia, refractory angina

REFERENCES

1. American College of Sports Medicine. 2000. *ACSM's guidelines for exercise testing and prescription.* Franklin, B.F., M.H. Whaley, and E.T. Howley, eds. 6th ed. Baltimore: Lippincott, Williams & Wilkins.

2. American Association of Cardiovascular and Pulmonary Rehabilitation. 1999. *Guidelines for cardiac rehabilitation programs.* 3rd ed. Champaign, IL: Human Kinetics, 281.

3. Southard, D.R., C. Certo, P. Comoss, N.F. Gordon, W.G. Herbert, E.J. Protas, P.M. Ribisl, S. Swails. 1994. Core competencies for cardiac rehabilitation professionals. *J. Cardiopul. Rehabil.* 14:87–92.

4. Herbert, W.G. 2000. Different purposes and values for allied healthcare professionals. *ACSM's Certified News* 10:1–4.

5. Siscovick, D.S., N.S. Weiss, and R.H. Fletcher. 1984. The incidence of primary cardiac arrest during vigorous exercise. *New Eng. J. Med.* 311:874–877.

6. Malinow, M.R., D.L. McGarry, and K.S. Kuehl. 1984. Is exercise testing indicated for asymptomatic active people? *J. Cardiopul. Rehabil.* 4:376–379.

7. Vander, L., B. Franklin, and M. Rubenfire. 1982. Cardiovascular complications of recreational physical activity. *Phys. and Sports Med.* 10:89–94.

8. VanCamp, S.P., and R.A. Peterson. 1986. Cardiovascular complications of outpatient cardiac rehabilitation programs. *J.A.M.A.* 256:1160–1163.

9. Vongvanich, P., M. Paul-Labrador, and C.N. Merz. 1996. Safety of medically supervised exercise in a cardiac rehabilitation center. *Am. J. Cardiol.* 77:1383–1385.

10. Franklin, B.A., K. Bonzheim, and S. Gordon. 1998. Safety of medically supervised outpatient cardiac rehabilitation exercise therapy: A 16-year follow-up. *Chest* 114:902–906.

11. Fletcher, G.A., G. Balady, V.F. Froelicher, L.H. Hartley, W.L. Haskell, M.L. Pollock. 1995. Exercise standards: A statement for health care professionals from the American Heart Association. *Circulation* 91:580–615.

12. Paul-Labrador, M., P. Vongvanich, and C.N. Merz. 1999. Risk stratification for exercise training in cardiac patients. Do the proposed guidelines work? *J. Cardiopul. Rehabil.* 19:118–125.

13. American Heart Association. 1997. Advanced Cardiac Life Support. Dallas: American Heart Association.

14. Livingston, M.D., and C. Dennis. 1999. Economic issues: The value and effectiveness of cardiac rehabilitation. In *Cardiac rehabilitation. A guide to the 21st century*, ed. N.K. Wenger, L.K. Smith, E.S. Froelicher, and P.M. Comoss. New York: Dekker.

15. Guralnik, D.B, and J.H. Friend, eds. 1966. *Webster's new world dictionary of the American language.* Coll. ed. Cleveland: World, 1724.

16. Herbert, D., and W. Herbert. 1998. Legal considerations. In *ACSM's resource manual for guidelines for exercise testing and prescription.* 3rd ed., ed. J.L. Roitman, 610–615. Baltimore: Lippincott, Williams & Wilkins.

17. Wenger, N.K., E.S. Froelicher, L.K. Smith, et al. 1995. *Cardiac rehabilitation. Clinical practice guidelines no. 17.* AHCPR pub. no. 96-0672, Oct. U.S. Department of Health and Human Services. Public Health Service. Agency for Health Care Policy and Research. National Heart, Lung, and Blood Institute.

INDEX

Note: The italicized *f* and *t* following page numbers refer to figures and tables, respectively.

ABOUT THE AUTHORS

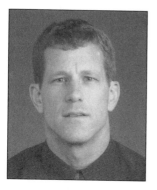

Peter H. Brubaker, PhD, has taught undergraduate and graduate courses in cardiovascular disease management for 15 years. Currently, he is director of cardiac rehabilitation and associate professor of health and exercise science at Wake Forest University. Dr. Brubaker has written more than 25 peer-reviewed manuscripts and 6 book chapters relating to cardiovascular disease management. He is vice president of the American Association for Cardiovascular and Pulmonary Rehabilitation (AACVPR) and past president of the North Carolina Cardiopulmonary Rehabilitation Association. He is certified by the American College of Sports Medicine (ACSM) as a Preventive/Rehabilitative Program Director and serves as Director of Certification for ACSM exams at Wake Forest and other institutions.

His scholarly work has earned him several awards, including one for excellence in research from Wake Forest, and one for professional service from the North Carolina Cardiopulmonary Rehabilitation Association. Additionally, Dr. Brubaker was named a fellow by the ACSM in 1997 and the AACVPR in 1993. He is a section editor for the ACSM and serves on the editorial board for the *Journal of Cardiopulmonary Rehabilitation* and the *Journal of Clinical Exercise Physiology*.

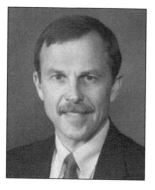

Leonard A. Kaminsky, PhD, is a professor specializing in clinical exercise physiology at Ball State University, and has taught undergraduate and graduate courses in exercise science for 17 years. He has directed adult fitness programs and cardiac and pulmonary rehabilitation programs for 15 years. Dr. Kaminsky holds both the Program Director and Exercise Test Technologist certifications from the ACSM, which named him to the first practice board for the Registry of Clinical Exercise Physiologists. He also chairs the ACSM academic standards and clinical competencies subcommittee, is a past president of the Midwest chapter of ACSM, and is editor of the organization's metabolic calculation software. Additionally, Dr. Kaminsky has authored or coauthored more than 35 research manuscripts, 4 book chapters, and hundreds of presentations and abstracts, the majority of which directly involved the work of graduate students in training. He serves on the editorial board of the *Journal of Cardiopulmonary Rehabilitation*. The ACSM named him a fellow in 1990.

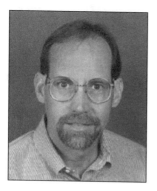

Mitchell H. Whaley, PhD, has taught undergraduate and graduate courses in clinical exercise physiology for the past 21 years. He has also directed or co-directed preventive and rehabilitation exercise programs for 18 of his 21 years of involvement in the field. Currently, he is professor of physical education at Ball State University. He is certified by the ACSM as both an Exercise Specialist$_{SM}$ and Exercise Program Director$_{SM}$. For the ACSM, Dr. Whaley serves on the board of trustees; is chair of the credentials committee; and has provided educational workshops and certification exams in the United States, Korea, and Belgium. He was associate clinical editor of the ACSM's *Guidelines for Exercise Testing and Exercise Prescription*, sixth edition.

Dr. Whaley's research interests include exercise/physical activity epidemiology and various topics related to exercise testing and prescription. He has coauthored 30 research articles and textbook chapters, has contributed more than 80 research-based presentations at professional meetings (many coauthored with his graduate students from Ball State) and has made more than 80 presentations to professional groups during the past decade. Dr. Whaley was honored in 1994 with the Visiting Scholar Award from the American College of Sports Medicine.